Physical Therapist Assistant Examination Review and Test-Taking Skills

Physical Therapist Assistant Examination Review and Test-Taking Skills

Mark Dutton, PT

Melissa Schneider, PTA, M.Ed

Janice Lwin, PT, DPT

Cassady Bartlett, PT, DPT

Annie Burke-Doe, PT, MPT, PhD

New York   Chicago   San Francisco   Athens   London   Madrid   Mexico City
Milan   New Delhi   Singapore   Sydney   Toronto

Physical Therapist Assistant Examination Review and Test-Taking Skills

1 2 3 4 5 6 7 8 9   LWI   27 26 25 24 23 22

ISBN 978-1-264-26888-7
MHID 1-264-26888-2

This book was set in Minion Pro by KnowledgeWorks Global Ltd.
The editors were Michael Weitz and Kim J. Davis.
The production supervisor was Richard Ruzycka.
Project management was provided by Revathi Viswanathan.
The cover designer was W2 Design.

This book is printed on acid-free paper.

Library of Congress Cataloging-in-Publication Data

Names: Dutton, Mark, author. | Schneider, Melissa, author. | Lwin, Janice,
    author. | Bartlett, Cassady, author. | Burke-Doe, Annie, author.
Title: Physical therapist assistant examination review and test-taking
    skills / Mark Dutton, Melissa Schneider, Janice Lwin, Cassady Bartlett,
    Annie Burke-Doe.
Description: New York : McGraw Hill, [2022] | Includes bibliographical
    references and index. | Summary: "This book will provide the necessary
    information to prepare for the National Physical Therapist Assistant
    Examination (NPTAE) including a breakdown of the NPTAE format, a
    comprehensive content review of all body systems, clinical tips, yellow
    and red flags to treatment, testing strategies, and sample questions"—
    Provided by publisher.
Identifiers: LCCN 2021037368 (print) | LCCN 2021037369 (ebook) | ISBN
    9781264268887 (paperback ; alk. paper) | ISBN 9781264268894 (ebook)
Subjects: MESH: Physical Therapy Modalities | Physical Therapist Assistants
    | Test Taking Skills | Study Guide
Classification: LCC RM725 (print) | LCC RM725 (ebook) | NLM WB 18.2 |
    DDC 615.8/2—dc23
LC record available at https://lccn.loc.gov/2021037368
LC ebook record available at https://lccn.loc.gov/2021037369

Contents

Authors

Cassady Bartlett, PT, DPT
Instructor
Hawkeye Community College
Waterloo, Iowa

Annie Burke-Doe, PT, MPT, PhD
Dean/Program Director
West Coast University
Los Angeles, California

Mark Dutton, PT
Senior Consultant
OrthoRecovery Specialists
Pittsburgh, Pennsylvania

Janice Lwin, PT, DPT
Program Director
American Career College
Anaheim, California

Melissa Scheider, PTA, M.Ed
Assistant Professor
Hawkeye Community College
Waterloo, Iowa

Preface

Congratulations on taking the next step toward becoming a licensed Physical Therapist Assistant! Passing the National Physical Therapist Assistant Examination (NPTAE) is a crucial step in obtaining licensure. This examination has reciprocity across the United States; therefore, you only need to pass it once to be licensed to practice in any state, although a separate state jurisprudence examination is necessary to complete requirements for licensure and to practice in each state. Check with your state Physical Therapy Board for more information.

Preparation to pass the NPTAE is a marathon, not a sprint. Your journey to success on this difficult, comprehensive examination should begin months before your test date. Proper time management, dedication to reviewing, and proficient knowledge of physical therapy principles are imperative to passing the NPTAE.

Physical Therapist Assistant Examination Review and Test-Taking Skills will provide the necessary information to prepare for the examination, including a breakdown of the NPTAE format, a comprehensive content review of all body systems, clinical tips, yellow and red flags to treatment, testing strategies, and sample questions.

In addition to studying content and understanding testing strategies, taking multiple practice examinations is a critical preparation step for success in the NPTAE. This book provides two 200-question practice examinations formatted in the style of the NPTAE.

We recommend using textbooks and review books, such as this one, when preparing for the examination. Lecture notes from your academic program will be less effective. The Federation of State Boards of Physical Therapy (FSBPT) establishes the NPTAE and has published a list of the most commonly used textbooks in PTA programs across the nation that they use to reference for examination questions. This list can be found at the following website: https://www.fsbpt.org/Secondary-Pages/Educators/Textbook-Survey-Data.

Good luck on your endeavors in this last step toward becoming a licensed Physical Therapist Assistant!

Introduction
What to Expect on the NPTAE: Content Outline, Examination Administration, and Format

JANICE LWIN

OVERVIEW

The National Physical Therapist Assistant Examination (NPTAE) is a 200-question, 4-hour multiple-choice examination designed to equitably test all candidates for entry-level knowledge of content and safety aspects in physical therapy to ensure only competent persons earn licensure to practice physical therapy. The examination is created through the Federation of State Boards of Physical Therapy (FSBPT).

Additional information regarding the examination and registration can be found at the FSBPT website: www.fsbpt.org.

■ QUICK SUMMARY OF THE NPTAE

The examination is 4 hours in length and comprises the following:

- 200-question examination
  - The examination is split into four separate sections of 50 questions. Once a 50-question section is submitted, the candidate cannot return to those questions.
  - One hundred and fifty questions are scored, 50 are unscored pretest questions and will not be included in the final calculation of the score. Candidates will not know which questions are pretest questions, and they will be embedded throughout the examination.
  - First two 50-question sections are allotted 2 hours; third and fourth sections are allotted 2 hours.
  - A scheduled 15-minute break is allowed between the second and third sections.

■ EXAMINATION SCORING

The passing score is 600.

- All jurisdictions and state licensing agencies have adopted FSBPT's criterion-referenced passing score.

- Questions are weighted, which means they do not equate to "one point per question," but scores are based on difficulty levels of questions.
- Criterion-based passing scores range from 95 to 108 questions correct out of the 150 scored questions.
- The candidate's scaled score reported by FSBPT ranges between 200 and 800, with a passing score of 600.

▣ APPLYING FOR ACCOMMODATIONS

- Candidates requesting accommodations (ie, additional examination time, specialized testing environment) for individual circumstances should contact their state licensing board at least 4 months before the test date for information on options available.

▣ APPLYING FOR THE EXAMINATION

The NPTAE is only offered four times per year, and registration closes approximately 1 month before the examination date. The candidate's academic institution must create an FSBPT profile, which provides the tester with instructions on creating an FSBPT ID and profile. Candidates must first register and be approved by the state licensing agency for where they plan to practice. Candidates can only apply to test and practice in one jurisdiction at a time. Each state has different criteria and requirements for application, and the candidate should contact their specific jurisdiction for more information. Following approval by the jurisdiction, the candidate can register for the NPTAE at www.fsbpt.org.

Specific test dates can be found at FSBPT's website www.fsbpt.org.

▣ EXAMINATION ADMINISTRATION

Candidates will take the NPTAE at a Prometric Testing Center located throughout the United States. Once a notice of testing eligibility is received from FSBPT, the candidate is encouraged to reserve a testing seat at www.prometric.com to ensure a convenient testing site is available. Demand is high for testing dates and times with Prometric; however, many options are available throughout the week, and appointments can be made in the morning or afternoon.

▣ RECEIVING YOUR SCORE

Generally, FSBPT releases a candidate's examination results 6 to 7 days after testing by logging in to your FSBPT account. Additional examination reports can be purchased through FSBPT. For specific examination result release dates, refer to FSBPT's website www.fsbpt.org.

▣ RETESTING

If you are unsuccessful at the NPTAE, you can reregister to retake the examination on the following test date offered. You are allowed three consecutive attempts at taking the NPTAE before skipping a test date in sequence. In most jurisdictions, there is a six-attempt lifetime limit taking the NPTAE.

▣ CONTENT OUTLINE SUMMARY

As you prepare for the NPTAE, it is important to be efficient and effective with your study time. The FSBPT, which provides an outline and description of each content area tested on the NPTAE, is available on the FSBPT website. This information is summarized in the following section. Pay close attention to which body systems and content areas make up the largest percentage of the examination. These areas are where you should spend most of your review to best prepare for success in this critical examination.

Additional information is available to the public, including an examination content outline can be found at www.fsbpt.org.

Body System	Question Range	Average Percentage of Examination
Musculoskeletal	36-41	28%
Neuromuscular and nervous	28-34	24%
Cardiovascular and pulmonary	21-26	18%
Integumentary	5-10	7%
Metabolic and endocrine	5-7	6%
System interactions	5-7	6%
Lymphatic	3-6	5%
Gastrointestinal	0-4	3%
Genitourinary	0-4	3%

% Questions per Body System on NPTAE

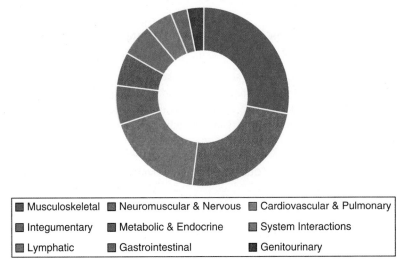

Musculoskeletal Neuromuscular & Nervous Cardiovascular & Pulmonary
Integumentary Metabolic & Endocrine System Interactions
Lymphatic Gastrointestinal Genitourinary

■ CONTENT AREAS

Each major body system will be broken down into questions based on content areas. This section describes the different content areas, questions per section, and sample NPTAE questions similar to the content areas. First, review the type of information included in each content area. Then, pay attention to which content areas will constitute most questions within the body system to help streamline your studying.

Content Area	Question Range	Average Percentage of Examination
Interventions	41-54	32%
Diseases/conditions that impact effective treatment	33-48	27%
Physical therapy data collection	29-37	22%
Equipment, devices, and technologies; therapeutic modalities	16-20	12%
Safety and protection; professional responsibilities; research	9-13	7%

% Questions per Content Area on the NPTAE

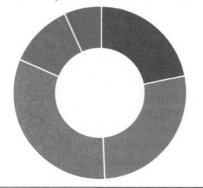

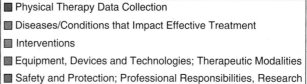

- ■ Physical Therapy Data Collection
- ■ Diseases/Conditions that Impact Effective Treatment
- ■ Interventions
- ■ Equipment, Devices and Technologies; Therapeutic Modalities
- ■ Safety and Protection; Professional Responsibilities, Research

■ PHYSICAL THERAPY DATA COLLECTION
29-37 QUESTIONS

Utilizing current best evidence, this section assesses the understanding and application of tests and measures. Using information gathered within this category, questions will cover the appropriate and effective application of knowledge to patient/client management through treatment and interventions while promoting health throughout the lifespan.

Questions per Body System

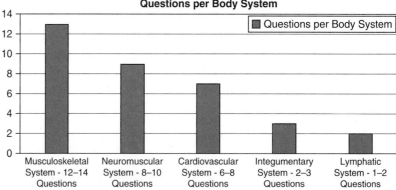

■ DISEASES/CONDITIONS THAT IMPACT
EFFECTIVE TREATMENT *33-48 QUESTIONS*

This section assesses the understanding of diseases and conditions of major body systems including the musculoskeletal, neuromuscular, cardiovascular, pulmonary, and integumentary system. Questions in this category cover the appropriate and effective application of knowledge to patient/client management through treatment and interventions while promoting health throughout the lifespan.

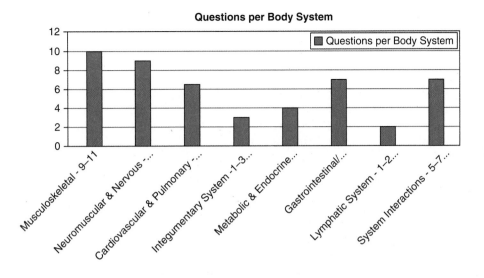

■ INTERVENTIONS *41-54 QUESTIONS*

According to current best practice, this section assesses the understanding and impact of interventions (including types, applications, responses and potential complications) for major body systems including the musculoskeletal, neuromuscular, cardiovascular, pulmonary, and integumentary system. Questions in this category cover the appropriate and effective application of knowledge to patient/client management through treatment and interventions while promoting health throughout the lifespan.

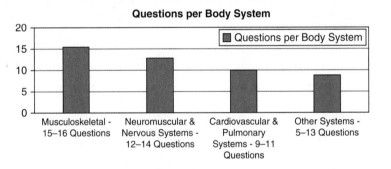

■ EQUIPMENT, DEVICES, AND TECHNOLOGIES *7-9 QUESTIONS*

According to current best practice, this section assesses the understanding and utilization of different equipment, devices and technologies incorporating safety and contextual determinants for their application and use. Questions in this category cover the appropriate and effective application of knowledge to patient/client management through treatment and interventions while promoting health throughout the lifespan.

■ THERAPEUTIC MODALITIES *9-11 QUESTIONS*

According to current best practice, this section assesses the understanding and utilization of different therapeutic modalities incorporating various safety and contextual determinants for their application and use. Questions in this category cover the appropriate and effective application of knowledge to patient/client management through treatment and interventions while promoting health throughout the lifespan.

The following information regarding the application, indications, contraindications, and precautions for the use of modalities that may appear on the NPTAE was taken from the FSBPT PTA Exam Content Outline:

- Thermal modalities.
- Iontophoresis.
- Electrotherapy (ie, neuromuscular electrical stimulation [NMES], transcutaneous electrical nerve stimulation [TENS], functional electrical stimulation [FES], interferential therapy, and high-voltage pulsed current).
- Phonophoresis.
- Ultrasound modalities.
- Mechanical modalities (ie, Mechanical motion devices, traction devices).
- Biofeedback.
- Intermittent compression.

■ SAFETY AND PROTECTION *4-6 QUESTIONS*

This section assesses the understanding of factors affecting patient/client protection and safety in addition to the role of the health care professional to provide safe and effective treatment. The following information regarding safety and protection that may appear on the NPTAE was taken from the FSBPT PTA Exam Content Outline:

- Factors influencing safety and injury prevention (eg, safe patient handling, fall prevention, equipment maintenance, environmental safety).
- Function, implications, and related precautions of intravenous lines, tubes, catheters, monitoring devices, and mechanical ventilators/oxygen delivery devices.
- Emergency preparedness (eg, cardiopulmonary resuscitation [CPR], first aid, disaster response).
- Infection control procedures (eg, standard/universal precautions, isolation techniques, sterile technique).
- Signs/symptoms of physical, sexual, and psychological abuse and neglect.

■ PROFESSIONAL RESPONSIBILITIES *3-4 QUESTIONS*

This section assesses the knowledge and role of health care professionals to provide a trustworthy environment for clinical decision-making. The following information regarding professional responsibilities that may appear on the NPTAE was taken from the FSBPT PTA Exam Content Outline: Standards of documentation.

- Patient–client rights (eg, ADA, IDEA, HIPAA, patient bill of rights).
- Human resource legal issues (eg, OSHA, sexual harassment).
- Roles and responsibilities of the physical therapist, physical therapist assistant, other health care professionals, and support staff.
- Standards of professional ethics.
- Standards of billing, coding, and reimbursement.
- Obligations for reporting illegal, unethical, or unprofessional behaviors (eg, fraud, abuse, neglect).
- State and federal laws, rules, regulations, and industry standards set by state and accrediting bodies (eg, state licensing entities, Joint Commission, CARF, CMS).
- Risk management and quality assurance (eg, policies and procedures, incident reports, peer chart review).
- Cultural factors and/or characteristics that affect patient–client management (eg, language differences, disability, ethnicity, customs, demographics, religion).
- Socioeconomic factors that affect patient–client management.
- Health information technology (eg, electronic medical records, telemedicine).

■ RESEARCH AND EVIDENCE-BASED PRACTICE *2-3 QUESTIONS*

This section assesses the knowledge and role of health care professionals to interpret and incorporate current research into evidence-based practice and clinical decision-making. Information includes the following content: The following information regarding research and evidence-based practice that may appear on the NPTAE was taken from the FSBPT PTA Exam Content Outline:

- Research methodology and interpretation (eg, qualitative, quantitative, levels of evidence).
- Data collection techniques (eg, surveys, direct observation).
- Measurement science (eg, reliability, validity).
- Techniques for accessing evidence (eg, peer-reviewed publications, scientific proceedings, guidelines, clinical prediction rules).

■ CONTENT THAT WILL NOT BE ON THE NPTAE

FSBPT has determined several content areas that are not deemed critical for entry-level PTAs to be tested on the NPTAE. **What follows is a list of those areas that will *NOT* be tested according to the FSBPT PTA Exam Content Outline**. Use this information to streamline your studying to include only pertinent information.

FSBPT has made the list of critical and noncritical PTA work activities available to the public at https://www.fsbpt.org/Free-Resources/NPTE-Development/Ensuring-Validity.

DATA COLLECTION

- Performing tests and measures of the following:
  - Body composition (ie, percent body fat, lean muscle mass).
  - Superficial reflexes and reactions (cremasteric and abdominal reflex).

INTERVENTIONS

- Performance of the following manual therapy techniques:
  - Manual lymphatic drainage.
  - Instrument-assisted soft tissue mobilization.
  - Peripheral joint manipulation (thrust) or spinal mobilization/manipulation (thrust).
  - Taping for lymphatic drainage.
- Application, adjustment, or training of the following equipment and devices:
  - Mechanical neuromuscular reeducation technologies (weighted vests, robotic exoskeletons, antigravity treadmills).
- Performance or training of the following integumentary techniques:
  - Selective enzymatic or autolytic debridement.
  - Sharp debridement.
  - Hyperbaric therapy.
  - Negative-pressure wound therapy.
- Utilization of the following therapeutic modalities:
  - Contrast bath/pools.
  - Phototherapy/laser light.
  - Infrared agents.
  - Fluidotherapy.
  - Diathermy.
  - Shockwave therapy.
- Application of the following research and evidence-based practice:
  - Design and/or direct research activities.
  - Participation in research activities.

Test-Taking Strategies for the NPTAE

JANICE LWIN

The National Physical Therapist Assistant Examination (NPTAE) is a challenging, comprehensive test of entry-level knowledge. The 200-question examination includes content from every major system requiring the student to focus for 4 hours to complete it.

Due to the nature of the NPTAE, many candidates have heightened anxiety during the examination, affecting their ability to work through the questions successfully. An effective method to combat test anxiety (in addition to proficient content knowledge) is understanding strategies to work through questions to arrive at the most logical answer. This section will provide testing strategies and tips to help you navigate the NPTAE.

EXAMINATION QUESTION BASICS

While solid content knowledge is crucial to success in the NPTAE, careful understanding of the format of NPTAE questions and strategies to eliminate wrong answers to arrive at the best choice is a key component to successful test-taking. These are some facts about the NPTAE to bear in mind:

- With only 4 hours to complete 200 questions, the candidate has 1.2 minutes per question.
- The questions do not test memorization skills but rather the application and clinical understanding of concepts. For example, a typical question will not ask, "What is the action of the iliopsoas muscle" but instead, "Which muscle might be affected if a patient has difficulty during the terminal swing phase of gait?"
- There is only ONE right answer. However, every other choice will *seem* attractive and reasonable.
- The NPTAE is a marathon, not a sprint. To prepare best for the examination, study in large blocks of time to mentally train the brain to replicate the examination duration. No extra points are awarded for finishing quickly; therefore, take your time.

DETERMINING THE BEST CHOICE

1. Read each question slowly, carefully, and twice.
2. Pick out keywords in the question stem to help understand the question.
3. Rephrase the question into your own words.
4. Formulate an answer before looking at the choices.
5. Read each answer choice slowly, carefully, and twice.
6. Do NOT read into the question or add details that are not already in the stem.
7. Eliminate the wrong answer choices one by one.
8. Eliminate similar answer choices since there can only be ONE best answer.

9. Refer back to your stem when in doubt or to confirm your answer selection.
10. Do not spend too much time deliberating on one question.
11. **Do NOT leave any questions blank.**
12. **Do NOT change your answers.**

1. **READ EACH QUESTION SLOWLY, CAREFULLY, AND TWICE**
   Candidates often read questions too quickly and miss pertinent information that changes the meaning of the question. For example, missing "EXCEPT" at the end of the statement or seeing "anterior" versus "posterior" when reading too fast. There is plenty of time to read each question and answer twice, and there will be some questions that you can answer quickly, leaving more time for the difficult questions. Pace yourself.

2. **PICK OUT KEYWORDS IN THE QUESTION STEM TO HELP UNDERSTAND THE QUESTION**
   Keywords can help clarify what the question asks and eliminate irrelevant information that may distract from the correct answer. For example, the underlined words in the sample question below would be keywords to clarify the question.

   During gait observation, the PTA notices a <u>lack of heel strike at initial contact</u>. Which of the following muscles should the PTA <u>strengthen to improve</u> this gait deviation?

   While the other words are helpful, the underlined words are *keywords* that differentiate what the candidate should be thinking to answer the question.

   "Lack of heel strike at initial contact" defines at what point during gait the candidate should be concerned.

   "Strengthen to improve" lets the candidate know the goal is to increase heel strike, and the focus should be on what muscle improves this motion.

3. **REPHRASE THE QUESTION INTO YOUR OWN WORDS**
   Before looking at the answer choices, rephrase the question into your words to clarify and simplify in your mind what the question is asking.

   During gait observation, the PTA notices a lack of heel strike at initial contact. Which of the following muscles should the PTA strengthen to improve this gait deviation?

   Rephrased question: Which muscle increases heel strike at initial contact?

4. **FORMULATE AN ANSWER BEFORE LOOKING AT THE CHOICES**
   Think about the possible answer choices before looking at the options. This approach can also clarify the direction the candidate should be thinking before getting confused by multiple options.

   During gait observation, the PTA notices a lack of heel strike at initial contact. Which of the following muscles should the PTA strengthen to improve this gait deviation?

   Formulating an answer: Heel strike at initial contact requires dorsiflexion of the foot. Dorsiflexion is the result of anterior tibialis muscle contraction.

5. **READ EACH ANSWER CHOICE SLOWLY, CAREFULLY, AND TWICE**
   Beware of similar choices that could be incorrect if read too quickly. For example, "anterior tibialis" and "posterior tibialis" can be erroneously mixed up if read too quickly.

   During gait observation, the PTA notices a lack of heel strike at initial contact. Which of the following muscles should the PTA strengthen to improve this gait deviation?

a. *Gastrocnemius*
b. *Anterior tibialis*
c. *Quadriceps*
d. *Posterior tibialis*

6. **DO NOT READ INTO THE QUESTION OR ADD DETAILS THAT ARE NOT ALREADY IN THE STEM**
Avoid adding your own words to the question stem. For example, in the previous question, the following thoughts would be erroneous in concluding as to why there is a lack of heel strike at initial contact:

• *If the patient has a SACH foot, dorsiflexion could be limited by a stiff heel cushion, therefore strengthening the quadriceps could be reasonable to increase knee extension and possibly stride length before the heel touches the ground.* There is no mention of the patient having a SACH foot.
• *Lack of heel strike might be because the person has a shortened stride length due to tight hamstrings, therefore, strengthening the quadriceps could be the right answer as the person tries to overcome lack of hip flexion and knee extension from a decreased length in the hamstrings.* There is no mention of tight hamstrings in the question.

7. **ELIMINATE WRONG ANSWER CHOICES**
Remember, all of the answer choices in the NPTAE will be *reasonable*, so there will not be an absurd answer completely out of place, but usually there are one or two choices that do not fit the question.

During gait observation, the PTA notices a lack of heel strike at initial contact. Which of the following muscles should the PTA strengthen to improve this gait deviation?

a. *Gastrocnemius*
b. *Anterior tibialis*
c. *Quadriceps*
d. *Posterior tibialis*

Using the assumption that one or two choices do not fit the question, the answer choice should immediately be centered around a muscle that performs dorsiflexion, which must also act on the ankle. Since choice "c," the quadriceps, does not act on the ankle, this choice can be eliminated with confidence.

At this point, the critical thinker would also have deduced that a correct heel strike requires dorsiflexion and that the gastrocnemius and posterior tibialis do not perform dorsiflexion (they are plantarflexors), allowing these options to be eliminated.

There is now only one option after eliminating the other three choices using the process of elimination, which is "b," anterior tibialis.

8. **ELIMINATE SIMILAR ANSWER CHOICES—THERE IS ONLY *ONE* BEST ANSWER**
Even if a candidate is not certain of the correct answer, eliminating incorrect answers can narrow down options for a better chance at determining the right answer. At times, the candidate may even be able to eliminate all other options, leaving only the correct answer.

• With a knowledge of muscles and actions, the tester should recognize the gastrocnemius and posterior tibialis both perform plantarflexion. Since there can only be ONE best answer, these choices can be eliminated since they perform the same motion.
• Even if a candidate is not certain of the correct answer, eliminating incorrect answers can narrow down options for a better chance at determining the right answer. At times, the candidate may even be able to eliminate all other options, leaving only the correct answer.

9. **REFER BACK TO YOUR STEM WHEN IN DOUBT OR TO CONFIRM YOUR ANSWER SELECTION**
   Once an answer has been chosen, reread the question to confirm it is the *best* choice.

10. **DO NOT SPEND TOO MUCH TIME DELIBERATING ON ONE QUESTION**
    If the above strategies do not produce a definitive answer, the most logical answer should be selected based on deductive reasoning. If necessary, the candidate can mark the question to return later for review but should not spend too much time on a difficult question to avoid running out of time.

11. **DO NOT LEAVE ANY QUESTION BLANK**
    The tester is not penalized for wrong answers; therefore, a "best guess" should be taken for every question.

12. **DO NOT CHANGE YOUR ANSWERS**
    Not changing your answers may be the most critical testing strategy! Many candidates second-guess their answer selections (especially when reviewing) and ultimately change answers from "correct" to "incorrect." This costly error can be the difference between passing and not passing the examination. **DO NOT** change an answer unless you are *absolutely certain* that the new answer is correct.

STUDY PEARL
The NPTAE can be overwhelming in terms of the amount of content the candidate must review. As a result, testers often claim they are "not good test-takers." The reality is that a candidate *must* pass the 200-question multiple-choice NPTAE to become a licensed Physical Therapist Assistant.

PRACTICE YOUR TEST-TAKING STRATEGIES

Sample Question 1
Which of the following exercises would be the MOST appropriate for a patient with right infraspinatus weakness?

1. Right sidelying internal rotation of the right shoulder
2. Left sidelying external rotation of the left shoulder
3. Right sidelying abduction of the right shoulder
4. Left sidelying external rotation of the right shoulder

Keywords: right, infraspinatus, weakness
Rephrase the question: Which exercise will strengthen the right infraspinatus muscle?
Formulate an answer: The right infraspinatus muscle performs right shoulder external rotation. Therefore, look for an answer choice that includes an external rotation movement of the right shoulder.
Eliminate wrong answers:
- Choice #1 can be eliminated because the infraspinatus does not perform internal rotation
- Choice #2 can be eliminated because the answer describes action occurring at the left shoulder, not right
- Choice #3 can be eliminated because the infraspinatus does not perform shoulder abduction
Refer back to the stem to confirm the answer choice:
- Is choice #4 the best choice to strengthen the infraspinatus muscle in the right shoulder? The answer is yes.

Sample Question 2
A patient with lumbar spinal stenosis is in physical therapy to strengthen the serratus anterior muscle. Which of the following exercises would be the MOST appropriate to perform with this patient?

1. Standing scapular protraction at 45 degrees shoulder flexion with a resistance band

2. Seated scapular protraction at 120 degrees shoulder flexion with resistance band

3. Prone scapular retraction at 90 degrees shoulder flexion with a hand weight

4. Seated scapular retraction at 45 degrees shoulder abduction with a hand weight

---

Keywords: lumbar spinal stenosis, strengthen, serratus anterior

Rephrase the question: Which exercise will strengthen the serratus anterior while still addressing the lumbar spinal stenosis diagnosis?

Formulate an answer: Patients with lumbar spinal stenosis prefer to be in a flexed posture at the spine. The serratus anterior muscle performs scapular protraction. Look for an answer choice that has the patient in a spinal flexed posture and includes scapular protraction exercises.

Eliminate wrong answers:

- Choice #1 can be eliminated because the standing position puts the spine in extension, and the serratus anterior is not effective at 45 degrees of shoulder flexion

- Choice #3 can be eliminated because prone position puts the spine in extension, and scapular retraction is not an action performed by the serratus anterior

- Choice #4 can be eliminated because scapular retraction is not an action performed by the serratus anterior even though a seated position puts the spine in flexion

Refer back to the stem to confirm the answer choice:

- Does choice #2 address the lumbar spinal stenosis diagnosis to have a patient in lumbar flexion and strengthen the serratus anterior into scapular protraction? The answer is yes.

Sample Question 3

Which of the following deformities would you expect to see in a patient with osteoarthritis?

1. Gout

2. Swan-neck deformity

3. Heberden nodes

4. Hallux valgus

Keywords: deformities, osteoarthritis

Rephrase the question: Persons with osteoarthritis often have which of the following deformities?

Formulate an answer: Osteoarthritis is a degenerative disorder of the joints due to wear down of articular cartilage

Eliminate wrong answers:

- Choice #1 can be eliminated because gout is a disorder that is the result of too much uric acid in the body and does not accompany osteoarthritis

- Choice #2 can be eliminated if the tester understands swan-neck and boutonniere deformities are symptoms of rheumatoid arthritis

- Choice #4 can be eliminated because it is a deformity of the foot that includes subluxation of the first metatarsophalangeal joint but not due to osteoarthritis

Refer back to the stem to confirm the answer choice:

- Is choice #3 associated with osteoarthritis? The answer is yes.

Sample Question 4

Which of the following steps should the PTA take when concluding treatment for a patient with orthopnea?

1. Place the patient in bed with the head elevated

2. Check blood pressure

3. Measure respiration rate

4. Provide oxygen via nasal cannula if the patient is short of breath

Keywords: concluding treatment, orthopnea

Rephrase the question: The PTA should provide which of the following actions before leaving a patient with orthopnea after treatment?

Formulate an answer: Even if the tester does not know what orthopnea is, the word can be broken down with an understanding of medical terminology. Ortho—meaning "upright" such as "orthostatic hypotension." Pnea—meaning "breath." It is reasonable to think the answer should involve concepts with positioning while breathing.

Eliminate wrong answers:

- Choice #2 can be eliminated because blood pressure is not associated with breathing or positioning
- Choice #3 may not want to be eliminated initially if the tester is unfamiliar with what orthopnea is but understands it has some association with breathing.
- Choice #4 can be eliminated because the question does not include information stating the patient is using supplemental oxygen; therefore, it is not within the PTA scope of practice to add oxygen via a nasal cannula at the end of treatment

Refer back to the stem to confirm the answer choice:

- The tester is left between choice #1 and #3 as reasonable options. Go back to the question and reread. As deduced earlier, "ortho" and "pnea" can be broken down into meaning a condition having to do with positioning and breathing.
- Respiration rate involves how many breaths a patient takes per minute. Although this is important in a patient with orthopnea who has difficulty breathing, the question specifically asks "what the PTA should do when concluding treatment," which would be positioning the patient with head of the bed elevated since "orthopnea" is difficulty breathing when in supine.

Does choice #1 address positioning for the patient who has difficulty breathing when supine? Yes, it does.

ADDITIONAL TESTING STRATEGIES

Besides proficient content knowledge and utilizing these testing strategies to think through answer choices carefully, some intangible factors can greatly influence success in the NPTAE. For example, stress and anxiety while studying and during the NPTAE can often sabotage success as candidates become occupied with negative thoughts. The following shifts in mindset and activities can help the candidate better prepare and perform during the NPTAE.

- Developing a *positive mental attitude* toward the NPTAE can change a negative mindset into a positive one and help the candidate become more confident and motivated in their review process.

Change the mindset from "I can't possibly learn all this information" to "I will spend the time studying to understand the material."

- Physical activity can decrease stress and anxiety as well as improve intellectual acuity
  - Even short bouts of exercise can re-focus the mind for more effective studying
- Proper nutrition can also support a positive mindset and mental sharpness
  - Foods high in trans-fats or sugar can have a negative effect of brain health

Neuromuscular and Nervous System

MELISSA SCHNEIDER · ANNIE BURKE-DOE

CHAPTER TABLE OF CONTENTS

▲ HIGH-YIELD TERMS

Neuroplasticity	An emerging body of research evidence supporting the hypothesis that brain remodeling throughout life is possible and is enhanced by the type and amount of practice related to skill acquisition.
Neurologic examination	An essential component of a comprehensive physical examination that includes the systems review and a comprehensive and systematic examination of both the central nervous system (CNS) and peripheral nervous system (PNS) in conjunction with other body systems. The examination should determine impairments in body function and structure, limitations in functional activities, and participation restrictions.
Cerebrovascular accident (CVA)/stroke	Occurs when blood flow interruption within brain blood vessels narrows or blocks a vessel (ischemia) or ruptures a vessel (hemorrhage).
Traumatic brain injury (TBI)	Results from a blow to the head and/or sudden acceleration-deceleration of the head, such as with motor vehicle accidents. TBIs can be closed or open in terms of whether or not the skull is fractured.
Mild TBI (mTBI)	A brain injury causing microscopic damage that may not be detectable on neuroimaging and may or may not involve a loss of consciousness.
Brain tumor	A mass or growth of abnormal cells in the brain.
Spinal cord injury (SCI)	An injury most commonly when there is fracture, dislocation, and/or subluxation of the vertebrae into the spinal cord.
Multiple sclerosis (MS)	A chronic, progressive, inflammatory disease that affects neurons in the CNS.
Parkinson disease (PD)	The second most common, progressive neurodegenerative disorder with deficits in the basal ganglia and its connections to movement and posturing, cognitive and psychiatric functions.
Huntington disease (HD)	A progressive neurodegenerative disorder caused by an autosomal dominant mutation where there is a severe loss of neurons in the caudate and putamen of the basal ganglia.
Amyotrophic lateral sclerosis (ALS)	A slow, progressive, asymmetric atrophy with muscular weakness and hyperreflexia.
Guillain–Barré syndrome (GBS)	A group of neuropathic conditions affecting the PNS, causing progressive weakness due to motor neuropathy and diminished or absent reflexes.

Postpolio syndrome (PPS)	A condition that affects people with a history of polio, followed by a period of neurologic stability, before developing new or exacerbated symptoms several years after the acute poliomyelitis infection.
Peripheral neuropathy	Damage to nerves leading to impaired sensation, movement, gland, or organ function.
Vestibular disorders	Categorized by their location as peripheral, central, or both. Peripheral vestibular disorders involve the peripheral sensory apparatus and/or inner ear structures and/or the vestibular nerve. Central vestibular disorders result from damage to the vestibular nuclei, the cerebellum, and the brainstem, including vestibular pathways within the brainstem that mediate vestibular reflexes.
Outcome measure	A type of test and measure that can be used in the patient management process to assist in the diagnosis and prognosis of patient care and tracking changes in human performance and health status.
Clinical practice guideline (CPG)	Recommendations based on the systematic review and evaluation of research evidence used to guide best practice for a specific condition.

■ ANATOMY AND PHYSIOLOGY OF THE NERVOUS SYSTEM

The nervous system is divided into the central nervous system (CNS) and the peripheral nervous system (PNS). The CNS contains the brain and spinal cord, while the PNS involves the spinal and cranial nerves and ganglia. Therefore, understanding neuroanatomy is critical to understanding brain functioning. Figure 2-1 illustrates the gross anatomical divisions of the CNS.

In the nervous system, it is important to understand the directional locations and planes of motion. Because the CNS bends around the closed system within the skull, planes are ventral-dorsal rather than anterior-posterior, as noted in musculoskeletal anatomy. See Figure 2-2 for the directional planes in the nervous system.

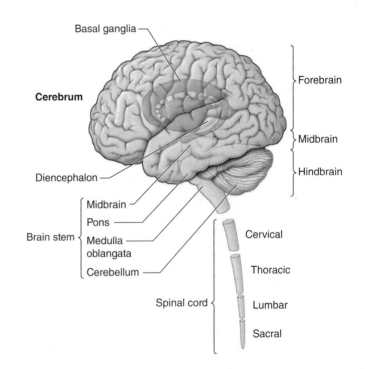

Figure 2-1. Gross anatomic divisions of the CNS. The cerebral hemispheres are found at the rostral end of the nervous system. The basal ganglia are contained within the cerebrum. The midbrain, pons, and medulla oblongata together are called the brainstem, and caudal to that is the spinal cord. Rostral to the midbrain is the diencephalon, the thalamus, and hypothalamus, which together with the cerebrum is called the forebrain. In this scheme (forebrain, midbrain, and hindbrain), the midbrain is itself, and the hindbrain is the pons, medulla, and cerebellum. (Adapted with permission from Kandel ER, Schwartz JH, Jessell TM, et al. *Principles of Neural Science*. 5th ed. 2013. Copyright © McGraw Hill LLC. All rights reserved. https://neurology.mhmedical.com.)

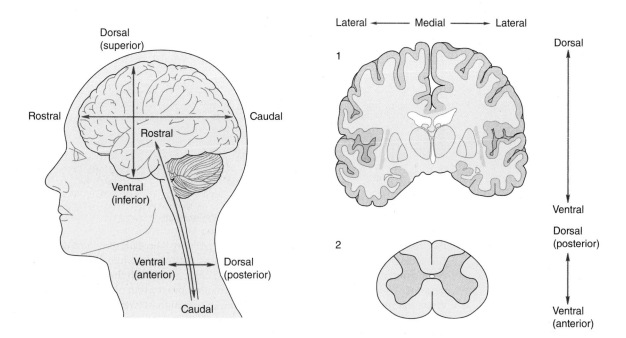

Figure 2-2. The directions used in the nervous system. The rostral direction is toward the nose and caudal is toward the tail. In the head of a person standing, rostral and anterior are roughly the same direction, and caudal and posterior are the same for the cerebral cortex. However, as the brainstem forms and descends into the spinal cord, the meanings of rostral and caudal shift. In the brainstem, rostral would be closer to the cerebrum and caudal would be closer to the spinal cord. Within the spinal cord, rostral would be toward the brainstem and caudal would be toward the coccygeal segments. In the person standing, for the spinal cord, rostral and superior are the same, and caudal and inferior are the same. The other directions used in the nervous system are dorsal, toward the back, and ventral, toward the front. The ventral side of the nervous system is the anterior part of the brainstem and spinal cord and the inferior part of the cerebrum. The dorsal part is the superior part of the cerebrum and the posterior part of the brainstem and spinal cord. Medial and lateral directions in the nervous system have the same meaning as in the regular cardinal planes. (Adapted with permission from Kandel ER, Schwartz JH, Jessell TM, et al. *Principles of Neural Science*. 5th ed. 2013. Copyright © McGraw Hill LLC. All rights reserved. https://neurology.mhmedical.com.)

Important distinctions exist between gray and white matter. Gray matter includes neurons, glial cells, axons, and their synapses into and out of tissues. White matter is made up of myelin, axons, and glial cells. See Figure 2-3 for a visual depiction of gray and white matter in the nervous system.

Neuroanatomy is clinically relevant when structure identification is paired with function. Therefore, understanding the basic terms is critical in how nervous system structures work together, and they are often repeated and used interchangeably. See Table 2-1 for common neuroscience terms. In addition, a list of the common terminology associated with the various neurologic diagnoses (Table A-3) can be found in the appendices at the end of this chapter.

CENTRAL NERVOUS SYSTEM

The CNS is composed of the brain and spinal cord. It is critical to understand how structures are connected for functional clinical significance. It is important to understand the types of neurons, physiology, and communication modes involved in how structures communicate with one another to command the PNS. Components of the CNS are identified in the following sections.

Cerebral Hemispheres

These involve left and right hemispheres and are collectively referred to as the cerebrum. The cerebral hemispheres support consciousness, memory, movement, sensation, emotion, and voluntary movement. The outermost layer is gray matter and is referred to as the cerebral cortex. Underneath this gray matter lie many gray matter structures, referred to as deep nuclei, such as the basal ganglia, interspersed with white matter structures to connect the cerebral hemispheres with other structures in the brain.

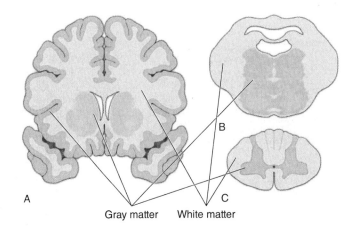

Gray matter   White matter

Figure 2-3. Brain, brainstem, and spinal cord sections showing gray and white matter. All levels of the CNS have a combination of gray matter and white matter. Gray matter is composed of the neurons and the supporting cells, along with the connections between neurons. The gray matter is where the information processing of the brain occurs. White matter is composed of axons carrying information between parts of the nervous system. In the cerebral hemispheres, there is white matter in the middle forming connections, and gray matter at the surface and in nuclei within the brain. In the brainstem and spinal cord, there is white matter on the outside, and gray matter within. (Part A: Reproduced with permission from Burke-Doe A, Dutton M, eds. *National Physical Therapy Examination and Board Review*. 2019. Copyright © McGraw Hill LLC. All rights reserved. https://accessphysiotherapy.mhmedical.com. Part B: Used with permission of John A. Buford, PT, PhD. Part C: Adapted with permission from Kandel ER, Schwartz JH, Jessell TM, et al. *Principles of Neural Science*. 5th ed. 2013. Copyright © McGraw Hill LLC. All rights reserved. https://neurology.mhmedical.com.)

Meninges

The meninges are a set of membranes that encase the CNS. From outermost to the innermost layer, they are as follows:

1. Dura mater, with its specialized infoldings of the falx cerebri and cerebellar tentorium, protects the brain and does not permit fluid to pass, except for exchange through blood vessels.

TABLE 2-1 • Common Terms in Neuroscience.	
Term	**General Usage**
Nucleus	A group of neurons in a gray matter structure that is anatomically relatively distinct from the surrounding tissue. A subnucleus would be a small nucleus that is a relatively distinct part of a larger nucleus.
Ganglion	Typically, a nucleus is located around the origin of a nerve; occasionally used instead of nucleus.
Cortex	The outer layer of the brain of both the cerebrum and the cerebellum, composed of gray matter.
Peduncle	A large bundle of axons that physically connects one structure to another.
Commissure	A group of axons traveling together to cross the midline.
Tract	A bundle of axons having a common origin, destination, and function.
Pathway	A route through which information travels, usually involving connections among multiple neurons. For example, there is a pathway from the cerebral cortex to the cerebellum that involves a connection with neurons in the brainstem. If the axons traveled directly from the cortex to the cerebellum, it would be called a tract, but because there is a connection to a neuron in the brainstem along the way, it is a pathway.
Lamina	A thin layer of white matter separating nuclei or subnuclei in gray matter.
Mesial	An inner surface formed by the apposition of two structures; in the nervous system, most commonly used along the midline where left and right parts of the brain are touching each other.

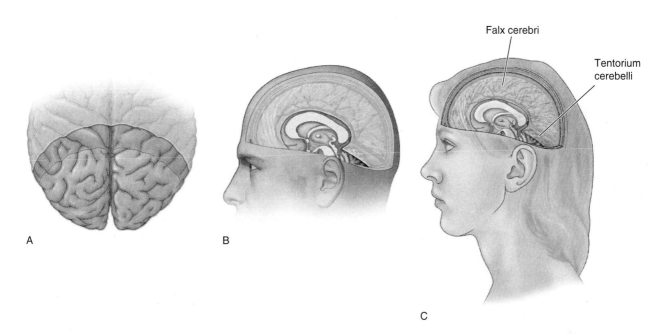

Falx cerebri

Tentorium
cerebelli

A   B

C

Figure 2-4. The meninges. **A** and **B.** This image of a brain shows layers of meninges removed, revealing the tough dura matter and the thinner arachnoid. The pia is continuous with the brain surface and cannot be distinguished without a microscope. **C.** The falx cerebri is a dura mater structure that separates the two cerebral hemispheres. (Part A and B: Reproduced with permission from Burke-Doe A, Dutton M, eds. *National Physical Therapy Examination and Board Review.* 2019. Copyright © McGraw Hill LLC. All rights reserved. https://accessphysiotherapy.mhmedical.com. Part C: Reproduced with permission from Martin JH. *Neuroanatomy Text and Atlas.* 4th ed. 2012. Copyright © McGraw Hill LLC. All rights reserved.)

2. Arachnoid mater is the middle layer and does not cover all brain surfaces, as does the dura mater; directly under the arachnoid mater are the cerebrospinal fluid (CSF) and dural sinuses.
3. Pia mater is the innermost layer of meninges. It also seals and protects the brain as a component of the blood–brain barrier; it is very thin and adherent to the nervous system within the deep crevices of the nervous tissue.

See Figure 2-4 for more details about the meninges.

Lobes of the Brain

The cerebral hemispheres can be divided into four major lobes: frontal, parietal, occipital, and temporal. Two additional regions, once considered lobes, are the limbic and insular regions. See Figure 2-5 for details regarding lobes of the brain.

Frontal Lobe. Begins at the central sulcus, and everything rostral is the frontal lobe. This lobe is responsible for thoughts, planning, decision-making, and actions. It is large in humans and typically sized in relation to intelligence.

Parietal Lobe. The rostral boundary is the central sulcus, and the caudal boundary is the parietal–occipital sulcus. The parietal lobe is responsible for sensation and perceptions from the somatosensory systems of the skin, muscles, and joints but not special senses such as vision and hearing. However, the parietal lobe does integrate information from the special senses relative to our overall sense of perception.

Occipital Lobe. Is bounded by the parietal lobe medially and the temporal lobe laterally. The occipital lobe's main function is for the special sense of vision. There are two specialized pathways for vision: the dorsal visual stream and the ventral visual stream. The dorsal visual stream is responsible for locating objected and integrating vision into perception and the parietal lobe's support. The ventral visual stream travels to the temporal lobe for object recognition and naming of objects.

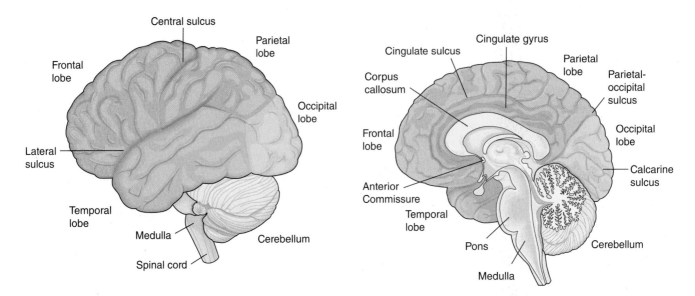

Figure 2-5. Lobes of the cerebral cortex and the landmark structures that form their boundaries. On the left, a lateral view of the brain shows the four major lobes. The central sulcus and the lateral sulcus are visible here. On the right, the medial view of the brain is shown, with the brain split in the sagittal plane, along the midline. The parietal–occipital sulcus is visible here, along with the cingulate gyrus. (Reproduced with permission from Martin JH. *Neuroanatomy Text and Atlas*. 3rd ed. 2003. Copyright © McGraw Hill LLC. All rights reserved.)

Temporal Lobe. Has no clear boundary between the temporal and occipital lobes; however, it is separated from the parietal and frontal lobes by the lateral sulcus. The temporal lobe is responsible for auditory processing as well as the identification of objects and memory.

Insular Region/Cortex. Is located deep in the lateral sulcus between the temporal and parietal lobes. The insular region is responsible for digestive and eating functions, autonomic functions, and sensations of pain or pleasure.

Limbic Region/Cortex. Specifically, the cingulate cortex can be located superior to the corpus callosum and is responsible for basic functions and motivation for hunger, emotions, and initiation.

Subcortical Structures

These include important white and gray matter structures, as listed below.

Thalamus. A major gray matter nucleus comprises multiple nuclei that serve as a major relay station for motor and sensory projections to and from the cerebral cortex.

Basal Ganglia. A collection of nuclei within the cerebral hemispheres that process and send information through the thalamus back to the cortex. See Figure 2-1. Specific basal ganglia nuclei include the caudate and putamen (together called the striatum), the globus pallidus, the subthalamic nucleus, and the substantia nigra. The latter is located in the dorsal midbrain rather than within the cerebral hemispheres, and the subthalamic nucleus sits just below the thalamus within the portion of the brain known as the diencephalon (eg, thalamus, hypothalamus, epithalamus, and subthalamus). The caudate nucleus borders and follows the lateral ventricles. The globus pallidus and putamen appear as a single nucleus, referred to as the lenticular nucleus, just medial to the insular region.

Hypothalamus. Located inferior to the thalamus and is where hormones are regulated by the brain for thirst and hunger and are detected based on physiologic signals, sleep-wake cycles are determined, and many other basic physiologic functions for homeostasis are regulated.

Hippocampal Formation.   Located in the medial aspect of the temporal lobe on the inferior surface of the brain. It is responsible for declarative memory, the ability to memorize information and experiences.

Amygdala.   A nucleus located in the temporal lobe can be found at the most rostral end of the hippocampal formation. It is responsible for creating memories, especially those related to intense emotions such as anger and fear.

Corpus Callosum.   Made up of axons that connect the right and left hemispheres primarily in the frontal and parietal lobes.

Anterior Commissure.   A white matter structure that links the left and right hemispheres.

Internal Capsule.   Another white matter pathway that sends and receives information to/from the cerebral cortex, connecting information from the spinal cord and brainstem.

Corona Radiate.   A significant amount of white matter comprises the majority of the subcortical white matter, and its spanning bulk is not typically pictured on images. Most axons communicate from one portion of the cortex to another without passing through the thalamus.

Ventricular System

The ventricular system consists of the "spaces," or cavities, inside the brain and includes the ventricles, passageways between the ventricles, and structures called the choroid plexus that secrete and reabsorb CSF. CSF is the filtrate of plasma that provides nourishment, waste removal, and brain and spinal cord protection. The choroid plexus can be located within the lateral and fourth ventricles. Thus, the ventricular system consists of two lateral ventricles, one in each cerebral hemisphere and a third and fourth ventricle. The third ventricle is a midline cavity located around the midbrain level, and the fourth ventricle is located between the brainstem and the cerebellum. CSF passes between the lateral and third ventricle through the interventricular foramen and between the third and fourth ventricles by the cerebral aqueduct.

CSF travels the path as described above and exits through one of the three major openings: the foramen of Magendie, which is a midline opening from the fourth ventricle to the posterior aspect of the medulla in the brainstem, and two lateral apertures, a left and a right, called the foramina of Luschka, coming out from each side of the fourth ventricle in the space between the cerebellum and pons. The central canal of the spinal cord, forming in the caudal medulla, is also a place for CSF to leave the fourth ventricle; however, this space is small compared to the three major openings described above.

Outside the ventricular system, CSF is in the subarachnoid space between the arachnoid and pia mater. Additionally, venous sinuses are located in the dura mater, called arachnoid villi, and they permit slow leaking of the CSF into the venous blood to allow the fluid to return to its circulatory path.

Cerebellum

Cerebellum means "little brain" and has a major role in motor learning and coordination of voluntary movement. Like the cerebral hemispheres, the cerebellum has an outer layer of gray matter and an inner layer of white matter that connects the nervous system through the pathways connecting the brainstem, spinal cord, and cerebrum.

Cerebellar Cortex.   Has three layers, each named by its structural features: a parallel fiber layer, a Purkinje layer, and a granular layer.

Deep Cerebellar Nuclei (DCN).   Deep gray matter structures that connect with specific areas of the cerebellar cortex. There are four specific DCN: the fastigial nucleus, the globose and emboliform nuclei, and the dentate nucleus.

Lobes of the Cerebellum. The cerebellum can be divided into three lobes. The anterior lobe is the part underneath the occipital lobe, rostral to a cerebellar cortex structure called the primary fissure. The posterior cerebellum is everything else, except for a small structure called the flocculonodular lobe, which is at the opposite end of the cerebellum from the anterior lobe and can be found on the anterior surface, opposed to the fourth ventricle.

Functional Divisions. The cerebellum can also be divided into functional divisions from a rehabilitation perspective. They are the vestibulocerebellum, the spinocerebellum, and the cerebrocerebellum.

Connections. Each of the DCN is connected mainly with a certain functional division of the cerebellum.

- Vestibulocerebellum is connected to the fastigial nucleus, and its function relates to vestibular control of eye movement, posture, and balance.
- Spinocerebellum is connected to the fastigial, globose, and emboliform nuclei, receiving postural sensory information via the spinocerebellar tracts and projecting to the medial descending system (rubrospinal, vestibulospinal, and reticulospinal tracts) to control postural stability.
- Cerebrocerebellum is connected to the dentate nucleus, sending efferents via the thalamus to the motor cortex and other cortical areas to participate in motor planning and motor control.

Cerebellar Peduncles. There are three white matter connections located on each side of the cerebellum and brainstem. Figure 2-6 shows that the three connections are the inferior, middle, and superior cerebellar peduncles.

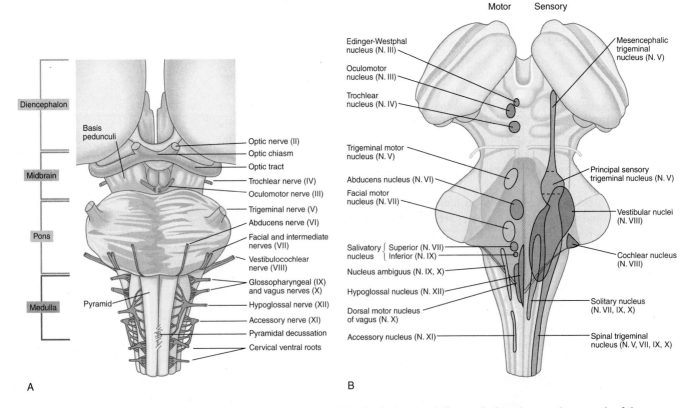

Figure 2-6. The cranial nerves. On the left **(A)**, a ventral view of the brainstem and diencephalon shows where each of the cranial nerves exits the brainstem. On the right **(B)**, a dorsal view shows where the cranial nerve nuclei are located for motor outputs and sensory inputs. (Reproduced with permission from Kandel ER, Schwartz JH, Jessell TM, et al., eds. *Principles of Neural Science*, 5th ed. 2013. Copyright © McGraw Hill LLC. All rights reserved. https://neurology.mhmedical.com.)

Brainstem

The brainstem involves the midbrain, pons, and medulla, and all the white matter communication between the brain and spinal cord passes through the brainstem. This major relay station is critical for many vital functions such as sensory, motor, and autonomic, and includes a role in more basic functions such as taste, eating, hearing, balance, and vision. In addition, the brainstem assists with the modulation of pain and supports functions such as posture, locomotion, and perception, along with arousal and cardiorespiratory function. See Figure 2-6.

Brainstem Structures. Some structures are isolated to a particular region of the brainstem, while others span the length of the brainstem in a rostrocaudal fashion.

- Trigeminal nucleus: Runs from the midbrain to the medulla to support the trigeminal nerve's sensory and motor functions.
- Reticular formation: A long column of gray matter found ventrolateral to the cerebral aqueduct and the fourth ventricle extending from the midbrain to the medulla that supports the reticulospinal tracts, key regulators for posture, locomotion, and gross limb movements.
- Raphe nuclei: Various functions that regulate the state of other parts of the nervous system, including arousal, the spinal cord circuits for control of walking, and the transmission and modulation of pain.

Midbrain. This is the most rostral level of the brainstem and contains the most visible white matter structures. The structures are called the cerebral peduncles, and they contain the axons from the cerebrum to the brainstem and the spinal cord. Also, within the midbrain are several important structures: substantia nigra, periaqueductal gray, red nucleus, superior colliculus, and the inferior colliculus.

Pons. The pons and medulla are distinguished from each other by the middle cerebellar peduncle. Within the pons, the ventral aspect contains the pontine nuclei, in which synapses occur as information enters the cerebellum. In the dorsal aspect of the pons, the trigeminal nuclei for the fifth cranial nerve (CN V), the nucleus for the sixth cranial nerve, abducens (CN VI), and the nucleus for the seventh cranial nerve, the facial nerve (CN VII) can be located. The vestibular nuclei are in the pons, slightly lateral to the midline and just ventral to the fourth ventricle.

Medulla. The medulla is the most caudal aspect of the brainstem, and its most prominent surface features anteriorly are the medullary pyramids and the inferior olives. In addition, there are other important nuclei, including the cranial nerve nuclei for nerves IX to XII (glossopharyngeal, vagus, spinal accessory, and hypoglossal) and the cardiorespiratory regulation centers.

Cranial Nerves. See Table 2-2.

Major Fiber Tracts. There are major tracts on the surface of the brainstem, including the cerebral and cerebellar peduncles, the medullary pyramids, and the dorsal columns. There are also certain internal white matter tracts of importance in rehabilitation (see Figure 2-7)

SPINAL CORD

The spinal cord is the direct source of connection between the brain and the body. Spinal nerves exit at both the left and right sides of each vertebral body that receive afferent sensory information and transmit efferent motor information. Like the CNS, the spinal cord is surrounded by meninges, including the dura, arachnoid, and pia mater. In addition, two special meningeal extensions of the spinal cord include the denticulate ligaments, which attach the spinal cord to the dura mater to assist with stability, and the filum terminale, which is an extension of the pia mater at the most caudal end of the cord. See Figure 2-8 for details.

TABLE 2-2 • Cranial Nerves.

	Nerve	Name	Cranial Foramina	Nucleus	Target	Function
Forebrain	I	Olfactory	Cribriform plate	Connects directly with forebrain	Nose: Olfactory mucosa	Smell
	II	Optic	Optic	Thalamus, lateral geniculate nucleus	Eye: Retina	Vision
Midbrain	III	Oculomotor	Superior orbital fissure	Oculomotor nucleus	Eyelid: Levator palpebrae superioris	Lid movements
					Eye muscles: Superior rectus, inferior rectus, medial rectus, inferior oblique	Eye movements
				Edinger–Westphal nucleus	Pupil: Sphincter pupillae	Pupillary constriction
					Intraocular lens: Ciliary muscles	Accommodation (focus of the eye)
	IV	Trochlear	Superior orbital fissure	Trochlear nucleus	Superior oblique muscle	Eye movement
	V	Trigeminal	V3, foramen ovale	Mesencephalic nucleus	Muscles of mastication	Proprioception
Pons	V	Trigeminal		Principal sensory nucleus	Face	Discriminative touch and vibration sense
				Motor nucleus	Muscles of mastication	Movement of mandible
	VI	Abducens	Superior orbital fissure	Abducens nucleus	Eye: Lateral rectus	Abduction of the eye
	VII	Facial	Internal auditory meatus	Facial nucleus	Face	Movement of muscles of facial expression; stylohyoid and posterior belly of digastric; stapedius
				Spinal nucleus of CN V	Ear	Sensation from external acoustic meatus and skin posterior to ear
				Superior salivatory nucleus	Lacrimal, sublingual, and submandibular glands	Lacrimation and salivation
				Nucleus solitarius	Anterior 2/3 of tongue	Taste
Medulla	VIII	Vestibulocochlear	Internal auditory meatus	Vestibular nuclear complex	Vestibulospinal tracts, vestibular nuclei, and cerebellum	Balance and reflex eye movements
				Cochlear nuclei	Inner ear: Organ of Corti	Hearing
	IX	Glossopharyngeal	Jugular	Spinal nucleus of V	Posterior 1/3 of tongue, tonsil, external ear, internal tympanic membrane, pharynx	Somatic sensation
				Nucleus solitarius	Tongue and pharynx	Gag reflex
					Carotid body	Chemoreceptors and baroreceptors
				Nucleus solitarius	Posterior 1/3 of tongue	Taste
				Nucleus ambiguus	Stylopharyngeus	Motor
				Inferior salivatory nucleus	Parotid gland	Salivation

Region	CN	Nerve	Foramen	Nucleus	Target	Function
Medulla	V	Trigeminal		Spinal nucleus of V	Face	Pain and temperature
	X	Vagus	Jugular	Spinal nucleus of CN V	Posterior meninges, external acoustic meatus, skin posterior to ear	Somatic sensation
				Nucleus solitarius	Larynx, trachea, esophagus, thoracic viscera, abdominal viscera	Somatic sensation
					Aortic arch	Stretch and chemoreceptors for cardiopulmonary system reflexes
				Nucleus solitarius	Taste buds in epiglottis	Taste
				Nucleus ambiguus	Pharyngeal muscles and intrinsic muscles of the larynx	Muscles of phonation and deglutition
				Dorsal motor nucleus of vagus	Cervical, thoracic, and abdominal viscera; ganglion neurons located in/near target organ	Smooth muscle and glands of pharynx, larynx, thoracic viscera, abdominal viscera
				Nucleus ambiguus	Cardiac muscle	Decrease heart rate and blood pressure
	XI	Accessory	Jugular	Spinal accessory nucleus; nucleus ambiguus	Sternocleidomastoid and trapezius	Shoulder and neck movement
	XII	Hypoglossal	Hypoglossal canal	Hypoglossal nucleus	Hyoglossus, genioglossus, styloglossus, intrinsic muscles of the tongue	Movement of the tongue

CN, cranial nerve.

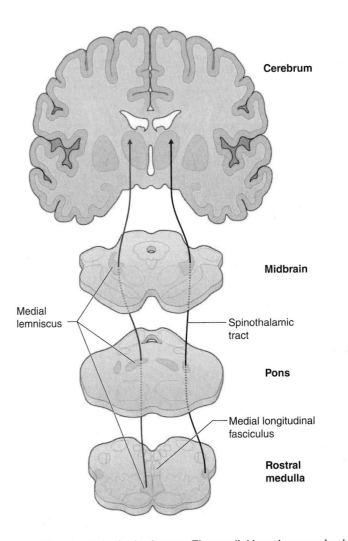

Figure 2-7. **Selected fiber tracts in the brainstem. The medial lemniscus and spinotha-lamic tracts carry sensory information upward toward the brain. The medial longitudinal fasciculus carries oculomotor control signals as well as commands for head and neck movements.** (Reproduced with permission from Nichols-Larsen DS, Kegelmeyer DA, Buford JA, et al. *Neurologic Rehabilitation: Neuroscience and Neuroplasticity in Physical Therapy Practice.* 2016. Copyright © McGraw Hill LLC. All rights reserved. http://accessphysiotherapy.mhmedical .com.)

When viewing the spinal cord, note the dorsal aspect containing the dorsal columns, which contain sensory fibers ascending toward the medulla. The ventral roots are formed by efferent axons of motor and autonomic projections from the spinal cord to the body. Two specialized spinal cord regions involve the cervical and lumbosacral regions; there is a lateral expansion of the ventral horns where limb muscle motoneu-rons are located.

The segmental organization of the spinal cord is organized for the vertebral bone that is formed alongside that particular segment during embryological development. Each seg-ment contains a combination of the dorsal and ventral roots; the first spinal nerve exits the intervertebral foramen above the first cervical vertebra, and the eighth spinal nerve exits below the seventh cervical vertebra (above T1). Thus, these segments are referred to as the eight cervical segments. From here, each spinal segment is named by the vertebra above the exit of its spinal nerve, so the first thoracic segment has a spinal nerve that exits below the first thoracic vertebra. In summary, there are 31 spinal segmental levels; 8 cervi-cal spinal segments, 12 thoracic, 5 lumbar, 5 sacral, and 1 coccygeal, with an equal number of spinal nerves accordingly on each side.

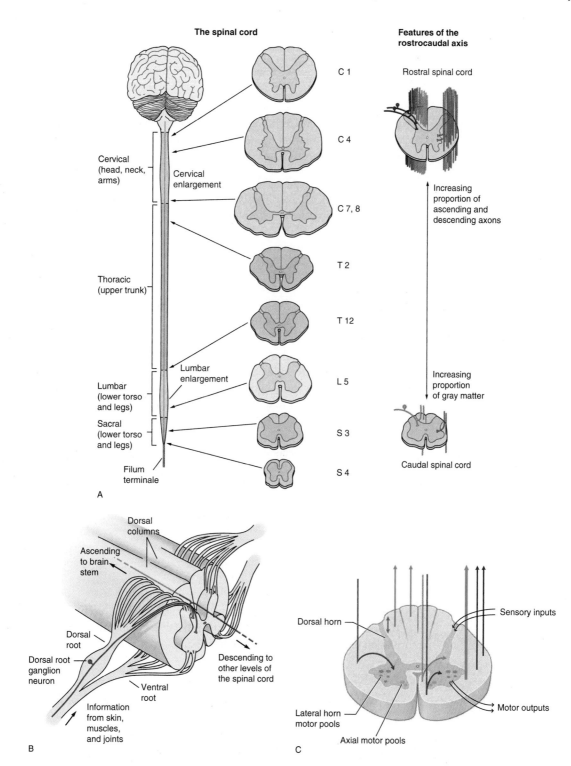

Figure 2-8. The spinal cord. **A.** The spinal cord carries all information between the brain and the body except that carried by the cranial nerves. There are enlargements at the cervical and lumbosacral levels to contain the extra gray and white matter for the arms and legs. Cross-sections representative of each segmental level are illustrated. Note how the relative proportion of white matter decreases at lower levels; few sensory axons have accumulated from below, and most motor axons have already terminated at levels above. **B.** The organization of a typical spinal segment is shown, including the dorsal roots, ventral roots, dorsal root ganglion, and spinal nerve. **C.** The general organization of information moving up and down the spinal cord is shown. Descending fibers (red) can travel in the lateral or ventral funiculus. Ascending fibers travel in the lateral and dorsal funiculus, some bound for the brain (green) and some for the cerebellum (purple). Special systems also descend to release neuromodulators that regulate spinal cord circuits (orange). (A, B: Reproduced with permission from Kandel ER, Schwartz JH, Jessell TM, et al., eds. *Principles of Neural Science*, 5th ed. 2013. Copyright © McGraw Hill LLC. All rights reserved. https://neurology.mhmedical.com. C: Reproduced with permission from Burke-Doe A, Dutton M, eds. *National Physical Therapy Examination and Board Review*. 2019. Copyright © McGraw Hill LLC. All rights reserved. https://accessphysiotherapy.mhmedical.com.)

The spinal cord supports complex communication within its own gray matter circuits for functions of flexor withdrawal, reflexive control of bowel and bladder function, and neural control of ambulation.

Sensory Pathways

Our sensation comprises complex networks, allowing humans to sense the perception of touch, muscle stretch and tension, joint pressure and motion, pain, pressure, temperature, vibration, and itch. The two essential sensory pathways, the dorsal column medial lemniscal system and the anterior lateral system, should be reviewed relative to Figure 2-9.

Motor Pathways

Each of the four major descending motor systems has specific functions to support motor control. These systems are the corticospinal system, the rubrospinal tract, the reticulospinal system, and the vestibulospinal system. They should be reviewed concerning the origin, decussation (the point at which fiber crosses) as appropriate, and termination. Please review Figure 2-9.

Spinal Tracts (Sensory Pathways and Motor Pathways)

To further understand the interneuron synapses within the spinal cord, one must further review the sensory and motor pathways.

The spinal sensory fibers (also known as ascending tracts or sensory pathways) are located variably within the white matter, and intrinsic neurons of the gray matter of the spinal cord receive primary sensory input and relay information to the cerebellum and cerebrum. The motor fibers (also referred to as ascending spinal tracts or motor pathways) supply information for voluntary muscle function, tone, reflexes, and equilibrium.

For example, if someone feels an uncomfortable pressure or stretch on the arm, this information is neurologically transmitted to the spinal cord, where the anterior spinothalamic tract carries information to the thalamus. Next, the thalamus relays this information to the cerebral cortex and cerebellum. Motor responses are then sent back out through the descending corticospinal tract within the spinal cord. Finally, the motor response leaves the spinal cord through the corresponding peripheral nerve, which innervates the arm and muscle tissue area where the pain and stretch first occurred. This process happens in microseconds but is an example of how the body moves and adapts continually to the environment.

There are multiple pathways within the spinal cord and are presented in Table 2-3. Please note the last portion of the tract name is indicative of whether the tract carries sensory information or motor responses and relates to the order of neuronal synapses.

PERIPHERAL NERVOUS SYSTEM

The PNS is composed of the sensory and motor axons traveling into and out of the CNS. In the PNS, Schwann cells create myelin. These cells cover only one segment of an axon. In most parts of the PNS, the spinal nerves exit the spinal cord and travel individually to innervate specific locations in the body; however, in both the lower cervical to include T1 and in the lumbosacral regions, spinal nerves are combined to form a bundle of plexus of spinal nerves that innervate the arms, legs, and skin (see Appendix C).

Cervical Plexus. Composed of the spinal nerves from C1 to C4. These nerves primarily provide innervation to the deep muscles of the neck, levator scapulae, superficial anterior neck muscles, and portions of the trapezius and sternocleidomastoid muscles. Additionally, the phrenic nerve is innervated through the branches formulated from the C3 to C5 spinal nerve roots.

Brachial Plexus. Formed of the anterior primary rami of C5 through T1. This plexus provides motor and sensory innervations. The five primary peripheral nerves of the brachial plexus include the musculocutaneous, axillary, radial, median, and ulnar nerves.

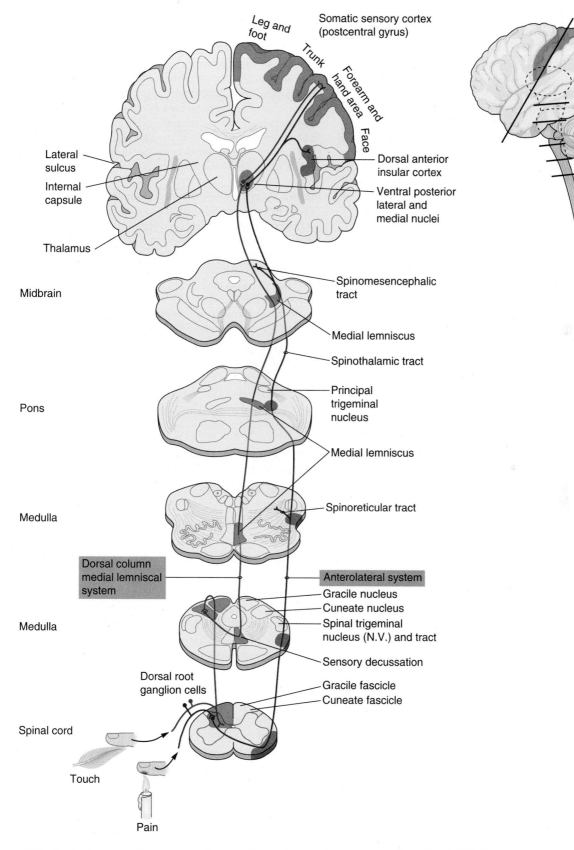

Figure 2-9. Ascending somatosensory pathways. (Reproduced with permission from Kandel ER, Schwartz JH, Jessell TM, et al. *Principles of Neural Science.* 5th ed. 2013. Copyright © McGraw Hill LLC. All rights reserved. https://neurology.mhmedical.com.)

TABLE 2-3 • The Multiple Pathways Within the Spinal Cord.	
Ascending Tracts (Sensory)	**Descending Tracts (Motor)**
Spinothalamic tract (lateral) Transmits pain and temperature sensations to the cerebral cortex by way of the thalamus *Spinothalamic tract (anterior)* Transmits light touch and pressure to the cerebral cortex by way of the thalamus *Spinoreticular tract* Reticular information affecting levels of consciousness *Spinocerebellar tract (ventral)* Ascends to the cerebellum for ipsilateral subconscious proprioception, muscle tension, joint space awareness, and assisting with posture for the trunk, upper and lower extremities *Spinocerebellar tract (dorsal)* Ascends to the cerebellum affecting ipsilateral subconscious proprioception, joint space awareness, muscle tension, trunk posture and extremity position awareness *Spinotectal tract* Carries information for reflexive and voluntary eye movements and responses to stimulus	*Corticospinal tract (lateral)* Contralateral voluntary fine movements *Corticospinal tract (anterior)* Primary motor pathway helping to control discrete and skillful movements of the extremities *Reticulospinal tract* Facilitates or inhibits either voluntary or reflexive activity of alpha and gamma motor neurons *Rubrospinal tract* Primary leads to innervation of the upper extremities. Facilitates flexor motor neurons and inhibits extensor neurons. Affects more proximal muscles than distal. *Vestibulospinal tracts (lateral and medial)* Lateral tract assists in postural adjustment, while the medial tract helps to facilitate proximal extensor muscles and regulates muscle tone in the neck and upper back *Tectospinal tract* Provides orientation of the head toward sound or a moving object

These five nerves provide muscle and sensory innervation for a majority of the upper extremities.

- The musculocutaneous nerve innervates the forearm flexors.
- The radial nerve innervates the elbow, wrist, and finger extensors.
- The ulnar nerve assists the median nerve with wrist and finger flexion, finger abduction, adduction, and opposition of the fifth finger.
- The median nerve alone provides innervation to the pronators and wrist and finger flexors. It also provides thumb abduction and opposition.
- The axillary nerve provides innervation to the deltoid muscle group.

Lumbosacral Plexus. Involves innervation from the L1 to S3 spinal nerves. Eight roots form six primary peripheral nerves. The sciatic nerve (common peroneal and tibial nerve) innervates the hamstrings before separating into its two components just above the knee. The femoral nerve located anteriorly provides innervation to the hip flexors and anterior thigh muscles. Hip adductors are supplied through the obturator nerve, and the tibial nerve supplies the ankle plantar flexors.

> **STUDY PEARL**
> All of the dermatomes and myotomes should be reviewed thoroughly.

AUTONOMIC NERVOUS SYSTEM

The autonomic nervous system (ANS) comprises two divisions: the sympathetic and parasympathetic divisions, which regulate vasculature, glands, and visceral organs. The sympathetic division is often known as the fight-or-flight response system because it responds to fear. The sympathetic division also contains the sympathetic chain ganglia, positioned along the length of the spinal cord to send efferent information to target organs. The parasympathetic division is often known as the rest-and-digest response system because it engages during relaxation, for example, when we are sleeping. In addition, the parasympathetic division also involves the cranial nerves, cranial nerve nuclei, and specialized structures in the sacral spinal cord. In the parasympathetic division, there are preganglionic neurons that project to target ganglia in the periphery and postganglionic neurons that project to the target organs. These two powerful PNS divisions work together in conjunction with the CNS.

Table 2-4 provides an overview of the major structures and landmarks in the nervous system.

TABLE 2-4 • Major Structures and Landmarks in the Nervous System, Emphasizing Function in Sensory and Motor Systems.

Structure	Functions
Meninges	Protect the brain and spinal cord
Lobes of the Cerebrum	
Frontal	Motor planning and initiation, language output, personality, problem-solving, insight, and foresight
Parietal	Sensory perception and integration, visual location, auditory location, music appreciation
Occipital	Vision (primary visual cortex and visual association cortex)
Temporal	Auditory processing, especially language, identification of objects, learning, and memory
Insular	Gustatory (taste) perception
Limbic	Emotional responses, drive-related behavior, and emotional memory
Major Cortical Landmarks	
Central sulcus	Divides frontal and parietal lobes
Parieto-occipital sulcus	Divides parietal and occipital lobes
Lateral sulcus	Superior border of temporal lobe
Cingulate sulcus	Superior border of limbic lobe
Precentral gyrus	Primary motor cortex
Postcentral gyrus	Primary sensory cortex
Posterior parietal association area	Integration of body awareness with visual perception
Subcortical Structures	
Lateral ventricle	C-shaped chambers in each cerebral hemisphere where most of the cerebrospinal fluid (CSF) is made; communicate with the third ventricle via the two interventricular foramen
Third ventricle	Midline cavity in diencephalon that connects with the fourth ventricle via the cerebral aqueduct
Fourth ventricle	Tent-like cavity between the cerebellum posteriorly and the pons and rostral medulla anteriorly that communicates with subarachnoid space
Choroid plexus	Vascularized tissue that secretes CSF
Cerebral aqueduct	Narrow channel through the midbrain that connects the third and fourth ventricles
Foramen of Magendie	Median aperture (opening) of the fourth ventricle through which CSF flows into the subarachnoid space
Foramina of Luschka	Two lateral apertures of the fourth ventricle through which CSF flows into the subarachnoid space
Basal ganglia	Initiation and selection of thoughts and especially actions
Caudate nucleus	Receives information primarily from association areas of the cerebral cortex; important for cognitive functions of the basal ganglia
Head	Rostral—main target for prefrontal cortex
Body	Superior—parietal areas
Tail	Wraps around into the temporal lobe—temporal areas
Putamen	Functionally and cellularly just like the caudate, but anatomically separated from caudate by fibers of the internal capsule. Receives information primarily from motor and somatosensory areas of the cerebral cortex; important for motor functions of the basal ganglia
Striatum	A name used to refer to the caudate and putamen in combination
Globus pallidus—external segment (GPe)	One target of output from striatum. Involved in intermediate stage of basal ganglia processing
Globus pallidus—internal segment (GPi)	Final output nucleus targeted by GPe and STN—has neurons with axons leaving basal ganglia to go to the thalamus and thereby influence cortex and the control of movement
Subthalamic nucleus	Works with GPe for intermediate steps in basal ganglia processing
Substantia nigra	The largest nucleus in the midbrain
Pars compacta (SNpc)	Location of dopamine-producing cells that project into the striatum (caudate and putamen) to control movement
Pars reticulata (SNpr)	Just like cells in GPi but SNpr cells control eye movements, while GPi cells are for the rest of the body
Internal capsule	Funnel-shaped region separating the thalamus from the basal ganglia; contains fiber tracts that relay almost all of the information going to and from the cerebral cortex and other (noncortical) parts of the brain

(Continued)

TABLE 2-4 • Major Structures and Landmarks in the Nervous System, Emphasizing Function in Sensory and Motor Systems. (Continued)

Structure	Functions
Hippocampus	Memory formation (declarative)
Amygdala	Emotions, learning whether something is "good" or "bad," aggression
Thalamus	Receives, filters, and distributes information bound for the cerebral cortex
Hypothalamus	Autonomic functions, drives, hormones
Cerebellum	Receives information from sensory systems, the cerebral cortex and other sites, and participates in the planning and coordination of movement
Cerebellar cortex	Three-layered structure that receives cerebellar inputs and projects them to the deep cerebellar nuclei
Folia	
Vermis	Repeated horizontal folds or gyri of the cerebellum
Flocculonodular lobe	Midline lobe of the cerebellum important for cerebellar control of body and posture
Spinocerebellum	Cerebellar control for vestibular responses and eye movements
	Consists of the vermis and medial parts of the lateral cerebellar hemispheres that receive spinal inputs; involved with regulation of posture and coordination of limb movements
Lateral cerebellar hemispheres	Main lobes of the cerebellum on each side of the vermis; medial part is part of spinocerebellum as stated above; lateral parts are part of the cerebrocerebellum, a functional division that communicates with the cerebral cortex for the coordination of motor planning and to some extent the coordination of higher-order thought processes
Deep cerebellar nuclei	Location for cells sends axons projecting out of the cerebellum to affect other parts of the nervous systems, especially the brainstem and (via the thalamus) the cortex
Brainstem	Consists of the midbrain, pons, and medulla
Midbrain	The most rostral of the three subdivisions of the brainstem
Cerebral peduncles	Two large cylindrical masses on ventral surface of midbrain containing descending motor fibers from the cortex
Red nucleus	Involved in cerebellar circuitry and in control of limb movements, especially shaping the hand during reaching
Cerebral aqueduct—PAG	Site of origin of a descending pain-control pathway
Superior colliculi	Involved in directing visual attention and controlling eye movements
Inferior colliculi	Major link in the auditory system
Pons	The second of the three parts of the brainstem, continuous rostrally with the midbrain and caudally with the medulla
Pontine nuclei	Nuclei in the basal pons that receive inputs from the cerebral cortex and project to contralateral cerebellum
Cerebellar peduncles	Three paired fiber bundles connecting the cerebellum and brainstem via cerebellar afferents and efferents
Vestibular nuclei	Involved in regulating posture and coordinating eye and head movements
Reticular formation	Complex network of nuclei involved in integrative functions such as control of complex movements, transmission of pain information, vital functions, and arousal and consciousness
Medulla	The most caudal of the three subdivisions of the brainstem
Pyramids	Two rounded masses on the ventral surface of the medulla containing motor fibers
Inferior olivary complex	Origin of "climbing fibers" to cerebellum that are involved in motor learning
Dorsal column nuclei	Nuclei for relay of proprioceptive and discriminative touch for dorsal column–medial lemniscus system
Vestibular nuclei	Involved in regulating posture and coordinating eye and head movements
Reticular formation	Complex network of nuclei involved in integrative functions such as control of complex movements, transmission of pain information, vital functions, and arousal and consciousness
Spinal cord	Conducts sensory/motor information to/from the brain; contains central pattern generators for control of walking
White matter	Fiber tracts (ie, myelinated axons) that carry information up and down
Gray matter	Contains neuronal cell bodies and reflex circuits
Cervical enlargement (C5-T1)	Expanded gray matter to control the arms, and expanded white matter for incoming and outgoing information

(Continued)

TABLE 2-4 • Major Structures and Landmarks in the Nervous System, Emphasizing Function in Sensory and Motor Systems. (*Continued*)

Structure	Functions
Lumbar enlargement (L2-S3)	Expanded gray area to control the legs, and expanded white matter for incoming and outgoing information
Dorsal roots	Incoming (sensory) information
Ventral roots	Outgoing (motor) commands
Spinal nerves	Where dorsal and ventral roots fuse before exiting the intervertebral foramina
Cauda equina	Spinal nerves in lower vertebral column on their way to their original foramina (vertebral column longer than spinal cord in adults)
Sympathetic chain	Series of interconnected ganglia that lie ventral and lateral to the vertebral column that contain cell bodies of postganglionic neurons in the sympathetic nervous system
Corpus callosum	White matter fiber tracts connecting left and right cerebral hemispheres

PAG, periaqueductal gray; STN, subthalamic nucleus.

EMBRYOLOGICAL DEVELOPMENT OF THE NERVOUS SYSTEM AND NEUROPLASTICITY

The nervous system arises from neural crest cells within the ectodermal layer of the developing embryo. The neural plate is altered by cell proliferation which then translates the neural plate into the neural tube. Further cell proliferation takes place and fosters the development of three vesicles into a five-vesicle structure identified by the telencephalon (cerebral hemispheres), diencephalon (retina, hypothalamus, thalamus, epithalamus, and subthalamus), mesencephalon (midbrain), metencephalon (pons, cerebellum), and myelencephalon (medulla), which is contiguous with the remainder of the neural tube that forms the spinal cord. The space or lumen of the neural tube eventually develops into the entire ventricular system and central spinal canal. See Figure 2-10 for identification of further developing cellular layers and further explanation. Additional terms related to developmental neuroplasticity are listed below.

- **Neurogenesis** refers to the development of neurons, and **gliogenesis** is the development of glial cells; these are interrelated processes.
- **Pruning** is the elimination of unnecessary axon collaterals.
- **Programmed cell death** is the destruction of neurons.
- **Long-term potentiation (LTP)** is associated with well-established connections in developing synapses and relates to axon survival and the entire strengthening of the neuronal network.

Adult Neurogenesis

Gliogenesis continues throughout the brain and spinal cord into adult life, while neurogenesis is mainly related to embryological and early postnatal development. The one noted exception is that neurogenesis does occur in adults near the hippocampus and olfactory bulb. Synaptogenesis in damaged pathways due to disease is unlikely.

Learning-Associated Neuroplasticity

There is an emerging body of research evidence to support the hypothesis that brain remodeling throughout life is possible and is enhanced by the type and amount of practice related to skill acquisition. LTP is mediated by several neurotransmitters and endogenous factors, along with brain-derived neurotrophic factor (BDNF) appearing to assist with synaptogenesis and supporting the synapse formation as related to the motor map reorganization. This then leads to angiogenesis, expansion of the capillary beds and permits an increased vascular density that supports the new synaptic communication.

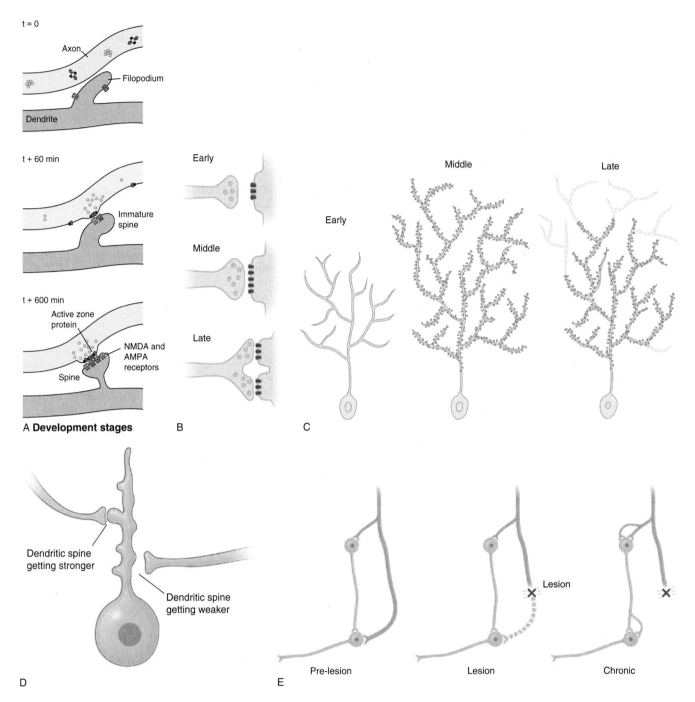

Figure 2-10. Synaptogenesis, pruning, and sprouting—mechanisms of neural development and injury repair. **A.** An axon passing by a cell can develop a new branch called a filopodium, which begins to form a synapse, and eventually becomes functional. The postsynaptic member begins to develop a synaptic spine. **B.** When a synapse strengthens over time, the presynaptic and postsynaptic elements can enlarge, and eventually, a second synapse can develop. **C.** As neurons develop, they initially lack synaptic spines. In the middle phase of development, they have an overabundance. As the connections mature, there is pruning, and some spines are eliminated. **D.** A dendritic spine can become stronger or weaker over time as the plasticity develops. **E.** In a circuit with alternative pathways, if one route is lesioned, the other can become stronger and replace the lost function. (A and C: Reproduced with permission from Kandel ER, Schwartz JH, Jessell TM, et al., eds. *Principles of Neural Science*, 5th ed. 2013. Copyright © McGraw Hill LLC. All rights reserved. https://neurology.mhmedical.com. Parts B, D, and E: Reproduced with permission of John A. Buford, PT, PhD.)

NEURONAL RESPONSE TO INJURY

Below are several important definitions related to CNS response to injury:

- *Focal degeneration*—Disruption of cellular function within the neuron's cell body and leads to cell death.
- *Remote neurodegeneration*—Commonly occurs after neural injury and leads to the loss of neurons in the area surrounding the focal injury and sites distal to but functionally related to the injured area.
- *Inflammation*—Occurs at the site of injury and in areas distant from the initial injury over approximately a 2-day to 8-week period; possibly longer dependent upon the neurological condition.
- *Excitotoxicity*—The excessive release of glutamate, dopamine, and norepinephrine that occurs due to CNS trauma or ischemia.
- *Apoptosis*—Programmed cell death that occurs in neural development but also in response to neural injury.
- *Autophagy*—A natural process to eliminate damaged proteins or organelles within the cell body to promote optimal cell functioning.

NEUROPLASTICITY AFTER CENTRAL NERVOUS SYSTEM INJURY

Plasticity Promoters

Postinjury, several neural changes work to support and strengthen the surviving neurons and their synapses to facilitate new axon and dendrite connections. The several known endogenous promotors of plasticity include neurotrophins such as BDNF and neurotrophin-3 (NT-3) that assist post-CNS injury. In addition, these endogenous neurotrophins can be enhanced by exercise both in the spinal cord and in the muscles.

Spontaneous Recovery

Spontaneous recovery is dependent on the integrity of the surrounding CNS tissue. After a neural shock, research has shown neuronal outgrowth, local sprouting, synaptogenesis, and angiogenesis. Sprouting is a mechanism by which axons grow additional distal projections to fill empty receptor sites.

Experience-Dependent Plasticity

This response depends on the activities of the patient postinjury and can be influenced by physical therapy interventions. The physical therapist (PT) must be aware that plasticity can be both adaptive and maladaptive.

Maladaptive Plasticity. Can be best described as learned nonuse. Nonuse is a process in which patients experience negative feedback—for example, when attempting to use their paretic arm after a stroke, and this experience discourages extremity use even though spontaneous recovery occurs. In addition, the patient will then use the less-involved extremity and is thus rewarded for completing compensatory strategies resulting in less and less use of the more involved extremity.

Adaptive Plasticity. Is best described through the research of constraint-induced movement therapy (CIMT). See Figure 2-11.

One of the seminal articles by Kleim and colleagues outlines the key principles related to adaptive plasticity. See outline in Box 2-1.

Physical therapist assistants (PTAs) and other rehabilitation team members play a critical role in neural recovery when, using research and theories of neuroplasticity, they directly targeted intervention programs. The potentially critical period postinjury is when the nervous system has the greatest opportunity for remodeling. Therefore, PTAs should emphasize task-specific training for new skill acquisition and translate the research regarding the importance of aerobic activity to raise BDNF, protein, and microRNA levels that support neuroplasticity mechanisms.

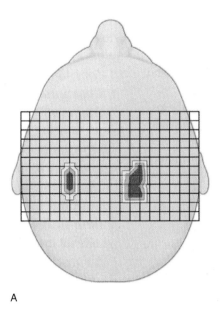

A

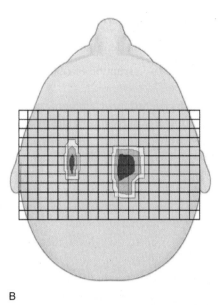

B

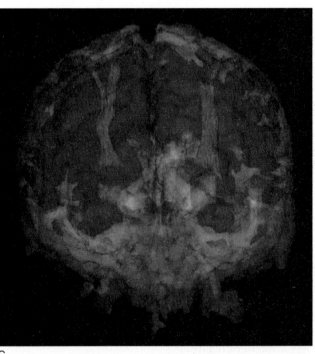

C

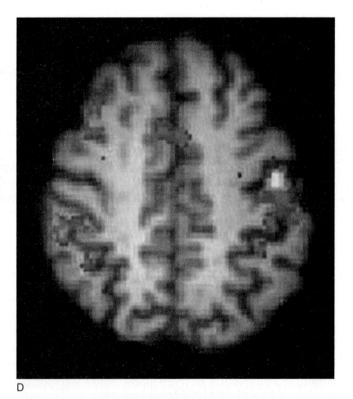

D

Figure 2-11. Imaging documentation of neural remodeling. **A.** Initial motor map of the paretic hand poststroke before treatment. **B.** Posttraining motor map illustrating expansion of the ipsilesional (right) motor cortex. **C.** Diffusion tensor imaging illustrates integrity of fibers within the internal capsule, associated with improved function, which could be the product of greater neuronal survival, enhanced sprouting, or a combination of the two. **D.** Demonstrates localized activity in the sensory discrimination network (ipsilesional primary sensory cortex, contralesional secondary sensory cortex, and right superior frontal cortex) of a left stroke survivor with full recovery of sensory ability (imaging view—right is anatomic left). (A and B: Reproduced with permission from Burke-Doe A, Dutton M, eds. *National Physical Therapy Examination and Board Review*. 2019. Copyright © McGraw Hill LLC. All rights reserved. https://accessphysiotherapy.mhmedical.com. C and D: Reproduced with permission from Deborah S. Nichols Larsen, PhD, FAPTA, FASAHP. The Ohio State University.)

CRITICAL FACTORS FOR ADAPTIVE NEURAL PLASTICITY

- Activity must target neural networks in which plasticity is desired.
- Activity can prevent secondary damage.
- Activity must target specific movements and skills salient to the patient to induce change in desired neural networks; saliency may activate critical emotional networks to facilitate plasticity.
- Neural plasticity requires repetition at an intensity that challenges the nervous system.
- The timing of activity is critical: (1) too much too early can exacerbate the lesion; (2) some early level of activity may be neuroprotective; (3) there may be a critical period or periods when plasticity is more likely; and (4) the window for plasticity is restricted and does not continue indefinitely.
- Older brains do not have the same capacity for remodeling that is available to younger brains.
- Plasticity in one neural network may facilitate (transference) or inhibit (interference) plasticity in other networks.

Data from Kleim JA, Jones TA. Principles of experience-dependent neural plasticity: implications for rehabilitation after brain damage. *J Speech Lang Hear Res.* 2008;51:S225–S239.

SPECIAL SENSES THAT INTERACT WITH CENTRAL NERVOUS SYSTEM

The special senses of vision, smell, taste, vestibular function, hearing, and proprioception and their interactions with the CNS are reviewed in the following sections.

Vision

The Eye. Figure 2-12 represents the anatomy of the eye, and Box 2-2 outlines the major functions.

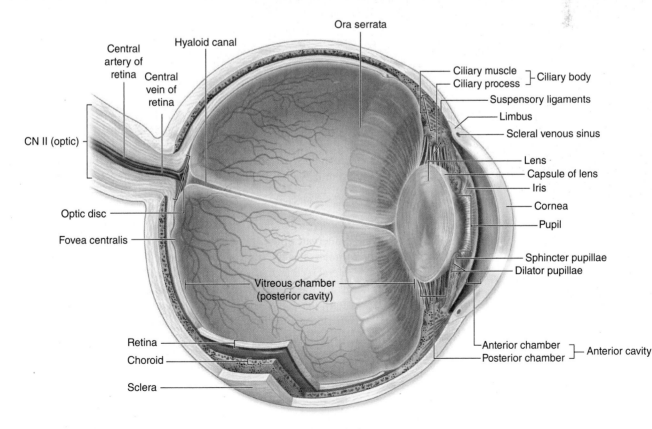

Figure 2-12. Anatomy of the eye. (Reproduced with permission from McKinley M, O'Laughlin VD. *Human Anatomy.* 3rd ed. 2012. Copyright © McGraw Hill LLC. All rights reserved.)

BOX 2-2 PUPIL AND LENS CONTROL

Pupillary Reflexes

Constriction: When a strong light hits the retina, it induces constriction of the pupil through a reflexive response. This reflex is mediated by sequential projections from the retina to the midbrain's pretectal nucleus, the Edinger–Westphal nuclei (also in the midbrain), to the ciliary ganglion, and ultimately to the ciliary muscles that constrict the pupil via parasympathetic fibers in CN III. Each Edinger–Westphal muscle connects to its counterpart on the opposite side such that pupillary constriction occurs bilaterally and symmetrically.

Dilation: Dilation can be achieved by inhibition of the reflexive loop that produces constriction or activation of the iris dilator muscle via the sympathetic nervous system component of the ciliary ganglion.

Accommodation

Changing the shape of the lens within the eye allows us to orient to near and far objects. To focus on objects in the distance, the lens becomes elongated, associated with ciliary muscle relaxation, while thickening of the lens achieves focus on near objects via ciliary muscle contraction; both of these changes serve to focus the image on the retina. The ciliary muscles of the lens create this change in lens shape through the same series of projections that control the pupillary reflexes; in fact, accommodation for near vision is also associated with pupil constriction and eye convergence (slight adduction), requiring integration via these brainstem nuclei.

Myopia (nearsightedness): Light is focused short of the retina, making distance vision poor, associated with poor elongation of the lens or an eye that is too long.

Hyperopia (farsightedness): Poor near vision caused by poor accommodation (inability of the lens to achieve a sufficiently round shape) or an eye that is too short.

Presbyopia: Age-induced change in the ability to accommodate, resulting in poorer near vision.

Visual Field(s). The view of the environment without eye movement. See Figure 2-13 for the schematic of visual fields.

Visual Receptors. Rod and cone cells, which are both photosensitive.

Visual Processing. A complex pathway, as visual projection is supported on the cornea, and the pathway eventually ends up at the visual cortex. Figure 2-14 represents this pathway.

Eye Movement and Visual Pursuit. The eye has six muscles innervated by cranial nerves III, IV, and VI. CN III innervates the superior rectus, inferior rectus, medial rectus, and inferior oblique. CN IV innervates the superior oblique, and CN VI innervates the lateral rectus. The medial and lateral recti produce medial (adduction) and lateral (abduction) horizontal movements. Similarly, the superior and inferior recti pull the eye upward (elevation) and downward (depression). Because of their oblique insertions on the eye, each also pulls the eyes inward. With superior rectus contraction, the eye moves up and in, and conversely, the inferior rectus contraction pulls the eye down and in to look at the tip of the nose. Both oblique muscles attach to the eye on the posterolateral surface; the superior oblique attaches to the eye's superior aspect and orients the eye downward and laterally, while the inferior oblique attaches on the inferior aspect orients the eye upward and laterally.

Smell

Olfaction. This is phylogenetically the oldest sensory system, and in nonhumans plays a critical survival role in locating food.

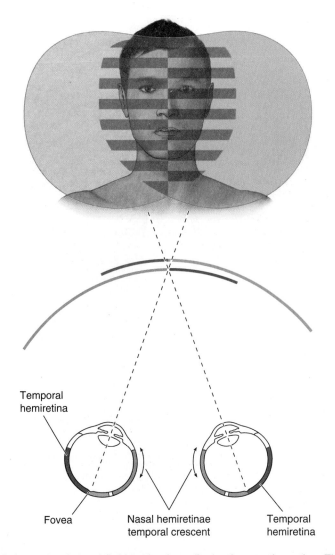

Temporal
hemiretina

Fovea

Nasal hemiretinae
temporal crescent

Temporal
hemiretina

Figure 2-13. Schematic of visual field projections. Projections to the retina: The central striped area illustrates the overlapping binocular visual field, conveyed to the temporal retina of each eye. The solid colored fields are unique to each eye. The right monocular visual field (green) is transmitted to the right nasal retina while the left (blue) is transmitted to the left nasal retina. This allows the projections from the right field to come together as the nasal fibers cross at the optic chiasm. (Reproduced with permission from Martin JH. *Neuroanatomy Text and Atlas*. 4th ed. 2012. Copyright © McGraw Hill LLC. All rights reserved. https://neurology.mhmedical.com.)

Olfactory Receptors. These are in the bipolar cells of the nasal epithelium and project multiple cilia into the mucosa that covers the epithelial layer. Only airborne chemicals that are soluble in the mucosa can activate the olfactory neurons, and these axons pass through the bony cribriform plate at the top of the nasal passage and form CN I, the olfactory nerve. A synapse occurs in the olfactory bulb and magnifies the olfactory communication. From here, the olfactory tract projects to the higher cortical centers for processing. See Figure 2-15 for more details.

Cortical Processing of Olfaction. This can be viewed in Figure 2-16.

Taste

Gustation. Like taste, it relies on the transduction of chemicals to perceive the sense of taste.

Taste Receptors. The five tastes that have been identified are salty, sweet, sour, bitter, and savory. Taste receptors die after about 10 days and are replaced with new cells. Taste is

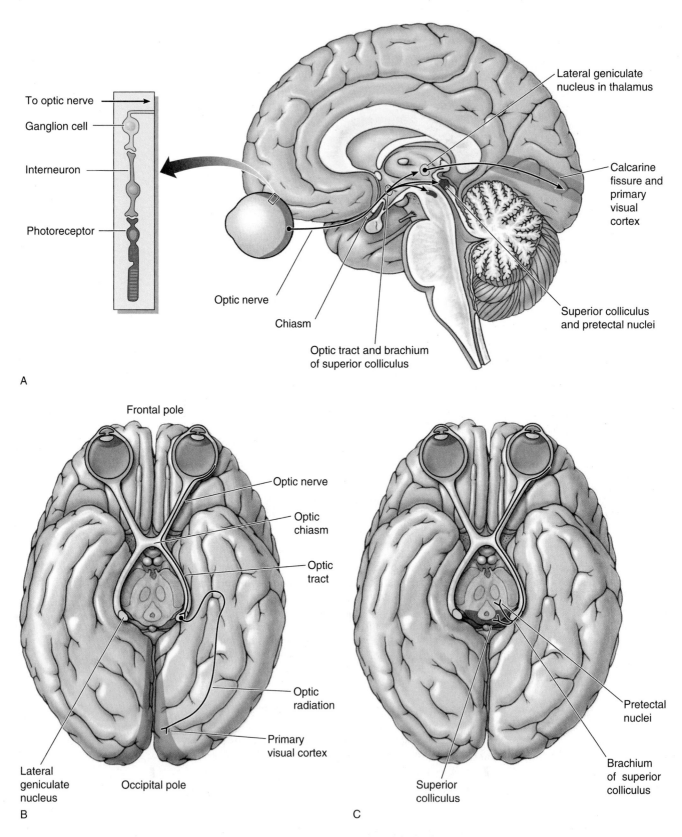

Figure 2-14. Visual projections from the retina to the visual cortex. (Reproduced with permission from Martin JH. *Neuroanatomy Text and Atlas*. 4th ed. 2012. Copyright © McGraw Hill LLC. All rights reserved. https://neurology.mhmedical.com.)

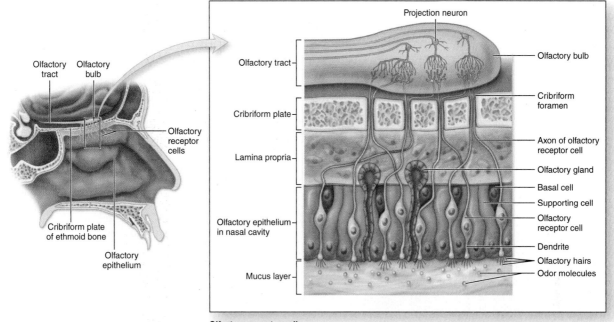

Olfactory receptor cells

Figure 2-15. **Olfactory receptors and projections.** Bipolar cells within the nasal epithelium project through the cribriform plate to the olfactory tubercle, activating mitral cells that project as the olfactory tract to the olfactory cortex in structures on the dorsum of the brain. (Reproduced with permission from McKinley M, O'Laughlin VD. *Human Anatomy*. 3rd ed. 2012. Copyright © McGraw Hill LLC. All rights reserved.)

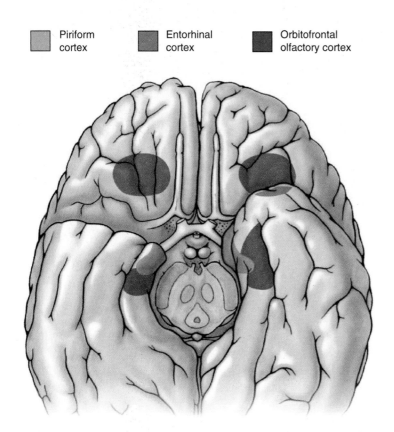

Figure 2-16. **Olfactory cortex.** (Reproduced with permission from Martin JH. *Neuroanatomy Text and Atlas*. 4th ed. 2012. Copyright © McGraw Hill LLC. All rights reserved. https://neurology.mhmedical.com.)

functionally important so that people can identify potentially dangerous poisons or impurities in food.

Central Processing of Taste. Three cranial nerves support this: VII (anterior two-thirds of the tongue), IX (posterior one-third of the tongue, pharynx), and X (epiglottis, larynx). Figure 2-17 illustrates the central processing of taste.

Vestibular Function and Hearing

Ear Anatomy. The ear has two functions: hearing and vestibular function. See Figure 2-18 for the components of the ear and Figure 2-19 for understanding central auditory processing.

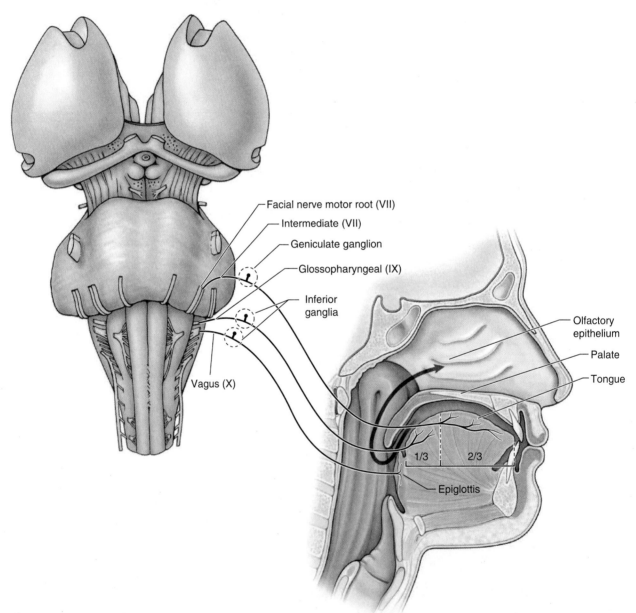

A

Figure 2-17. Cranial nerve projections of taste. **A.** The three cranial nerves (VII, IX, and X) innervate the oral cavity through long dendritic projections from the cells within the peripheral ganglia (inferior, geniculate) with axonal projections to the solitary nucleus. **B.** Gustatory projections from the solitary nucleus project to the ventral posterior medial nucleus of the thalamus. (Reproduced with permission from Martin JH. *Neuroanatomy Text and Atlas.* 4th ed. 2012. Copyright © McGraw Hill LLC. All rights reserved. https://neurology.mhmedical.com.)

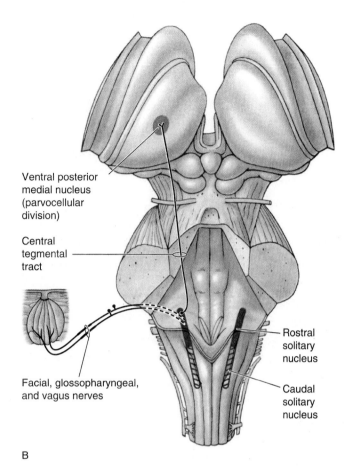

Ventral posterior
medial nucleus
(parvocellular
division)

Central
tegmental
tract

Facial, glossopharyngeal,
and vagus nerves

Rostral
solitary
nucleus

Caudal
solitary
nucleus

B

Figure 2-17. (Continued)

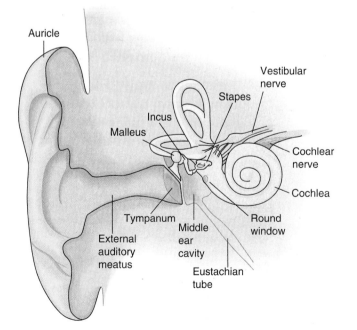

Auricle

Vestibular
nerve

Stapes

Incus

Malleus

Cochlear
nerve

Cochlea

Tympanum

Middle
ear
cavity

Round
window

External
auditory
meatus

Eustachian
tube

Figure 2-18. The three components of the ear. The ear has three functional components:
(1) the external ear (auricle, external acoustic meatus, and tympanic membrane) that
funnels sound to the interior of the ear; (2) the middle ear (auditory ossicles—malleus,
incus, and stapes) that transmits vibration to the eardrum; and (3) the inner ear (cochlea)
that allows the transduction of sound to neural signals. (Reproduced with permission
from Kandel ER, Schwartz JH, Jessell TM, et al. *Principles of Neural Science*. 5th ed. 2013.
Copyright © McGraw Hill LLC. All rights reserved. https://neurology.mhmedical.com.)

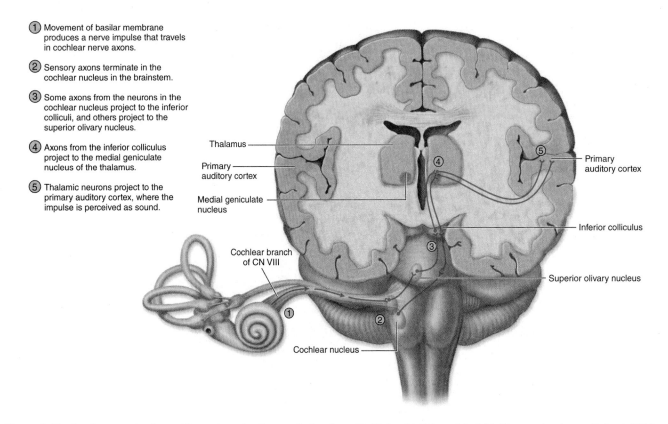

① Movement of basilar membrane produces a nerve impulse that travels in cochlear nerve axons.

② Sensory axons terminate in the cochlear nucleus in the brainstem.

③ Some axons from the neurons in the cochlear nucleus project to the inferior colliculi, and others project to the superior olivary nucleus.

④ Axons from the inferior colliculus project to the medial geniculate nucleus of the thalamus.

⑤ Thalamic neurons project to the primary auditory cortex, where the impulse is perceived as sound.

Figure 2-19. Auditory projections. (Reproduced with permission from McKinley M, O'Laughlin VD. *Human Anatomy*. 3rd ed. 2012. Copyright © McGraw Hill LLC. All rights reserved.)

Vestibular System. Detects motion and position of the head through several receptors. The labyrinths comprise three semicircular canals and two otolithic organs called the utricle and the saccule. The outermost labyrinth is called the bony labyrinth and is filled with perilymphatic fluid, and the innermost labyrinth, called the membranous labyrinth, is filled with endolymphatic fluid. Figure 2-20 illustrates the cochlea and vestibular labyrinth.

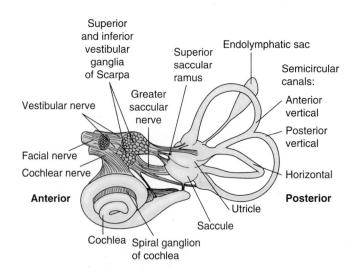

Figure 2-20. Vestibular labyrinths: This schematic illustrates the relationship of the cochlea and the components of the vestibular labyrinth: the vestibule with its saccule and utricle and the three semicircular canals. (Reproduced with permission from Kandel ER, Schwartz JH, Jessell TM, et al. *Principles of Neural Science*. 4th ed. 2000. Copyright © McGraw Hill LLC. All rights reserved.)

Receptors.   The sensory cells in each of the organs named above contain hair cells, translating signals into neural fining.

Semicircular Canals.   These sense angular acceleration, such as rotations, tilting, or turning of the head. There are three semicircular canals: horizontal, anterior, and posterior. The semicircular canals are oriented with the extraocular eye muscles.

Utricle and Saccule.   These detect linear acceleration and static head position, such as leaning to one side or riding in an elevator.

Vestibular Pathways.   The primary afferents have cell bodies in Scarpa ganglion, and from here, information travels along CN VIII and enters the brainstem at the pons–medulla junction. The target areas for this information are the vestibular nuclei and the cerebellum. From here, projections are sent to the oculomotor nuclei (CN III, IV, and VI), which regulate the vestibular-ocular reflex (VOR). The VOR allows humans to maintain an image stable on the retina's fovea during the presence of head movement. In addition, efferent projections are communicated to the spinal cord in the form of the medial and lateral vestibulospinal tracts to support the activation of muscles for postural responses. See Figure 2-21 for a schematic of the vestibular pathway.

Balance/Postural Control.   The ability of the body to maintain an upright position requires adequate balance and use of perception. Perception is the integration of sensory information to assess the position and motion of the body in space, involving sensory and higher-level cognitive processes. The three main specialized sensory systems used for balance are the visual, somatosensory, and vestibular systems.

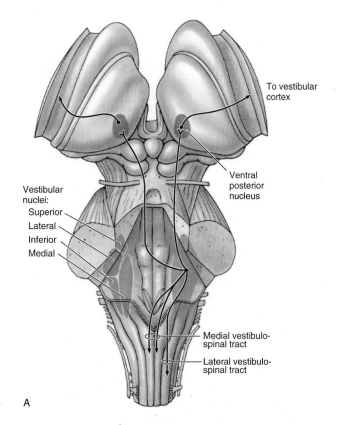

Figure 2-21. **A and B. The vestibular nuclei. The four vestibular nuclei can be visualized in this diagram along with their projections to the thalamus and spinal cord.** (Reproduced with permission from Martin JH. *Neuroanatomy Text and Atlas*. 4th ed. 2012. Copyright © McGraw Hill LLC. All rights reserved. https://neurology.mhmedical.com.)

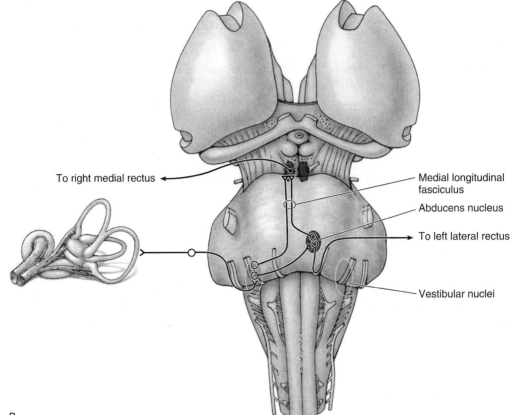

To right medial rectus

Medial longitudinal fasciculus

Abducens nucleus

To left lateral rectus

Vestibular nuclei

B

Figure 2-21. (*Continued*)

SPECIALIZED FUNCTIONS OF THE CENTRAL NERVOUS SYSTEM—COGNITION AND LANGUAGE

Cognition is an expansive term used to describe our ability to perceive the world around us, interact with it, remember our past experiences in it, and imagine potential experiences with it; the concepts of thinking, memory, imagery, problem-solving, and decision-making are all included within the term cognition. These complex skills involve multiple neural pathways.

Executive Function

Executive function refers to a spectrum of abilities, including attention, working memory, inhibition, task switching, abstract thought, behavioral regulation, decision-making, sequence planning, and initiation.

Attention. The ability to focus awareness on visual, auditory, tactile, or other sensory stimuli, but also involves the ability to prioritize attention on one among competing stimuli and switch attention from one stimulus to another.

Task Switching. The ability to focus on one task and then immediately switch to another task.

Perseveration. Failure to switch attention to a new appropriate cue and instead continue the current task.

Memory. The concepts of learning and memory coexist. Implicit and explicit memory systems are organized in Figure 2-22. Working memory is the ability to retain or manipulate information cognitively for immediate use.

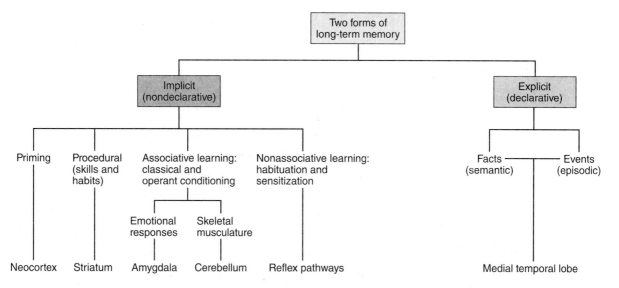

Figure 2-22. **Schematic of implicit and explicit memory systems. Long-term memory can be divided into explicit (semantic—facts; episodic—events) and implicit (procedural) memories. Explicit memories are encoded by the medial temporal lobe structures and their connections to the anterior cingulate and prefrontal cortices. Implicit memories are generated within an array of networks, including the sensory cortices (priming), striatum of the basal ganglia and cerebellum (motor skills, habits), the cerebellum and amygdala (classical and operant conditioning), and reflex networks of the brainstem.** (Reproduced with permission from Kandel ER, Schwartz JH, Jessell TM, et al. *Principles of Neural Science.* 5th ed. 2013. Copyright © McGraw Hill LLC. All rights reserved. https://neurology.mhmedical.com.)

Emotions. Complex learned responses elicited by sensory stimuli that produce a motor response, physiologic changes, and/or motivate us to some type of action. Emotions, along with memory, are controlled and regulated by the limbic system.

Language. A higher-level skill that differentiates humans from other animals. Our language abilities are usually divided into receptive and expressive language skills. The anatomic language centers are identified as the Broca's area and the Wernicke's area. These locations are depicted in Figure 2-23.

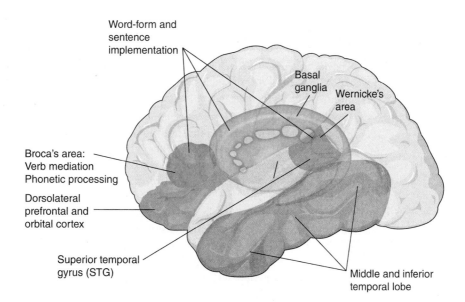

Figure 2-23. Language centers. The historic Broca's and Wernicke's areas are depicted in association with the surrounding areas that contribute to language skills (dorsolateral and orbitofrontal cortex, middle and inferior temporal lobes, basal ganglia). (Reproduced with permission from Kandel ER, Schwartz JH, Jessell TM, et al. *Principles of Neural Science.* 5th ed. 2013. Copyright © McGraw Hill LLC. All rights reserved. https://neurology.mhmedical.com.)

■ NEUROLOGIC EXAMINATION

The examination of the neurologic system is an essential component of a comprehensive physical examination performed by the PT. It includes the systems review or screening and a comprehensive and systematic examination of both the central and peripheral nervous system in conjunction with other body systems. In addition, the examiner should determine impairments in body function and structure, limitations in functional activities, and participation restrictions consistent with the World Health Organization's International Classification of Functioning, Disability, and Health (ICF). The PTA plays an important role throughout the episode of care by providing treatment interventions, collecting data through continual assessment testing, providing thorough documentation, and regular communication with the PT.

COMPONENTS OF THE NEUROLOGIC ASSESSMENT BY THE PHYSICAL THERAPIST ASSISTANT

The PTA provides treatment interventions relative to the Plan of Care (POC), or evaluation, developed by the PT. While providing a prescribed regimen, the PTA continually monitors the patient, considering the following.

- *Patient goals*—Provide and create a treatment session specific to the goals developed within the POC.
- *Medications*—Identify prescribed medications and supplements and stay informed on what each medication is used for, along with potential side effects that may be exhibited.
- *Communication*—Provide thorough communication through monitoring the patient's mental status, alertness, orientation, memory, and individual communicative abilities. Standardized outcome measures that include communication should be reviewed in this chapter's appendices (Table A-1).
  - Can the client communicate? Does the patient have word-finding problems consistent with expressive aphasia or trouble enunciating consistent with dysarthria?
  - Note voice quality; is volume adequate?
  - Does the individual understand language or show signs of aphasia?
- *Integumentary*—Assess the potential presence of skin abnormalities, inflammation, and incision or wound drainage or abnormalities.
- *Cardiovascular/pulmonary*—Monitor patient vital signs, including pain ratings and exertion levels. Watch for adversities through exhibited body movements, fatigue, or facial expressions.
- *Musculoskeletal*—Familiarize oneself with the patient's capability of participating in the treatment intervention. Assess strength and range of motion (ROM).
- *Neuromuscular*—Screen for muscle tone, strength, functional movement, and coordination. Note any discrepancies with mental status, reflexes, sensory response, posture, and mobility. Details regarding the mental status of the neurologic patient can be found in Table 2-5.
- *Muscle tone*—An increase in tone (hypertonicity) that is often seen with increased resistance to passive movement. There are two types of hypertonicity: spasticity and rigidity. Spasticity is characterized by increased resistance to passive movement, as the velocity of the movement is increased (velocity-dependent), and by hyperreflexia (exaggerated monosynaptic reflexes). Rigidity is increased resistance throughout the ROM that is independent of the velocity of the movement; reflexes are typically normal with rigidity. The causes of spasticity and rigidity are different and will be discussed in later sections specific to neurologic diagnoses. A limb that feels heavy or "floppy" is hypotonic, demonstrating limited resistance to passive movement and poor ability to sustain power or maintain a given posture. Hypotonia can be caused by both central and peripheral nervous system disorders. Reflexes can be decreased (hyporeflexia), normal, or exaggerated (hyperreflexia), depending on the cause of the hypotonia. It is important to note that tone can fluctuate depending on the time of day and other environmental and personal stimuli; therefore, testing should be performed at the same time each day and with the same clinician. Standardized outcome measures for tone and spasticity should be reviewed in the appendices of this chapter (Table A-1).

TABLE 2-5 • Mental Function Assessment.		
Area to Be Examined	**What to Look for**	**Insight**
Appearance	Clothes, posture, grooming, alertness	Ability to take care of themselves; mood/affect
Behavior	Impulse control, fidgeting, overall movements	
Speech	Volume/rate Coherence	Mood (eg, loud and fast speech—related to mania; soft and slow—related to depression) Indication of higher-level processing
Mood/affect	Flat—minimal or absent affective response to situation Labile—shifting emotional outbursts (eg, crying/laughing) Blunted—some emotional response but less than would be expected for the situation Constructed/Inappropriate—responses that are inconsistent with the situation (eg, laughing at a sad situation)	Signs of mental illness or cortical disease
Thought processing	Word usage Thought stream Continuity—coherence of thought and idea association Content—complete/incomplete responses	Language issues (agnosia, expressive aphasia) Slow versus overabundant gives an indication of mood and cognition Ability to follow the discussion and respond accordingly—higher-level cognition or receptive language problems Higher-level cognition/language issues, delusions suggest mental disorders
Perception	Screening of vision, hearing, touch, taste, and smell	General system integrity/dysfunction; potential medication side effects
Attention/concentration	Ability to stay focused on a task	Frontal lobe dysfunction; anxiety
Memory	Long-term and current episodic memory (client's history and current events); immediate memory (naming 3 objects immediately and then in 5 and 15 minutes)	Temporal and frontal lobe function/dysfunction
Judgment	Decision-making in complex situations (safe vs unsafe)	Executive function (frontal lobe function)
Intelligence	Requires specific testing but a general sense can be obtained by responses to questions, general language used, etc.	Overall ability to participate in treatment/cortical deficits
Insight	Understanding of the current illness and potential limitations	Executive function

Reproduced with permission from Nichols-Larsen DS, Kegelmeyer DA, Buford JA, et al., eds. *Neurologic Rehabilitation: Neuroscience and Neuroplasticity in Physical Therapy Practice.* 2016. Copyright © McGraw Hill LLC. All rights reserved. https://accessphysiotherapy.mhmedical.com.

- *Reflexes*—Review the POC, which will provide any reflexive deficits. Deep tendon reflexes are typically documented using a numerical scale. Refer to Table 2-6.
- *Cranial nerves*—Cranial nerves originate in the brainstem and support the facial muscles and eyes, sensory receptors, and specialized senses such as hearing, vision, smell, taste, and vestibular function. See Table 2-7 for further detail regarding cranial nerve function and screening.
- *Sensory*—Review the POC to provide patient sensory deficits and associated ability.

TESTS OF PROPRIOCEPTION

- *Movement sense (kinesthesia)*—The therapist has the patient close their eyes and then moves the extremity through a small ROM. The patient is asked to verbally indicate the direction of movement while the extremity is in motion. Before performing the test, the therapist should demonstrate the examination to the patient with their eyes open to establish understanding. Communication should be simple, for example, "up," "down," or "in" and "out." Hold the patient's extremities using bony prominences to minimize additional sensory input.

TABLE 2-6 · Deep Tendon Reflex Grades.

Reflex Grade	Evaluation	Response Characteristics
0	Absent	No visible or palpable muscle contraction
1+	Hyporeflexia	Slight or sluggish muscle contraction with little or no joint movement Reinforcement may be required to elicit a reflex response
2+	Normal	Slight muscle contraction with slight joint movement
3+	Hyperreflexia	Clearly visible, brisk muscle contraction with moderate joint movement
4+	Abnormal	Strong muscle contraction with one to three beats of clonus Reflex spread to contralateral side may be noted
5+	Abnormal	Strong muscle contraction with sustained clonus Reflex spread to contralateral side may be noted

TABLE 2-7 · Cranial Nerve Function and Screening Methods.

Cranial Nerve	Name	Function	Screening
I	Olfactory	Smell	Have patient identify familiar smells (vanilla); there are vials that can be purchased or therapists can make their own.
II	Optic	Vision	Reading close and distant items.
III	Oculomotor	Eye movement, pupillary reflexes	Eye tracking in all directions, pupillary response to light; at rest, eye will be slightly depressed and rotated toward the nose when damaged.
IV	Trochlear	Superior oblique eye muscle innervation	Observe eye position at rest; will be elevated if there is a problem.
V	Trigeminal	Muscles of mastication and sensation of the face	Observe jaw motion (resistance to motion, opening, side-to-side mobility), temporalis muscles can be palpated.
VI	Abducens	Lateral rectus of the eye innervation	Look at eye movement; if damaged, there will be an inability to look outward (abduct the eye).
VII	Facial	Muscles of facial expression, taste for the anterior 2/3 of tongue	Look for facial asymmetries, observe motions (raising eyebrows, wrinkling forehead, closing eyes, frowning/smiling, lip pursing, etc). Taste with common liquids (lemon juice, honey) can also be tested.
VIII	Vestibulocochlear	Hearing and vestibular	Can use the "rub test"—rub thumb and forefinger together next to the ear. Ask the patient to point to which ear they hear it in. Check both. Look for differences. You can use a tuning fork, which tests for air conduction and structural problems that can occur inside the ear—strike tuning fork on your hand and place behind the ear on the bony surface. Observe balance.
IX	Glossopharyngeal	Sensation and taste for posterior tongue and pharynx	Ask about swallowing, which may be impaired; have patient say "ahh" and watch for palatal-uvula movement; unilateral nerve damage can yield asymmetric motion; absent gag reflex is also a sign of damage (stimulate with tongue depressor).
X	Vagus	Innervates epiglottis and larynx, parasympathetic innervation of internal organs	Voice hoarseness with increased heart and respiration rate are signs of CN X damage.
XI	Accessory	Trapezius and sternocleidomastoid muscle innervation	Observe ability to shrug shoulders and turn head to both sides.
XII	Hypoglossal	Tongue muscles	Observe tongue protrusion and mobility; unilateral lesions will result in lateral movement when protruding tongue.

- *Position sense*—Place the patient's extremity in a position, and the patient is then asked to communicate the position verbally.
- *Vibration testing*—The most reliable and valid way to test the dorsal column–medial lemniscal system. A 250-Hz tuning fork is suggested. Strike the fork against the palm of their hand and then place it on a bony prominence while asking the patient what they feel.
- *Cutaneous sensation* is commonly tested by (1) monofilament testing for sensory threshold; (2) pinprick for pain; and (3) water vials for hot and cold modalities. This can be achieved by applying a light touch across the surface of both upper/lower limbs, and the individual is asked if they "can feel it" and "does it feel the same." Then the same assessment should be completed with the patient's eyes closed and asked to identify the location of the randomly applied stimulus. If deficits are found, a more thorough sensory examination should be completed, including pinprick and temperature. Additional tests include identifying common objects, shapes of varying weight, etc. See Table 2-8 for common sensory deficits and options for testing and documenting each.
- *Coordination and balance*—A patient's functional mobility is relative to coordination and balance and is continually assessed by the PTA.
  - *Coordination*—Is the ability to execute smooth, accurate, and controlled movements. It is characterized by appropriate speed, distance, direction, rhythm, muscle tension, and synergistic movements accomplished via orchestrated reversals of opposing muscle group activations. Proximal stabilization is critical to achieving distal movement when performing many of these tests. Coordination involves nonequilibrium, which involves assessing the extremities, and equilibrium, which involves upright postural control. Typically, nonequilibrium tests are completed first, followed by the equilibrium tests. Observing the quality of movement, noted time to complete the test, monitoring the patient's speed, and whether adjustments are needed to succeed with the task at hand. In addition, nonequilibrium tests should include unilateral and bimanual tasks with eyes open and closed and with altering speeds. Nonequilibrium tests are outlined in Box 2-3. Equilibrium testing begins with observing the patient's standing

TABLE 2-8 • Common Sensory Impairments and Assessment Methods.		
Name of Sensory Impairment	**Definition of Sensory Impairment**	**Assessment**
Abarognosis	Inability to recognize weight	Hold objects of varying weights in each hand and have patient state which is heavier (or the same)
Allodynia	Pain is caused by nonpainful stimuli such as light touch	Uncovered in the sensory examination when light touch or other nonpainful stimuli elicit pain
Analgesia	Complete loss of pain sensitivity	Lack of pinprick sensation along with findings from the history
Astereognosis	Inability to use touch to recognize the shape or form of an object	Have patient identify shapes of objects while eyes are closed; use common shapes like square and ball
Atopognosia	Inability to localize a sensation	During light touch testing, ask patient to localize the touch with eyes closed
Dysesthesia	Abnormal touch sensation that may be experienced as unpleasant or painful	Typically determined during cutaneous testing (touch localization)
Hyperalgesia	Increased sensitivity to pain	Senses pinprick as being more painful than is typical and discovered through the history
Hyperesthesia	Increased sensitivity to sensory stimuli	Noted throughout the examination as an increased sensitivity to stimuli as compared to normal
Hypoalgesia	Decreased response to pain	Identified with the pinprick testing
Paresthesia	Abnormal sensation such as prickling or burning feeling that has no apparent cause	Noted during the history or when asked if they have any burning or prickling sensations

BOX 2-3   NONEQUILIBRIUM COORDINATION TESTS

Most of these tests should be performed first with eyes open and then closed to examine the influence of vision on the individual's coordination. After doing each test at a comfortable pace, instruct the client to move faster and examine the influence of speed on coordination:

1. *Finger to nose:* With the shoulder in a flexed position, bring the finger to the tip of the nose and back out to the examiner's hand or just straight out in front, repeating several times.

2. *Finger to therapist's finger:* The therapist sits in front of the client and has them alternately touch the therapist's fingertip. The therapist places their fingertip at nose height, arm's length away from the client. The movement is alternated. The therapist can also try moving their finger so that the client has to contact the finger in different locations by moving their finger. The therapist should observe how easily and smoothly the client can change the trajectory of this movement in response to a moving target.

3. *Opposition of fingers:* The thumb is touched to the tip of each finger on the same hand, moving in order from the index finger to the pinky and back down to the index finger. Be sure the client is instructed to fully abduct the thumb after each digit is touched.

4. *Grasp:* The hand is opened and closed with gradually increasing speed. Encourage the client to fully open the hand with each repetition. Failure to fully open the hand or progressive shrinking of movement may be indicative of basal ganglia disorder.

5. *Alternating pronation and supination:* The client is asked to alternately pronate and supinate with the arms held at the sides and elbows flexed (hands can be placed on legs while seated so that the palms and back of the hands alternately touch the thighs).

6. *Tapping (hand and/or foot):* The arm is placed on a table or the client's leg, and the client is instructed to tap the hand on the table or knee. For the foot, the client is seated with the knee flexed and foot flat on the floor, then asked to tap their toe on the ground.

7. *Rebound test:* The client is positioned with the elbow in 90 degrees of flexion, and the therapist applies resistance to elbow flexion. The client is instructed to maintain the flexed posture. The therapist then suddenly releases their resistance and observes the response; since the elbow flexors are active, the arm will begin to flex when the resistance is released. A normal response involves the opposing muscle group (triceps) rapidly checking the flexion movement with little motion occurring. Abnormal tests involve a large flexion of the elbow or a loss of trunk control in response to the sudden change in resistance.

8. *Heel on shin:* In supine or sitting, the client is asked to slide the heel up the shin from the ankle to the knee and back down again. Any movement off of the shin is considered a coordination deficit.

9. *Toe to examiner's finger:* Examiner holds their finger out, and the client is asked to point to it with their great toe. This motion can be alternated.

10. *Drawing a circle:* The client is asked to draw a circle on the floor with the big toe. A figure of eight can also be used. In supine, they can be asked to draw the figure in the air. This test can also be done with the upper extremity, using the finger to draw an imaginary circle in the air.

posture and progresses as described in Box 2-4. Table 2-9 outlines common movement and coordination abnormalities and their assessment methods.

- *Balance*—A composite impairment and involves a systematic aspect of the examination due to the complexity. Therapists should examine static and dynamic balance in a seated and standing position. Balance is best assessed using standardized outcome measures that capture various aspects of the feedforward and feedback postural control systems under various functional and environmental conditions. Standardized outcome measures for balance should be reviewed in the appendices of this chapter

BOX 2-4	EQUILIBRIUM COORDINATION TESTS

Tests are listed from least to most difficult

1. Standing in a normal, comfortable posture
2. Standing, feet together (narrow base of support)
3. Standing, with one foot directly in front of the other in tandem position (toe of one foot touching the heel of other foot)
4. Standing on one foot
5. Arm position may be altered in each of the above postures (ie, arms at side, overhead, hands on the waist, and so forth)
6. Displacing balance unexpectedly (while carefully guarding the patient, wearing gait belt)
7. Standing, alternate between forward trunk flexion and return to neutral
8. Standing, laterally flex trunk to each side
9. Standing; eyes open to eyes closed; ability to maintain an upright posture without visual input is referred to as a *positive Romberg sign*
10. Standing in tandem position, eyes open to eyes closed—*sharpened Romberg*
11. Walking, placing the heel of one foot directly in front of the toe of the opposite foot (tandem walking)
12. Walking along a straight line drawn or taped to the floor, or placing feet on floor markers while walking
13. Walking sideways, backward, or cross-stepping
14. Marching in place
15. Altering the speed of ambulatory activities; observe patient walking at normal speed, as fast as possible, and as slow as possible
16. Stopping and starting abruptly while walking
17. Walking and pivoting (turn 90, 180, or 360 degrees)
18. Walking in a circle, alternate directions
19. Walking on heels and then on toes
20. Walking with horizontal and vertical head turns
21. Stepping over or around obstacles
22. Stair climbing with and without using handrail; one step at a time versus step over step
23. Performing agility activities (coordinated movement with upright balance)—jumping jacks; alternate flexing and extending the knees while sitting on a Swiss ball

(Table A-1). Further resources in the appendices should assist in the decision-making process for both balance and gait standardized outcome measures concerning the patient diagnosis and clinical practice setting.

- *Transfers*—The PTA is instrumental in providing treatment interventions related to improving the transition safely from varied surfaces. Transfers include the patient's ability to change positions in bed and transitioning from sitting to standing and standing to sitting from a variety of support surfaces. The PTA should note and document the level of assistance, movement strategies that are unsafe or inefficient, the environment in which the activity is taking place, and any assistive devices or adaptive equipment. Refer to Table 2-10 for descriptions of assistance levels. In addition, standardized outcome measures for transfers and functional mobility should be reviewed in the appendices of this chapter (Table A-1).
- *Gait/locomotion*—Consists of many components such as power, coordination, sensation, and balance, working together in a coordinated fashion to achieve this complex process. Observational gait analysis can assist in detecting a variety of diagnoses. For

TABLE 2-9 • Movement and Coordination Impairments with Assessment Methods.

Impairment	Definition	Sample Test
Dysdiadochokinesia	Impaired alternating movements	Finger to nose Alternate nose to finger Pronation/supination Knee flexion/extension Walking, alter speed or direction
Dysmetria	Uncoordinated movement, characterized by over- or undershooting intended position	Pointing to a target Drawing a circle or figure eight Heel on shin Placing feet on floor markers while walking
Dyssynergia	Movement decomposition and loss of coordination	Finger to nose Finger to therapist's finger Alternate heel to knee Toe to examiner's finger
Hypotonia	Diminished muscle tone	Passive movement Deep tendon reflexes
Tremor (resting)	Oscillating movements at rest	Observation of patient at rest Observation during functional activities (tremor will diminish or disappear with movement)
Tremor (intentional)	Oscillating movements with movement	Observation during functional activities Alternate nose to finger Finger to finger Finger to therapist's finger Toe to examiner's finger
Tremor (postural)	Oscillating trunk movements	Observation of steadiness of normal standing posture
Asthenia	Diminished strength	Fixation or position holding (UE and LE) Application of manual resistance to assess muscle strength
Rigidity	Hypertonia with normal reflexes	Passive movement Observation during functional activities Observation of resting posture(s)
Bradykinesia	Slowness of movement and loss of associated movements (eg, arm swing)	Walking, observation of arm swing and trunk motions Walking, alter speed and direction Request that a movement or gait activity be stopped abruptly Observation of functional activities; timed tests
Disturbances of posture	Inability to maintain a given position, react to displacement, or adjust one's posture to changing expectations	Fixation or position holding (UE and LE) Displace balance unexpectedly in sitting or standing Standing—alter base of support (eg, one foot directly in front of the other; standing on one foot)
Disturbance of gait	Any change in the ability to walk under varying conditions	Walk along a straight line Walk sideways, backward March in place Alter speed and direction of ambulatory activities Walk in a circle

LE, lower extremity; UE, upper extremity.

example, an ataxic gait with a wide base of support indicates involvement of the cerebellum. Therefore, the patient's gait should be carefully analyzed using each subphase: initial contact, stance (early, mid, and late), push-off, and swing. Some considerations during the gait analysis should include the following:

- Assistance, assistive device, use of an orthotic device
- Description of the gait pattern on a variety of support surfaces, directions, and incorporating turns and velocity at a comfortable, self-selected speed
- Loss of balance and direction if appropriate

TABLE 2-10 • Terminology for Levels of Assistance.

Independence	Completes the activity with no assistance and is safe while doing it.
Modified independence	Completes the activity with no assistance and is safe but requires the use of an assistive device or orthosis.
Supervision	Completes the activity with no assistance but is not safe < 50% of the time. The level of safety risk is minimal. Assistance provided is that of the therapist being in close proximity in order to assist if needed, but not touching the client.
Contact guard assist (CGA)	Completes the activity with no assistance but there are consistent safety concerns or periodic losses of balance requiring light assistance to regain balance.
Minimal assistance (Min)	Assistance is required but no more than 25% of the work is done by the person helping, during times of assistance.
Moderate assistance (Mod)	Assistance is required but no more than 75% of the work is done by the person helping, during times of assistance.
Maximal assistance (Max)	The majority of the work is done by the person helping (> 75%).
Total assist	The patient does not do anything and all work is done by the person(s) helping.

Additional items to document: Number of helpers should be included. Typically this is documented as +1 Min assist, meaning only one person helped. +2 Mod assist would mean that two people helped. Any assistive device that is used should also be documented; ie, +1 Min assist with walker.

Reproduced with permission from Nichols-Larsen DS, Kegelmeyer DA, Buford JA, et al., eds. *Neurologic Rehabilitation: Neuroscience and Neuroplasticity in Physical Therapy Practice.* 2016. Copyright © McGraw Hill LLC. All rights reserved. https://accessphysiotherapy.mhmedical.com.

- Stair climbing
- Use of a wheelchair on a variety of support surfaces

Further resources in the appendices of this chapter (Table A-1) should be used to assist in the clinical decision-making process for both balance and gait standardized outcome measures concerning the patient diagnosis and clinical practice setting.

■ ADULT NEUROLOGIC DEFICITS/DIAGNOSES

STROKE

Pathophysiology

Stroke, or cerebrovascular accident (CVA), is the leading cause of adult disability and represents the greatest rehabilitation diagnosis. There are three stroke classifications.

- An ischemic stroke occurs when blood flow interruption occurs within the brain blood vessels, which can narrow or block the vessel. An ischemic stroke results from either an embolism (a moving thrombus), or a thrombus, which is the blockage of an artery. Ischemic strokes are seven times more common than hemorrhagic strokes.
- A hemorrhagic stroke refers to a rupture of a vessel within the brain. Hemorrhagic strokes are more typical with poorly controlled and long-term hypertension, which cause the weakening of the vascular wall. Hemorrhage within the cerebral vessels is referred to as an **intracerebral hemorrhage**, and hemorrhage in the subarachnoid space is referred to as **subarachnoid hemorrhage**. Hemorrhagic strokes often result in increased disability and death as compared to ischemic strokes.
- Transient ischemic attacks (TIAs) are the final classification, yet they differ slightly as TIAs present with temporary stroke-like symptoms. TIAs result from brief blockages with associated stroke symptoms that resolve quickly (< 24 hours) and are not associated with permanent consequences; however, TIAs indicate negative changes in circulation and should be further evaluated by the medical team.

Stroke risk factors and their cardiovascular consequences are listed in Table 2-11.

Cerebral Circulation and Why Results of Stroke Are Variable

The brain is supported by a complex arterial system that involves two components: anterior and posterior circulation. A schematic of major blood vessels of the brain can be viewed in

TABLE 2-11 • Stroke Risk Factors and Their Cardiovascular Consequences.	
Risk Factor	**Explanation of Relationship with Stroke[a-d]**
Age	With increasing age, the frequency and severity of many other risk factors increase and multiple comorbidities are common, thus increasing the risk for stroke.
Gender	Men are more likely to have strokes at younger ages, but more women than men have strokes annually, perhaps due to the greater number of women living longer.
Race	Stroke is more common in African, Asian, and Hispanic Americans than in Caucasians. This partially reflects disparities in health care and the delay in diagnosis and treatment of risk factors in these racial groups. It may also relate to differences in diet or access to health literature.
Hypertension	Uncontrolled hypertension stresses blood vessels, decreasing their pliability and causing thickening of the arterial walls, which in turn makes them susceptible to clot formation and hemorrhage.
High cholesterol	Cholesterol is an essential lipid for cell maintenance; cholesterol, specifically low-density lipoproteins (LDL), contributes to plaque formation in vessel walls.
Obesity	Stresses the cardiovascular system and is often associated with hypertension, high cholesterol, and diabetes (metabolic syndrome).
Atrial fibrillation (AF)	AF is associated with a high incidence of embolism formation and subsequent embolic stroke.
Congenital heart anomaly	A high incidence of stroke has been associated with a patent foramen ovale (PFO), which is the persistence of the fetal connection between the right and left atria that typically closes at birth. PFO is associated with embolitic stroke.
Atherosclerosis	Plaque buildup in blood vessels (atherosclerosis) throughout the body is associated with both embolitic and thrombotic stroke.
Diabetes	Vascular changes are common in type 2 diabetes, increasing the stiffness of the vascular wall and resulting in decreased capacity for vasodilation.
Alcohol abuse	Excessive alcohol consumption is associated with increased clotting and thereby stroke.
Smoking	Smoking increases the likelihood of blood clots and contributes to the development of atherosclerosis.
Drug abuse	Many drugs (cocaine, LSD, amphetamines, heroin, opiates, Ecstasy, PCP) are associated with risk of stroke, often associated with induced hypertension, vasospasm with/without tachycardia. Heroin/opiates/LSD are more likely to induce stroke by cardioembolism.

[a]Ihle-Hansen H, Thommassen B, Wyllar TB, Engedal K, Fure B. Risk factors for and incidence of subtypes of ischemic stroke. Funct Neurol. 2012;27(1):35-40.

[b]Roda L, McCrindle BW, Manlhiot C, et al. Stroke recurrence in children with congenital heart disease. Ann Neurol. 2012;72:103-111.

[c]Esse K, Fossati-Bellani M, Traylor A, Martin-Schild S. Epidemic of illicit drug use, mechanisms of action/addition and stroke as a health hazard. Brain Behav. 2011;1(1):44-54.

[d]Parry CD, Patra J, Rehm J. Alcohol consumption and non-communicable diseases: epidemiology and policy implications. Addiction. 2011;106:1718-1724.

Figure 2-24. In this figure, it is important to identify the carotid artery system consisting of the internal carotid arteries, the anterior, middle, and posterior arteries. The anterior circulation is further supported by the anterior and the posterior communicating arteries. The second component of the perfusion system, referred to as posterior circulation, begins with identifying the vertebral arteries, the basilar artery, the anterior inferior cerebellar artery, the **superior cerebellar artery**, and finally, the **posterior cerebral artery**.

Stroke Syndromes

Specific stroke symptoms are associated with the damaged vasculature distribution outlined in Table 2-12, and Figure 2-25 demonstrates deficits and corresponding impairments at the brainstem level. Patients present with varying numbers and degrees of these symptoms based on the amount of damage in the circulation.

Acute Management

Ischemic Stroke. A comprehensive history should be taken to discover the time of onset of stroke symptoms. If medically appropriate, the patient will receive a tissue-type plasminogen activator (rTPA or TPA) to break down the clot and open the narrowed vessel. There are important inclusion and exclusion criteria as to if the patient should receive this

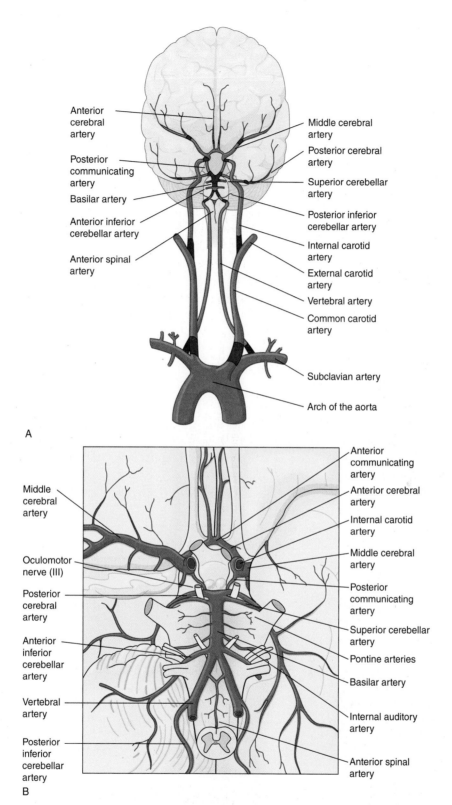

Figure 2-24. Schematic of the major blood vessels of the brain and the circle of Willis. **A.** The brain is supplied by two networks, arising from the aorta: the internal carotid network, branching into the anterior and middle cerebral arteries that supply the anterior two-thirds of the cerebral hemispheres and the vertebral artery system that supplies the posterior one-third and the brainstem and cerebellum. **B.** The circle of Willis comprises the anterior cerebral arteries, the anterior communicating arteries, and the internal carotid arteries (components of the carotid artery system), as well as the posterior communicating arteries and the posterior cerebral arteries (components of the vertebral artery system). The vertebral artery distribution, illustrated on the dorsal surface of the brainstem, supplies the brainstem and cerebellum as well as the posterior cerebrum. (Adapted with permission from Kandel ER, Schwartz JH, Jessell TM, et al. *Principles of Neural Science.* 5th ed. 2013. Copyright © McGraw Hill LLC. All rights reserved. https://neurology.mhmedical.com.)

TABLE 2-12 · Stroke Syndromes and Associated Symptoms.

Artery	Areas of Damage	Common Symptoms
Anterior cerebral **A**[a] Labels: Superior frontal gyrus; Anterior cerebral artery infarct; Cingulate gyrus; Corpus callosum; Insular cortex; Putamen; Globus pallidus; Thalamus; Third ventricle	Frontal lobe Medial surface Anterior and superior aspect of primary motor area Anterior and superior aspect of premotor cortex Parietal lobe Medial surface Superior aspect of lateral surface	Apathy/lack of spontaneity Contralateral motor dysfunction of the lower leg and foot Bladder incontinence Gait apraxia Contralateral sensory dysfunction of leg and foot
Middle cerebral **B**[c] Labels: Cingulate gyrus; Caudate nucleus, head; Internal capsule, anterior limb; External capsule; Putamen; Insular cortex; Claustrum; Globus pallidus; Anterior commissure; Optic tract; Middle cerebral artery infarct	Lateral surface of frontal lobe Primary motor area Premotor area Broca's area Lateral surface of parietal lobe Parietal lobe projections to frontal lobe and contralesional parietal lobe Internal capsule (posterior limb) Optic radiations Superior (parietal lobe) Inferior (temporal lobe, "Meyer loop") Both Temporal lobe (Wernicke's area)	Contralateral hemiparesis (UE > LE) Apraxia Expressive aphasia (left)[b] Contralateral hemisensory loss Contralateral neglect syndrome (right) Bilateral sensory discrimination loss Contralateral hemiparesis and hemisensory loss Inferior quadrantanopia Superior quadrantanopia Homonymous hemianopia Receptive aphasia (left)[b]
Carotid artery	Distribution of both anterior and middle cerebral arteries	Combination of anterior and middle cerebral artery symptoms
Posterior cerebral	Occipital lobe Thalamus Hippocampus (temporal lobe) Cerebral peduncle/midbrain Lateral geniculate Cranial nerve III	Contralateral hemianopia or quadrantanopia Cortical blindness (bilateral) Visual agnosia, agraphia (dominant) Prosopagnosia—loss of facial recognition Contralateral hemisensory loss Memory loss (dominant hemisphere) Hemianopia/quadrantanopia Ophthalmoplegia: Ipsilateral gaze deviation—down and out (unopposed pull of superior oblique and lateral rectus) Double vision, lack of accommodation

Artery	Structure	Symptoms
Basilar	Medulla	Death is common due to loss of medullary centers associated with respiration control
	Reticular activating system	Loss of consciousness, coma
	Cranial nerve disruption	
	Cranial nerve IX and XII	Tongue paresis, loss of taste, swallowing deficits (dysphagia) and vocal loss (dysphonia)—ipsilateral/bilateral
	Pons	
	Cranial nerve III	Dilated pupil(s)—ipsilateral/bilateral
	Cranial nerves V and VII	Facial muscle paresis and sensory loss (dysarthria)—ipsilateral/bilateral
	Cranial nerve VI	Horizontal gaze paresis: bilateral eye turns in—ipsilateral
	Descending motor fibers	Contralateral hemiparesis or quadreparesis (pure motor stroke)
	Ascending sensory fibers	Contralateral hemisensory loss
	Cerebellum	Ipsilateral/bilateral ataxia, vertigo, nystagmus (ipsilateral/bilateral)
	Distribution of posterior cerebral artery	Same symptoms as above
Anterior inferior cerebellar	Lateral pontine syndrome	
	Vestibular nuclei	Vertigo, nystagmus, nausea, ipsilesional falling
	Cochlear nucleus	Ipsilateral tinnitus and deafness
	Trigeminal nucleus	Ipsilateral sensory loss to face; ipsilateral paresis of muscles of mastication (dysarthria, dysphagia)
Posterior inferior cerebellar[d]	Wallenberg syndrome (lateral medulla)	
	Cerebellum/peduncles	Ipsilateral limb and gait ataxia
	Vestibular nuclei	Vertigo, nystagmus, nausea
	Cranial nerve IX	Dysphagia
	Cranial nerve X	Dysphonia
	Horner syndrome	
	Postganglionic sympathetic neuron damage	Ipsilateral ptosis, miosis, and anhidrosis
	Cranial nerve V—sensory portion	Ipsilateral facial sensory loss
	Second-order spinothalamic neurons	Contralateral loss of pain and temperature in extremities
Superior cerebellar	Cerebellum/peduncles	Ipsilateral ataxia (mild trunk, severe limb and gait), vertigo/dizziness, nausea, vomiting, dysarthria, dysmetria, optokinetic nystagmus
	Medial lemniscus/spinal lemniscus (midbrain)	Contralateral sensory loss (touch, pain, and temperature)
	Corticospinal fibers (pons)	Contralateral paresis

[a] Strokes of the anterior cerebral artery are uncommon, most likely due to the redundancy of circulation from the right and left systems.

[b] Damage to both areas results in global aphasia (both expressive and receptive).

[c] Reproduced, with permission, from Afifi AK, Bergman RA. Functional Neuroanatomy. 2nd ed. New York, NY: McGraw-Hill; 2005, Fig 28–2, pg. 361.

[d] Reproduced with permission from Nichols-Larsen DS, Kegelmeyer DA, Buford JA, et al, eds. Neurologic Rehabilitation: Neuroscience and Neuroplasticity in Physical Therapy Practice. 2016. Copyright © McGraw Hill LLC. All rights reserved. https://accessphysiotherapy.mhmedical.com and Reproduced with permission from Afifi AK, Bergman RA. Functional Neuroanatomy: Text and Atlas, 2nd ed. 2005. Copyright © McGraw Hill LLC. All rights reserved.

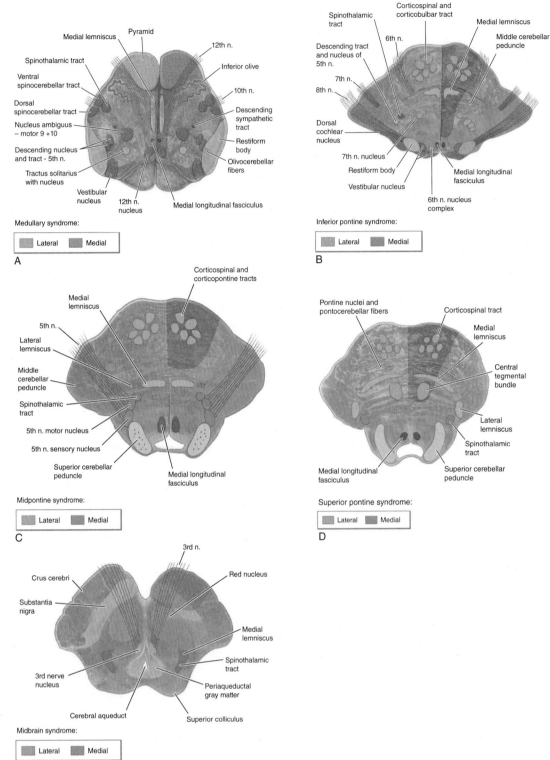

Figure 2-25. A-E. Brainstem circulation and stroke syndromes. Ascending syndromes **A-E**, from the medulla (**A**) to the midbrain (**E**), illustrate the complexity of structures damaged with lateral and medial stroke syndromes at each level. Damage to the corticospinal tracts, medial lemniscus, and spinothalamic tract results in loss of function contralateral to the lesion; damage at the level of the lower medulla often results in bilateral loss of corticospinal and medial lemniscal function because of the decussation of these fibers at this level. Typically, cranial nerve, spinocerebellar or cerebellar peduncle or medial longitudinal fasciculus symptoms are ipsilateral to the lesion. Thus, brainstem syndromes often present with contralateral or bilateral changes in the limbs, ipsilateral or bilateral changes in balance/proprioception, and ipsilateral or bilateral changes in cranial nerve function. (Reproduced with permission from Jameson JL, Fauci AS, Kasper DL, et al, eds. *Harrison's Principles of Internal Medicine.* 20th ed. 2013. Copyright © McGraw Hill LLC. All rights reserved. https://accessmedicine.mhmedical.com.)

drug, and the medical team synthesizes the current and past medical history to make this determination. TPA is most effective if given within the first 4.5 hours of the onset of stroke symptoms. Imaging is used to rule out a hemorrhage before administering TPA.

Hemorrhagic Stroke. A pooling of blood, which results in cerebral edema and potentially hydrocephalus. Hemorrhagic stroke is more likely to cause the patient to lose consciousness, and often intracranial pressures are increased. Therefore, these patients require careful monitoring and support to minimize demise.

Measuring Stroke Severity. This can be achieved using a variety of standardized outcome measures; however, in the acute setting, it is most common for the medical team to use the NIH Stroke Scale (NIHSS) or its **modified version**, the mNIHSS, the modified Rankin, and the Glasgow Coma Scale (GCS). These measures can be located using the resources outlined in the appendices of this chapter (Table A-1).

Initial Stroke Outcomes

About 20% of individuals admitted into an acute care hospital will die because of a stroke, and another 20% will return home. It is estimated that 60% of individuals who survive their stroke often require rehabilitation support at varying levels of care; this may be a skilled rehabilitation and nursing facility or an inpatient rehabilitation hospital, depending on the ability of the individual to participate in 3 hours of therapy each day and expected prognosis.

Acute Neuroplasticity Poststroke

The brain attempts to heal itself to return to a state of homeostasis. This neuroplasticity term is referred to as **spontaneous reorganization**. The stroke itself causes neuronal cell death, and the area surrounding the cell death, called the ischemic penumbra, is further susceptible to cause an increase in cell death. Early medical interventions attempt to minimize the penumbra and support **angiogenesis** for increased healing and work toward homeostasis. Minimizing the cascade of inflammatory processes is dependent on the activity of surviving neurons and a balance of excitatory and inhibitory connections.

TRAUMATIC BRAIN INJURY

Traumatic brain injury (TBI) is a leading cause of long-term disability. Concussions are more common in men between 17 and 24 years of age yet are becoming more gender-neutral in the current population.

TBI can result from a blow to the head and/or sudden acceleration-deceleration of the head, such as in a motor vehicle accident. TBIs can be closed or open in terms of whether or not the skull is fractured. Closed TBIs are more common due to car accidents, falls, and blows to the head from falls or assaults. Injuries penetrating the skull can occur from anything that will penetrate the skull, for example, a bullet. TBIs are classified as mild, moderate, or severe, depending on the initial clinical presentation and the length of time the person is unconscious. The GCS, seen in Box 2-5, is most often used to capture initial clinical presentation.

Pathophysiology of TBI

TBIs are either focal or diffuse. The **focal injury** occurs in the area of contact between the brain and the skull. Focal damage is characterized by (1) **contusions**—bruising of the brain surface, (2) **lacerations**—tearing of the pia or arachnoid matter, or the brain tissue, and/or (3) **hematomas**—bleeding within the subdural or epidural spaces or the brain tissue, referred to as **intraparenchymal**. These hemorrhages occur due to rupture of the blood vessels within these areas: (1) subdural—tearing of cerebral arteries or veins that bleed into the space between the dura and arachnoid matters, (2) epidural—tearing of meningeal arteries of the dura with bleeding into the space between the dura and the skull, and (3) intraparenchymal—tearing of the penetrating intracerebral arteries with bleeding into the brain tissue.

Diffuse axonal injury (DAI) results from the tearing of axons that comprise the white matter due to rotational forces as the brain moves within the cranium. Most often, DAI occurs

---

BOX 2-5   GLASGOW COMA SCALE

The Glasgow Coma Scale (GCS) was developed in the 1970s and assesses eye movements, verbal responses, and motor behavior, looking for spontaneous versus responsive activity, with each scale recorded numerically as indicated here.

Score	Eye Opening	Verbal Responsiveness	Motor Behavior
1	None	None	None
2	Opens in response	Makes sounds	Limbs in extension to deep pressure
3	Opens to verbal stimulation	Saying words	Limbs in flexion
4	Spontaneously opens	Confused but talking	Flexor withdrawal of limb to stimulus
5	N/A	Oriented	Localized response to stimulus
6	N/A	N/A	Moves to commands

Data from Teasdale G, Maas A, Lecky F, et al. The Glasgow Coma Scale at 40 years: standing the test of time. *Lancet Neurol.* 2014;13(8):844-854.

---

with motor vehicle accidents; however, it is also becoming more common with minor TBI or concussions. DAI is most common in white matter structures of the brainstem, corpus callosum, and some white matter projections in lateral hemispheres.

The degree of severity and consequences of TBI depends on the areas of focal damage and the amount of white matter damage.

TBI Consequences

Coma, Posttraumatic Amnesia, and Executive Dysfunction. As noted with the GCS, there is a loss of consciousness initially after TBI, lasting for seconds to weeks. When the loss of consciousness exceeds 6 hours, it is defined as a coma, which is characterized by a lack of responsiveness, volitional movement, and the normal sleep-wake cycle. After sustaining a severe TBI, some people will enter what is known as a **vegetative state**, characterized by an emergence of a sleep-wake cycle and a generalized response to stimuli. A patient may move through this state to one of minimal consciousness, indicated by specific responses to stimulation but no ability to speak.

Patients who recover from coma after a moderate to severe TBI progress through the vegetative state to a gradual state of responsiveness and severe confusion, abnormal behavior, and memory deficits, defined as **posttraumatic amnesia**. As the patient moves through the recovery process and the posttraumatic amnesia decreases, the patient often has impairment of multiple systems. A tool frequently used to characterize, and document behavior, memory, and awareness changes is the Rancho Los Amigos (RLA) Cognitive Recovery Scale. Additional outcome measures are available in the appendices at the end of this chapter (Table A-1).

Secondary Impairments Following TBI

Respiratory Distress Syndrome. A common secondary complication of TBI is acute respiratory distress syndrome (ARDS), which occurs in up to 31% of TBI admissions and ultimately is the leading cause of death after TBI. ARDS is defined as inflammation of the lung lining, disruption of gas exchange, and hypoxia.

Interventions involve respiratory support for those with a GCS of less than or equal to 8. Those patients who can breathe independently may require continuous positive airway pressure (CPAP), provided through a mask, or positive pressure support, provided through a nasal cannula.

Intracranial Hypertension. Posttraumatic intracranial hypertension (ICH) occurs from hematomas that may increase pressure or shift the brain tissue across the midline. Also, if there is compromised blood perfusion, this will exacerbate ICH and cause an increase in intracranial pressure (ICP). Therefore, it is critical to monitor the patient's ICP when a hematoma has been diagnosed, and this is typically performed with an ICP monitor. If the hematoma is large, it may require immediate surgical removal to decrease the secondary effects.

Epilepsy.   Approximately 25% of patients with severe TBI will develop posttraumatic epilepsy (PTE). The epilepsy may occur within the first week of the injury and up to a year or more postinjury. The cause of PTE is unknown, and many theories exist to support these clinical findings. Many patients who experience PTE are supported with antiepileptic medications. Use and weaning off these medications depends on seizure activity and is accomplished with the support of the physician.

Dysautonomia/Paroxysmal Sympathetic Hyperactivation.   Dysautonomia, more recently renamed paroxysmal sympathetic hyperactivation (PSH), is a dysregulation of autonomic function that presents in 10% to 12% of TBI hospital admissions. It is noted to occur more frequently with severe TBI and fractures, infections, or prolonged ventilation. The theory is that PSH occurs as a result of damage between the hypothalamus and cortex, which causes a loss of inhibition and hypersensitivity to stimuli, and the patient has periods from minutes to hours of tachycardia, hyperpyrexia (fever), elevated blood pressure, extensor posturing (decorticate or decerebrate), and excessive sweating. Medications, such as baclofen, β-blockers, benzodiazepine, and morphine, are the most common intervention.

Neuropsychiatric Changes.   Some of the most debilitating secondary effects after TBI are the neuropsychiatric changes. Two common behavioral syndromes are emotional and behavioral dyscontrol. **Emotional dyscontrol** manifests as agitation, irritability, restlessness, pathologic laughing/crying, and/or emotional lability. **Behavioral dyscontrol** is characterized by disinhibition and sometimes aggression; this can result in the pulling out of intravenous (IV) lines and feeding tubes, fighting and swearing early in recovery, as well as hypersexual behavior and excessive risk-taking in later recovery. In addition, many TBI survivors will experience additional psychiatric conditions, especially depression.

The most effective intervention for the common neuropsychiatric diagnoses is behavior modification and management. However, in some cases, pharmacologic management is considered or required.

Mild TBI and Concussion.   Mild TBI (mTBI) and concussion are discussed as one category, as a concussion is defined as a mild form of a TBI. In both conditions, microscopic damage may not be detectable on neuroimaging, and the injury may or may not involve a loss of consciousness.

It is more common to see mTBI and concussions in the younger population, of which many are still developing brain function and capacity. Therefore, the public must be educated on preventing mTBI and concussions related to athletic events. Screening instruments can be found using the resources outlined in the appendices of this chapter (Table A-1). Table 2-13 details the symptoms of concussion.

TABLE 2-13 • Symptoms of Concussion or mTBI.			
Cognitive	**Physical**	**Emotional**	**Sleep**
Poorer concentration	Blurred vision	Irritability	Drowsiness/lethargy
Memory disturbance	Headache	Depression	Increased sleepiness
Slower processing	Nausea/vomiting Noise and/or light sensitivity Poor balance/coordination	Hyperemotionality Anxiety	Insomnia

BRAIN TUMOR

Types of Primary Brain Tumors

Primary brain tumors are most common in children, second to the childhood diagnosis of leukemia. Primary brain tumors are defined as abnormal cell proliferation of neurons or glia within the brain, meninges, vasculature, or pituitary or pineal glands.

Glioma. This is the most common type of tumor in adults and children and can be further subdivided into astrocytomas, oligodendrogliomas, ependymomas, and mixed gliomas (which typically involve both astrocytes and oligodendrocytes). Gliomas are staged from I (least benign) to stage IV (malignant) based on their growth rate and whether they have penetrated the surrounding tissue. Table 2-14 describes tumor locations and characteristics.

Tumor Symptoms

Symptoms are often specific to the neuroanatomic location of the tumor itself; however, an increase in ICP is often the first indication of a tumor. Like TBI, tumors may cause nausea, headaches, blurred vision, and fatigue. Many tumors may cause seizures and ultimately epilepsy due to the irritation and eventual death of adjacent cells. Memory or executive function changes occur when the temporal or frontal lobe is involved. Tumors of the posterior frontal/parietal lobe can present with contralateral sensorimotor disturbances such as a stroke. It is common for these symptoms to be initially mild and progress as the tumor increases in size. Tumors located in the posterior fossa disrupt the cerebellum and brainstem, leading to clinical presentations similar to brainstem strokes that include lack of coordination, dizziness, ataxia, and deficits in the cranial nerves.

Tumor Diagnosis

Imaging is the best diagnostic tool to identify the presence of a tumor. Tumors on a computed tomography (CT) scan appear as areas of hypointensity (lighter than the normal

TABLE 2-14 • Tumor Locations and Characteristics.

Tumor Type	Common Locations	Characteristics
Ependymoma	Usually infratentorial but can be supratentorial (parietal or temporal lobe)	Arise from ventricular ependymal cells (lining of the ventricles); infratentorial tumors are typically Stage III, while supratentorial tumors are typically Stage II.
Gliomas	Anywhere	Arise from glial cells—astrocytes (astrocytoma), oligodendrocytes (oligodendrocytoma); can range from grade I to IV glioblastomas. Stage IV astrocytoma stimulates abnormal angiogenesis, creating highly vascularized tumors. Prognosis is poor.
Glioneuronal	Temporal or frontal lobes; cerebellum	Tumor comprises both glial cells and neuronal components, arising from neuroepithelial tissues; most common in temporal lobe. Associated with epilepsy that is pharmacologically resistant.
Medulloblastoma	Cerebellum and vermis	Fast-growing malignant posterior fossa tumor in children < 7 years; associated with hydrocephalus.
Meningioma	Arachnoid matter	Stages I to III (most are Stage I); multiple genetic contributions. Stages I and II are effectively treated with surgery and radiation.
Pituitary adenoma	Pituitary gland	Benign tumors of one of the six cell types of the pituitary, leading to abnormal secretion of the respective secretory hormones (adenocorticotropic, growth, prolactin, thyroid-stimulating, follicle-stimulating, and luteinizing) with associated symptomatology. Tumor growth may disrupt pituitary function. Commonly treatable with gamma knife surgery.
Primitive neuroectodermal tumors (PNETs)	Supratentorial—often within pineal gland	Metastasize easily, so staged according to: 0 = no metastases; 1 = cells in CSF; 2 = supratentorial metastases; 3 = spinal metastases. Fatal in almost 50% (only 20% if in pineal gland), especially once metastasized. Treated with surgery and radiation, sometimes with chemotherapy.

CSF, cerebrospinal fluid.

surrounding tissue), and therefore, a magnetic resonance imaging (MRI) is used for tumor identification.

Medical Treatment of Brain Tumors

Medical treatment needs to be aggressive to minimize secondary neuronal damage. Medical interventions could include surgical resection, radiation, and chemotherapy, depending on the tumor type and location.

SPINAL CORD INJURY

Pathophysiology

Spinal cord injuries occur most commonly when a fracture, dislocation, and/or subluxation of the vertebrae impinge on the spinal cord. In addition, neurologic damage from a spinal cord injury (SCI) may occur due to primary (or direct) injury and secondary injury. The primary injury is at the site of dysfunction occurring initially, and the **secondary injury** occurs because of inflammation and an increased level of toxicity from the primary injury. The average age for an injury occurrence is 43 years. However, about half of all SCIs occur in people under 30, and more SCIs occur in men than women. Additional causes of SCI include transverse myelitis, spinal stenosis, spinal abscess, or tumor.

Classifications of Spinal Cord Injury

Spinal cord injuries are classified as either complete or incomplete. A complete injury means the patient has complete loss of sensory or motor function below the level of injury and in the S4 and S5 sacral segments. Incomplete injuries have partial preservation of motor or sensory function below the level of neurologic injury and in the S4 and S5 segments. SCI classifications by the level and severity of the primary pathology using the ASIA Impairment Scale (AIS) are summarized in Table 2-15. The Asia Motor Score Scale (which identifies key muscles for greatest functional improvement) and the International Standards for Neurological Classification of SCI (ISNCSCI) can be located in the appendices at the end of this chapter (Tables A-1 and A-2).

Clinical Syndromes of Spinal Cord Injury

Brown-Sequard Injury. An injury to primarily one side of the cord, leaving the other side relatively intact. See Figure 2-26 for details. A patient with a Brown-Sequard injury most commonly loses motor function, proprioception, and vibration on the same side of the body as the injury, while losing pain and temperature sensations on the opposite side of the body.

Central Cord Syndrome. It is caused by a lesion of the center core of the gray matter and occurs with trauma, tumors, or syrinxes, and presents with lower motor neuron (LMN) signs of the upper extremities, with less severe impairments of the lower extremities. See Figure 2-27 for details.

TABLE 2-15 • Classification of SCI.	
AIS A	Complete; no sensory or motor function below the level of the injury
AIS B	Incomplete; no motor function but some sensation below the injury, including in the anal sphincter region (S4-S5)
AIS C	Incomplete; some sensory and motor function below the injury but most of these muscles score below 3 on MMT
AIS D	Incomplete; sensory and motor function with at least half of the muscle groups scoring 3 or higher on MMT
AIS E	Normal motor and sensory function

ASIA, American Spinal Injury Association; AIS, ASIA Impairment Scale; MMT, manual muscle test; SCI, spinal cord injury.

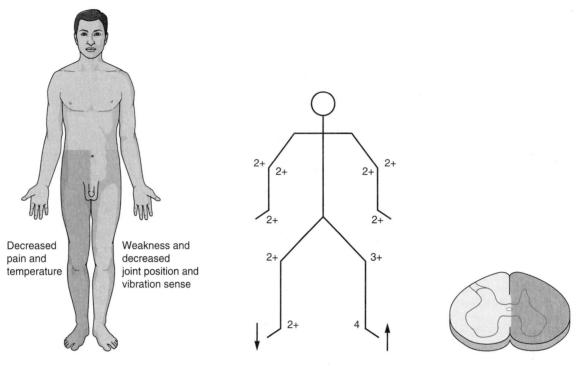

Figure 2-26. **Brown-Sequard pattern of injury. The primary symptoms of a Brown-Sequard pattern are ipsilesional motor and somatosensory dysfunction with contralesional loss of pain and temperature (A); hyperreflexia in the ipsilesional leg (B); and a lesion confined to one side of the spinal cord (C).** (Reproduced with permission from Kandel ER, Schwartz JH, Jessell TM, et al. *Principles of Neural Science.* 5th ed. 2013. Copyright © McGraw Hill LLC. All rights reserved. https://neurology.mhmedical.com.)

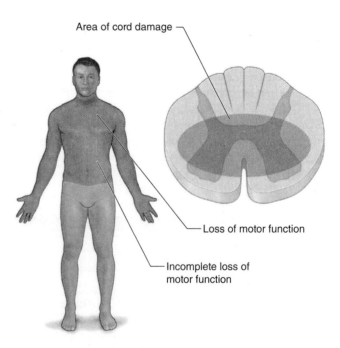

Figure 2-27. **Central cord syndrome. This shows a lesion in the central gray matter, sparing a peripheral rim of white matter (right). The shaded areas (left) show the regions with complete loss of motor function (dark) and incomplete, mild loss of motor function (light).** (Reproduced with permission from Nichols-Larsen DS, Kegelmeyer DA, Buford JA, et al., eds. *Neurologic Rehabilitation: Neuroscience and Neuroplasticity in Physical Therapy Practice.* 2016. Copyright © McGraw Hill LLC. All rights reserved. https://accessphysiotherapy.mhmedical.com.)

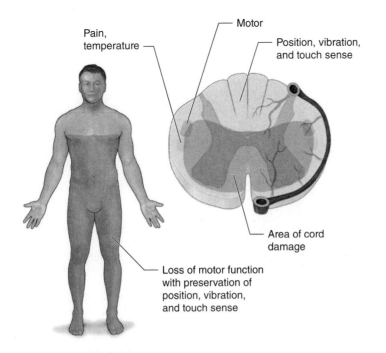

Figure 2-28. Anterior spinal cord injury. The lesion location in the ventral gray and white matter is shown on the right image of the cord. The shaded regions on the left show loss of motor function and pain and temperature sensation. Vibration and position sense remain. (Reproduced with permission from Nichols-Larsen DS, Kegelmeyer DA, Buford JA, et al., eds. *Neurologic Rehabilitation: Neuroscience and Neuroplasticity in Physical Therapy Practice.* 2016. Copyright © McGraw Hill LLC. All rights reserved. https://accessphysiotherapy .mhmedical.com.)

Anterior Spinal Cord Syndrome. It is a lesion of the anterior two-thirds of the spinal cord and is caused by damage or infarction of the anterior spinal artery. See Figure 2-28 for details. Flexion injuries to the spine are commonly associated with anterior spinal cord syndrome, and loss of motor, pain, and temperature sensations will occur.

Posterior Spinal Cord Syndrome. It is a lesion in the posterior part of the spinal cord and can be caused by a penetrating wound to the back or hyperextension that fractures the vertebral arch. See Figure 2-29 for details.

Conus Medullaris. An injury to the conus medullaris occurring at the L1 vertebral level, where the spinal cord tapers to an end. See Figure 2-30 for details. Patients will present with back pain, flaccid paralysis, and areflexic bowel and bladder function.

Cauda Equina Syndrome. Similar to a conus medullaris injury, and is named as such because of damage to the nerves below the L2 vertebral level. See Figure 2-30 for details.

Medical Management

Acute medical management begins with the emergency response teams. The care will continue in the emergency department for both traumatic and nontraumatic SCIs. The medical team will make an early decision regarding spinal stabilization and whether surgery is indicated. Once the patient has been stabilized and medically cleared, the interprofessional rehabilitation process begins.

The PTA must be mindful of several body systems that can pose life-threatening conditions if not managed. These systems include (1) cardiovascular and pulmonary system, (2) bladder and bowel functioning, (3) respiratory system, and (4) integumentary system. Therefore, significant attention should be paid to these systems and the possible deficits with persons after sustaining an SCI. Below is a list of possible medical complications common for individuals with SCI that should be considered and reviewed in further detail.

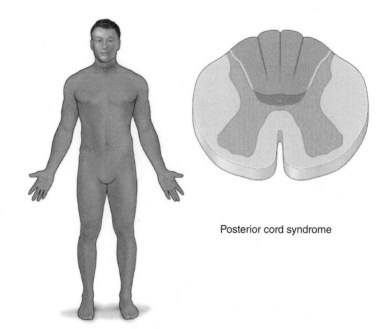

Posterior cord syndrome

Figure 2-29. **Posterior cord syndrome. The shaded region depicted in the right image of the cord shows the lesion located in the dorsal columns. The affected body regions are shown on the left which have loss of vibration and position sense.** (Reproduced with permission from Nichols-Larsen DS, Kegelmeyer DA, Buford JA, et al., eds. *Neurologic Rehabilitation: Neuroscience and Neuroplasticity in Physical Therapy Practice.* 2016. Copyright © McGraw Hill LLC. All rights reserved. https://accessphysiotherapy.mhmedical.com.)

- Autonomic dysfunction and autonomic dysreflexia.
- Cardiac and vasomotor changes—hypotension, bradycardia, arrhythmia.
- Deep vein thrombosis (DVT).
- Bladder and bowel dysfunction.

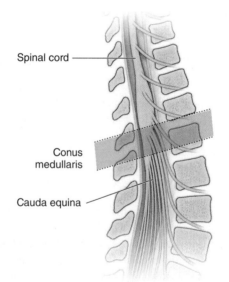

Spinal cord

Conus medullaris

Cauda equina

Figure 2-30. **Conus medullaris and cauda equina injuries The conus medullaris injury damages the distal portion of the spinal cord at L1; the cauda equina injury damages the spinal nerves, located in the spinal segments below the end of the cord.** (Reproduced with permission from Nichols-Larsen DS, Kegelmeyer DA, Buford JA, et al., eds. *Neurologic Rehabilitation: Neuroscience and Neuroplasticity in Physical Therapy Practice.* 2016. Copyright © McGraw Hill LLC. All rights reserved. https://accessphysiotherapy.mhmedical.com.)

- Mental and emotional support.
- Pressure ulcer and skin integrity.

MULTIPLE SCLEROSIS

Multiple sclerosis (MS) is a chronic, progressive, debilitating demyelinating disease that affects neurons in the CNS. MS typically affects people between the ages of 20 and 50 and is one of the most common causes of neurologic disability in young adults. MS is two to three times more common in women than in men, and whites of European descent have a higher incidence of MS than any other ethnicity. An increased risk of MS is also associated with smoking and low blood levels of vitamin D.

Pathophysiology

Environmental agents specific to certain viruses are believed to be possible triggers for MS; however, the exact cause is unknown. Although specific genes have not been directly linked to MS, there is one gene, human leukocyte antigen (HLA), located on chromosome 6, strongly associated with the development of the disease.

MS is an autoimmune disease that attacks the CNS, mediated in part by activated T cells that travel through the blood–brain barrier. This immune response results in inflammatory damage to the myelin covering as well as the axons themselves. See Figure 2-31 for details.

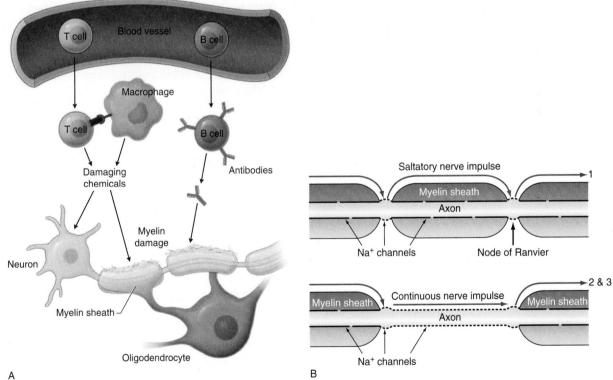

Figure 2-31. **A.** Autoimmune process of myelin damage: activated T cells and potentially B cells, followed by macrophage activity, induce myelin inflammation that can damage the myelin. During the inflammatory phase, conduction is impaired, producing symptoms associated with the involved axons; as inflammation recedes, recovery of symptoms occurs if remyelination is achieved. **B.** Schematic representation of demyelination and axonal degeneration in MS. (1) schematic of normal neural function in a myelinated axon; (2) in acute demyelination, action potentials cannot cross the open space due to low numbers of voltage-gated sodium channels in the internodal axonal regions and stop; (3) in a demyelinated axon, conduction can take place if voltage-gated sodium channels are added to the axon membrane through neuroplasticity, but is much slower; (4) with further loss of myelin, axon degeneration occurs (not shown). (A: Reproduced with permission from Burke-Doe A, Dutton M, eds. *National Physical Therapy Examination and Board Review*. 2019. Copyright © McGraw Hill LLC. All rights reserved. https://accessphysiotherapy .mhmedical.com. B: Reproduced with permission from Hauser SL, ed. *Harrison's Neurology in Clinical Medicine*. 3rd ed. 2013. Copyright © McGraw Hill LLC. All rights reserved.)

BOX 2-6	TYPES OF MULTIPLE SCLEROSIS

The clinical disease course varies widely and is unpredictable from person to person and within a particular person over time. However, four main subtypes describe the most frequent clinical course for multiple sclerosis (MS).

Relapsing-Remitting MS

Most individuals (about 85%) diagnosed with MS are initially diagnosed with relapsing-remitting MS (RRMS). People with RRMS have clearly defined relapses, also called attacks, flareups, or exacerbations, during which neurologic function worsens. These relapses are followed by remissions, defined as periods during which the disease does not progress, and individuals experience complete or incomplete recovery of neurologic function. Incomplete recovery leads to incremental worsening of disability over time. Relapse rates for untreated RRMS are about one to two relapses a year and are correlated with disability.

Secondary Progressive MS

Following an initial period of RRMS, many people develop a secondary progressive MS (SPMS) course, in which the disease steadily worsens, with or without notable relapses and remissions or plateaus. Approximately 50% of people with RRMS developed SPMS within 10 years of diagnosis before the advent of disease-modifying medications. Unfortunately, long-term data are not yet available to determine if this transition is delayed in treated individuals.

Primary Progressive MS

Primary progressive MS (PPMS) affects approximately 10% of people and is characterized by slowly worsening neurologic function from diagnosis with no distinct relapses or remissions. The rate of progression may vary over time, with occasional plateaus and temporary minor improvements. Individuals with PPMS tend to be older (ie, around 40 years old) at the onset.

Progressive-Relapsing MS

Progressive-relapsing MS (PRMS) includes about 5% of people with MS who experience steadily worsening disease from the beginning, with superimposed relapses followed by no or little recovery along the way. In contrast to RRMS, the disease continues to progress, and disability increases even during relapses.

In rare cases, individuals with MS experience a very mild disease course called benign MS, in which full neurologic function is preserved 15 years after disease onset. On the other extreme, some individuals experience a very rapid disease course called malignant MS (Marburg disease), leading to death within a short time of onset.

Various types of MS exist. Box 2-6 describes the clinical presentation of each MS subgroup.

MS has a variety of symptoms and lacks a definitive diagnostic test. An MS diagnosis remains a clinical diagnosis whereby the practitioner considers the patient's history after a clinical neurologic examination. Neurologic symptoms related to the demyelinated anatomic locations in the CNS are separated in time and space. Imaging and other diagnostic tests help confirm an MS diagnosis. Box 2-7 provides a list of common symptoms associated with MS, and these symptoms should be explored in further detail.

Medical Management

Medical management is best achieved with a multidisciplinary approach, with long-term management supported with disease-modifying immunomodulatory pharmacologic drugs. Acute symptoms and relapses are most notably treated with high-dose intravenous corticosteroids for a period of 3 to 5 days. Drug side effects of both types of intervention should be considered. Pain management is usually managed with anticonvulsant medications, including gabapentin, pregabalin, and carbamazepine. In addition, medications and many rehabilitation interventions are often used to support varying levels of spasticity, fatigue, ataxia and tremor, cognition, emotion, bowel, bladder, and sexual issues.

| BOX 2-7 | COMMON SYMPTOMS OF MULTIPLE SCLEROSIS |

Sensory Symptoms
- Hypoesthesia, numbness
- Paresthesias

Pain
- Dysesthesias
- Optic or trigeminal neuritis
- Lhermitte sign
- Chronic pain

Visual Symptoms
- Blurred or double vision
- Diminished acuity/loss of vision
- Scotoma
- Internuclear ophthalmoplegia
- Nystagmus

Motor Symptoms
- Weakness or paralysis
- Fatigue
- Spasticity
- Impaired balance
- Ataxia and intention tremor
- Impaired gait and mobility
- Impaired speech and swallowing

Cognitive Symptoms
- Decreased information processing speed
- Short-term memory problems
- Decreased attention and concentration
- Executive function problems
- Impaired visual-spatial processing
- Impaired verbal fluency

Emotional/Behavioral Symptoms
- Depression
- Pseudobulbar affect
- Euphoria
- Lack of insight
- Adjustment disorders
- Obsessive-compulsive disorders

Cardiovascular Dysautonomia

Bladder and Bowel Symptoms
- Urinary urgency, frequency
- Nocturia
- Urinary hesitancy, dribbling
- Constipation
- Diarrhea
- Incontinence

Sexual Symptoms
- Erectile and ejaculatory dysfunction
- Decreased vaginal lubrication
- Decreased libido
- Decreased ability to achieve orgasm

Life expectancy is near normal for most people with MS, and most persons with MS do not become severely disabled. The prognostic indicators for MS vary from person to person; however, the guidelines below are suggested for the most accurate prognosis.

- Gender.
- Age.
- Symptom.
- Progression of disease.
- Neurologic findings at 5 years.
- MRI findings.

PARKINSON DISEASE

Parkinson disease (PD) is the second most common progressive neurodegenerative disorder, with deficits in the basal ganglia and its connections to movement and posture regulation, cognitive and psychiatric functions.

PD is estimated to affect 1 million Americans and 7 to 10 million people worldwide. There are approximately 60,000 new cases of PD annually in the United States, with an average age of onset of 62 years. PD affects men 1.5 times more than women, with the highest incidence among Hispanics.

Etiology and Risk Factors

Parkinsonism is a group of disorders that includes slowing movement, tremor, rigidity or stiffness, and balance problems. Parkinsonism includes idiopathic PD and secondary parkinsonism. **Parkinson-plus syndromes** mimic PD in some ways but are caused by other neurodegenerative disorders.

Idiopathic Parkinson Disease. Idiopathic PD is the most common form of parkinsonism, affecting 78% of individuals. Most scientists believe PD is caused by an interaction between genetic and environmental factors, although the exact cause remains unknown.

Secondary Parkinsonism. Toxins, trauma, multiple strokes, infections, metabolic disorders, and drugs are the known causes of secondary parkinsonism. **Toxic parkinsonism** can be caused by such toxins as carbon monoxide, mercury, and cyanide poisoning. **Posttraumatic parkinsonism** can be caused by severe or frequent head injuries and is also associated with dementia. **Vascular parkinsonism** is caused by one or more small, sudden strokes to the basal ganglia.

Pathophysiology

PD is caused by degeneration of nigrostriatal dopamine-containing neurons whose cell bodies are in the **substantia nigra pars compacta** (SNpc) of the midbrain and project primarily to the putamen. The loss of dopamine causes numerous motor deficits; however, by the time the patient experiences any clinical symptoms, approximately 60% of the SNpc neurons have already been lost. The effects produce increased activity in the indirect motor pathway and decreased activity in the direct pathway. As a result, the patient will experience stiffness, muscle rigidity, and an inability to activate and relax muscles needed for functional activities. In addition, a patient with PD experiences symptoms of slow movement (bradykinesia) and a reduction in the amplitude of movement (hypokinesia).

Clinical Presentation

Primary Motor Symptoms

- **Tremor** is the initial symptom for patients with PD in approximately 70% of individuals and typically presents as an involuntary slow oscillation in the hand or fingers on one side of the body, defined as resting tremor and often referred to as a pill-rolling tremor.
- **Bradykinesia** is defined as slowness of voluntary movement, and typically poses challenges when individuals attempt initiation of movements. A reduction of movement

amplitude (hypokinesia) affects all movements and is a primary cause of reduced gait speed and step length.

- **Rigidity**, which can be cogwheel or lead pipe, affects the proximal musculature of the shoulders and neck and later progresses to the muscles of the face and extremities.
- **Postural instability** typically occurs in the later stages of PD and will worsen over time. Declining balance poses an increase in fall risks and loss of overall independence and function. Postural instability in patients with PD causes (1) reduced limits of stability, (2) reduced magnitude of postural responses, (3) impaired postural adaptations, and (4) altered anticipatory postural adjustments. Many of these deficits cause postural deformities as the disease progresses. This posture is characterized by rounded shoulders and a forward head with increased trunk, hip, and knee flexion.

Secondary Motor Symptoms. Muscle performance and strength of both the upper and lower extremities have been noted to decline over time in persons with PD.

Gait deficits are more common in the middle to late stages of PD and contribute to falls, loss of independence, and hospitalization. PD will cause slower gait velocity, shorter step length, an increased step variability, and an increased time in double-limb support. In addition, trunk rotation is decreased, which then causes a reduction in arm swing. **Dystonia**, involuntary sustained muscle contractions that cause abnormal movements and/or postures, often interfere with gait with the foot and ankle involvement. Additional characteristics of a parkinsonian gait include **festination** and freezing, which may increase the number of falls.

> **Freezing of gait** is a manifestation of akinesia, and a person with PD will have the appearance that their feet are glued to the floor.
>
> **Dual-tasking** during gait is also impaired in persons with PD because of the decreased gait speed and increased gait variability.

Other Motor Symptoms. Patients with PD often have speech disorders and dysphagia due to bulbar dysfunction. These occur because of the rigidity and bradykinesia of the orofacial and laryngeal muscles.

- **Motor learning**—Because the striatum is involved in all stages of motor learning, most importantly when learning new skills that consist of a sequence of movements, research has shown that learning new motor skills or fine-tuning skills is preserved in the early stages of PD for those without dementia. Individuals with PD generally take longer to learn motor tasks than healthy controls. In patients with PD, motor learning with gait training has been shown to benefit from external auditory or visual cueing.

Nonmotor Symptoms. Nonmotor symptoms are common for individuals with PD. These include autonomic dysfunction, cognitive/behavioral disorders, and sensory and sleep abnormalities.

Medical Diagnosis and Progression

PD is generally based on the patient's clinical presentation; however, differentiation of PD from other forms of parkinsonism is essential. PD usually progresses slowly in the first 5 years, followed by a gradual increase in symptoms for approximately 13 years. The average rate of progression can be seen in Table 2-16.

Two outcome measures widely used to measure disease progression and severity of symptoms are the Unified Parkinson's Disease Rating Scale (UPDRS) and the Hoehn–Yahr Classification of Disability Scale. Please view the appendices at the end of this chapter (Table A-1) for additional resources.

Medical Management

Pharmacological Management. There is no cure for PD. Medical management aims to slow down the progression of the disease through neuroprotective strategies and

TABLE 2-16 • Progression of Symptoms Across Disease Stages in Parkinson Disease (PD) and Huntington Disease (HD).

Disease	Premanifest	Early	Middle	Late
PD	• Hyposmia • Constipation • Depression/anxiety • Rapid eye movement (REM) sleep behavior disorder • Reduced arm swing • Mild motor function changes	• Unilateral tremor • Rigidity • Mild gait hypokinesia • Micrographia • Reduced speech volume	• Bilateral bradykinesia, axial and limb rigidity • Balance and gait deficits/falls • Speech impairments • May need assistance toward end of stage	• Severe voluntary movement impairments • Pulmonary function and swallowing compromised • Dependence in mobility, self-care, and activities of daily living
HD	• Mild motor symptoms (rapid alternating movements, fine coordination, gait) • Difficulty with complex thinking tasks • Depression, aggression, irritability	• Mild chorea (mainly hands) • Mild balance problems (turns) • Abnormal extraocular movements • Mild visuospatial and cognitive deficits • Depression, irritability	• Chorea, dystonia • Voluntary movement abnormalities • Balance and gait deficits/falls • Cognitive/behavioral problems • Weight loss • Difficulties with self-care	• Bradykinesia, rigidity • Severe dysarthria, dysphagia • Chorea (may be less) • Global dementia • Psychosis • Dependence in mobility, self-care, and activities of daily living

Reproduced with permission from Nichols-Larsen DS, Kegelmeyer DA, Buford JA, et al., eds. *Neurologic Rehabilitation: Neuroscience and Neuroplasticity in Physical Therapy Practice.* 2016. Copyright © McGraw Hill LLC. All rights reserved. https://accessphysiotherapy.mhmedical.com.

treatment of motor and nonmotor symptoms. A wide range of first-line medications supports the neuroprotective aspects and assists with symptom management. See Table 2-17 for details.

Deep Brain Stimulation. Deep brain stimulation (DBS) can be used to change the firing of the brain circuits; however, it does not slow down the progression of the disease. Therefore, DBS is reserved for patients who do not have success with pharmacologic management.

TABLE 2-17 • Medications for Parkinson Disease.

Drug	Action	Side Effects	Brand Names
Levodopa/carbidopa	L-dopa converted to dopamine in the brain to restore DA levels	Orthostatic hypotension, dyskinesias, hallucinations, sleepiness	Sinemet, immediate and sustained release; Parcopa
Dopamine agonists	Directly stimulate postsynaptic dopamine receptors	Nausea, sedation, dizziness, constipation, hallucinations Linked to impulse control disorders (eg, pathologic gambling, compulsive shopping, hypersexuality)	Pramipexole (Mirapex), ropinirole (Requip), piribedil (Trivastal), rotigotine transdermal patch (Neupro), apomorphine (Uprima)
Anticholinergics	Block acetylcholine receptors and may inhibit dopamine reuptake in striatum	Blurred vision, dry mouth, dizziness, and urinary retention; toxicity causes impaired memory, confusion, hallucinations, and delusions	Trihexyphenidyl HCl (Artane), benztropine mesylate (Cogentin), procyclidine hydrochloride (Kemadrin)
Catechol-O-methyl transferase (COMT) inhibitors	Inhibits enzyme COMT to prevent degradation of dopamine	Dyskinesia, nausea, vomiting, orthostatic hypotension, sleep disorders, hallucinations, diarrhea, liver damage with tolcapone	Entacapone (Comtan), entacapone and levodopa (Stalevo), tolcapone (Tasmar)
Monoamine oxidase B (MAO-B) inhibitors	Inhibits enzyme MAO-B to prevent degradation of dopamine	Mild nausea, dry mouth, dizziness, orthostatic hypotension, confusion, hallucinations, insomnia	Selegiline hydrochloride (Eldepryl), rasagiline (Azilect)
Amantadine	Increases release of dopamine presynaptically; blocks acetylcholine receptors	Dizziness, nausea, and anorexia; livedo reticularis (ie, purplish red blotchy spots on skin), leg edema, confusion, hallucinations	Amantadine hydrochloride (Symmetrel), Symadine

Reproduced with permission from Nichols-Larsen DS, Kegelmeyer DA, Buford JA, et al., eds. *Neurologic Rehabilitation: Neuroscience and Neuroplasticity in Physical Therapy Practice.* 2016. Copyright © McGraw Hill LLC. All rights reserved. https://accessphysiotherapy.mhmedical.com.

HUNTINGTON DISEASE

Huntington disease (HD) occurs in the United States in about 1 in every 10,000 people and approximately a total of 30,000 people diagnosed with the disease. The onset is typically between the ages of 30 and 50. HD affects females slightly more than men and is more common in white people of Western European descent than in Asian or African ancestry.

Etiology and Risk Factors

HD is caused by an autosomal dominant mutation in the huntingtin (HTT) gene mapped to chromosome 4. Any child from a person having HD has a 50% chance of inheriting the disease.

Pathophysiology

There is severe loss of neurons in the caudate and putamen nuclei of the basal ganglia with the diagnosis of HD. These areas have a decreased size and an increase in the ventricular space.

Clinical Presentation

Symptoms typically evolve slowly over time and vary from person to person, even within the same family. There are motor, cognitive, and behavioral deficits.

Motor Symptoms. Patients with HD typically have involuntary movements such as **chorea** and **dystonia**. Choreic movements start as general restlessness and progress to involve the face, head, lips, tongue, and trunk and cause flailing movements called **ballismus**.

Voluntary motor impairments may present in the form of apraxia and the persistence of nonfunctional movements. In addition, there are musculoskeletal impairments related to muscle performance, posture, and tone that can negatively impact activity and participation for the patient.

Speech and swallowing impairments develop over time for persons with HD, and patients have difficulty with articulation, alternations in pitch, and a reduction in the rate of speech. In addition, dysphagia will appear as the disease progresses.

Changes in motor learning are similar to those with PD.

Cognitive Symptoms. In the early stages of HD, cognitive problems arise. These may include impaired perception of time, decreased processing speed, impaired visuospatial perception, short-term memory decline, and executive function deficit; however, in later stages, patients with HD often have global dementia.

Behavioral Symptoms. With HD, emotional and behavioral changes often present before the onset of motor symptoms; these include depression, anxiety, and apathy.

Other Symptoms. Sleep disturbances are common with HD, and often sleep studies are warranted.

Sensory disturbances typically present in the form of pain from dystonias and the alterations in muscle imbalances.

Cardiovascular and respiratory function is compromised due to declines in abnormal changes in metabolic and physiologic responses to aerobic exercise. In addition, inactivity causes long-term deconditioning and negative changes in overall endurance.

Falls are very common due to the degree of involuntary movements and changes in muscle performance and the musculoskeletal system.

Weight loss is often common with HD, and although the causes are not clearly understood, referrals to a registered dietician should be made for further support.

TABLE 2-18 • Total Functional Capacity Staging of Huntington Disease.

Stage	TFC Scores	Description
Stage I (early)	11-13	No limitations in any area
Stage II (middle)	7-10	Some problems with work and financial capacity but still able to meet responsibilities at home and complete all ADLs
Stage III (middle)	3-6	Limited work ability, needs assistance with finances and home responsibilities; some difficulty with ADLs but still living at home
Stage IV (late)	1-2	No longer working or able to take care of finances or home chores; increased difficulty with ADLs and may no longer be living at home
Stage V (late)	0	Requires a total care facility and is unable to care for self

ADLs, activities of daily living.

Diagnosis

An HD diagnosis is typically made with genetic testing to determine whether a person carries the HD gene. In addition, if there is the presence of motor signs and positive family history, a clinical diagnosis can be made.

Clinical Course

The clinical course of HD can be divided into five approximate stages: premanifest, prediagnostic, early, middle, and late. Typical progression of HD across the disease stages can be viewed in Table 2-18.

The Unified Huntington's Disease Rating Scale (UHDRS) is the standardized outcome measure used to quantify disease severity and to track symptom changes over time. Please see the appendices at the end of this chapter (Table A-1) for further details.

Medical Management

Pharmacologic management assists in supporting motor, cognitive, and emotional/behavioral symptom management. Typical medications and their side effects used for symptom management are summarized in Table 2-19.

TABLE 2-19 • Medications Used to Treat Huntington Disease.

Subclass of Drug	Example Medications	Potential Side Effects
Antichoreic Drugs		
Dopamine-depleting medication	Tetrabenazine (Xenazine)	Depression, extrapyramidal symptoms, drowsiness, akathisia
Atypical antipsychotics	Olanzapine (Zyprexa), risperidone (Risperdal)	Extrapyramidal symptoms, drowsiness, akathisia
Neuroleptics (dopamine-blocking agents)	Haloperidol (Haldol), fluphenazine (Prolixin)	Extrapyramidal symptoms, sedation, akathisia
Antidepressants (used for depression and sometimes for irritability and anxiety)		
Selective serotonin reuptake inhibitors (SSRIs)	Fluoxetine (Prozac), citalopram (Celexa), sertraline (Zoloft), paroxetine (Paxil)	Insomnia, gastrointestinal upset, restlessness, weight loss, dry mouth, anxiety, headache
Tricyclic antidepressant	Amytriptyline (Elavil), nortriptyline (Pamelor)	Same as SSRIs
Other medications	Bupropion (Wellbutrin), venlafaxine (Effexor)	Insomnia, headache
Antipsychotics (used for psychosis and sometimes for irritability or for chorea suppression)		
Atypical antipsychotics	Olanzapine (Zyprexa), quetiapine (Seroquel), ziprasidone (Geodon), aripiprazole (Abilify)	Extrapyramidal symptoms, drowsiness, akathisia
Neuroleptics (dopamine-blocking agents)	Haloperidol (Haldol), fluphenazine (Prolixin)	Extrapyramidal symptoms, sedation, akathisia

MOTOR NEURON DISEASE AND NEUROPATHY

Motor neuron disease and neuropathies involve diseases that affect the neurons and affect how the nerves and muscles are activated. Therefore, the initial examination is typically with electrophysiologic studies. These may be various tests, including nerve conduction studies to detect demyelination and a reduced conduction velocity and clinical electromyography, determining if the axons themselves are injured.

Amyotrophic Lateral Sclerosis

Amyotrophic lateral sclerosis (ALS) is classified as a rare disease; however, it is the most common motor neuron disease. There are approximately 2 cases per 100,000 every year. In the United States, non-Hispanic Caucasians are twice as likely as African American and Hispanic populations to develop ALS.

Known risk factors for ALS include age, gender, family history, disease-causing mutations, and living in geographic areas where clusters of patients with ALS have been reported. ALS primarily affects adults between the ages of 40 and 70 and is more frequent in men than women. In addition, there is some research to suggest links to lifestyle behaviors. However, there is currently insufficient evidence to determine if any lifestyle influences increase the risk of ALS.

ALS is named for atrophy of the muscle fibers and the hardening of the corticospinal neurons in the spinal cord. The etiology of ALS remains unknown. Several suspected neurodegenerative processes, such as genetic mutations, glutamate excitotoxicity, mitochondrial dysfunction, neurofilament aggregation, neurotrophic factor deficits, ribonucleic acid (RNA) metabolism disorders, autoimmune reaction, and programmed cell death (apoptosis), may play a role. By the time most patients report motor deficits, they have already lost as much as 50% of the motor neurons.

ALS has slow, progressive asymmetric atrophy with muscular weakness and hyperreflexia. For most patients, symptoms begin in the extremities, with 20% to 30% of patients presenting with bulbar symptoms (ie, bulbar-onset ALS). See Table 2-20 for details.

The ALS diagnosis is made on clinical presentation, as there are no biological markers or definitive diagnostic tests. Often neuroimaging and electrophysiologic studies are used to support the clinical diagnosis and rule out other disorders.

The medical prognosis is harsh, as death occurs due to respiratory failure within 3 to 5 years of diagnosis due to the progressive nature.

Medical management should involve an interprofessional team of health care practitioners. Unfortunately, there is no cure for ALS; however, research trials using various medications to slow down the progression of the disease and assist with managing symptoms are utilized.

TABLE 2-20 • Motor Neuron Pathology and Associated Signs and Symptoms in Amyotrophic Lateral Sclerosis.

Motor Neuron Type	Affected Neurons	Associated Signs and Symptoms
Upper motor neurons (UMNs)	Pyramidal Betz motor neurons in the cerebral cortex, corticospinal, and corticobulbar tracts	Loss of dexterity or the ability to coordinate movements; muscle paresis; spasticity; Hoffmann and Babinski reflexes; hyperreflexia; spastic dysarthria
Brainstem motor neurons (bulbar)	Cranial nerve nuclei: V (trigeminal), VII (facial), IX (glossopharyngeal), X (vagus), and XII (hypoglossal)	Difficulty with chewing; dysphagia; flaccid dysarthria/anarthria
Lower motor neurons (LMNs)	Ventral horn cells in the spinal cord	Muscle paralysis and atrophy; fasciculations; flaccid tone; hyporeflexia; respiratory problems

The physical therapy clinician will facilitate exercise regimens specific to the patient during the stage of the disease progression. General suggestions include (1) avoiding heavy eccentric exercises, (2) moderate resistance strengthening exercises for tested 3/5 muscle strength, and (3) monitoring overuse as the disease progresses.

Guillain–Barré Syndrome

Guillain–Barré syndrome (GBS) is a group of neuropathic conditions that affect the PNS, causing progressive weakness due to motor neuropathy and diminished or absent reflexes. Autonomic and sensory deficits are also possible.

The incidence of GBS is about 2 per 100,000 persons, and an estimated 100,000 people develop GBS each year worldwide. The incidence of GBS increases with age, and people over age 50 are at the greatest risk for developing GBS, with males being more likely than females to develop GBS.

Many patients with GBS have respiratory and gastrointestinal types of infections that precede the onset of the disease by 1 to 3 weeks. A clinical diagnosis of GBS is related to the following two pathologies: acute inflammatory demyelinating polyradiculoneuropathy (AIDP) and acute motor axonal neuropathy (AMAN), with AIDP being more common. See Table 2-21 for details.

GBS is characterized by weakness, numbness, tingling, pain in the limbs, or some combination of these symptoms. With AIDP, symptoms progress rapidly and are fairly symmetric. Respiratory failure is common in patients with rapid progression of the disease. This weakness can continue and progress for up to 1 to 3 weeks after GBS onset, followed by a plateau

TABLE 2-21 • Guillain–Barré Syndrome Subtypes.			
Type	**Pathologic Features**	**Clinical Features**	**Nerve Conduction Studies**
Acute inflammatory demyelinating polyradiculoneuropathy (AIDP)	• Multifocal peripheral demyelination • Slow remyelination • Probably both humeral and cellular immune mechanisms	• Progressive, symmetrical weakness; hyporeflexia or areflexia • Often accompanied by sensory symptoms, CN weakness, and autonomic involvement	Demyelinating polyneuropathy
Acute motor axonal neuropathy (AMAN)	• Antibodies against gangliosides GM1, GD1a/b, GalNAc-GD1a in peripheral motor nerve axons; no demyelination	• Strongly associated with *Campylobacter jejuni* infection; more common in the summer, in younger patients, and in eastern Asia • Only motor symptoms; CN involvement uncommon • Deep tendon reflexes may be preserved	Axonal polyneuropathy, normal sensory action potential
Acute motor and sensory axonal neuropathy (AMSAN)	• Mechanism similar to AMAN, but with sensory axonal degeneration	• Similar to those of AMAN, but with predominantly sensory involvement	Axonal polyneuropathy, reduced or absent sensory action potential
Miller Fisher syndrome	• Antibodies against gangliosides GQ1b, GD3, and GT1a • Demyelination	• Bilateral ophthalmoplegia • Ataxia • Areflexia • Facial, bulbar weakness occurs in 50% of cases • Trunk, extremity weakness occurs in 50% of cases	Generally normal, sometimes discrete changes in sensory conduction or H-reflex detected
Pharyngeal-cervical-brachial variant	• Antibodies against mostly gangliosides GT1a, occasionally GQ1b, rarely GD1a; no demyelination	• Weakness particularly of the throat muscles, face, neck, and shoulder muscles	Generally normal, sometimes axonal neuropathy in arms

CN, cranial nerve.

of symptoms. It is estimated that 20% of patients cannot walk after 6 months from the onset of symptoms. Additional symptoms include cranial neuropathies, sensory disturbances, pain, and autonomic disturbances.

Diagnosis of GBS is based on the clinical presentation of progressive, relatively symmetrical weakness with decreased or absent deep tendon reflexes. In addition, electrodiagnostic and hemodynamic studies and CSF analysis assist in supporting a definitive diagnosis.

The prognosis for GBS is usually very good. Overall mortality is estimated to be 5% related to sepsis conditions, pulmonary emboli, or unexplained cardiac arrest, possibly related to dysautonomia. The degree of recovery will depend on the degree of remyelination and axonal regrowth.

Patients with GBS should be hospitalized to support cardiac, respiratory, and bowel and bladder functions relative to evidence of clinical disease progression. Medical treatments to assist recovery and/or eliminate symptoms of GBS include plasma exchange and intravenous immunoglobulin (IVIg). The patient will be monitored through three phases of recovery: (1) acute phase, (2) plateau phase, and (3) recovery phase. The use of nonfatiguing exercise protocols is indicated for patients with GBS.

Myasthenia Gravis

Myasthenia Gravis is a condition where there is a neurologic communication breakdown between nerves and muscles. It is characterized by weakness and quick fatigue of any voluntary muscle group.

The immune system produces antibodies that block or destroy muscle receptor sites for the neurotransmitter acetylcholine (ACh). ACh is required with effective muscle contraction. With less ACh, fewer receptor sites are available, so muscles do not receive nerve signals for voluntary contraction. Fewer receptor sites progressively lead to increased muscle weakness.

Antibodies can also block the function of tyrosine kinase, a protein involved with forming the neuromuscular junction.

Other causes of myasthenia gravis include an enlarged thymus in adults, possibly due to tumors (thymomas), which can trigger the production of the antibodies that block ACh. Additionally, some people with a specific form of myasthenia gravis, called antibody-negative myasthenia gravis, have antibodies that fight against another protein called lipoprotein-related protein 4.

This disease is most common in women younger than 40 years and men older than 60 years. Myasthenia gravis presents with inconsistent muscle weakness; however, muscle strength and control usually worsen with use. Symptoms normally reach their worst within a few years after disease onset.

The disease has some characteristic signs and symptoms:

Eye Muscles
- The first signs and symptoms involve eye problems such as drooping of one or both eyelids (ptosis).
- Diplopia.

Face and Throat Muscles
- Impaired speaking with a soft or nasal sounding speech.
- Difficulty with swallowing, causing problems with swallowing pills, eating, and drinking.
- Chewing is difficult and might wear out when eating a meal.
- Facial expressions may change due to muscle weakness.

Neck and Limb Muscles

- Causes weakness in the neck, arms, and legs, affecting walking and the ability to hold the head upright.

People with myasthenia gravis are more likely to have hypothyroidism or hyperthyroidism and autoimmune conditions such as lupus and rheumatoid arthritis. The PTA should also be aware of the patient's potential to experience a myasthenic crisis, a life-threatening condition when the patient experiences the inability to breathe adequately due to respiratory muscle weakness. Medical emergency treatment is required, and the patient may require mechanical ventilation, medications, and blood filtering therapies.

Acute Poliomyelitis and Postpolio Syndrome

Acute anterior poliomyelitis is a viral disease in which the *poliovirus* enters the body by oral ingestion and multiplies in the intestine. The majority of infected individuals (95%-99%) remain asymptomatic; however, 1% to 5% of persons develop fever, fatigue, headache, vomiting, stiffness in the neck, and pain in the limbs, similar to viral meningitis. It can strike at any age but affects mainly children under 3 (over 50% of all cases). It has largely been eradicated through vaccination programs, but 416 cases were reported in 2013. Polio leads to asymmetric, flaccid paralysis, with the legs more commonly involved than the arms. In 10% to 15% of all paralytic cases, severe bulbar weakness occurs. After the initial infection, the virus is shed in feces for several weeks and can spread if donning and doffing of proper personal protective equipment (PPE) does not occur.

The pathologic findings consist of inflammation of meninges and anterior horn cells, with loss of spinal and bulbar motor neurons. Less common findings include abnormalities in the cerebellar nuclei, basal ganglia, reticular formation, hypothalamus, thalamus, cortical neurons, and dorsal horn. Recovery begins in weeks and reaches a plateau in 6 to 8 months. Three major factors determine the extent of neurologic and functional recovery:

1. The number of motor neurons that recover and resume their normal function.
2. The number of motor neurons that sprout axons to reinnervate muscle fibers left denervated by the death of motor neurons (ie, collateral sprouting).
3. The degree of muscle hypertrophy wherein muscle fibers may increase in size from two to three times the normal size.

Due to collateral sprouting, a single motor neuron that normally innervates 100 muscle fibers might eventually innervate 700 to 2000 fibers. As a result, survivors of acute polio have a few significantly enlarged motor units doing the work previously performed by many units. Fiber type grouping occurs in the reinnervated muscle, and the normal mosaic interspersion of type I and type II fibers will be diminished or absent. Compensation by collateral sprouting and muscle hypertrophy may result in normal manual muscle tests even though more than half the original anterior horn cells are destroyed in some patients.

Postpolio syndrome (PPS) is a condition that affects people who have a history of polio, followed by a period of neurologic stability, and then develop new or exacerbated symptoms several years after the acute poliomyelitis infection. The exact incidence of PPS is unknown. However, evidence suggests that PPS affects 25% to 40% of polio survivors.

Patients with PPS identify fatigue as their most debilitating symptom. In addition, PPS causes weakness in the muscles that were involved in the initial infection of polio. Often muscle weakness is asymmetrical, and pain is a common complaint with PPS.

The diagnosis of PPS first rules out other diagnoses, and the physician will order a blood test to determine if the creatine kinase level is elevated. Unfortunately, the cause of PPS remains unknown.

Management is directed at treating the symptoms, as there is no specific pharmaceutical treatment for the diagnosis. PPS has periods of stability or a plateau and is a very slowly progressing condition. In addition, electromyography (EMG) studies are typically ordered and will display chronic denervations.

PERIPHERAL NEUROPATHIES

Peripheral neuropathy is defined as damage to nerves, leading to impaired sensation, movement, gland, or organ function. If the damage involves one nerve, it is defined as **mononeuropathy**. If it involves multiple nerves, it is defined as **polyneuropathy**. Neuropathies occur in 3% to 4% of persons over 55 years due to the common nature of diabetes. Neuropathies also occur due to trauma, infection, autoimmune disorders, and inherited disorders. See Table 2-22 for causes of peripheral neuropathies.

Effects of Muscle Denervation

If muscles become denervated (ie, atrophy of type I and type II fibers), they undergo several structural changes, including the proliferation of extrajunctional acetylcholine receptors normally found only at the neuromuscular junction. As a result, surgical repair may be indicated and may involve a nerve graft.

PERIPHERAL AND CENTRAL VESTIBULAR DISORDERS

It is estimated that as many as 35% of adults aged 40 years or older in the United States have experienced some form of vestibular dysfunction. In addition, up to 65% of individuals older than 60 years of age experience dizziness or loss of balance, often daily.

Vestibular disorders can be categorized by their location as peripheral, central, or both. Peripheral vestibular disorders involve the peripheral sensory apparatus and/or inner ear structures and/or the vestibular nerve. Central vestibular disorders result from damage to the vestibular nuclei, the cerebellum, and the brainstem, including vestibular pathways within the brainstem that mediate vestibular reflexes.

Peripheral Vestibular Disorders

Peripheral vestibular disorders, based on the anatomy involved, can be further divided into the following three types: (1) acute unilateral vestibular hypofunction (UVH), (2) bilateral vestibular hypofunction (BVH), and (3) recurrent pathologic excitation or inhibition of the peripheral vestibular system.

Unilateral Vestibular Hypofunction. UVH is a decrease in peripheral vestibular function that can be caused by viral or bacterial infections, head trauma, vascular occlusion, and unilateral vestibulopathy. It can also occur following some surgical procedures. Individuals with UVH experience symptoms of acute vertigo, nystagmus, oscillopsia, postural instability, nausea and vomiting, and impaired vestibular ocular reflex (VOR).

Vestibular Neuritis. It is the second most common cause of peripheral vestibular pathologies. It typically affects people between 30 and 60 years of age, with a higher incidence in women in their fourth decade of life and men in their sixth decade of life. Vestibular neuritis can be unilateral or bilateral and often occurs after a viral infection. Patients will have severe symptoms of rotational vertigo for 48 to 72 hours (while hearing remains intact), but note gradual improvement over 6 weeks. Medications are only indicated initially, and physical therapy interventions are recommended for those who remain with impairments in their postural control and gaze abilities.

Vestibular Labyrinthitis. It is an inflammatory disorder where the deficit occurs in the membranous labyrinth, typically caused by viral and bacterial infections. This condition affects individuals of all ages but is more common in adults in their fourth to seventh decades of life. The patient experiences vertigo, nystagmus, postural instability, nausea, tinnitus, and hearing loss. Medical intervention attempts to decrease the infection, and if residual symptoms persist, physical therapy is indicated.

TABLE 2-22 • Causes of Peripheral Neuropathies.

Category	Mechanism of Nerve Damage	Examples
Trauma		
Stretch injury	Severance or tearing of the nerve due to a traction force	• Brachial plexus damage at birth (Erb palsy) • Radial nerve injury secondary to a humeral fracture
Lacerations, stab wounds, and penetrating trauma	Partial or complete severing of the nerve	• May be a cleancut (surgical incision, glass) or • Irregular (blunt instruments, knife stabbings)
Compression	Mechanical deformation and ischemia	• "Saturday night palsy" in which the radial nerve is compressed while sleeping either from a partner laying on the arm or from placement of the arm under the body; known as "Saturday night palsy" because it is thought to be more common when the person is impaired by alcohol • Bone displacement from fracture • Hematoma • Compartment syndrome—swelling within the facial sheath following severe trauma
Repetitive stress injury	Repetitive flexing of a joint leads to irritation and swelling When swelling is in a constricted area through which a nerve passes, the nerve becomes compressed	• Carpal tunnel is a well-known condition thought to be caused by repetitive stress such as typing or working with a jackhammer
Systemic Disease		
Diabetes 1 and 2	Most common form in the United States; mechanism is usually loss of peripheral blood flow leading to ischemia of the distal nerve endings	• Usually a symmetrical distal polyneuropathy • Sensorimotor neuropathy found in up to 50% of patients involves paresthesia, hyperesthesia, sensory loss of vibration, pressure, pain and temperature; presence of a foot ulcer may clue physician into diagnosis • Acute diabetic mononeuropathy (carpal tunnel, cranial nerves): common nerves compressed are the median at the wrist (carpal tunnel), ulnar at the elbow, peroneal at the fibular head, and lateral cutaneous nerve of the thigh at the inguinal ligament • Diabetic autonomic neuropathy is a widespread disorder of the cholinergic, adrenergic, and peptidergic autonomic fibers that leads to dysregulation of one or more of the following systems: cardiac, sexual, gastrointestinal, sudomotor (sweating), pupillomotor (blurred vision), and bladder dysfunction
Kidney disorders	Leads to high levels of ammonia in the blood	• Caused by uremic toxicity
Autoimmune diseases	• Sjogren syndrome • Lupus • Rheumatoid arthritis and other connective tissue disorders • Acute inflammatory demyelinating neuropathy (Guillain–Barré syndrome) • Chronic inflammatory demyelinating polyradiculopathy (CIDP) • Multifocal motor neuropathy	• Immune system attacks the body's own tissues, leading to nerve damage • Inflammation in tissues around nerves can spread directly into nerve fibers • Over time, these chronic autoimmune conditions can destroy joints, organs, and connective tissues, making nerve fibers more vulnerable to compression injuries and entrapment • Guillain–Barré syndrome can damage motor, sensory, and autonomic nerve fibers • CIDP usually damages sensory and motor nerves, leaving autonomic nerves intact • Multifocal motor neuropathy affects motor nerves exclusively; it may be chronic or acute
Vitamin deficiencies and alcoholism	• Deficiencies of vitamins E, B_1, B_6, B_{12}, niacin, and thiamine • Alcohol abuse	• Damage to the nerves associated with long-term alcohol abuse may not be reversible when a person stops drinking alcohol • Chronic alcohol abuse also frequently leads to nutritional deficiencies (including B_{12}, thiamine, and folate) that contribute to the development of peripheral neuropathy

(Continued)

Category	Mechanism of Nerve Damage	Examples
TABLE 2-22 • Causes of Peripheral Neuropathies. (*Continued*)		
Systemic Disease (cont.)		
Vascular disease	Lack of blood to the nerves, most commonly the terminal nerve endings leads to ischemia	• Vasculitis leads to loss of distal blood supply and anoxic damage to distal nerve fibers
Cancers	Neuroblastomas, tumors, paraneoplastic syndromes	• Cancer can infiltrate nerve fibers or exert damaging compression forces on nerve fibers • Tumors also can arise directly from nerve tissue cells • Paraneoplastic syndromes can indirectly cause widespread nerve damage • Toxicity from the chemotherapeutic agents and radiation used to treat cancer also can cause peripheral neuropathy
Infections	• Herpes varicella zoster (shingles), Epstein-Barr virus, West Nile virus, cytomegalovirus, and herpes simplex members of the large family of human herpes viruses • Lyme disease, diphtheria, and leprosy are bacterial diseases • Human immunodeficiency virus (HIV) leading to AIDs • Lyme disease, diphtheria, and leprosy	• The viruses can severely damage sensory nerves, causing attacks of sharp, lightning-like pain; postherpetic neuralgia is long-lasting, particularly intense pain that often occurs after an attack of shingles • The bacterial infections are characterized by extensive peripheral nerve damage • A rapidly progressive, painful polyneuropathy affecting the feet and hands is often the first clinically apparent sign of HIV infection • Bacterial diseases characterized by extensive peripheral nerve damage
Inherited neuropathies	• Charcot-Marie-Tooth disease • Mutations in genes that produce proteins involved in the structure/function of the peripheral nerve axon or the myelin sheath	• Symptoms include: • Extreme weakening and wasting of muscles in the lower legs and feet • Foot deformities, such as high arches and hammertoes • Gait abnormalities: foot drop and a high-stepped gait • Loss of tendon reflexes and numbness in the lower limbs • Decreased or increased sensation • Dutonomic changes: decreased sweating; edema; uncontrolled BP, HR; bowel and bladder problems • Motor changes: weakness or paralysis; muscle atrophy • Trophic changes: shiny skin, brittle nails, neurogenic joint damage
Toxins		
Heavy metals and environmental toxins	Lead, mercury, arsenic, insecticides, and solvents	
Drugs	• Anticonvulsants • Antiviral agents • Antibiotics • Some heart and blood pressure medications • Chemotherapy drugs	• In most cases, the neuropathy resolves when these medications are discontinued or dosages are adjusted. • About 30%-40% of people who undergo chemotherapy develop peripheral neuropathy, and it is a leading reason why people with cancer stop chemotherapy early • The severity of chemotherapy-induced peripheral neuropathy (CIPN) varies from person to person

Reproduced with permission from Nichols-Larsen DS, Kegelmeyer DA, Buford JA, et al., eds. *Neurologic Rehabilitation: Neuroscience and Neuroplasticity in Physical Therapy Practice.* 2016. Copyright © McGraw Hill LLC. All rights reserved. https://accessphysiotherapy.mhmedical.com.

Vestibular Schwannoma of an Acoustic Neuroma. It is the slowest growing tumor in the human body. Vestibular Schwannomas are usually benign. They originate from the Schwann cells and are located along the vestibular portion of CN VIII. However, when the tumor grows, it causes additional impairments involving other cranial nerves and causes compression of the brainstem or cerebellum.

Bilateral Vestibular Hypofunction. Typically caused by persons taking ototoxic medications but can also occur after an infection, with autoimmune disorders, and with normal aging. Patients typically report disequilibrium, severe postural instability that results in gait ataxia, and oscillopsia with head movement.

Recurrent Vestibular Disorders

These include benign paroxysmal positional vertigo (BPPV), Ménière disease (endolymphatic hydrops), and perilymphatic fistula. These disorders are characterized by periods of normal functioning with intermittent periods of vestibular symptoms.

Benign Paroxysmal Positional Vertigo. BPPV is the most common peripheral vestibular disorder. It typically affects women more than men in their fourth and fifth decades of life and is the cause of approximately 50% of complaints of dizziness in older people. BPPV occurs because otoconia detach from the otolithic membrane in the utricle and move into one of the semicircular canals (SCCs). BPPV has two forms: **canalithiasis**, where otoconia are free-floating in the SCC, or **cupulolithiasis**, where the otoconia are attached to the cupula. Posterior SCC canalithiasis accounts for 81% to 90% of all cases. Physical therapy for assessment and intervention consists of head maneuvers and vestibular rehabilitation exercises as the first choice of treatment.

Ménière Disease. Ménière disease is a disorder of the inner ear, also known as **idiopathic endolymphatic hydrops**, and involves increased pressure caused by malabsorption of the endolymph in the duct and sac, which inappropriately excites the nerve. It more commonly affects women than men in their fourth and fifth decades of life. An attack involves aural fullness, a reduction in hearing, and tinnitus, followed by rotational vertigo, postural imbalance, nystagmus, nausea, and vomiting after a few minutes. Typically, an attack lasts 24 to 72 hours, followed by improvement of symptoms. Medical treatment supports fluid buildup along with dietary restrictions of salt, caffeine, and alcohol. Pharmacologic treatments include vestibular suppressants, antiemetics, and antinausea medications during acute episodes. In addition, many long-term patients with Ménière disease benefit from psychological support to manage the lifestyle changes.

Perilymphatic Fistula. A perilymphatic fistula (PLF) is commonly caused by a tear or defect in the oval and/or round windows that separate the air-filled middle ear and the fluid-filled perilymphatic space of the inner ear. Because of this small opening, perilymph leaks into the middle ear. A PLF is usually caused by minor head trauma, excessive intracranial or atmospheric pressure changes (as in rapid airplane descent or scuba diving), extremely loud noises, objects perforating the tympanic membrane, ear surgery (stapedectomy), or vigorous straining (as in lifting a heavy object). Physical therapy is contraindicated. Medical treatment involves bed rest with the head elevated for 5 to 10 days, and if symptoms persist, surgery is indicated. Table 2-23 outlines and compares peripheral vestibular symptoms and conditions.

Central Vestibular Disorders

Central vestibular disorders occur because of vertebrobasilar ischemic disease, traumatic head injury, migraine-associated dizziness, and conditions that affect the brainstem and cerebellum. Vertebrobasilar ischemic stroke and insufficiency relate to the insufficient blood supply to the brainstem, cerebellum, and inner ear. Symptoms could include vertigo, Wallenberg syndrome, blurred vision or diplopia, drop attacks, syncope (fainting) or weakness, ataxia, and headaches depending on the vasculature involved.

Traumatic Brain Injury. This was discussed previously as a neurologic diagnosis. The incidence of central vestibular pathology occurs in about 50% to 70% of all individuals sustaining an mTBI, and almost all moderate TBIs report varying levels of vertigo.

Migraine-Associated Dizziness (Vestibular Migraine). Involves 10% of all Americans and affects women more than men aged between 25 and 55 years. These individuals could

TABLE 2-23 • Symptomatology of Peripheral Vestibular Disorders.

	UVH	BVH	BPPV	Ménière Disease	Perilymphatic Fistula
Vertigo	+	−	+	+	+
Nystagmus	+	−	+	+	−/+
Duration of vertigo	Days to weeks	N/A	30 seconds-2 minutes	30 minutes-24 hours	Seconds to minutes
Nausea	+	−	−/+	+	−/+
Postural imbalance	+	++	+	+	+
Specific symptoms	Acute onset, tinnitus, hearing loss with labyrinthitis	Gait ataxia	Onset latency, adaptation	Fullness of ear, tinnitus, hearing loss	Loud tinnitus, Tullio phenomenon
Precipitating event	Upper respiratory or gastrointestinal infection	Treatment with antibiotics (gentamicin, streptomycin)	Looking up, turning in bed		Head trauma, ear surgery, coughing, sneezing, straining
Outcome	Resolution of most symptoms by 1 year; dark vertigo may be permanent	Symptoms are typically permanent	Resolved with PT or surgery in most people	Vertigo severity diminishes but hearing loss is often permanent	Usually resolves in 4 weeks

BVH, bilateral vestibular hypofunction; BPPV, benign paroxysmal positional vertigo; UVH, unilateral vestibular hypofunction; −, absent; +, present; ++, very strong.
Reproduced with permission from Nichols-Larsen DS, Kegelmeyer DA, Buford JA, et al., eds. *Neurologic Rehabilitation: Neuroscience and Neuroplasticity in Physical Therapy Practice.* 2016. Copyright © McGraw Hill LLC. All rights reserved. https://accessphysiotherapy.mhmedical.com.

experience episodic symptoms of vertigo, dizziness, imbalance, and motion sickness that can last minutes to hours, which may or may not involve headaches.

Conditions Affecting the Brainstem and Cerebellum. Include diagnoses such as Friedreich ataxia, cerebellar atrophy, brain tumor, and multiple sclerosis.

Central Versus Peripheral Vestibular Pathology. Differentiating peripheral from central vestibular pathology is critical for assessment and intervention. Table 2-24 provides key features to differentiate peripheral from central vestibular pathologies.

TABLE 2-24 • Common Symptoms Differentiating Central Versus Peripheral Vestibular Pathology.

Central Vestibular Pathology	Peripheral Vestibular Pathology
Uncommon to have hearing loss	Symptoms may include hearing loss, fullness in ears, tinnitus
Nystagmus direction is purely vertical or torsional	Nystagmus is horizontal and torsional
Pendular nystagmus (eyes oscillate at equal speeds)	Jerk nystagmus (nystagmus has slow and fast phases)
Nystagmus either does not change or reverses direction with gaze	Nystagmus increases with gaze toward the direction of the fast phase (ie, away from the side of the lesion)
Nystagmus either does not change or it increases with visual fixation	Nystagmus is decreased with visual fixation
Symptoms of acute vertigo not usually suppressed by visual fixation	Symptoms of acute vertigo usually suppressed by visual fixation
Nausea/vomiting more mild	Nausea/vomiting usually severe
Oscillopsia is severe	Oscillopsia is mild unless lesion is bilateral
Abnormal performance on smooth pursuit and/or saccades	Smooth pursuit tracking and saccade performance normal
If sudden onset, patient likely not able to stand and walk even with assistance (severe ataxia)	If sudden onset, patient can stand and walk with assistance (mild ataxia)
Other neurologic symptoms are present	Other neurologic symptoms are rare
Symptoms may recover slowly or never resolve	Symptoms usually resolve within 7 days in people with UVH

UVH, unilateral vestibular hypofunction.
Reproduced with permission from Nichols-Larsen DS, Kegelmeyer DA, Buford JA, et al., eds. *Neurologic Rehabilitation: Neuroscience and Neuroplasticity in Physical Therapy Practice.* 2016. Copyright © McGraw Hill LLC. All rights reserved. https://accessphysiotherapy.mhmedical.com.

TABLE 2-25 • Common Drugs Used to Treat Acute Vertigo and Associated Nausea and Emesis.

Medication	Class	Sedation	Antiemesis	Side Effects
Dimenhydrinate (Dramamine)	Antihistamine; phosphodiesterase inhibitor	+	++	Dry mouth, tinnitus, blurred vision, coordination problems
Diphenhydramine (Benadryl)	Antihistamine	+	++	Tachycardia, urinary retention
Promethazine (Phenergan)	Antihistamine; anticholinergic; phenothiazine	++	++	Dry mouth, constipation, blurred vision
Meclizine (Antivert, Bonine)	Antihistamine; anticholinergic	++	+	Dry mouth, tiredness
Prochlorperazine (Compazine)	Antihistamine; anticholinergic; phenothiazine	+	+++	Dry mouth, blurred vision, constipation
Scopalamine (Transderm Scop)	Anticholinergic (nonselective muscarinic)	+	++	Dry mouth, dilated pupils, blurred vision
Ondansetron (Zofran)	Serotonin 5-hydroxytryp-tamine$_3$ (5-HT$_3$) receptor antagonist		+++	Headache, constipation, blurred vision
Lorazepam	Benzodiazepine	++	+	Addiction, effects increased with other sedative drugs

+, mild; ++, moderate; +++, prominent.

Reproduced with permission from Nichols-Larsen DS, Kegelmeyer DA, Buford JA, et al., eds. *Neurologic Rehabilitation: Neuroscience and Neuroplasticity in Physical Therapy Practice.* 2016. Copyright © McGraw Hill LLC. All rights reserved. https://accessphysiotherapy.mhmedical.com.

Additional Vestibular Diagnoses. Other diagnoses involving the vestibular system that should be reviewed in further detail include motion sickness and cervicogenic dizziness.

Vestibular Function Tests—Medical Assessment and Management

Testing for individuals with vestibular dysfunction could involve the following:

- Electronystagmography/videonystagmography.
- Rotational chair testing.
- Vestibular-evoked myogenic potential.
- Computerized dynamic posturography.
- Visual perception tests.
- Hearing tests.
- Neuroimaging—MRI and/or CT.

Pharmacologic treatment may be indicated in the acute phases of recovery. See Table 2-25 for a list of common medications.

CEREBELLAR DISORDERS

Disorders of the cerebellum typically involve the clinical presentation of ataxia. Table 2-26 outlines acquired and hereditary causes.

Clinical Manifestations of Cerebellar Damage

The primary sign of cerebellar damage is ataxia, related to gait and balance and/or the limbs themselves. Table 2-27 outlines cerebellar impairments.

Medical Management of Cerebellar Damage

There is no cure for patients who suffer from cerebellar damage, and pharmacologic interventions to date have had limited success in reducing symptoms or slowing or stopping disease progression.

TABLE 2-26 • Selected Causes of Cerebellar Damage.	
Acquired Causes	**Hereditary Causes**

• Stroke (ischemic, hemorrhagic)
• Toxicity (alcohol, heavy metals [mercury, lead, thallium], medications, organic solvents [toluene, benzene], phencyclidine [PCP])
• Tumor (primary cerebellar tumor, metastatic disease)
• Immune-mediated (multiple sclerosis, celiac disease, vasculitis [Behçet disease, lupus], paraneoplastic cerebellar degeneration)
• Congenital and developmental (Chiari malformation, agenesis, hypoplasias [Joubert syndrome, Dandy–Walker cyst], dysplasias)
• Infection (cerebellitis, abscess)
• Metabolic (hypothyroidism, acute thiamine [B$_1$] deficiency, chronic vitamin B$_{12}$ and E deficiencies)
• Trauma
• Degenerative nonhereditary diseases (multiple system atrophy [MSA], idiopathic late-onset cerebellar ataxia [ILOCA])
	• Autosomal recessive:
	  • Friedreich ataxia (FA)
	  • Early-onset cerebellar ataxia (EOCA)
	  • Ataxia telangiectasia
	• Autosomal dominant:
	  • Spinocerebellar ataxias (SCAs)
	  • Episodic ataxias (EAs)
	  • Dentato-rubral-pallidoluysian atrophy (DRPLA)
	  • Gerstmann-Straussler-Scheinker (GSS) disease
	• X-linked disorders:
	  • Mitochondrial disease
	  • Fragile X–associated tremor/ataxia syndrome

Reproduced with permission from Nichols-Larsen DS, Kegelmeyer DA, Buford JA, et al., eds. *Neurologic Rehabilitation: Neuroscience and Neuroplasticity in Physical Therapy Practice.* 2016. Copyright © McGraw Hill LLC. All rights reserved. https://accessphysiotherapy.mhmedical.com.

TABLE 2-27 • Signs and Symptoms of Cerebellar Damage.			
Symptom/Sign	**Area of Cerebellar Damage**	**Functional Manifestation**	**Examination Findings**
• Limb ataxia • Dysmetria • Dyssynergia • Dysdiadochokinesia • Decomposition • Rebound	Lateral cerebellum, deep cerebellar nuclei (globose, dentate nuclei)	Uncoordinated movement of ipsilateral arm and/or leg	• Impaired FTN and HTS • Impaired rapid alternating movements • Slow, effortful fine finger movements • Impaired limb rebound
Tremor	Cerebellar efferent pathways to the red nucleus and inferior olivary nucleus, deep cerebellar nuclei	• Postural tremor • Kinetic tremor • Intention tremor (<5 Hz)	• Side-to-side tremor of outstretched arms or tremor when standing still • End-point tremor on FTN or HTS test
Hypotonia	Vermis, flocculonodular lobe	Decreased ability to maintain a steady force	• Ipsilateral hypotonia of limbs • Pendular deep tendon reflexes
Balance and gait dysfunction	Anterior lobe, vermis, fastigial nucleus	• Wide-based stance • Uncoordinated gait • Difficulty with stopping or turning • Frequent falls	• Impaired sharpened Romberg test • Impaired spatiotemporal/kinematic gait parameters • Unsteady tandem gait • Impaired stopping and turning
Oculomotor dysfunction	Flocculonodular lobe, vermis, fastigial nucleus	• Oscillopsia • Blurred or double vision	• Nystagmus • Impaired slow pursuit • Impaired shift of gaze/saccades • Impaired VOR cancelation
Speech impairments	Rostral paravermal region of the anterior lobes	• Dysarthria • Slurred speech	• Impaired articulation and prosody • May be slow, hesitant, or accentuate some syllables
Cognitive and psychiatric impairments	Bilateral posterior lobes (cognitive), vermis (emotional)	• Memory problems, difficulty functioning at work or in home • Impaired communication skills • Personality changes	• Impaired executive functions • Impaired visuospatial function • Agrammatism, dysprosodia • Blunted affect or disinhibited, inappropriate behavior

FTN, finger-to-nose, HTS, heel-to-shin; VOR, vestibulo-ocular reflex.

Reproduced with permission from Nichols-Larsen DS, Kegelmeyer DA, Buford JA, et al., eds. *Neurologic Rehabilitation: Neuroscience and Neuroplasticity in Physical Therapy Practice.* 2016. Copyright © McGraw Hill LLC. All rights reserved. https://accessphysiotherapy.mhmedical.com.

■ INTERVENTIONS FOR ADULT NEUROMUSCULAR DEFICITS

Treatment interventions are formulated and relative to the short-term and long-term goals for each patient.

STROKE

Physical Therapy Management in Acute Care

The rehabilitation team has an early role in assessing and preventing any additional hospital complications that would affect the prognosis. Acute care management typically lasts 24 to 72 hours with a plan for discharge to a skilled rehabilitation and nursing facility, an inpatient rehabilitation hospital/unit, or home.

Early intervention is essential for long-term improvement in addition to preventing **learned nonuse**. There is limited time for the rehabilitation team in acute care to return the patient to their highest level of independence. Often, there is an emphasis on compensatory interventions that typically encourage using the less involved extremities to complete functional tasks. Research has shown that early compensatory strategies create learned nonuse, and although it can be beneficial in functional mobility, it is the responsibility of the PT and PTA to translate the evidence and keep the long-term goals in mind. Interventions shown to be effective focus on the following:

1. Assessment.
2. Early intervention and prevention of complications.
3. Task-oriented practice.
4. Intensive repetitive practice.

See the appendices at the end of this chapter (Table A-1) to view the ANPT stroke evidence database to guide effectiveness (EDGE) recommendations for stroke and acute care.

Early Intervention and Prevention of Complications

The goal is to minimize acute medical complications so early mobilization and therapy can begin. Therefore, the PTA needs to monitor vital signs during this phase of rehabilitation. Early sessions should focus on preventing contractures and postural hypotension and minimizing the risk of pneumonia and skin breakdown. If able, patients and family members should be trained with ROM techniques to be performed three times a day. Hypertonicity can lead to contractures; thus, it is important to emphasize proper positioning and ROM, especially for the ankle plantarflexors, hip extensors, and the hemiplegic upper extremity.

Task-Oriented Practice

Physical therapy should be salient and encourage activities to facilitate the benefits of motor control principles. Likewise, acute care interventions should be meaningful and encourage activities or tasks to retrain motor control. For example, early acute therapy should involve functional mobility in the hospital bed and exercise to manage fatigue.

Upright Activities

Once the patient is medically stable, interventions should include transfers, gait, and imagery to facilitate mobility. Exercise might start with eccentric activation, depending on the degree of weakness. Box 2-8 provides some suggestions for upright activities in the acute setting.

Assistance Levels

When documenting, it is essential to identify the appropriate level of assistance required for patient safety.

Physical Therapy Management in the Rehabilitation Setting

As the inpatient rehabilitation setting begins, the stroke survivor is still in the acute stage of recovery. Interventions need to consider neuroplasticity as a critical component in the

BOX 2-8	TECHNIQUES FOR TEACHING TRANSFERS AND GAIT IN THE ACUTE SETTING

- **Keys to working on transfers**
  - Encourage the individual to be an active participant.
  - The therapist should not provide any more assistance than is absolutely necessary.
  - Positioning of the extremities in positions that lead into the movement can help obtain success.
- **Supine to sidelying**
  - Utilize passive positioning to minimize therapist assistance: make sure that the bottom arm is flexed so that it does not end up trapped under the body; if moving onto the nonparetic side, cross the paretic leg over the nonparetic leg to position for rolling (the client should be encouraged to assist with this positioning, as able).
  - The therapist can then place hands at the shoulder and pelvis to assist the client in using momentum to rock twice and then roll over on the third try.
  - Encourage head turning with the roll for additional momentum.
- **Sidelying to sitting edge of the bed**
  - Roll to sidelying facing the edge of the bed, using the techniques above.
  - Drop the legs off of the side of the bed from the sidelying position. Encourage the client to use the nonparetic leg to get the paretic leg off of the bed but with as much active movement as possible from the paretic leg.
  - To make the move from sidelying to sitting easier, the head of the bed may be placed in a slightly elevated position.
  - Instruct to push on the bed with both arms as the legs are dropped over the edge of the bed.
  - The therapist should assist at the shoulder and pelvis only as needed.
  - If the paretic arm is "on top," the therapist may wish to assist by placing the hand in a weight-bearing position.
  - The therapist then places a hand on the client's hand to stabilize it in weight-bearing and places their other hand on the posterior aspect of the elbow to encourage active weight-bearing through the paretic arm.
- **Sit-to-stand from bed**
  - First, ensure that the feet are flat on the floor with the hips and knees flexed to 90 degrees (or elevate the bed and place with hips and knees in a less flexed posture to make the transfer easier).
  - Both arms should be placed in weight-bearing during the transfer to encourage active movement and provide proprioceptive input in the early stages of recovery.
  - The bedside table can be utilized to provide a stable surface for weight-bearing through bilateral arms. Bedside tables allow you to start with the table at a lower level and raise the table as the client comes to standing, and then provide a stable surface for standing activities that allow for the use of both arms.
  - If there is reasonable function in the paretic hand, the client can push off the bed with bilateral upper extremities and then place the hands on a walker. Unilateral assistive devices should not be used for standing activities, as they encourage learned nonuse of the involved upper extremity and lower extremity and do not promote equal weight-bearing bilaterally.
- **Early gait activities: acute care**
  - Equal weight-bearing and use of the paretic leg should be a focus at this stage in rehabilitation.
  - During gait, devices that allow the use of bilateral upper extremities post-cerebrovascular accident (CVA) are parallel bars, wheeled walkers with arm trough attached, and the bedside table.
  - Early gait and standing activities should focus on upright trunk control, encouraging the use of the paretic limbs during gait, and using a step-through pattern bilaterally.
  - Therapist assistance with the paretic extremities can be provided as needed to advance the leg and brace the extremities for weight-bearing support.
  - Regardless of ability, the client should actively participate in all movements to encourage recovery of movement, even in flaccid extremities.

recovery process. Inpatient rehabilitation should focus on relearning functional mobility and managing impairments as a component of mobility training.

Intensive Practice: Upper Extremity. The focus of the upper extremity should be to minimize learned nonuse, as this is associated with a poor long-term outcome. The involved upper extremity should be incorporated with all functional tasks, and hand shaping should be considered. See Box 2-9 for a list of upper extremity rehabilitation suggestions.

BOX 2-9	KEYS TO REHABILITATION OF THE UPPER EXTREMITY

1. The hand shapes the activation of the entire upper extremity.
2. Use meaningful tasks.
3. Lower physical demands by
   a. Placing the extremity in a gravity eliminated position for the key musculature
   b. Providing support to the trunk and proximal musculature to minimize degrees of freedom and focus on one joint motion
4. Choose functional tasks that will produce the movements that are the focus of that client's therapy session. Examples are as follows:
   a. For hand opening, have them reach for a 12-oz soda can or small ball to encourage finger and wrist extension to lift a relatively light object. This activity can also focus on elbow extension in combination with shoulder flexion (moving out of synergy patterns).
   b. For coordination, have the individual reach for a small target and push on it.
   c. For fine motor control, have the client reach for a small object, remove it, and place it in another location. Example: Remove thumbtack from bulletin board and place in a small container for storage.

Reproduced with permission from Nichols-Larsen DS, Kegelmeyer DA, Buford JA, et al., eds. *Neurologic Rehabilitation: Neuroscience and Neuroplasticity in Physical Therapy Practice.* 2016. Copyright © McGraw Hill LLC. All rights reserved. https://accessphysiotherapy.mhmedical.com.

Bilateral task training is another successful method for retraining upper extremity function after stroke successfully returning function to the upper extremity after CVA.

Both **functional electrical stimulation** (FES) and mirror activities can be beneficial for upper extremity recovery.

Intensive Practice: Gait. Gait should be practiced with all rehabilitation team members to ensure the high, intensive practice needed in this stage of recovery. Whether overground or on the treadmill, gait training should focus on the quality of the gait pattern. Gait needs to include training as a component of the task-oriented approach and involve walking over and around obstacles and on/off different surfaces. The patient can begin to utilize problem-solving and motor learning at an optimal level. Lastly, as the patient works toward mastery during dynamic gait activities, it is essential to encourage dual-tasking conditions, only if they are safe, so patients practice walking in conditions similar to real-world environments.

Assistive Devices. Assistive devices with wheels offer more support for a step-through gait pattern. Unilateral devices, unfortunately, encourage more of a compensatory gait pattern by permitting patients to spend more time on their stronger or less involved side. The PT initially prescribes the proper assistive device for each patient.

Spasticity: Medical Management in the Chronic Phase

When not responsive to conservative physical therapy interventions, chronic spasticity may require the use of pharmaceuticals by the physician. These medications include, but are not limited to, **botulinum toxin (Botox)** as an intramuscular injection and intrathecal or oral baclofen or oral diazepam, dantrolene, and tizanidine.

Physical Therapy Management in the Home Health and Outpatient Environments

The PTA must engage the patient in an intensive task-specific intervention program relative to the POC short-term and long-term goals in outpatient and home care environments. These interventions should include walking on uneven surfaces, including stairs and transfers from various surfaces, and should involve functional practice specific to the patient's environment. For example, transfer training might include car, toilet, tub, and kitchen chair transfers. In addition, once common tasks and skills have been achieved, physical therapy interventions should include other treatment paradigms such as virtual

TABLE 2-28 • Proprioceptive Neuromuscular Facilitation (PNF) diagonal patterns.				
Upper Extremity	**D₁ Flexion Pattern**	**D₁ Extension Pattern**	**D₂ Flexion Pattern**	**D₂ Extension Pattern**
Scapula	Anterior elevation	Posterior depression	Posterior elevation	Anterior depression
Shoulder	Flexion Adduction Lateral rotation	Extension Abduction Medial rotation	Flexion Abduction Lateral rotation	Extension Adduction Medial rotation
Elbow	Extension	Extension	Extension	Extension
Radioulnar joint	Supination	Pronation	Supination	Pronation
Wrist	Flexion Radial deviation	Extension Ulnar deviation	Extension Radial deviation	Flexion Ulnar deviation
Fingers	Flexion	Extension	Extension	Flexion
Lower Extremity	**D₁ Flexion Pattern**	**D₁ Extension Pattern**	**D₂ Flexion Pattern**	**D₂ Extension Pattern**
Pelvis	Anterior elevation	Posterior depression	Anterior Depression	Posterior Elevation
Hip	Flexion Adduction Lateral rotation	Extension Abduction Medial rotation	Flexion Abduction Medial rotation	Extension Adduction Lateral rotation
Knee	Flexion	Extension	Flexion	Extension
Ankle and foot	Dorsiflexion Inversion	Plantarflexion Eversion	Dorsiflexion Eversion	Plantarflexion Inversion

reality, robotics, circuit and strength training, proprioceptive neuromuscular facilitation (PNF) techniques, and constraint-induced movement therapy (CIMT). The various PNF techniques and the methods by which they can be used to assist the patient in a progression through increased motor control and return of optimal functional mobility are outlined in Tables 2-28 and 2-29.

TABLE 2-29 • Proprioceptive Neuromuscular Facilitation (PNF) Techniques.	
Stage of Motor Control	**PNF Techniques Used with the Progression of Motor Control**
Stage 1—mobility In the adult patient, mobility is referring to the available range of motion to assume a posture. Having sufficient motor unit activity to initiate a movement.	• Joint distraction • Hold relax[a] • Contract relax[a] • Hold relax with active movement[a] • Rhythmic initiation[a] • Rhythmic rotation • Repeated contractions[a]
Stage 2—stability The ability to maintain a steady position in a weight-bearing, antigravity posture. Sometimes thought of as maintaining static postural control.	• Alternating isometrics • Rhythmic stabilization[a] • Slow reversal hold[a]
Stage 3—controlled mobility Mobility superimposed on the previously developed postural stability by moving within the posture. The limbs are weight-bearing and the body moves.	• Agonistic reversals[a] • Slow reversal[a] • Slow reversal hold[a]
Stage 4—skillful movement Mastered movement which follows controlled mobility. The trunk of the body is performing work and motion along with the movement of extremities, together maintaining safe, dynamic mobility. Can be used for strengthening when the patient exhibits proximal stability and distal mobility.	• Agonistic reversals[a] • Slow reversal[a] • Slow reversal hold[a] • Resisted progression (used with gait and locomotion) • Timing for emphasis[a] • Normal timing[a]

[a]*PNF diagonal flexion and extension directional patterns for the upper extremity, lower extremity, pelvic and scapular regions, are often performed in conjunction with a variety of the PNF techniques. Use of PNF patterns and techniques are prescribed by the physical therapist.*

Physical Therapy Management of Special Cerebrovascular Accident Syndromes

Neglect Syndrome. Physical therapy aims to increase the patient's awareness of the "neglected" aspect of their environment and their paretic limb. Treatment involves various interventions that incorporate spatial organization training and increased visual scanning, and overall sensory awareness.

Pusher Syndrome. The goal of physical therapy should be to ensure patients have accurate visual information vertically and encourage their active movements to achieve vertical alignment. The focus should first be on achieving vertical alignment and then practicing other motor tasks while sustaining vertical alignment.

TRAUMATIC BRAIN INJURY

Physical Therapy Management

Physical therapy intervention needs to focus on the three unique aspects of the TBI population: physical, cognitive, and behavioral. Many interventions for CVA are appropriate and evidence-based for TBI, with the additional considerations of possible bilateral involvement, peripheral nerve injuries, and musculoskeletal injuries. The interventions below focus on the cognitive and behavioral aspects of intervention for TBI.

Cognition/Memory. Cognition includes attention, memory, initiation, judgment, and speed of processing. Each of these aspects should be evaluated separately, as all relate to long-term and overall rehabilitation outcomes. Therefore, it is essential to use standardized outcome measures to quantify the patient's cognition and memory at initial evaluation, during reevaluations, and again at discharge. For full details, see the appendices at the end of this chapter (Table A-1) for TBI measures specific to each clinical practice setting.

Early Management. Early care is focused on saving the person's life. After a moderate to severe TBI, the patient will be in an intensive care unit (ICU), and the team focuses on determining the severity of the injury, preserving life, and preventing further damage. As the patient is stabilized, early mobility can occur, including strength and ROM. The PTA is helping monitor the level of arousal, defining the patient's cognitive state using the RLA stages of cognitive function, and beginning to understand the extent of neuromuscular and musculoskeletal deficits. Table 2-30 describes common behaviors following TBI and suggestions for intervention. While in the ICU, the therapist needs to minimize contractures with splinting, ROM, and/or serial casting.

Assessment and Management Based on Rancho Los Amigos Levels of Cognitive Functioning. The first three RLA levels are often called the coma levels, as the patient is quite unresponsive. At Level I, the patient does not respond to any stimuli; progression to a generalized response is defined as Level II. Once the responses to stimuli are stimulus-specific, this is defined as Level III. Management in Levels I through III focuses on skin integrity and proper positioning. A variety of stimuli—for example, auditory and tactile—are appropriate components of the intervention, and family members should be educated to communicate with their loved ones, despite their inability to hold a conversation.

As the patient progresses into RLA Level IV, the PT can initiate the motor examination, and the therapy clinicians should utilize standardized outcome measures, as outlined in the appendices of this chapter (Table A-1). For example, in RLA Level IV (confused and agitated), the intervention is more about a behavior strategy than a learning strategy, as the patient in this stage is not capable of new learning.

In RLA Levels V and VI, patients continue to have varying agitation levels and other behaviors such as confusion, apathy, lack of initiation, impulsivity, and disinhibition. Therefore, PTs and PTAs should offer several options for interventions and engage the patient in positive feedback to reinforce participation in therapy sessions.

TABLE 2-30 • Common Behaviors s/p Traumatic Brain Injury (TBI) and Their Management.

Behavior Description	Key to Management	Management Strategies
Agitation is common s/p TBI and is defined as excesses of behavior. Typical agitated behaviors include restlessness, inability to focus or maintain attention, irritability, and, at higher levels of agitation, combativeness.	Prevent escalation of agitation and modify the environment and staff behavior to avoid the use of both physical and medical restraints.	• Be calm both verbally and in your physical and nonverbal actions. • Treatment session goals should be flexible to allow adjustment to the level of agitation. • Treatment environment should be quiet, with minimal external stimuli. • Be aware of tension building up in the client; stop the external stimulation before agitation becomes combative. • Redirect the patient's attention and move them to a location with less stimulating or frustrating activities until agitation is reduced. • Do not attempt to discuss agitation logically or elicit guilt for the behavior. • Do not leave the patient unsupervised or alone during agitation. • Try to maintain consistency in the personnel who interact with the patient so as to promote familiarity and decrease novel stimuli. • To the extent possible, permit moving about or verbalization during periods of increased agitation.
Confusion results from the inability of patients to recall minute-to-minute, hour-to-hour, or day-to-day events in their life. As a result, they are unable to understand their current situation in light of what has or what will occur. Associated problems include diminished attention, learning, and orientation.	Increase and even provide the external structure for the individual, particularly in regard to time, place, and activities.	• Place calendars in client's rooms with a schedule of daily activities posted in their room; also have one that they can take with them throughout the day. • Post the steps for them to follow for their ADLs in their room. • At the start of each treatment session, review your name, what day and date it is, what time of day it is, and where they are. Use calendars, clocks, name tags, and building signage to reinforce this information. • Maximize consistency and establish routines within and between treatment sessions. • To increase client awareness, start each activity with a short and easy-to-understand explanation of what is expected of them. • At the end of the session, use the client's schedule to elicit from him or her the next activity in which he or she will engage.
Impulsivity is a tendency to act without thinking. It is common in people s/p TBI and often seen along with agitation and confusion.	Provide consistency across caregivers and visitors, and have the client verbally rehearse strategies for each treatment activity.	• The entire team should attempt to use the same strategy with a patient; inconsistency will only create confusion. • Verbally review the steps for each activity before allowing the patient to start. • Use a written list of steps that the patient reviews (out loud or to himself) before starting. • The patient verbally rehearses aloud the steps needed to complete the task. • The patient waits a few seconds before beginning a task, and is instructed to think about how to complete the task before doing it. • Aloud, verbal rehearsal should be consistently implemented, in all treatment sessions and throughout the day. As a patient demonstrates increased control, this can be gradually shaped into rehearsing to oneself and then simply pausing before starting the task.
Disinhibition is an inability to stop oneself from acting on one's thoughts. *Sexually inappropriate behavior* is a special case of lack of inhibition.	Remain calm and provide concrete feedback about the behavior.	• Initially, focus on addressing simple situations that may be easiest for the patient to learn to manage. • Identify the issue as "self-control" and use this as the key word for cueing the patient, when they need to be controlling their behaviors. • When delaying gratification is the issue, start with short increments between the behavior and the reward, lengthening the increment as the patient improves. Using a watch or timer for specific cueing may be helpful in this regard. • It is important to provide the patient with feedback on the inappropriateness of sexual behavior in this situation, and not to regard its presence with negative attention. • Avoid emotional responses such as anger or embarrassment; this can reinforce the behavior. • Ignoring the behavior or passing it off with a humorous comment also may reinforce its presence and not provide the patient with the adequate information to understand that the behavior is inappropriate. • The best approach is an immediate, unemotional, straightforward expression of the inappropriateness of the behavior. Be certain the patient knows what behavior is being referred to, such as "your sexual hand gesture is inappropriate and won't be appreciated by most women/men."

(Continued)

TABLE 2-30 • Common Behaviors s/p Traumatic Brain Injury (TBI) and Their Management. (Continued)

Behavior Description	Key to Management	Management Strategies
Perseveration is a person's repetition of certain behaviors, either actions or verbalizations. Some individuals perseverate on a consistent theme, while others repeat external stimuli or their own immediately preceding responses.	Use cueing and pacing to interrupt the repetitive behavior and provide a stimulus to move on to the next step.	• Pace interactions with the client to allow disengagement from one activity before proceeding to the next. • Provide a highly structured environment. • Use cues to redirect the client from the perseverative behavior to the next step. • Do not attempt to use logic to "discuss away" a repetitive theme.
Confabulation is the creation of false memories and is frequent in confused patients, sometimes reflecting the inability to find another explanation for what is happening.	It is important to keep in mind that confabulation may be serving a purpose for the patient, including reducing anxiety.	• For lower functioning, more confused patients, ignore the confabulation and do not challenge its veracity. • For higher functioning patients, provide nonthreatening feedback on the inaccuracy of the memory, then redirect attention to another task.
Inability to self-reflect is due to a lack of insight into the effects of ones behavior on others. The client is not aware of their capabilities or limitations and typically overestimates their ability to perform any given task. These patients will often blame others for their frustration and may exhibit paranoia.	Use concrete goals that are posted within easy access of the person with TBI, and note on the posted goal form as progress is made.	• Include the client in goal setting. • Goals should be concrete and progress should be recorded, where the client can monitor their own progress. • Consistently attempt to elicit the client's insight into their deficits. Be nonjudgmental and express expectations that the deficit will be overcome. • Videotape can provide concrete feedback. • Only make the client aware of deficits that can be worked on in rehabilitation and for which you expect to see improvement. • Continual reinforcement is necessary, after insight is accomplished, to change the behavior.
Apathy can be differentiated from resistance by the presence of lethargy with a bland affect, an absence of agitation, and low motivation. *Depression* is sometimes evident as a patient's self-awareness improves. It may show itself in tears, but also may be evident in social withdrawal, self-degrading comments, anxiety, irritability, and catastrophizing.	Treatment should target choices and acknowledge accomplishments.	• Staff and family should encourage participation. • You may need to remind the patient of the consequences of their injury and the impact of the lack of participation in rehabilitation. • Graphs or other concrete ways of showing progress may be useful to elicit motivation. • Be firm in presenting activities and do not present yes/no choices. Offer two or more alternatives for a given activity. • Working in conjunction with other patients may be motivating. • Activities that the patient spontaneously shows interest in should be used to meet rehabilitation goals. • Ask the client to choose the activity to elicit motivation. • Identify short-term goals and be explicit about the relationship between therapy activities and these goals. • Review progress to date. • Redirect the patient's attention from catastrophic or anxious thoughts. • Inform the psychology staff of the nature of the patient's depressive or anxious thoughts.
Lack of initiation differs from apathy in that the patient is motivated to perform an activity but is unable to determine how to carry it out. Lack of initiation may be evident in problems determining the correct sequence of steps or simply not knowing the first step. It is important to keep in mind that the patient is not always aware of this shortcoming and may provide other excuses for why an activity is not initiated or carried out.	Cueing at the start of or next step in an activity is the key to facilitating initiation.	• Cueing is the primary means of assisting a person who lacks initiation. Cues should be external. • Do not perform or passively assist them to initiate the activity. • Verbal cues should be used initially. Using the same word to cue the same behaviors will assist the patient in moving to the next step. • As independence increases, replace verbal cues with other external cues that do not require another person to present the cue. Examples of external cues are lists posted in the room for ADLs routines. External cues should be succinct, readily visible, and free of distracting content. • Clients whose improvement continues should be weaned from external cues to simple verbal statements that can be said aloud or thought to oneself as the patient completes the activity. These self- reminders should be succinct and easy to learn. • While in the inpatient setting, begin to train the patient and family in techniques for establishing a daily routine.

ADLs, activities of daily living.

RLA Levels VII and VIII should focus on return to the community and involve school or work retraining as indicated in the setting of long-term goals and expectations.

Goal setting when working with patients who have sustained a TBI should include body function and structure impairments and activity and participation restrictions, in addition to behavioral and cognitive components.

mTBI AND CONCUSSION

Controversy exists in terms of treatment of mTBI and concussion. There is research to support early rest to improve the overall physical, and cognitive impairment initially sustained with mTBI, and there is also research that supports moderate physical activity to improve cognitive performance. In addition, there is evidence to support the view that intense physical activity, when introduced too early, will delay recovery. Returning to full play in a sport or returning to usual physical and cognitive activity should only occur after neuropsychological testing has been completed and return to full activity is indicated.

Most individual's symptoms will resolve after a few weeks; however, up to 30% of people will suffer from symptoms that persist for a greater amount of time—referred to as a post-concussive syndrome, with impairments similar to those outlined with TBI.

BRAIN TUMOR

A patient's physical therapy management with a brain tumor is similar to those interventions outlined in stroke and/or focal brain injury. Interventions for patients with a brain tumor diagnosis should note the increased fatigue, cognitive dysfunction with impairments in processing speed, working memory or attention, and diminished respiratory capacity, which often occurs after radiation therapy. PTs and PTAs, along with the rehabilitation team, should consider this specific area of oncology as a specialty area of practice whereby the team should focus on specific body function and body structure impairments, along with activity and participation restrictions related to general physical conditioning. Physical therapy improves functional outcomes with early intervention and minimizes sequelae associated with postradiation therapy.

SPINAL CORD INJURY

Physical Therapy Management in the Acute Setting

The patient who sustains an SCI will undergo careful observation in the ICU, and the team goals are to minimize further medical complications. The PT will begin their assessment once the patient is medically stable. The standardized assessment for the SCI diagnosis uses the ISNCSCI/AIS examination, which many members of the rehabilitation team can complete. The earlier sensory and motor return exhibited by the patient, the better the overall prognosis.

Acute Physical Therapy Management

The goal in acute care is to prevent complications such as pneumonia, skin breakdown, and DVT. Patients with tetraplegia are at risk for upper extremity contracture and joint pain, so careful consideration should be paid to positioning and ROM.

The patient may have precautions due to spinal stabilization or fracture; however, active exercise should incorporate partially or fully innervated muscles during functional tasks and basic mobility. Once medically stable, a sitting program should be initiated to learn to adjust to the cardiovascular changes since the injury. An abdominal binder and/or lower extremity support hose may be indicated to prevent postural hypotension.

Management of the Patient in the Inpatient Rehabilitation Setting

General Approach. The focus of inpatient and outpatient therapy for complete SCI focuses on a compensatory approach and seeks to use principles of neuroplasticity when supported by the evidence. Compensatory interventions involve movement strategies such as momentum and muscle substitution and adaptive equipment and bracing to replace the muscles and aspects of the patient's body that are not functioning. There should be a delicate balance between the timing of the compensatory strategies and the use of neuroplasticity evidence. Under principles of plasticity, the patient should be encouraged to use maximal effort when performing tasks, engage in making errors to encourage learning, and involve a high number of repetitions for activity training. Restorative approaches to rehabilitation may replace or supplement compensatory approaches for individuals with incomplete SCI.

Physical therapy intervention needs to be cautious and communicate with and refer to other team members regarding spasticity, heterotopic ossification, and osteoporosis.

The level and type of SCI injury predict the expected functional abilities of the patient once the spinal shock has resolved. These levels should be reviewed in Table 2-31; note that these levels are simply guidelines, and patients after SCI may have unique recovery patterns.

The goal of inpatient rehabilitation is to prepare the patient to return home. Therefore, emphasis is placed on managing bowel and bladder care, bed mobility, management and protection of the upper extremities, transfers, skin protection, and wheelchair use.

Physical Therapy Management of the Patient in the Outpatient Rehabilitation Setting

In the outpatient setting, the emphasis for physical therapy management of SCI is on maximizing patient independence and functional mobility. In addition, continued medical and psychological support may be needed to manage neuropathic pain and spasticity and address sexuality, depression, and adjustment issues to SCI. Research has shown that the greatest changes in motor return occur within the first year after SCI, and recovery seen in the first 6 months is optimal.

Gait training after SCI may follow either a compensatory or restorative approach. The compensatory approach typically involves the use of an assistive device and lower extremity bracing. A restorative approach to locomotor training may involve using a body weight support system, task training, and overground walking to approximate normal walking mechanics and speed to promote muscle activation. Individuals with motor incomplete SCI have the best potential for locomotor recovery following a restorative approach.

TABLE 2-31 • Prediction of Mobility and Outcomes by Level of SCI.			
SCI Level	**Expected Active Muscles**	**Potential Functional Outcome**	**Required Equipment**
C1-C4	Neck and facial muscles Diaphragm-C4	*Bed mobility*: dependent *Transfers*: dependent *Pressure relief*: independent with power WC *Eating*: dependent *Dressing*: dependent *Grooming*: dependent *Bathing*: dependent *WC propulsion*: independent with power WC *Standing*: dependent *Walking*: not expected	Hospital bed Transfer board and/or lift Tilt or recliner WC; WC cushion — — — Rolling shower/commode chair Tilt table; standing frame ventilator

C5	Muscles listed for C1-C4
	Biceps, brachialis,
	  brachioradialis
	Deltoid
	Infraspinatus
	Subscapularis
		Bed mobility: min–mod assist
		Transfers: min assist
		Pressure relief: independent with power WC
		Eating: min assist
		Dressing: dependent
		Grooming: min assist
		Bathing: dependent
		WC propulsion: independent with power WC
		Standing: dependent
		Walking: not expected
			Hospital bed
			Transfer board; lift
			Tilt or recliner WC; WC cushion
			Splints and equipment to
			  assist eating, dressing, and
			  grooming
			Rolling shower/commode chair
			Tilt table; standing frame

(Continued)

SCI Level	Expected Active Muscles	Potential Functional Outcome	Required Equipment
	TABLE 2-31 • Prediction of Mobility and Outcomes by Level of SCI. (*Continued*)		
C6	Muscles for C1-C5 Extensor carpi radialis Serratus anterior	*Bed mobility*: min assist *Transfers*: min assist *Pressure relief*: independent with power WC *Eating*: independent *Dressing*: independent upper body; min–mod assist lower body *Grooming*: independent *Bathing*: independent upper body; min–mod assist lower body *WC propulsion*: independent with power WC; manual: independent indoors; min–mod assist outdoors *Standing*: dependent *Walking*: not expected	Hospital bed Transfer board; lift Tilt or recliner WC; WC cushion Splints Splints Splints Rolling shower/commode chair Tilt table; standing frame
C7-C8	Muscles for C1-C6 Triceps, flexor carpi ulnaris, finger extensors Finger flexors C8	*Bed mobility*: independent *Transfers*: independent *Pressure relief*: independent with power WC *Eating*: independent *Dressing*: independent *Grooming*: independent *Bathing*: independent upper body; min assist lower body *WC propulsion*: manual independent indoors and outdoors *Standing*: min assist *Walking*: not expected	Hospital bed or standard bed With or without transfer board WC cushion Adaptive devices Adaptive devices Adaptive devices Shower/commode chair Tilt table; standing frame
T1-T9	Muscles for C1 to level of injury Intrinsics of hand Intercostals Erector spinae Abdominals T6	*Bed mobility*: independent *Transfers*: independent *Pressure relief*: independent *Eating*: independent *Dressing*: independent *Grooming*: independent *Bathing*: independent *WC propulsion*: manual independent *Standing*: independent *Walking*: not functional	Standard bed With or without transfer board WC cushion Shower/commode chair Standing frame
T10-L1	Muscles C1 to level of injury Intercostals, external and internal oblique Rectus abdominus L1 partial hip flexor	*Bed mobility*: independent *Transfers*: independent *Pressure relief*: independent *Eating*: independent *Dressing*: independent *Grooming*: independent *Bathing*: independent *WC propulsion*: manual independent *Standing*: independent *Walking*: functional; independent to min assist	Standard bed WC cushion Padded tub bench Standing frame Walker, forearm crutches, braces
L2-S5	Muscles C1 to level of injury Iliopsoas, quadratus lumborum, piriformis, obturators	*Bed mobility*: independent *Transfers*: independent *Pressure relief*: independent *Eating*: independent *Dressing*: independent *Grooming*: independent *Bathing*: independent *WC propulsion*: manual independent *Standing*: independent *Walking*: functional; independent to min assist	Standard bed WC cushion Padded tub bench Standing frame Forearm crutches, braces

WC, wheelchair.

MULTIPLE SCLEROSIS

Physical therapy interventions for MS will depend on the area of deficit and disease stage and should include further assessment of fatigue levels, spasticity, sensory changes and pain complaints, motor deficits, and overall functional losses. Interventions are generally presented for relapsing-remitting multiple sclerosis (RRMS), except where otherwise stated.

If a patient is in an acute exacerbation, exercise is not recommended. Often, patients take high doses of corticosteroids to minimize the inflammatory process; however, these medications have side effects that contraindicate exercise.

Once the patient is past their attack or acute flareup, the PTA should monitor blood pressure and check for swelling in the ankles before initiating exercise. Some individuals with MS experience Uhthoff sign when they become overheated. *Uhthoff sign* is a temporary worsening of neurologic symptoms, such as increased weakness, spasticity, or blurred vision, when the body gets overheated.

The therapist should be mindful of fatigue, sensory changes, spasticity, and ataxia during physical therapy interventions.

Interventions should include static and dynamic balance training and exercises for ataxia and coordination. These are seen in Box 2-10 and are pertinent to supporting patients with MS; however, they are not MS-specific.

BOX 2-10   EXTREMITY EXERCISES FOR ATAXIA AND COORDINATION

Instructions: *I want you to copy the motion that I demonstrate, focusing on doing it slowly and smoothly.* Typically, these are initially done with the individual in a position to watch what they are doing to use visual feedback. To work on proprioception, they can be progressed to being done without visual feedback.

Upper Extremities

Alternate Flexion and Extension—Flex the right elbow while extending the left elbow and then reverse. Also, do this with the wrist and shoulder.

Supination and Pronation—Alternately supinate and pronate the forearm. The difficulty is increased by first going progressively faster, supinating and pronating in sync, and then to make it even harder, do it bilaterally and out of sync (ie, the right forearm is supinated while the left forearm is pronated). This can also be done with shoulder external and internal rotation.

Finger Dexterity—Touch the first digit to the thumb and then extend, touch the second digit to the thumb and extend, and continue to the third and fourth digits. The difficulty is increased by going progressively faster.

Rock, Paper, Scissors—Make a pattern using the motions of fist to the palm of the opposite hand, palm to palm of the opposite hand, and ulnar side of hand to the palm of the opposite hand. Start with a combination of two motions, then progress to combinations of three motions. Have the individual with MS copy the pattern that you make. Then, you can have them practice doing the pattern repetitively.

Lower Extremities

Flexion and Extension—While in supine, slide the heel toward the buttocks, then straighten the leg back out slowly, alternately flexing and then extending the hips and knees. To make this more difficult, place the heel on the shin at knee level, trace the shin bone down to the ankle, and trace it back up. Again, focus on making a smooth motion.

Dorsiflexion and Plantarflexion—Alternate dorsiflexion and plantarflexion of the ankle.

Bilateral Ankle Dorsi- and Plantarflexion—While seated, first dorsiflex both feet (up on heel), then plantarflex both feet (up on toes) and repeat.

BOX 2-11 **PRINCIPLES OF EXERCISE PROGRESSION IN MULTIPLE SCLEROSIS**

1. Exercise should be prescribed on an intermittent basis with a pattern of a brief bout of exercise followed by rest, and then another bout until the desired exercise is completed. Training benefits, using this type of exercise–rest pattern, are similar to the outcomes of continuous exercise with an equal duration.

2. For resistance exercise, the rate of overload progression should be addressed with caution, and full recovery between training sessions should be allowed to prevent musculoskeletal overuse injuries.

3. Resistance can be safely increased by 2% to 5% when 15 repetitions are correctly performed in consecutive training sessions.

4. Cardiorespiratory and resistance programs should alternate training on separate days of the week, with 24 to 48 hours of recovery between training sessions.

5. Watch for Uhthoff sign and provide rest and cooling strategies when this occurs.

6. Given the impact of fatigue and weakness on performing activities of daily living (ADLs), the exercise program progression should include the following:

   - Start by building up participation in ADLs
   - Progress to building in inefficiencies to normal daily tasks such as parking a little further away to increase walking distance
   - Move to participation in active recreation that the individual enjoys or typically participates in
   - Finally, progress to a structured aerobic training program

Interventions Aimed at Functional Deficits

Interventions to treat changes in functional performance are similar to those identified in the stroke intervention section. Body function and structure impairments should be addressed, and functional training should involve task-specific and task-oriented actives. Physical therapy interventions should include aerobic conditioning because of improved cognition, strengthening, and balance exercises. Box 2-11 provides exercise progression principles for patients with MS. To manage the fatigue factor with MS, patients need to be educated and participate in energy conservation techniques. As the disease progresses, FES and/or lower extremity bracing may be indicated to address the distal weakness. Additionally, assistive devices, adaptive equipment, and wheelchair recommendations may be required.

PARKINSON DISEASE

Physical therapy interventions for individuals with PD may include various treatments to promote motor learning, strength, flexibility and ROM, functional mobility, balance, gait, use of assistive devices, and cardiorespiratory function. Interventions always include patient and family education.

Patients with PD benefit from stretching and ROM activities to minimize the indirect impairments of decreased ROM, stooped posture, and the development of contractures. Relaxation techniques, stretching, and ROM can be targeted for muscle groups frequently affected by rigidity, such as hip flexors, knee flexors, ankle plantarflexors, pectoralis muscles, and cervical flexors. The therapist should promote axial rotation due to the lack of upper and lower trunk disassociation resulting from PD-associated rigidity. Patients with PD can benefit from strengthening exercises targeting weak extensor muscle groups to counteract the active ROM losses in hip extension, knee extension, ankle dorsiflexion, scapular retraction, and cervical extension. The cardiovascular decline in patients with PD can contribute to decreased functional mobility and participation restrictions. Aerobic training can improve maximal oxygen consumption in individuals with PD.

To address limitations in functional mobility, functional, task-specific training should be incorporated, including repeated sit-to-stand from a variety of surfaces, stair climbing, upper extremity overhead reaching activities, and rolling in bed to emphasize trunk disassociation. In addition to functional strength training, patients with PD benefit from education related to restorative and compensatory approaches to functional mobility, including bed mobility, transfers, sit-to-stand, gait training, and fall recovery. A therapeutic approach designed to improve movement perception and increase movement scaling in patients with PD is called LSVT BIG. This exercise approach is based on the Lee Silverman Voice Treatment LSVT LOUD, a treatment approach used in increasing voice production for patients with PD experiencing hypophonia. The LSVT BIG approach focuses on high-amplitude movements, multiple repetitions, high intensity, and increasing difficulty. This treatment intervention is typically performed for 1 hour, four times per week for 4 weeks.

Gait training and assistive device prescription is an important component of physical therapy management for patients with PD. Common gait deviations include reduced stride length, reduced velocity, cadence abnormalities, increased double-limb support time, insufficient dorsiflexion, insufficient hip and knee extension, difficulty turning, festinating gait, freezing of gait, and difficulty with motor and cognitive dual tasking. Gait training in patients with PD can be enhanced using rhythmic auditory stimulation (RAS), visual cues, and body weight–supported treadmill training.

Patient and family education is an integral part of the PTA's role in caring for a patient with PD. PTAs provide education to patients, families, and caregivers related to disease progression, symptom management, movement strategies, energy conservation, strategies to perform ADLs and recreational activities, fall prevention strategies, fall recovery strategies, and additional PD resource identification. Individuals with PD often experience psychosocial problems such as depression, anxiety, social isolation, loss of control, and difficulty coping with disability. PTAs need to be mindful of medications and their potential side effects. Therapy should be scheduled when medications are optimally dosed.

HUNTINGTON DISEASE

In HD, patients often resort to limited activity and participation due to their apathy and lack of insight into their deficits. Therefore, interventions in the early stages of the disease should include the following:

- ROM and stretching similar to PD.
- Transfers with a focus on forward weight shifts.
- Gait training similar to PD—research suggests that a rolling walker provides the safest and most organized gait pattern.
- Stair training to include definite stops before ascending and descending stairs and use of the railing.

Late-stage disease should involve physical therapy interventions for prescribing a custom wheelchair for optimal alignment and supporting a safe home environment with modification as indicated.

AMYOTROPHIC LATERAL SCLEROSIS

Creating and supporting interventions for patients with ALS may be challenging due to the disease's progressive nature. The research supports individualized interventions and the inclusion of exercise and activity at all stages of the disease. The general goals of physical therapy intervention are to maintain optimal independence throughout the disease process. Physical therapy goals should include (1) maintaining safe and independent mobility, (2) maintaining maximal muscle strength and endurance, (3) preventing and minimizing secondary impairments such as skin breakdown and contractures, (4) preventing or managing pain, (5) educating on energy-conservation techniques to prevent unnecessary fatigue and respiratory discomfort, and (6) providing adaptive, assistive, and orthotic equipment to maximize functional independence.

BOX 2-12	GENERAL EXERCISE GUIDELINES FOR INDIVIDUALS WITH AMYOTROPHIC LATERAL SCLEROSIS

- Start exercise interventions when individuals are in the early stages of the disease so that they have sufficient strength, respiratory function, and endurance to exercise without excessive fatigue.
- Strengthening exercise programs should emphasize concentric rather than eccentric muscle contractions, at moderate resistance and intensity (eg, one to two sets of 8-12 reps or three sets of 5 reps), in muscles that have antigravity strength (ie, > 3 grade strength) exclusively.
- Endurance exercise programs should emphasize moderate-intensity activities (50%-80% peak heart rate [HR], 11-13 rating of perceived exertion [RPE], three times per week) as tolerated without inducing excessive fatigue. Rest periods are recommended, especially if the continuous activity goes beyond 15 minutes.
- Individuals with ALS should be advised to have adequate oxygenation, ventilation, and intake of carbohydrates and fluids before exercising.
- Use available technology (eg, assistive devices, body weight–supported systems) to optimize exercise program effectiveness without causing excessive fatigue.
- Exercise compliance can be improved by integrating enjoyable physical activities and a formal exercise program, providing opportunities for socialization and providing rewards for accomplishing goals.

Reproduced with permission from Nichols-Larsen DS, Kegelmeyer DA, Buford JA, et al., eds. *Neurologic Rehabilitation: Neuroscience and Neuroplasticity in Physical Therapy Practice*. 2016. Copyright © McGraw Hill LLC. All rights reserved. https://accessphysiotherapy.mhmedical.com.

Exercise prescriptions must carefully consider and balance the current activity level, from disuse atrophy, from overuse activity with continual monitoring of fatigue level. Historically, there is controversy regarding the depth and degree of exercise programs for individuals with ALS. However, there is a building body of evidence that supports moderate, individualized exercise programs that improve neuronal plasticity and enhance the cardiovascular and pulmonary systems. Box 2-12 displays the current practice and evidence in prescribing exercise programs for persons with ALS.

Physical Therapy Management

Dal Bello-Haas proposed a three-stage model for ALS progression as a framework for physical therapy clinical management. See Table 2-32 for details.

GUILLAIN–BARRÉ SYNDROME

Physical Therapy Management

Limited evidence exists to support exercise and rehabilitation in people with GBS. However, several studies support the benefits of high-intensity inpatient or outpatient interprofessional rehabilitation to decrease disability and improve the overall quality of life.

Acute/Progressive Stage. Initially, many patients with GBS will be in an ICU on ventilation with varying degrees of paralysis and sensory dysfunction. Physical therapy interventions can include education on positioning and prevention of skin breakdown, respiratory care, facilitation of speech and swallowing functions, pain management, bed positioning, ROM exercises, gentle stretching, massage, and functional activities in sitting and standing as tolerated.

Chronic/Recovery Stage. Once symptoms have plateaued, strength will begin to return over weeks to months, typically following a descending pattern, with arm function returning before leg function. As the patient is recovering, the PTA can progress exercise and functional mobility training while being mindful of fatigue levels. Repetitions should remain low, with a high frequency of short intervals of activity. Most patients require a wheelchair for locomotion for several months. Gait training is often initiated in the parallel bars and eventually progresses to a rolling walker, Lofstrand crutches, or a cane. Patients with GBS may also benefit from using an ankle-foot orthosis to support distal weakness in the lower extremities. Lastly, energy conservation strategies and being mindful of fatigue levels throughout all stages of rehabilitation should continually guide the intervention.

TABLE 2-32 • ALS Disease Stages and Common Intervention Strategies.

Stage	Common Impairments and Activity Limitations	Interventions

Early	• Mild-to-moderate weakness in specific muscle groups
	• Difficulty with ADLs and mobility toward the end of this stage
		• Restorative/preventative
		  • Strengthening exercises[a]
		  • Endurance exercises
		  • ROM (active, active-assisted) and stretching exercises
		• Compensatory
		  • Assess potential need for appropriate adaptive and assistive devices
		  • Assess potential need for ergonomic modifications of the home/workplace
		  • Educate patient about the disease process, energy conservation, and support groups

Middle	• Severe muscle weakness in some groups; mild-to-moderate weakness in other groups
	• Progressive decrease in mobility and ADLs throughout this stage
	• Increasing fatigue throughout this stage
	• Wheelchair needed for long distances; increased wheelchair use toward end of stage
	• Pain (especially shoulders)
		• Compensatory
		  • Support weak muscles (assistive devices, supportive devices, adaptive equipment, slings, orthoses)
		  • Modify the workplace/home (eg, install ramp, move bedroom to first floor)
		  • Prescribe wheelchair
		  • Educate caregivers regarding functional training
		• Preventative
		  • ROM (active, active-assisted, passive) and stretching exercises
		  • Strengthening exercises (early middle)
		  • Endurance exercises (early middle)
		  • Assess need for pressure-relieving devices (eg, pressure-distributing mattress)

Late	• Wheelchair dependent or restricted to bed
	• Complete dependence with ADLs
	• Severe weakness of UE, LE, neck, and trunk muscles
	• Dysarthria, dysphagia
	• Respiratory compromise
	• Pain
		• Preventative
		  • Passive ROM
		  • Pulmonary hygiene[a]
		  • Hospital bed and pressure-relieving devices
		  • Skin care, hygiene[a]
		  • Educate caregivers on prevention of secondary complications
		• Compensatory
		  • Educate caregivers regarding transfers, positioning, turning, skin care
		  • Mechanical lift

ADLs, activities of daily living; LE, lower extremity, ROM, range of motion; UE, upper extremity.

[a]May be restorative.

Reproduced with permission from Nichols-Larsen DS, Kegelmeyer DA, Buford JA, et al., eds. *Neurologic Rehabilitation: Neuroscience and Neuroplasticity in Physical Therapy Practice*. 2016. Copyright © McGraw Hill LLC. All rights reserved. https://accessphysiotherapy.mhmedical.com.

POSTPOLIO SYNDROME

Physical Therapy Management

Physical therapy interventions need to be mindful of the major complaint from PPS patients of fatigue. Aerobic exercises that might include using the treadmill, bike, walking, swimming, and resistive activities should be prescribed at a low-to-moderate intensity. Exercise programs should avoid the overworked muscle groups and should be in alignment with muscle strength testing. Patients with PPS should be encouraged to use the Borg rating of perceived exertion to determine appropriate exercise intensity for aerobic exercise. Programs can be progressed at a slow rate under the supervision and direction of the PT. In addition, patients with PPS should be educated in behavior modification related to energy conservation and efficiency. Exercise guidelines are listed in Box 2-13.

Psychosocial Considerations

Many patients managing their PPS benefit from psychological support to manage their chronic stress, depression, anxiety, compulsiveness, and type A behavior. Referrals to other members of the interprofessional team or attending a support group may be indicated.

BOX 2-13	GENERAL PRINCIPLES FOR DESIGNING EXERCISE PROGRAMS

- Use a low-to-moderate exercise intensity.
- Slowly progress the exercise, especially if muscles have not been exercised for a while and/or have obvious chronic weakness from acute poliomyelitis.
- Strengthening exercises should only be attempted with muscles that can move against gravity.
- Pace exercise to avoid fatigue (intermittent periods of rest and exercise).
- Rotate exercise types, such as stretching, general (aerobic) conditioning, strengthening, endurance, or joint ROM exercises.
- Exercise should not cause muscle soreness or pain.
- Exercise should not lead to fatigue that prevents participation in other activities that day or the days following.

Reproduced with permission from Nichols-Larsen DS, Kegelmeyer DA, Buford JA, et al., eds. *Neurologic Rehabilitation: Neuroscience and Neuroplasticity in Physical Therapy Practice*. 2016. Copyright © McGraw Hill LLC. All rights reserved. https://accessphysiotherapy.mhmedical.com.

PERIPHERAL NEUROPATHY

Physical Therapy Management

The best physical therapy intervention is prevention, and for those with prediabetes and diabetes, this involves long-term control of blood glucose levels through appropriate diet, oral drugs, or insulin injections to prevent further damage. Exercise can be an effective modality for prevention and treatment. For pain management, medications may be indicated. However, the PTA should be mindful of the side effects and potential for variable effectiveness.

Functional Training. To support patients with diabetic peripheral neuropathy, research indicates that exercise improves balance, trunk proprioception, strength, 6-minute walk (6MW) distance, and habitual physical activity.

Denervated Muscle. The use of electrical stimulation is indicated for certain patients expected to have nerve regrowth after complete denervation. Galvanic current has been used to maintain the connective tissue mobility within the denervated muscle. However, there is controversy in the research about the use of electrical stimulation in denervated muscle, as it has been found to slow but does not prevent muscle atrophy.

Sensory Impairment. Treatment for sensory impairment should be focused on teaching the client that they are at a high risk of injuring their extremities since they cannot feel painful stimuli. The PTA should teach the patient to perform frequent skin inspections, avoid tight or restrictive clothing, and test water temperatures when performing basic ADLs.

VESTIBULAR DISORDERS

Benign Paroxysmal Positional Vertigo

Physical therapy goals and expected outcomes for patients with BPPV are (1) removal of otoconia from the SCCs, (2) eliminating complaints of vertigo with head movement, (3) improved balance, and (4) independence in all functional activities involving head motions. The greatest efficacy for interventions utilizes particle repositioning head maneuvers that move the displaced otoconia out of the affected SCC. The three main maneuvers used to treat posterior and anterior SCC BPPV are (1) the canalith repositioning maneuver (CRM), (2) the liberatory maneuver, and (3) Brandt–Daroff habituation exercises.

The **canalith repositioning maneuver** (also called the Epley maneuver) is used to treat canalithiasis and can be viewed in Figure 2-32.

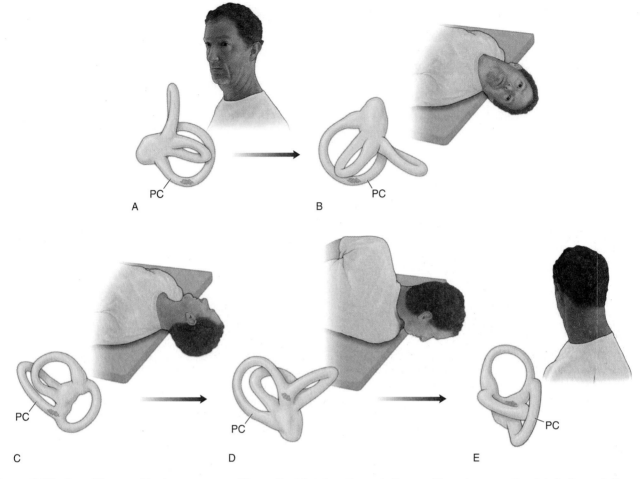

Figure 2-32. Canalith repositioning maneuver. The patient is taken through five positions to move the debris through the canal: (A) long-sitting with the head rotated 45 degrees toward the affected side; (B) quickly moved to supine with head extended 30 degrees while maintaining the 45-degree rotation to the affected side, then maintained for 1 to 2 minutes; (C) turn head to the opposite side while maintaining extension over the end of the table; (D) roll to side without moving the head, again maintained for 1 to 2 minutes; (E) return to sitting on the side of the plinth. (Reproduced with permission from Nichols-Larsen DS, Kegelmeyer DA, Buford JA, et al., eds. *Neurologic Rehabilitation: Neuroscience and Neuroplasticity in Physical Therapy Practice.* 2016. Copyright © McGraw Hill LLC. All rights reserved. https://accessphysiotherapy.mhmedical.com.)

The **Liberatory maneuver** (also called the Semont maneuver) is the most common maneuver to treat cupulolithiasis and can be viewed in Figure 2-33.

Brandt–Daroff exercises are repeated movements into and out of positions that cause vertigo and can be viewed in Figure 2-34.

The **Bar-B-Que roll maneuver** (BBQ roll) (Figure 2-35) is the most common intervention for horizontal SCC cupuolithiasis and canalithiasis. Often the BBQ roll is followed by forced prolonged positioning (FPP) when the maneuver is not initially successful. FPP involves lying on the more involved side for 30 to 60 seconds and then slowly rolling into sidelying with the unaffected ear down and remaining in this position overnight.

Unilateral Vestibular Hypofunction

Physical therapy goals for patients with UVH and expected outcomes are to (1) improve gaze stability during functional activities (2) decrease the patient's complaints of disequilibrium and oscillopsia with head motions, (3) improve static and dynamic balance, and (4) return the patient to his or her previous level of activity and participation level. Recovery is based on static and dynamic compensations along the vestibular nerves and firing along the vestibular nuclei. Mechanisms include these compensations and the use

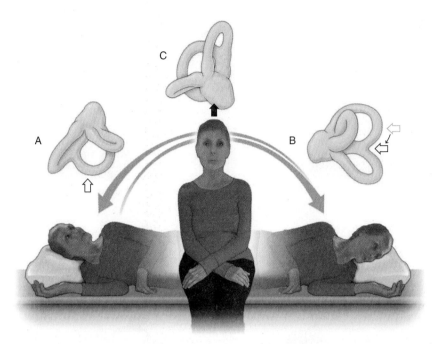

Figure 2-33. Liberatory maneuver. The liberatory maneuver is used to dislodge the debris within the cupula by **(A)** patient is initially in sidelying; **(B)** patient is rapidly brought to sitting on the side of the plinth; and **(C)** patient is rapidly brought to sidelying on the opposite side. This is done by a fluid movement from one side to the other. (Reproduced with permission from Nichols-Larsen DS, Kegelmeyer DA, Buford JA, et al., eds. *Neurologic Rehabilitation: Neuroscience and Neuroplasticity in Physical Therapy Practice.* 2016. Copyright © McGraw Hill LLC. All rights reserved. https://accessphysiotherapy.mhmedical.com.)

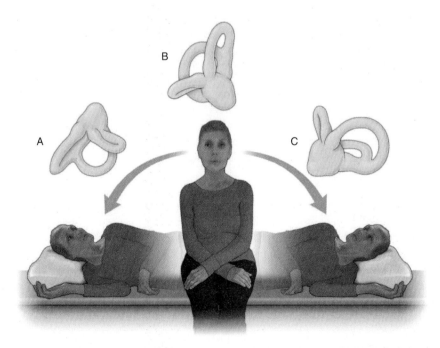

Figure 2-34. Brandt–Daroff exercises. The patient begins by sitting sideways on the bed, then quickly lies down on her side with her head turned 45 degrees toward the ceiling. She returns to upright and then quickly lies down on the other side, again with the head turned 45 degrees toward the ceiling. (Reproduced with permission from Nichols-Larsen DS, Kegelmeyer DA, Buford JA, et al., eds. *Neurologic Rehabilitation: Neuroscience and Neuroplasticity in Physical Therapy Practice.* 2016. Copyright © McGraw Hill LLC. All rights reserved. https://accessphysiotherapy.mhmedical.com.)

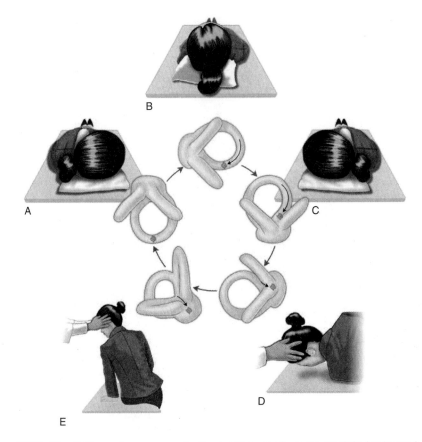

Figure 2-35. Bar-B-Que roll maneuver for the treatment of geotropic right horizontal SCC-BPPV. Turn head toward the involved ear while lying supine (**A**), then turn head 270 degrees toward the unaffected side through a series of stepwise 90-degree turns (**B-D**); then resume the sitting position (**E**). Each position should be maintained for at least 1 or 2 minutes, or until the induced nystagmus and vertigo are resolved. The corresponding illustrations demonstrate the orientation of the semicircular canals and the location of the otolithic debris in the horizontal canal. (Reproduced with permission from Nichols-Larsen DS, Kegelmeyer DA, Buford JA, et al., eds. *Neurologic Rehabilitation: Neuroscience and Neuroplasticity in Physical Therapy Practice*. 2016. Copyright © McGraw Hill LLC. All rights reserved. https://accessphysiotherapy.mhmedical.com.)

of substitution strategies and habituation. Research supports vestibular rehabilitation of UVH for less than 6 weeks, as long as patients are compliant with their exercise programs.

Gaze Stabilization or Adaptation Exercises. Patients who suffer from visual blurring and dizziness will benefit from individualized exercises that cause a retinal slip to create an error signal, which causes the brain to adapt to the incoming vestibular input. Exercises used to induce adaptation have the patient maintain visual fixation of an object while the head is moving with both a stationary and moving target. See Figure 2-36. These exercises should be progressed in terms of body position, speed of head movement, and overall endurance to continually move the head. Additional adaptation exercises include (1) active eye movements between two targets and (2) between imaginary targets.

Habituation Exercises. Habituation exercises can be used to treat patients who report motion-provoked dizziness. These exercises are based on the early Cawthorne and Cooksey exercise and the more recent motion sensitivity quotient. The purpose of the exercises is to provoke symptoms with rests in between to allow the patient's symptoms to return to baseline.

Postural Stability Exercises. Balance exercise should be a component of the intervention to prevent falls and improve the patient's balance. The PT should consider all balance

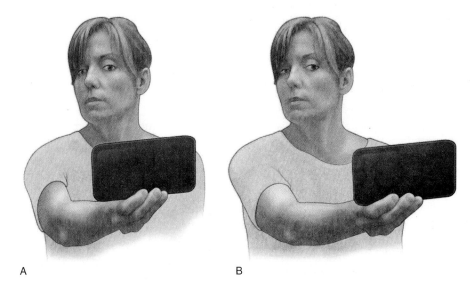

A   B

Figure 2-36. Gaze stability exercise. **A.** X1 Paradigm—Patient moves head back and forth while maintaining gaze on stable target. **B.** X2 Paradigm—Patient moves head back and forth while moving target in the opposite direction. (Reproduced with permission from Nichols-Larsen DS, Kegelmeyer DA, Buford JA, et al., eds. *Neurologic Rehabilitation: Neuroscience and Neuroplasticity in Physical Therapy Practice.* 2016. Copyright © McGraw Hill LLC. All rights reserved. https://accessphysiotherapy.mhmedical.com.)

systems and under both static and dynamic conditions. Box 2-14 provides treatment progressions for balance.

Bilateral Vestibular Hypofunction

Physical therapy goals for patients with BVH and expected outcomes are to (1) improve the gaze stability, (2) decrease the patient's complaints of disequilibrium and oscillopsia with head motions, (3) improve static and dynamic balance, and (4) prevent physical deconditioning by engaging in an aerobic program.

For patients with BVH who have some remaining function, gaze stability exercises should be used to tolerance and similar to UVH.

Balance exercises for individuals with BVH should enhance the substitution of visual and somatosensory information, as they are at risk of falls. Exercises should aim to improve postural stability and develop compensatory strategies that can be used in situations where balance is compromised.

Patients with BVH may have a significant decrease in their activity, become deconditioned, and have an increased fear of falling. Therefore, patients should engage in an aerobic program in the community that could include walking or aquatics.

Central Vestibular Disorders

Physical therapy goals and expected outcomes for patients with central vestibular disorders include (1) fall prevention strategies, (2) compensatory strategies for gaze stability, and (3) prevention of physical deconditioning. Recovery from central vestibular pathologies is often more than 6 months and may require adaptive mechanisms due to the damage.

Physical therapy interventions for individuals with central vestibular pathology will depend on the patient's signs and symptoms and the location of the lesion. Treatment interventions will be similar to those for UVH when there is involvement of the vestibular nuclei. When patients have complaints of dizziness, interventions should focus on gaze stability and/or habituation exercises. Lastly, gait and balance exercises that promote

BOX 2-14 **POSTURAL STABILITY EXERCISES AND INTERVENTIONS**

Static Balance Control

To promote static balance control, the patient can start by maintaining a standing posture on a firm surface. More challenging activities include practice in the tandem and single-leg stance, lunge, and squat positions. Progress these activities by standing on soft surfaces (eg, foam, sand, and grass), narrowing the base of support, moving the head, or closing the eyes. Add a secondary task (ie, catching a ball or mental calculations) to further increase the level of difficulty.

Dynamic Balance Control

To promote dynamic balance control, interventions may involve the following:

- Maintain equal weight distribution and upright trunk postural alignment while standing on a soft surface (eg, carpeting, foam, wobble boards). Progress the activities by superimposing movements such as shifting the body weight, rotating the trunk, rotating the head side to side or up and down.
- Perform standing bends and squats on firm surface. Progress to narrow base of support, eyes closed, soft surface, reaching to touch floor.
- Transitions into and out of chair or on and off floor. Progress to without arm support, eyes closed.
- March in place on a firm surface with eyes open. Progress to marching with eyes closed, on soft surfaces, and with head turns.
- Walk and turn suddenly or walk in a circle while gradually decreasing the circumference of the circle, first in one direction and then in another.

Anticipatory Balance Control

To practice anticipatory balance control, the patient can perform the following:

- Reach in all directions to touch or grasp objects, catch a ball, or kick a ball.
- Bend and pick up objects off of lower surfaces.
- Perform step-up and -down exercises or lunges in multiple directions.
- Maneuver through an obstacle course.

Reactive Balance Control

To train reactive balance control, the patient can perform the following activities:

- Work to gradually increase the sway in standing in different directions while on a firm, stable surface.
- Practice forward walking with abrupt stops. Progress to backward walking.
- To emphasize training of the *ankle strategy*, practice swaying while standing on one leg with the trunk erect.
- To emphasize training of the *hip strategy*, walk on lines drawn on the floor, perform tandem stance, perform single-leg stance with trunk bending, or stand on a rocker balance board.
- To emphasize the *stepping strategy*, practice stepping up onto a stool or curb or over progressively larger obstacles (ie, electric cord, shoe, phone book) or practice stepping with legs crossed in front or behind the other leg (eg, weaving or braiding).
- To increase the challenge during these activities, add anticipated and unanticipated external forces. For example, have the patient lift boxes that are identical in appearance but of different weights, throw and catch balls of different weights and sizes.

Sensory Organization

Many of the activities previously described can be utilized while varying the reliance on specific sensory systems.

- To reduce or destabilize the *visual inputs*, have the patient close the eyes or practice in low lighting or darkness, or move the eyes and head together during the balance activity.
- To decrease reliance on *somatosensory cues*, patients can narrow the base of support, stand on a soft surface, or stand on an unstable surface (ie, rocker or incline board).

Examples of these types of activities might include the following:

- Walking backward, side-stepping, and braiding performed with the eyes closed.
- Walking while watching a ball being tossed from one hand to the other.
- Walking with head and eye movements.
- Standing or marching in place on foam performed first with eyes open and later with eyes closed.
- Walking across an exercise mat or mattress in the dark.

Balance During Functional Activities

Clinicians should focus on activities similar to the activity limitations identified in the evaluation. For example, if reaching is limited, the patient should work on activities such as reaching for a glass in the cupboard, reaching behind (putting an arm in a sleeve), or catching a ball off-center. Having the patient perform two or more tasks simultaneously increases the level of task complexity. In addition, practicing recreational activities that the patient enjoys, such as golf, increases motivation for practice while challenging balance control.

Safety During Gait, Locomotion, or Balance

To emphasize safety, clinicians should have the patient practice postural sway activities within the person's actual stability limits and progress dynamic activities, emphasizing promoting function. If balance deficits cannot be changed, environmental modifications (eg, better lighting, installation of grab bars, removal of throw rugs), assistive devices, and increased family or external support may be required to ensure safety.

the integration of somatosensory, visual, and vestibular inputs are often effective with these patients.

CEREBELLAR DISORDERS

Recovery and interventions should depend on the cause and specific regions of the CNS and cerebellum involved. Overall prognosis may be more favorable for causes involving only a portion or specific location of the cerebellum than a poorer prognosis when the cause is cerebellar degeneration.

Physical therapy goals and expected outcomes for individuals with cerebellar ataxia include (1) improvement of static and dynamic postural stability during functional activities, (2) development of appropriate fall prevention strategies and precautions for safe functioning in daily life, and (3) prevention of physical deconditioning by engaging in aerobic exercise and/or resistance training.

Interventions should focus on stretching, strengthening, aerobic exercise, balance exercises, gait training, and vestibular rehabilitation if the patient experiences vertigo, nystagmus, or oculomotor complaints. Examples of static and dynamic balance exercises commonly pre-scribed can be found in Table 2-33.

■ PEDIATRIC NEUROLOGY

Pediatric physical therapy is a specialty practice that addresses the needs of the child and family. Care is provided through support, guidance, and family-centered, cultur-ally appropriate, age-appropriate (0-21 years) interventions to improve quality of life and function. Pediatric treatment settings can vary among the acute neonatal ICU, the acute hospital, an outpatient setting, school, and home, to address a few. Pediatric PTAs

TABLE 2-33 • Exercises for Cerebellar Ataxia.

Exercise Type	Variations
Static balance activities	Single-limb stance Quadruped weight shift—lift one arm, lift one leg, lift one arm and the opposite leg
Dynamic balance Kneeling Standing	• Alternately put one foot in front and then the other (half-kneeling position) • Alternately put one foot to the side and then the other • Alternately come to standing, using a half-kneel position and return to kneeling • Swing arms • Step in each direction—front, side, back • Braiding stepping • Stair climbing • Overground walking on different surfaces
Whole-body movements Quadruped Kneeling	• Raise one arm and the opposite leg; flex them to touch elbow and knee under the trunk and then extend (repeat multiple times then complete with opposite arm and leg) • Crouch to floor, bending knees, arms and trunk; then extend back up into a kneeling position • Move into side-sitting to one side, return to kneeling and then to side-sitting on the opposite side
Fall prevention activities Standing Walking Trunk and shoulder mobility	• Therapist disturbs balance in forward, backward, and lateral positions • Toe-touches—bends to touch toes and returns to upright; therapist may introduce a balance displacement • Repeatedly move to quadruped from standing and return to upright; therapist may introduce a balance displacement • When pushed in upright, patient practices flexing forward to the floor • Therapist provides balance displacement while the patient is walking • From prone lying, push up into extended arms position to stretch upper back • Spine rotation: supine lying—bend knees and alternately rotate the knees to the right and left side • Flexion of the shoulder: supine lying—lift the arms in the direction of the head

treat infants and children with disabilities, typically developing children, adolescents, and young adults with and without disabilities. Some unique aspects of pediatric physical therapy include understanding child development related to behavior management, developmental models, family interactions, social trends, reimbursement issues, and the requirements of working in diverse areas. Table 2-34 describes typical development which must be understood in treatment.

DATA COLLECTION

The PT and the PTA participate in data collection using tests/measures, including outcome measures. Tests and measures for the pediatric population are vast and can include assessment in behavior, intelligence, gross and fine motor, and adaptability to various environments, and are often norm- or criterion-referenced.[1] Norm-referenced tests (NRTs) are standardized tests on groups of individual populations designed to test and allow the clinician to determine the exact developmental age of the child compared to performance typically expected. Criterion-referenced tests measure the child's development of skills in terms of absolute mastery levels. These tests have reference points that may not be dependent on a reference group—the child is competing against himself or herself rather than a reference group.

Signs and symptoms of atypical development in the neurologic pediatric population may include, but are not limited to, the following:

- Impairment of body function and structures (physiology and anatomical structures).
- Changes in muscle tone (hypotonic, hypertonic).
- Presence of spasticity.
- Impaired age-appropriate development (delay in gaining milestones).
- Quiet, unresponsive baby.
- Lack of language development.
- Comprehension limitations.
- Limitations in social interactions.

TABLE 2-34 • Developmental Charts.

1-2 months	6-8 months
Activities to be observed: • Holds head erect and lifts head. • Turns from side to back. • Regards faces and follows objects through visual field. • Drops toys. • Becomes alert in response to voice. **Activities related by parent:** • Recognizes parents. • Engages in vocalizations. • Smiles spontaneously.	**Activities to be observed:** • Sits alone for a short period. • Reaches with one hand. • First scoops up a pellet, then grasps it using thumb opposition. • Imitates "bye-bye." • Passes object from hand to hand in midline. • Babbles. **Activities related by parent:** • Rolls from back to stomach. • Is inhibited by the word *no*.
3-5 months	**9-11 months**
Activities to be observed: • Grasps cube—first ulnar then later thumb opposition. • Reaches for and brings objects to mouth. • Makes "raspberry" sound. • Sits with support. **Activities related by parent:** • Laughs. • Anticipates food on sight. • Turns from back to side.	**Activities to be observed:** • Stands alone. • Imitates pat-a-cake and peek-a-boo. • Uses thumb and index finger to pick up pellet. **Activities related by parent:** • Walks by supporting self on furniture. • Follows one-step verbal commands; eg, "Come here," "Give it to me."

(Continued)

TABLE 2-34 • Developmental Charts. (*Continued*)

1 year

Activities to be observed:
- Walks independently.
- Says "mama" and "dada" with meaning.
- Can use a neat pincer grasp to pick up a pellet.
- Releases cube into cup after demonstration.
- Gives toys on request.
- Tries to build a tower of two cubes.

Activities related by parent:
- Points to desired objects.
- Says one or two other words.

18 months

Activities to be observed:
- Builds tower of three to four cubes.
- Throws ball.
- Seats self in chair.
- Dumps pellet from bottle.

Activities related by parent:
- Walks up and down stairs with help.
- Says 4-20 words.
- Understands a two-step command.
- Carries and hugs doll.
- Feeds self.

24 months

Activities to be observed:
- Speaks short phrases, two words or more.
- Kicks ball on request.
- Builds tower of six to seven cubes.
- Points to named objects or pictures.
- Jumps off floor with both feet.
- Stands on either foot alone.
- Uses pronouns.

Activities related by parent:
- Verbalizes toilet needs.
- Pulls on simple garment.
- Turns pages of book singly.
- Plays with domestic mimicry.

30 months

Activities to be observed:
- Walks backward.
- Begins to hop on one foot.
- Uses prepositions.
- Copies a crude circle.
- Points to objects described by use.
- Refers to self as *I*.
- Holds crayon in fist.

Activities related by parent:
- Helps put things away.
- Carries on a conversation.

3 years

Activities to be observed:
- Holds crayon with fingers.
- Builds tower of 9-10 cubes.
- Imitates three-cube bridge.
- Copies circle.
- Gives first and last name.

Activities related by parent:
- Rides tricycle using pedals.
- Dresses with supervision.

3-4 years

Activities to be observed:
- Climbs stairs with alternating feet.
- Begins to button and unbutton.
- "What do you like to do that's fun?" (Answers using plurals, personal pronouns, and verbs.)
- Responds to command to place toy *in*, *on*, or *under* table.
- Draws a circle when asked to draw a person.
- Knows own sex. ("Are you a boy or a girl?")
- Gives full name.
- Copies a circle already drawn. ("Can you make one like this?")

Activities related by parent:
- Feeds self at mealtime.
- Takes off shoes and jacket.

4-5 years

Activities to be observed:
- Runs and turns without losing balance.
- May stand on one leg for at least 10 seconds.
- Buttons clothes and laces shoes. (Does not tie.)
- Counts to four by rote. "Give me two sticks." (Able to do so from pile of four tongue depressors.)
- Draws a person. (Head, two appendages, and possibly two eyes. No torso yet.)
- Knows the days of the week. ("What day comes after Tuesday?")
- Gives appropriate answers to: "What must you do if you are sleepy? Hungry? Cold?"
- Copies + in imitation.

Activities related by parent:
- Self-care at toilet. (May need help with wiping.)
- Plays outside for at least 30 minutes.
- Dresses self except for tying.

5-6 years

Activities to be observed:
- Can catch ball.
- Skips smoothly.
- Copies a + already drawn.
- Tells age.
- Concept of 10 (eg, counts 10 tongue depressors), may recite to higher number by rote.
- Knows right and left hand.
- Draws recognizable person with at least eight details.
- Can describe favorite television program in some detail.

Activities related by parent:
- Does simple chores at home (eg, taking out garbage, drying silverware).
- Goes to school unattended or meets school bus.
- Good motor ability but little awareness of dangers.

6-7 years

Activities to be observed:
- Copies a Δ.
- Defines words by use. ("What is an orange?" "To eat.")
- Knows if morning or afternoon.
- Draws a person with 12 details.
- Reads several one-syllable printed words. (My, dog, see, boy.)

(*Continued*)

TABLE 2-34 • Developmental Charts. (*Continued*)

7-8 years

Activities to be observed:
- Counts by 2s and 5s.
- Ties shoes.
- Copies a ◊.
- Knows what day of the week it is. (Not date or year.)
- No evidence of sound substitution in speech (eg, *fr* for *thr*).
- Draws a man with 16 details.
- Reads paragraph #1 Durrell:

Reading:
- Muff is a little yellow kitten. She drinks milk. She sleeps on a chair. She does not like to get wet.

Corresponding arithmetic:

```
  7     6     6     8
 +4    +7    −4    −3
```

Adds and subtracts single-digit numbers.

8-9 years

Activities to be observed:
- Defines words better than by use. ("What is an orange?" "A fruit.")
- Can give an appropriate answer to the following:
- "What is the thing for you to do if …
  - —you've broken something that belongs to someone else?"
  - —a playmate hits you without meaning to do so?"
- Reads paragraph #2 Durrell:

Reading:

A little black dog ran away from home. He played with two big dogs. They ran away from him. It began to rain. He went under a tree. He wanted to go home, but he did not know the way. He saw a boy he knew. The boy took him home.

Corresponding arithmetic:

```
        67
 67    16    14    −84
 +4   +27    −8    −36
```

Is learning borrowing and carrying processes in addition and subtraction.

9–10 years

Activities to be observed:
- Knows the month, day, and year.
- Names the months in order. (15 seconds, 1 error.)
- Makes a sentence with these three words in it (item 1 or 2 below; can use words orally in proper context):
  - work … money … men
  - boy … river … ball
- Reads paragraph #3 Durrell:

Reading:
- Six boys put up a tent by the side of a river. They took things to eat with them. When the sun went down, they went into the tent to sleep. In the night, a cow came and began to eat grass around the tent. The boys were afraid. They thought it was a bear.

Should comprehend and answer the question: "What was the cow doing?"

Corresponding arithmetic:

```
 5204    23    837
 −530    ×3     ×7
```

Learning simple multiplication.

10-12 years

Activities to be observed:
- Should read and comprehend paragraph #5 Durrell:

Reading:
- In 1807, Robert Fulton took the first long trip in a steamboat. He went one hundred and fifty miles up the Hudson River. The boat went five miles an hour. This was faster than a steamboat had ever gone before. Crowds gathered on both banks of the river to see this new kind of boat. They were afraid that its noise and splashing would drive away all the fish.
- Answer: "What river was the trip made on?"
- Ask to write the sentence: "The fishermen did not like the boat."

Corresponding arithmetic:

```
 420    9)72   31)62
× 89
```

Should do multiplication and simple division.

12-15 years

Activities to be observed:
- Reads paragraph #7 Durrell:

Reading:
- Golf originated in Holland as a game played on ice. The game in its present form first appeared in Scotland. It became unusually popular and kings found it so enjoyable that it was known as "the royal game." James IV, however, thought that people neglected their work to indulge in this fascinating sport so that it was forbidden in 1457. James relented when he found how attractive the game was, and it immediately regained its former popularity. Golf spread gradually to other countries, being introduced in America in 1890. It has grown in favor until there is hardly a town that does not boast of a private or public course.
- Ask to write a sentence: "Golf originated in Holland as a game played on ice."
- Answers questions:
  - "Why was golf forbidden by James IV?"
  - "Why did he change his mind?"

Corresponding arithmetic:

```
 4762÷536     □      7 1/6
             +□     −3 1/6
```

Reduce fractions to lowest forms.
Does long division, adds and subtracts fractions.

Data from Leavitt SR, Gofman H, Harvin D, Hutchings JJ. Use of developmental charts in teaching well-child care. *J Pediatr.* 1963;62:278-279.

▲ HIGH-YIELD TERMS

Intraventricular hemorrhage (IVH)	Also known as **intraventricular** bleeding; it is bleeding into the brain's ventricular system, where the cerebrospinal fluid is produced and circulates toward the subarachnoid space. It can result from physical trauma or from **hemorrhaging** in stroke.
Periventricular leukomalacia (PVL)	A type of brain injury that affects infants. The condition involves the death of small areas of brain tissue around fluid-filled areas called ventricles. The damage creates "holes" in the brain.
Norm-referenced test (NRT)	A type of **test**, assessment, or evaluation that yields an estimate of the position of the **tested** individual in a predefined population concerning the trait being measured.
Standardized tests	Any form of test that (1) requires all test-takers to answer the same questions, or a selection of questions from a common bank of questions, in the same way, and that (2) is scored in a "standard" or consistent manner, which makes it possible to compare the relative performance of individual students or groups of students. While different tests and assessments may be "standardized" in this way, the term is primarily associated with large-scale tests administered to large populations of students, such as a multiple-choice test given to all the eighth-grade public school students in a particular state, for example.
APGAR score	An objective score of the condition of a baby after birth. This score is determined by scoring the heart rate, respiratory effort, muscle tone, skin color, and response to a catheter in the nostril.
Retinopathy of prematurity (ROP)	A potentially blinding disease caused by abnormal development of retinal blood vessels in premature infants. The retina is the inner layer of the eye that receives light and turns it into visual messages sent to the brain.
Hyperbilirubinemia	A condition in which there is too much bilirubin in the blood. When red blood cells break down, a substance called bilirubin is formed. Babies cannot easily get rid of the bilirubin, and it builds up in the blood and other tissues and fluids of the baby's body.
Sensory processing disorder (SPD)	A condition that exists when multisensory integration is not adequately processed to provide appropriate responses to the demands of the environment. It is still debated whether SPD is an independent disorder or the observed symptoms of various other, more well-established disorders.
Respiratory distress syndrome (RDS)	A breathing disorder that affects newborns. RDS rarely occurs in full-term infants. Instead, the disorder is more common in premature infants born about 6 weeks or more before their due dates.
Cyanosis	A bluish color of the skin and the mucous membranes due to insufficient oxygen in the blood. For example, the lips can develop cyanosis when exposed to extreme cold. Cyanosis can be present at birth, as in a "blue baby," an infant with a heart malformation that permits into the arterial system blood that is not fully oxygenated.
Baclofen	A muscle relaxer and an antispastic agent. Baclofen is used to treat muscle symptoms caused by multiple sclerosis, including spasms, pain, and stiffness. Baclofen is sometimes used to treat muscle spasms and other symptoms in people with injury or disease of the spinal cord.
Diazepam	First marketed as Valium, it is a medication of the benzodiazepine family that typically produces a calming effect. It is commonly used to treat a range of conditions, including anxiety, alcohol withdrawal syndrome, benzodiazepine withdrawal syndrome, muscle spasms, seizures, trouble sleeping, and restless legs syndrome.
Dantrolene	**Dantrolene** sodium is a postsynaptic muscle relaxant that lessens excitation-contraction coupling in muscle cells. It achieves this by inhibiting Ca^{2+} release from sarcoplasmic reticulum stores by antagonizing ryanodine receptors.
Tizanidine	A short-acting muscle relaxant to treat spasticity.
Botox	A highly purified preparation of botulinum toxin A, a toxin produced by the bacterium *Clostridium botulinum*. Botox is injected in very small amounts into specific muscles as a treatment for spasticity.
Antalgic	Counteracting or avoiding pain, as a posture or gait assumed to lessen pain.
Tonic seizures	During a tonic seizure, the individual's muscles initially stiffen, and they lose consciousness. The eyes roll back into the head as the muscles (including those in the chest, arms, and legs) contract and the back arches. As the chest muscles tighten, it becomes harder for the individual to breathe—the lips and face may take on a bluish hue, and the individual may begin to make gargling noises.
Clonic seizures	During a **clonic seizure**, the individual's muscles begin to spasm and jerk. The elbows, legs, and head will flex and then relax rapidly at first, but the frequency of the spasms will gradually subside until they cease altogether. As the jerking stops, it is common for the person to let out a deep sigh, after which normal breathing resumes.
Gowers sign	A medical sign indicating weakness of the proximal muscles, namely those of the lower limb. The sign describes a patient who must use their hands and arms to "walk" up their own body from a squatting position due to lack of hip and thigh muscle strength.

Tests, measures (Table 2-35), and screening that may be relevant to the pediatric population will be based on history and systems review and may include, but are not limited to, the following:

- Impairment level measures (joint motion, muscle function).
- Functional limitations (activity-based measures, often standardized measures).
- Disability (participation assessment).
- Reflexes (Table 2-36 describes primitive reflexes).
- Determination of developmental age (Table 2-34)
- Infant assessments
  - APGAR score—a measure of the physical condition of a newborn infant.
  - Behavioral assessment—Brazelton Neonatal Behavioral Assessment Scale.
  - General movements assessment.
  - Movement Assessment of Infants (MAI).
  - Alberta Infant Motor Scale.
- Comprehensive developmental assessments.
  - Bayley Scales of Infant Development II.
  - Peabody Development Motor Scales (PDMS-2).
  - Bruininks Oseretsky Test of Motor Proficiency (BOT-2).
- Assessments designed for children with disabilities.
  - Gross Motor Function Measure (cerebral palsy).
  - Pediatric Evaluation of Disability Inventory (PEDI).
- School-based.
  - School Function Assessment.
  - Hawaiian Early Learning Profile.

TABLE 2-35 • Test and Measure in Pediatrics.	
Test and Measure	**Relevance to Pediatric Physical Therapy**
Aerobic capacity/endurance	Children with respiratory conditions such as bronchopulmonary dysplasia or cystic fibrosis, or who have ventilation-assist needs should be tested in this area. In addition, those children whose movement is severely restricted by neuromotor conditions or musculoskeletal conditions such as juvenile chronic arthritis (JCA), osteogenesis imperfecta, or arthrogryposis may warrant testing in this area.
Anthropometric characteristics	Cartilage models of the long bones appear by the 6th week of gestation and primary centers of ossification appear in almost all bones of the limbs by the 12th week, and in the vertebrae by the 7th or 8th week. Children with conditions that affect growth such as pituitary gland dysfunction or bone disease such as osteogenesis imperfecta will have bone growth impairments. Indirectly, cardiac or renal conditions can also retard growth. Growth can also fall below norms in children with cerebral palsy. Growth charts with plots of height, weight, and frontal-occipital circumference are maintained by physicians and nurses. Body composition, the ratio of fat mass to fat-free mass, impacts performance on tests of aerobic and muscular fitness. Obesity in American children is a growing concern and points to a community health role of the pediatric physical therapist to improve fitness in children. Baseline measurement may include girth and body fat tests.
Arousal, attention, and cognition	This aspect is commonly addressed by other disciplines using tests such as the Brazelton Neonatal Assessment of Behavior Scale (BNABS), the Assessment of Preterm Infant Behavior (APIB), and the Movement Assessment of Infants (MAI).
Assistive and adaptive devices	Children with all types of conditions and varying severity of involvement can have assistive device needs ranging from temporary crutches to sophisticated power-driven wheelchairs. Adaptive devices may be needed at certain times for children who experience pain associated with JCA, or for children with spinal cord injuries, traumatic brain injuries, or severe cerebral palsy. Some standardized tests include testing with and without equipment, such as found on the Gross Motor Function Measure (GMFM), the Pediatric Evaluation of Disability Inventory (PEDI), and the School Function Assessment (SFA).

(Continued)

TABLE 2-35 • Test and Measure in Pediatrics. (*Continued*)

Test and Measure	Relevance to Pediatric Physical Therapy
Circulation	Testing in this area is important for children with cardiac conditions, lymphatic conditions, respiratory conditions including bronchopulmonary dysplasia, diabetes, and certain genetic syndromes involving the circulatory or lymphatic systems. In addition, children with obesity should have baseline measures of at least pulse rate and blood pressure completed.
Cranial and peripheral nerve integrity	The pediatric physical therapist does not routinely examine cranial nerve integrity in children, as this is often done by other disciplines with whom the physical therapist collaborates. Nonetheless, the pediatric physical therapist should be aware of the clinical signs and symptoms that may indicate cranial and peripheral nerve involvement. For example, absence or asymmetry of smiling, or other facial reactions may indicate facial nerve problems. Testing is also important for children who have severe neurologic involvement following traumatic brain injury or near drowning, or in later stages of progressive disorders.
Environmental, home, and work (job/school/play) barriers	Results of these tests are often used to suggest modifications to the environment. Specific examples in pediatric physical therapy are the PEDI and the SFA.
Ergonomics and body mechanics	For children, consideration includes classroom placement for listening, attending, or functioning, as well as the height of the seat in class and whether or not foot support is provided. This section may also include assessment of safety at school; dexterity in coordination for pointing to objects on the language board, or using hand controls on a power wheelchair; analyzing preferred postures for performance of tasks and activities; and how varied body or equipment placement improves performance or posture, or minimizes fatigue.
Gait, locomotion, and balance	Once walking has begun, clinicians will most often use observation to describe the gait pattern. The 30-second walk test is an example of a quick appraisal of a child's functional performance with gait, specifically the distance the child can walk in 30 seconds.[a] Balance testing may be done using the original or Modified Functional Reach test, or the Pediatric Clinical Test for Sensory Interaction in Balance (PCTSIB). The Bruininks Oseretsky Test of Motor Proficiency has a subtest on balance. Similarly, the Gross Motor Scale of the Peabody Developmental Motor Scales (PDMS) has five categories, of which "balance" is one.
Integumentary integrity	The assessment of skin integrity in children is particularly important in cases of suspected abuse.
Joint integrity/mobility	Joint integrity measurements of children are mostly subjective. Two tests of hip joint integrity in infants under age 6 months are used to detect hip dysplasia associated with subluxation or dislocation.
Motor function (motor control and motor learning)	Recently, the functional-ecological theories of motor control addressing function, practicality, culture, and environment seem to have attracted the greatest attention clinically. Testing of motor control may be subjective or objective, and typically focuses on a very specific aspect of motor performance. Motor learning cannot be measured directly; instead, it is inferred from behavior.
Muscle performance (including strength, power, and endurance)	Muscle tone abnormalities are common in children with impaired neuromotor development and range from hypertonicity, spasticity, and rigidity to hypotonicity, hypotonia, and flaccidity. Muscle tone can be judged subjectively by observation of posture and movement as well as by hands-on examination of a muscle's response to stretch. The muscle tone section of the MAI can also be used. Methods of strength testing in children include manual muscle testing, or the appraisal of functional skills that require strength.
Neuromotor development and sensory integration	A number of standardized tests exist for the assessment of motor milestone development, most of which are based on knowledge of normal development. For example, the Alberta Infant Motor Scale (AIMS) provides motor milestone information and is extremely valuable for describing motor function in the child who is under 19 months old or who has not yet achieved walking.
Orthotic, protective, and supportive devices	Children with cerebral palsy and myelomeningocele commonly use orthotic devices. Children who incur burns may wear compression garments. Infants with congenital club foot deformity may undergo serial casting.
Pain	The pain-o-meter, in which children are asked to show on a scale their level of pain, has been employed with children with JCA. Visual analogue scales for pain have also been employed so children can judge their own pain levels. In pediatrics, managing pain and other sensations under one category—sensory integrity—is common for most reporting purposes.

(Continued)

TABLE 2-35 • Test and Measure in Pediatrics. (*Continued*)	
Test and Measure	**Relevance to Pediatric Physical Therapy**
Posture	Postural control shows a distinct, continuous developmental progression and is a critical component of skill acquisition. The development of postural control appears to follow a cephalocaudal sequence starting with the head. Delayed or abnormal development of postural control limits a child's ability to develop age-appropriate motor skills, including independent mobility and manipulation skills. Causes of poor postural control can include spasticity, insult to the motor or sensory component of the central and peripheral nervous system, Down syndrome, cerebral palsy, abnormalities of muscle structure and function, and decreased strength. *Note:* Resting posture in recumbent, sitting, and standing positions may result in contractures. Parents can be asked about the duration of time that the child spends in postures such as supine lying so that recommendations can be made.
Prosthetic requirements	Children with congenital amputations comprise the largest percentage of children with limb deficiencies. The examination should describe the child's level of accommodation to the prosthetic device and the time spent with or without the device.
Range of motion	Atypical neuromuscular activity during the years of musculoskeletal growth can result in modeling errors that can cause joint dysfunction and disability. Lower limb rotational deformities are also common in children with neuromuscular disorders. Range of motion may be tested passively, by moving the child's limb, or actively, by letting the child perform the movement. For example, children with JCA are often tested actively to concurrently judge the effective range of motion, whereas children with cerebral palsy (CP) are often tested passively or by both means to distinguish true available motion from poor control, spasticity, or weakness.
Reflex integrity	In pediatrics, reflexes may be classified as diagnostic or developmental. Diagnostic reflexes include reflexes that might be used in a neurologic examination at any age such as muscle stretch reflexes, clonus, Babinski, or variations of the Babinski reflex. Developmental reflexes tend to be more specific to neurologic examination of the developing infant and young child. This cluster of reflexes include attitudinal, righting, protection, and equilibrium reactions. Rather than specifically testing the primitive reflexes, many clinicians use visual appraisal of posture and movement to ascertain their persistence or influence.
Self-care and home management (including activities of daily living [ADLs] and instrumental activities of daily living [IADLs])	A tool such as the Transdisciplinary Play-Based Assessment[b,c] can be used. In addition, two standardized functional tests in pediatrics provide information pertinent to this area: the PEDI and the SFA. Another test, the Canadian Occupational Performance Measure,[d-g] is designed to help establish goals by identifying functional limitations in daily life and rating them in importance to reducing disability in daily roles.
Sensory integrity (including proprioception and kinesthesia)	In very young children, sensation cannot be tested in the same way it is tested in adults. Rather, the examiner must look at the child's facial expression or other body reactions to judge sensory integrity. For older children, more sophisticated tests of sensation and sensory perception are embedded in the Sensory Integration and Praxis Test (SIPT). This test, which requires special training and advanced clinical skills, evaluates sensory processing deficits related to learning and behavior problems, including visual, tactile, and kinesthetic perception as well as motor performance.
Ventilation and respiration (gas exchange)	The majority of clinical tests in this area produce objective data on pulmonary function such as obtained with a spirometer (measures air volume after maximal inspiration), and the oximeter (measures oxygen saturation in the blood). Infants with respiratory distress syndrome (RDS) or bronchopulmonary dysplasia (BPD), children with cystic fibrosis or asthma, children with cardiac conditions, and those who are ventilator dependent definitely should be examined in this area.

[a]Data from Campbell SK, Kolobe TH, Osten ET, et al. *Construct validity of the test of infant motor performance.* Phys Ther. 1995;75:585-596.

[b]Data from Lotan M, Manor-Binyamini I, Elefant C, et al. *The Israeli Rett Syndrome Center. Evaluation and transdisciplinary play-based assessment.* Sci World J. 2006;6:1302-1313.

[c]Data from Linder TW. Transdisciplinary Play-Based Assessment. *Baltimore, MD: Paul H Brookes; 1996.*

[d]Data from Verkerk GJ, Wolf MJ, Louwers AM, et al. *The reproducibility and validity of the Canadian Occupational Performance Measure in parents of children with disabilities.* Clin Rehabil. 2006;20:980-988.

[e]Data from Eyssen IC, Beelen A, Dedding C, et al. *The reproducibility of the Canadian Occupational Performance Measure.* Clin Rehabil. 2005;19:888-894.

[f]Data from Carswell A, McColl MA, Baptiste S, et al. *The Canadian Occupational Performance Measure: a research and clinical literature review.* Can J Occup Ther. 2004;71:210-222.

[g]Data from Law M, Baptiste S, McColl M, et al. *The Canadian occupational performance measure: an outcome measure for occupational therapy.* Can J Occup Ther. 1990;57:82-87.

TABLE 2-36 • Primitive Reflexes.

Reflex	Description
Rooting	Response to light tactile stimulation near the mouth. Infant moves head in direction of the stimulus and opens the mouth. Usually disappears around 9 months of age.
Sucking	Response to nipple or finger in mouth. Can be assessed as to whether it is sustainable and consistent.
Moro	One hand supports the infant's head in midline, the other supports the back. The infant is raised to 45 degrees and the head is allowed to fall through 10 degrees. Mature response is abduction then adduction of the limbs. Usually disappears around 3-6 months of age.
Palmar/plantar grasp	Stimulus applied to palm of hand or soles of feet. The response is a grasping of the digits. Usually disappears around 2-3 months of age.
Tonic labyrinthine	Prone position facilitates flexion. Supine position facilitates extension.
Asymmetric tonic neck reflex (ATNR)	Related to position of head turn: • Extension of extremities on face side. • Flexion of extremities on skull side. Usually disappears around 2-7 months of age.
Babinski	The foot twists in and the toes fan out in response to a stroke of the sole of the foot. Usually disappears around 6-9 months of age.
Symmetric tonic neck reflex (STNR)	Infant positioned in quadruped. Arm and head do the same thing, legs do the opposite; eg, head is extended, arms extend, and legs flex.
Crossed extension	Pressure applied to sole of the foot produces flexion and extension of the opposite leg.
Proprioceptive placing	Pressure applied to dorsum of the foot or hand. Response is flexion, followed by extension of the extremity to bring the foot/hand on top of the stimulating surface. Usually disappears around 1 month of age.
Positive supporting	Pressure applied to sole of the foot produces extension of the extremity for weight-bearing. Also known as primary standing.
Neonatal stepping	Walking motion produced as the infant is moved along a surface while being held under the arms. Also known as automatic walking.

Data from Capute AJ, Palmer FB, Shapiro BK, et al. Primitive reflex profile: a quantitation of primitive reflexes in infancy. *Dev Med Child Neurol.* 1984;26:375-383; Damasceno A, Delicio AM, Mazo DF, et al. Primitive reflexes and cognitive function. *Arq Neuropsiquiatr.* 2005;63:577-582; Schott JM, Rossor MN. The grasp and other primitive reflexes. *J Neurol Neurosurg Psychiatry.* 2003;74:558-560; Zafeiriou DI. Primitive reflexes and postural reactions in the neurodevelopmental examination. *Pediatr Neurol.* 2004;31:1-8.

- Sensory integration.
  - Pediatric Clinical Test of Sensory Interaction for Balance.
  - Sensory Integration and Praxis tests.
- Pain scales.
  - Faces pain scale.
  - Neonatal infant pain scale.
  - Faces, legs, activity, cry, consolability behavioral pain scale (FLACC).
- Visual assessment.
  - Developmental Test of Visual-Motor Integration.
  - Developmental Test of Visual Perception.

DISEASE/CONDITIONS THAT IMPACT EFFECTIVE INTERVENTION

Prematurity

Clinical Significance Prematurity is defined as neonates born at less than 37 weeks' gestation (40 is typical gestation). Most of the difficulties associated with prematurity (preterm) occur in infants with birth weights of 1500 g (3 lb, 5 oz) or less, usually in those born

TABLE 2-37 • Determination of Gestational Age.
• Menstrual age: The age of a fetus or newborn, in weeks, from the first day of the mother's last normal menstrual period.
• Gestational age: Also known as fetal age, is the time measured from the first day of the woman's last menstrual cycle to the current date—the time inside the uterus. A pregnancy of normal gestation is approximately 40 weeks, with a normal range of 38-42 weeks.
• Preterm: Born before 37 weeks of gestational age.
• Post term: Born after 42 weeks.
• Conceptional age: The age of a fetus or newborn in weeks since conception.
• Chronological age: The time elapsed from date of birth to present day.
• Corrected age: Based on the age the child would be if the pregnancy had actually gone to term. The corrected age, generally used for the first 2 years of life, can be calculated as the chronological age minus the number of weeks/months premature.

at less than 32 weeks of gestational age. Causes of prematurity include, but are not limited to, poor prenatal care, multiple fetuses, complications (eg, placental abnormalities, preeclampsia), increased maternal age, comorbidity, and mother's lifestyle. Therefore, gestational age and birth weight should be assessed and interpreted (Table 2-37).

Diagnostic Tests and Measures

Laboratory Tests. Laboratory tests are completed to improve the outcome. Tests include blood glucose to maintain proper glucose levels, complete blood count for red cell measurement (anemia, polycythemia, infection), Coombs test for blood type, electrolyte levels, and metabolic screening.

Imaging. Chest radiographs, cranial ultrasonography.

Clinical Findings, Secondary Effects, Complications

1. Intraventricular hemorrhage
2. Periventricular leukomalacia
3. Retinopathy of prematurity (ROP)
4. Hyperbilirubinemia
5. Global hypotonia, with the level of hypotonia related to the degree of prematurity
6. Posturing of the extremities in extension and abduction, with decreased flexor patterns and midline orientation
7. Absent, reduced, or inconsistent primitive reflexes
8. Minimal spontaneous movement
9. Dysfunction of sensory organization
10. Difficulty moving between states of deep sleep, light sleep, alertness
11. Thermoregulation problems
12. Respiratory distress syndrome (RDS) (lack of surfactant)
13. Fluid, electrolyte, and glucose management

Interventions/Treatment

Medical. Medical treatment, based on a needs assessment, can include stabilization in the delivery room with prompt respiratory and thermal management. In addition, the American Academy of Pediatrics has established guidelines that include skincare, fluid and electrolyte management, and feeding.

Pharmacologic. Prematurity is not a specific illness. Medications will be prescribed for a purpose.

Physical Therapy. The PTA can provide consultation and education to the health care team, caregivers, and families. Education on positioning, handling, carrying the preterm infant, and safety related to baby on their back for sleep and tummy time for play. The PTA observes the infant and monitors handling tolerance and behavioral states of alertness, drowsiness, and sleep. Muscle tone, symmetry, reflexes, feeding, and breathing are assessed, and once the PT examination and evaluation are completed, interventions will be determined based on the infant's individual needs. Interventions may include facilitation to master skills such as head control, reciprocal movement, and other developmentally age-appropriate activities and strengthening activities to improve functional movement such as breathing. PTAs can offer hands-on training for movement, feeding, play, and home modifications to encourage movement, communication, hearing, vision, and play skills. Other major interventions include ROM techniques, active movement, illness prevention, and equipment needs, use, and monitoring as appropriate.

SELECTED OVERVIEW OF COMMON CONDITIONS RELATED TO THE NEONATE PULMONARY SYSTEM

Cyanosis

Newborns with significant cyanosis should be evaluated by the appropriate medical staff expeditiously. The numerous reasons for cyanosis in neonates and infants include pulmonary, hematologic, toxic, and cardiac causes.[2] Diminished pulses in all extremities indicate poor cardiac output or peripheral vasoconstriction. Absent or diminished femoral pulses suggest the presence of ductal-dependent cardiac lesions (eg, coarctation of the aorta). Although hypertension is uncommon in newborns, it is rarely idiopathic.

Respiratory Distress Syndrome

Originally described in adults, acute respiratory distress syndrome (ARDS), also known as *hyaline membrane disease*, occurs in all ages. The clinical signs depend on the type, acuity, and severity of the initial insult but include dyspnea/tachypnea, flaring of the nostrils, use of accessory muscles, and diffuse rales. The prognosis of infants with RDS varies with the severity of the original disease.

Bronchopulmonary Dysplasia

Bronchopulmonary dysplasia (BPD) is a chronic lung disease of infancy, which begins with the destruction of the respiratory tract cilia followed by necrosis of the respiratory epithelium cells as distal as the bronchioles. In addition, the chronic lack of oxygenation often impairs neuromotor development.

Bronchiolitis

Bronchiolitis is an acute, infectious, inflammatory disease of the upper and lower respiratory tract resulting in obstruction of the small airways. Although it may occur in all age groups, the larger airways of older children and adults better accommodate mucosal edema, and severe symptoms are usually only evident in young infants. Respiratory syncytial virus (RSV) is the most commonly isolated agent. The disease is highly contagious. Viral shedding in nasal secretions continues for 6 to as long as 21 days after developing symptoms. Hand washing and the use of disposable gloves and gowns may reduce nosocomial spread. Eighteen to twenty percent of hospitalized infants with RSV bronchiolitis develop apnea. Diagnosis is based on the infant's age, seasonal occurrence, and physical findings. Physical examination often reveals otitis media, retractions, fine rales, and diffuse, fine wheezing. The severity of the disease is directly related to postconceptual age. Infants younger than 6 months are the most severely affected due to smaller, more easily obstructed airways and a decreased ability to clear secretions. First infections are usually most severe, with subsequent attacks generally milder.

Periventricular Leukomalacia

Periventricular leukomalacia (PVL), a bilateral white matter lesion, may result from hypotension, ischemia, and coagulation necrosis at the border or watershed zones of deep penetrating arteries of the middle cerebral artery. Decreased blood flow affects the white matter at the superolateral borders of the lateral ventricles. The site of injury affects the descending corticospinal tracts, visual radiations, and acoustic radiations. Initially, most premature infants are asymptomatic. If symptoms occur, they usually are subtle. Symptoms may include decreased tone in lower extremities, increased tone in neck extensors, apnea and bradycardia events, irritability, pseudobulbar palsy with poor feeding, and clinical seizures.

Periventricular Hemorrhage-Intraventricular Hemorrhage

Periventricular hemorrhage-intraventricular hemorrhage (PVH-IVH) remains a significant cause of morbidity and mortality in infants born prematurely. PVH-IVH is thought to be caused by capillary bleeding. Two major factors contributing to the development of PVH-IVH are (1) loss of cerebral autoregulation and (2) abrupt alterations in cerebral blood flow and pressure. Sequelae of PVH-IVH include lifelong neurologic deficits, such as cerebral palsy (CP), mental retardation, and seizures. PVH-IVH is diagnosed primarily using brain imaging studies, usually cranial ultrasonography. As PVH-IVH can occur without clinical signs, serial examinations are necessary for the diagnosis.

SELECTED OVERVIEW OF COMMON CONDITIONS RELATED TO THE NEONATE CARDIOVASCULAR SYSTEM

Patent Ductus Arteriosus

Patent ductus arteriosus (PDA) is the fifth or sixth most common congenital cardiac defect. It involves the persistence of a normal fetal structure between the left pulmonary artery and the descending aorta beyond 10 days of life. Signs and symptoms include, but are not limited to, tachypnea, tachycardia, diaphoresis, and cyanosis.

Tetralogy of Fallot

Tetralogy of Fallot (TOF) is a complex of anatomic abnormalities arising from the maldevelopment of the right ventricular infundibulum. Cyanosis develops within the first few years of life, or at birth, which may demand surgical repair. However, the rare patient may remain marginally and imperceptibly cyanotic, or acyanotic and asymptomatic, into adult life.

SELECTED OVERVIEW OF COMMON CONDITIONS RELATED TO THE NEONATE NEUROLOGIC SYSTEM

Hydrocephalus

Hydrocephalus is an abnormal accumulation of cerebrospinal fluid (CSF) within the ventricles inside the brain. Intracranial pressure (ICP) rises if CSF production exceeds absorption due to CSF overproduction, increased resistance to CSF flow, or increased venous sinus pressure. Congenital hydrocephalus is thought to be caused by a complex interaction of environmental and perhaps genetic factors. Acquired hydrocephalus may result from intraventricular hemorrhage, meningitis, head trauma, tumors, and cysts. Symptoms in infants include poor feeding, irritability, reduced activity, and/or vomiting. In addition, the symptoms in children include a slowing of mental capacity, drowsiness, headaches, neck pain, visual disturbances, and gait disturbance.

Arthrogryposis

Arthrogryposis, or arthrogryposis multiplex congenita, encompasses nonprogressive neurologic conditions characterized by multiple joint contractures and rigid joints found throughout the body at birth. The pathogenesis of arthrogryposis has not been determined but is thought to be due to a combination of fetal abnormalities, maternal disorders (eg, infection, drugs, trauma, and other maternal illnesses), and genetic inheritance. Although joint contractures and associated clinical manifestations vary from case to case, there are several common characteristics: the involved extremities are fusiform or cylindrical with thin layers of subcutaneous tissue and absent skin creases. The deformities are usually symmetric, and the severity increases distally, with the hands and feet typically being the most deformed. In addition, the patient may have joint dislocations, especially the hips, and occasionally at the knees.

Brachial Plexus Injury

Brachial plexus injury occurs most commonly in larger babies during delivery. Associated injuries include fractured clavicle, fractured humerus, subluxation of the cervical spine, cervical cord injury, and facial palsy. Erb palsy (C5-C6) is the most common and is associated with a lack of shoulder motion. The involved extremity lies adducted, prone, and internally rotated. Moro, biceps, and radial reflexes are absent on the affected side. The grasp reflex is usually present. Five percent of patients have an accompanying (ipsilateral) phrenic nerve paresis. Klumpke paralysis (C7-C8, T1) is rare, resulting in weakness of the intrinsic muscles of the hand; grasp reflex is absent. If cervical sympathetic fibers of the first thoracic spinal nerve are involved, Horner syndrome is present.

Spina Bifida

Spina bifida includes a continuum of congenital anomalies of the spine due to insufficient neural tube closure and failure of the vertebral arches to fuse. Spina bifida is classified into aperta (visible or open) and occulta (not visible or hidden). The three main types of spina bifida are listed in Table 2-38. Spina bifida aperta is often used interchangeably with myelomeningocele, an open spinal cord defect that usually protrudes dorsally. The neurologic complications associated with spina bifida are outlined in Table 2-39. Interventions are based on clinical findings and may include ROM techniques, strengthening, positioning, handling, mobility, ambulation, equipment assessment, and family and caregiver education.

Cerebral Palsy

CP is nonprogressive damage to the cerebral cortex and other parts of the brain during prenatal, perinatal, or postnatal periods. CP is diagnosed when a child does not reach motor milestones while also exhibiting abnormal muscle tone or movement pattern dysfunctions such as asymmetry. Despite advances in neonatal care, CP remains a significant clinical problem. In most cases of CP, the exact cause is unknown but is most likely multifactorial. CP can be classified in several ways, including a diagnosis based on the area of the body exhibiting motor impairment: monoplegia (one limb), diplegia (lower limbs), hemiplegia (upper and lower limbs on one side of the body), and quadriplegia (all limbs). Other classifications and manifestations are represented in Table 2-40.

TABLE 2-38 • The Three Main Types of Spina Bifida.	
Type	**Description**
Spina bifida occulta	"Occulta" means hidden; thus the defect is not visible. Rarely linked with complications or symptoms. Usually discovered accidentally during an x-ray or MRI for some other reason.
Meningocele (spina bifida aperta)	The membrane that surrounds the spinal cord may enlarge, creating a lump or "cyst." This is often invisible through the skin and causes no problems. If the spinal canal is cleft, or "bifid," the cyst may expand and come to the surface. In such cases, since the cyst does not enclose the spinal cord, the cord is not exposed. The cyst varies in size, but it can almost always be removed surgically if necessary, leaving no permanent disability.
Myelomeningocele (spina bifida aperta)	The most complex and severe form of spina bifida. A section of the spinal cord and the nerves that stem from the cord are exposed and visible on the outside of the body, or, if there is a cyst, it encloses part of the cord and the nerves. Usually involves neurologic problems that can be very serious or even fatal. This condition accounts for 94% of cases of true spina bifida. The most severe form of spina bifida cystica is myelocele, or myeloschisis, in which the open neural plate is covered secondarily by epithelium and the neural plate has spread out onto the surface.

TABLE 2-39 • Neurologic Complications Associated with Spina Bifida.

Complication	Description
Syringomeningocele	The Greek word *syrinx*, meaning tube or plate, is combined with *meninx* (membrane) and *kele* (tumor); the term thus describes a hollow center with the spinal fluid connecting with the central canal of the cord enclosed by a membrane with very little cord substance.
Syringomyelocele	Protrusion of the membranes and spinal cord leads to increased fluid in the central canal, attenuating the cord tissue against a thin-walled sac.
Diastematomyelia	From the Greek root *diastema* (interval) and *myelon* (marrow). Accompanied by a bony septum in some cases.
Myelodysplasia	From the Greek term *myelos*, meaning spinal cord, with *dys* for difficult and *plasi* for molding. This is a defective development of any part of the cord.
Arnold-Chiari deformity	Malformation of the cerebellum with elongation of the cerebellar tonsils. The cerebellum is drawn into the fourth ventricle. The condition also is characterized by the smallness of the medulla and pons and internal hydrocephalus. In fact, all patients with spina bifida cystica (failure to close caudally) have some form of Arnold-Chiari malformation (failure to close cranially). The Chiari II malformation is a complex congenital malformation of the brain, nearly always associated with myelomeningocele. This condition includes downward displacement of the medulla, fourth ventricle, and cerebellum into the cervical spinal canal, as well as elongation of the pons and fourth ventricle, probably due to a relatively small posterior fossa. Signs and symptoms include stridor, apnea, irritability, cerebellar ataxia, and hypertonia.
Craniorachischisis (total dysraphism)	A condition in which the brain and spinal cord are exposed. This often results in early spontaneous abortion, often associated with malformations of other organ systems.
Tethered cord	A longitudinal stretch of the spinal cord that occurs with growth resulting in progressive loss of sensory and motor function, long tract signs, and changes in posture and gait. Presence may be signaled by foot deformities previously braced easily, new onset of hip dislocation, or worsening of a spinal deformity, particularly scoliosis. Progressive neurologic defects in growing children may suggest a lack of extensibility of the spine or that it is tethered and low lying in the lumbar canal with the potential for progressive irreversible neurologic damage and requiring surgical release.
Hydrocephalus	Characterized by a tense, bulging fontanel and increased occipital frontal circumference. Signs and symptoms include decreased upper extremity coordination, disturbed balance, strabismus, and ocular problems. Medical intervention involves placement of a shunt between ventricle and heart/abdomen.
Neurogenic bowel and bladder	Incontinence.

Data from Ali L, Stocks GM. Spina bifida, tethered cord and regional anaesthesia. *Anaesthesia.* 2005;60:1149-1150; Dias L. Orthopaedic care in spina bifida: past, present, and future. *Dev Med Child Neurol.* 2004;46:579; Mitchell LE, Adzick NS, Melchionne J, et al. Spina bifida. *Lancet.* 2004;364: 1885-1895; Shaer CM, Chescheir N, Erickson K, et al. Obstetrician-gynecologists' practice and knowledge regarding spina bifida. *Am J Perinatol.* 2006;23: 355-362; Spina bifida. *Nurs Times.* 2005;101:31; Verhoef M, Barf HA, Post MW, et al. Functional independence among young adults with spina bifida, in relation to hydrocephalus and level of lesion. *Dev Med Child Neurol.* 2006;48:114-119; Woodhouse CR. Progress in the management of children born with spina bifida. *Eur Urol.* 2006;49:777-778.

Disturbances include the following:

1. Primary impairments of the muscular system include insufficient muscle force generation, spasticity, abnormal extensibility, and exaggerated or hyperactive reflexes.
2. Primary impairments of the neuromuscular system include poor selective control of muscle activity, reduced anticipatory regulation, and a decreased ability to learn distinctive movements.

Medical. Diagnosis will consist of observation, history, and a neurologic examination. Pharmacologic, neurosurgical, and orthopedic surgeries may be recommended at some point. In addition, orthotic interventions may be recommended.

Pharmacologic

- Skeletal muscle relaxants (baclofen, diazepam, dantrolene, tizanidine).
- Antispasticity medications (baclofen, diazepam, dantrolene, tizanidine, Botox).

TABLE 2-40 • Cerebral Palsy Classifications and Manifestations.				
	Spastic	**Athetoid**	**Ataxic**	**Hypotonic**
Muscle stiffness	Excessively stiff and taut, especially during attempted movement	Low	Variable	Diminished resting muscle tone and decreased ability to generate voluntary muscle force
Posture	Abnormal postures and movements; mass patterns of flexion/extension	Poor functional stability, especially in proximal joint	Low postural tone with poor balance	Variable
Visual tracking	Some deficits	Poor visual tracking	Poor visual tracking, nystagmus	Variable
Muscle tone	Increase in antigravity muscles Imbalance of tone across joints that can cause contractures and deformities	Fluctuates, but generally decreased—floppy baby syndrome	Slightly decreased	Minimal to none
Initiating movement	Difficult	No problems	No problems	Difficult
Sustaining movement	Able to in some	Unable	No problems	Unable
Terminating movement	Unable	Variable	No problems	Uncontrolled
Muscle coactivation	Abnormal	Poorly timed	No problems	None
ROM limitations	Passive ROM decreased overall	Hypermobile	In spine	Hypermobile

Reproduced with permission from Dutton M. *McGraw-Hill's NPTE (National Physical Therapy Examination),* 2nd ed. 2012. Copyright © McGraw Hill LLC. All rights reserved. https://accessphysiotherapy.mhmedical.com.

Physical Therapy. PTs and PTAs play an important role with this condition and have a strong potential to influence children's lives. Children with CP have variable, but significant disruptions in recreation, community roles, personal care, education, mobility, housing, and nutrition and are most associated with locomotion capabilities. Therefore, the clinician must identify the abilities and participation restrictions, activity limitations, and impairment of body structure and function of the patient. At all ages, examination of impairment involves qualitative, and when possible, quantitative assessment of single-system and multisystem impairments. Common physical therapy equipment is described in Table 2-41.

SELECTED OVERVIEW OF OTHER COMMON CONDITIONS RELATED TO THE CHILD

Cystic Fibrosis

Cystic fibrosis (CF), an autosomal recessive disorder involving multiple organ systems (lungs, liver, intestine, pancreas) and exocrine gland dysfunction, can result in chronic respiratory infections, pancreatic enzyme insufficiency, and associated complications in untreated patients. The root cause of CF is a malfunction of the epithelial cells' ability to conduct chloride that results in water transport abnormalities, resulting in viscous secretions occurring in the respiratory tract, pancreas, gastrointestinal tract, sweat glands, and other exocrine tissues. This increased viscosity makes the secretions difficult to clear. The clinical characteristics of CF are listed in Table 2-42. Sweat chloride analysis is critical to distinguish CF from other causes of severe pulmonary and pancreatic insufficiencies. CF is a disorder that often requires management by a multidisciplinary team. The goals of the interventions are maintenance of adequate nutritional status, prevention of pulmonary and other complications, encouragement of physical activity, and provision of adequate psychosocial support. Physical therapy assistants may participate in pulmonary function tests, especially FEV_1, sputum analysis, auscultation, airway clearance techniques, physical exercise, and postural care. Intensive chest therapy, including massage, postural drainage, percussion, shaking and vibrations, and monitoring during treatment, is essential as the patient may require supplemental oxygen, especially in advanced stages of the disease.

TABLE 2-41 • Pediatric Adaptive Equipment.		
Equipment	Type	Description
Standers	*Supine version:* User enters the device on their backs, then strapped in and brought upright. Used when more support is needed posteriorly. *Prone version:* Loads from the chest and the patient is strapped from behind. Used for cases when greater head and trunk control is needed.	Promotes weight-bearing and stretching and, depending on the child's diagnosis, can help with the proper formation of the hip joint and building bone density. Promotes bone mineralization and respiratory, bowel, and bladder function. Helps teach mobility skills. Allows the child to gain important emotional and social support by enabling them to interact with the rest of the world from a "normal" position.
Sidelyers		Used in cases when the patient has a tonic labyrinthine reflex (TLR), which can elicit more extensor tone in supine, and more flexor tone in prone.
Adaptive seating		Seating can be customized to meet the specific support and posture needs of the individual. As a general rule, seating systems should be customized to maintain the head in a neutral position, the trunk upright, and the hips, knees, and ankles in correct alignment. For children with cerebral palsy, seating systems can be designed with a sacral pad and kneeblock to correct pelvic tilt, decrease pelvic rotation, and abduct/derotate the hip joint.
Orthoses	Various	Orthoses are frequently required to maintain functional joint positions, especially in nonambulatory or hemiplegic patients. Frequent reevaluation of orthotic devices is important, as children quickly outgrow them and can undergo skin breakdown from improper use. AFOs are commonly used. Submalleolar orthosis is used for forefoot and midfoot malalignment.

AFO, ankle-foot orthosis.

TABLE 2-42 • Clinical Manifestations of Cystic Fibrosis.	
System	Signs and Symptoms
Gastrointestinal tract	Intestinal, pancreatic, and hepatobiliary Meconium ileus Recurrent abdominal pain and constipation Diabetes Patients may present with a history of jaundice or gastrointestinal tract bleeding Minimal weight gain—failure to thrive (FTT)
Integumentary	Salty perspiration ("Kiss your Baby week" for early detection) Clubbing of nail beds Central and peripheral cyanosis
Respiratory tract	Wheezing, rales, or rhonchi Chronic or recurrent cough, which can be dry and hacking at the beginning and can produce mucoid (early) and purulent (later) sputum Recurrent pneumonia, atypical asthma, pneumothorax, and hemoptysis are all complications and may be the initial manifestation Dyspnea on exertion, history of chest pain, recurrent sinusitis, nasal polyps, and hemoptysis may occur Pulmonary artery hypertension Cor pulmonale Bronchospasm
Urogenital tract	Males are frequently sterile because of the absence of the vas deferens Undescended testicles or hydrocele may exist

Regular exercise, including aerobic training, resistive training, anaerobic training, and strengthening, will assist in maintaining the quality of life.

In the neonate, because the lungs are morphologically normal at birth, the most frequently seen symptoms are meconium ileus, malabsorption of nutrients, and failure to thrive, all of which are associated with the gastrointestinal tract. In addition, some infants may develop signs of impaired respiratory function.

Down Syndrome (Trisomy 21)

The extra chromosome 21 in Down syndrome (DS) affects almost every organ system and results in a wide spectrum of phenotypic consequences. Impairments and/or conditions associated with DS include hypotonia, decreased force generation of muscles, congenital heart defects, visual and hearing losses, cognitive deficits (intellectual disability), thyroid dysfunction, diabetes, obesity, digestive problems, low bone density, and depression. In addition, a person with DS achieves developmental milestones at a later age, often with less refinement due to poor balance, reduced strength, sensory difficulties, and reduced physical activity levels. Therefore, interventions focus on improving developmental milestones, balance, strength, physical activity, sensory integration, and emotional well-being.

Seizure Disorders

Seizures can be defined as neurologic manifestations of involuntary and excessive neuronal discharge. The symptoms depend on the part of the brain involved and may include an altered level of consciousness, tonic-clonic movements of some or all body parts, or visual, auditory, or olfactory disturbance. Differential diagnosis includes epilepsy, drugs (noncompliance with prescription, withdrawal syndrome, overdose, multiple drug abuse), hypoxia, brain tumor, infection (eg, meningitis), metabolic disturbances (eg, hypoglycemia, uremia, liver failure, electrolyte disturbance), and head injury. Most seizures in children involve loss of consciousness and tonic-clonic movements, but auditory, visual, or olfactory disturbance, behavioral change, or absences in attention may also occur. The various types of seizures are outlined in Table 2-43. A person with seizure disorders should be encouraged to exercise and participate in healthy activities in the community.

TABLE 2-43 • Seizure Disorders.	
Type	**Description**
Generalized	Affects both hemispheres Characterized by a change in the level of consciousness Bilateral motor involvement
Simple partial	Affects only part of the brain (focal, motor, or sensory) Formerly called focal seizures May progress to generalized seizures The history is important because the anticonvulsants used for partial seizures differ from those used for generalized seizures
Complex partial	Partial seizure with affective or behavioral changes
Febrile	Associated with temperature > 38°C Occurs in children < 6 years old (prevalence is 2%-4% among children < 5 years old) No signs or history of underlying seizure disorder Often familial Uncomplicated and benign if the seizure is of short duration (< 5 minutes) Involves tonic-clonic movements

Data from Camfield P, Camfield C. Advances in the diagnosis and management of pediatric seizure disorders in the twentieth century. *J Pediatr.* 2000;136:847-849; Nelson LP, Ureles SD, Holmes G. An update in pediatric seizure disorders. *Pediatr Dent.* 1991;13:128-135; Sanger MS, Perrin EC, Sandler HM. Development in children's causal theories of their seizure disorders. *J Dev Behav Pediatr.* 1993;14:88-93; Tharp BR. An overview of pediatric seizure disorders and epileptic syndromes. *Epilepsia.* 1987;28(suppl 1):S36-S45.

Duchenne Muscular Dystrophy

The muscular dystrophies associated with defects in dystrophin range greatly, from the very severe Duchenne muscular dystrophy (DMD) to the far milder Becker muscular dystrophy (BMD). DMD, the best-known form of muscular dystrophy, is due to a mutation in a gene on the X chromosome that prevents dystrophin production, a normal protein in muscle. DMD affects boys, and very rarely, girls. DMD typically manifests with weakness in the pelvis and upper limbs, resulting in frequent falling, an inability to keep up with peers while playing, and an unusual gait (waddling). Around the age of 8 years, most patients notice difficulty climbing stairs or rising from the ground. Because of this proximal lower back and extremity weakness, parents often note that the child pushes on his knees to stand (Gowers sign). The posterior calf is usually enlarged due to fatty and connective tissue infiltration or compensatory hypertrophy of the calves secondary to weak tibialis anterior muscles. Respiratory muscle strength begins a slow but steady decline. The forced vital capacity gradually wanes, leading to symptoms of nocturnal hypoxemia such as lethargy and early morning headaches. As DMD progresses, a wheelchair may be required. Most patients with DMD die in their early twenties because of muscle-based breathing and cardiac problems. Management of the person with DMD often includes stretching to improve ROM and to delay the onset of contracture development. Activities at school and in the community may include swimming, riding a bicycle, but care is taken to decrease participation in strenuous or fatiguing activities as they can cause more muscle damage. Breathing exercises and the use of spirometry may improve respiratory function. Modification may be required for ADLs.

■ RELEVANT PHARMACOLOGY

In addition to the expanded pharmacology section in Appendix D, Tables 2-44 to 2-51 outline the more common drugs prescribed for patients with neurologic conditions.

TABLE 2-44 • Drugs for Parkinson Disease.	
Therapeutic class: Antiparkinson drugs	
Pharmacology class: Dopaminergic drugs	**Indications:**[a] Parkinsonism **Adverse effects:** Uncontrolled and purposeless movements, involuntary movements, loss of appetite, nausea, vomiting, and orthostatic hypotension
Medications: Generic names (trade names)	
Amantadine (Symmetrel) Apomorphine Bromocriptine (Parlodel) Entacapone (Comtan) Levodopa–carbidopa (Parcopa, Sinemet) Amantadine (Symmetrel) Levodopa–carbidopaentacapone (Stalevo) Pramipexole (Mirapex) Rasagiline (Azilect) Ropinirole (Requip) Rotigotine (Neupro) Selegiline (Eldepryl, Zelapar) Tolcapone (Tasmar)	
Pharmacology class: Anticholinergic drugs	**Indications:**[b] Parkinsonism **Adverse effects:** Uncontrolled and purposeless movements, involuntary movements, loss of appetite, nausea, vomiting, and orthostatic hypotension
Medications: Generic names (trade names)	
Benztropine (Cogentin)	
Biperiden (Akineton)	
Diphenhydramine (Benadryl)	
Trihexyphenidyl (Artane)	

[a]Dopaminergic drugs prescribed varies by diagnosis; [b]anticholinergic drugs prescribed varies by diagnosis.

TABLE 2-45 • Drugs Used for Alzheimer Disease.

Therapeutic class: Drugs used for Alzheimer disease	
Pharmacology class: Acetylcholinesterase inhibitors	**Indications:**[a] Alzheimer disease, dementia **Adverse effects:** Vomiting, diarrhea, dark urine, weight loss
Medications: Generic names (trade names)	
Galantamine (Razadyne) Rivastigmine (Exelon)	

[a]Acetylcholinesterase inhibitors prescribed varies by diagnosis.

TABLE 2-46 • Drugs Used for Multiple Sclerosis.

Therapeutic class: Drugs used for multiple sclerosis (MS)	
Pharmacology class: Immunosuppressant, potassium channel blockers, immune modulator	**Indications:**[a] MS **Adverse effects:** Flu-like symptoms, anxiety, discomfort at the injection site, redness, pain, nausea, joint pain, muscle stiffness
Medications: Generic names (trade names)	
Alemtuzumab (Lemtrada)	
Dalfampridine (Ampyra)	
Dimethyl fumarate (Tecfidera)	
Fingolimod (Gilenya)	
Glatiramer (Copaxone)	
Interferon beta-1a (Avonex, Rebif)	
Interferon beta-1b (Betaseron, Extavia)	
Mitoxantrone (Novantrone)	
Natalizumab (Tysabri)	
Peginterferon beta-1a (Plegridy)	
Teriflunomide (Aubagio)	
Drugs Used for MS Symptoms	
Pharmacology class: Dopaminergic, antiseizure, central adrenergic, corticosteroids	**Indications:**[b] MS **Adverse effects:** Flu-like symptoms, anxiety, discomfort at the injection site, redness, pain, nausea, joint pain, muscle stiffness
Medications: Generic names (trade names)	
Amantadine (Symmetrel) Gabapentin (Neurontin) Modafinil (Provigil) Methylprednisolone (Solu-Medrol)	

[a]Immunosuppressants, potassium channel blockers, immunomodulators prescribed varies by diagnosis;
[b]dopaminergic, antiseizure, central adrenergic, corticosteroids prescribed varies by symptoms.

TABLE 2-47 • Centrally Acting Antispasmodic Drugs.	
Therapeutic Class: Centrally acting antispasmodic drugs	
Pharmacology class: Skeletal muscle relaxants	**Indications:**[a] Muscle spasms, stiffness, and rigidity **Adverse effects:** Drowsiness, blurred vision, dizziness, dry mouth, rash, tachycardia
Medications: Generic names (trade names)	
Baclofen (Lioresal) Carisoprodol (Soma) Chlorzoxazone (Paraflex, Parafon Forte) Cyclobenzaprine (Amrix, Flexeril) Metaxalone (Skelaxin) Methocarbamol (Robaxin) Orphenadrine (Banflex, Myolin, Norflex) Tizanidine (Zanaflex)	
Pharmacology class: Benzodiazepines	**Indications:**[b] Muscle spasms **Adverse effects:** Drowsiness, sedation, amnesia, weakness, disorientation, ataxia, sleep disturbance, blood pressure changes, blurred vision, nausea, vomiting
Medications: Generic names (trade names)	
Clonazepam (Klonopin) Diazepam (Valium) Lorazepam (Ativan)	

[a]Skeletal muscle relaxants prescribed varies by diagnosis;
[b]benzodiazepines prescribed varies by diagnosis.

TABLE 2-48 • Direct-Acting Antispasmodic Drugs.	
Therapeutic class: Direct-acting antispasmodic drugs	
Pharmacology class: Drugs blocking the release of acetylcholine	**Indications:**[a] Cervical dystonia, involuntary blinking eyelids, cosmetic procedures, spasticity **Adverse effects:** Extreme weakness, pain at the injection site
Medications: Generic names (trade names)	
Abobotulinumtoxin A (Dysport) Incobotulinumtoxin A (Xeomin) Onabotulinumtoxin A (Botox) Rimabotulinumtoxin B (Myobloc)	
Pharmacology class: Drugs reducing muscle tension	**Indications:**[b] Muscle spasms **Adverse effects:** Muscle weakness, drowsiness, dry mouth, dizziness, nausea, erratic blood pressure, photosensitivity, and urinary retention
Medications: Generic names (trade names)	
Dantrolene (Dantrium)	

[a]Drugs blocking the release of acetylcholine varies by diagnosis;
[b]drugs reducing muscle tension prescribed varies by diagnosis.

TABLE 2-49 • Drugs for Pain Management.

Therapeutic Class: Drugs for pain management

Pharmacology class: Opioid agonist	**Indications:**[a] Moderate-to-severe pain that cannot be controlled with other classes of analgesics **Adverse effects:** Respiratory depression, sedation, nausea, constipation, vomiting

Medications: Generic names (trade names)

Fentanyl (Abstral, Actiq, Duragesic, Fentora, Lazanda, Onsolis)
Hydromorphone (Dilaudid, Exalgo)
Levorphanol (Levo-Dromoran)
Meperidine (Demerol)
Methadone (Dolophine)
Morphine (Astramorph PF, Duramorph)
Oxymorphone (Opana)
Codeine
Hydrocodone (Hycodan)
Oxycodone (OxyContin, Oxecta); oxycodone
Terephthalate (Percocet-5, Roxicet)

Pharmacology class: Opioid antagonist	**Indications:**[a] For opioid overdoes and postoperative depression, opioid or alcohol dependence **Adverse effects:** Rapid loss of analgesia, increase blood pressure, tremors, hyperventilation, nausea, vomiting, and drowsiness

Medications: Generic names (trade names)

Naloxone (Evzio, Narcan)
Naltrexone (ReVia, Vivatrol)

Pharmacology class: Opioids with missed agonist-antagonist effects	**Indications:**[b] Moderate-to-severe pain **Adverse effects:** Respiratory depression, sedation, nausea, constipation, vomiting

Medications: Generic names (trade names)

Buprenorphine (Buprenex, Butrans, Suboxone)
Butorphanol (Stadol)
Nalbuphine (Nubain)
Pentazocine (Talwin Nx, Talwin)

Pharmacology class: Nonopioid analgesics NSAIDs: Ibuprofen and similar drugs	**Indications:**[c] Pain, fever, inflammation **Adverse effects:** Gastric discomfort and bleeding, hepatotoxicity

Medications: Generic names (trade names)

Aspirin (acetylsalicylic acid)
Salsalate (Disalcid)
Diclofenac (Cambia, Cataflam, Voltaren XR, Zipsor)
Diflunisal
Etodolac
Fenoprofen (Nalfon)
Flurbiprofen (Ansaid, Ocufen)
Ibuprofen (Advil, Motrin)
Indomethacin (Indocin, Tivorbex)
Ketoprofen
Ketorolac (Acular, Sprix, Toradol)
Mefenamic acid (Ponstel)
Meloxicam (Mobic)
Nabumetone (Relafen)
Naproxen (Naprosyn, Naprelan)
Naproxen sodium (Aleve, Anaprox)
Oxaprozin (Daypro)
Piroxicam (Feldene)
Sulindac (Clinoril)
Tolmetin (Tolectin)

(Continued)

TABLE 2-49 • Drugs for Pain Management. (*Continued*)

Pharmacology class: NSAIDS: Selective cox-2 inhibitors	Indications:[d] Pain and inflammation Adverse effects: Respiratory depression, sedation, nausea, constipation, vomiting
Medications: Generic names (trade names)	
Celecoxib (Celebrex)	
Pharmacology class: Centrally acting analgesics	**Indications:**[e] Pain and inflammation **Adverse effects:** vertigo, dizziness, headache, nausea, vomiting, constipation, and lethargy
Medications: Generic names (trade names)	
Acetaminophen (Tylenol) Tramadol (Ultram) Ziconotide (Prialt)	

[a]*Opioid agonists prescribed varies by diagnosis;*

[b]*opioid mixed agonists and antagonists prescribed varies by diagnosis;*

[c]*NSAIDs prescribed varies by diagnosis;*

[d]*selective cox-2 inhibitors prescribed varies by diagnosis;*

[e]*centrally acting analgesics prescribed varies by diagnosis.*

TABLE 2-50 • Drugs for Anxiety and Insomnia.

Therapeutic class: Antidepressant, anxiolytic

Pharmacology class: Selective serotonin reuptake inhibitor (SSRI)	Indications:[a] Depression, anxiety disorders, obsessive-compulsive disorder (OCD), panic disorders, posttraumatic stress, premenstrual dysphoric disorder Adverse effects: Serious reactions include dizziness, nausea, insomnia, somnolence, confusion, seizure, serotonin syndrome
Medications: Generic names (trade names)	
Citalopram (Celexa) Escitalopram (Lexapro) Fluoxetine (Prozac) Fluvoxamine (Luvox) Paroxetine (Paxil) Sertraline (Zoloft)	
Pharmacology class: Atypical antidepressants	**Indications:**[b] Depression, anxiety disorders, neuropathic pain, fibromyalgia **Adverse effects:** Headache, insomnia, nervousness, dry mouth, dizziness, weight gain, sexual dysfunction, and chills
Medications: Generic names (trade names)	
Duloxetine (Cymbalta) Mirtazapine (Remeron) Trazodone (Oleptro) Venlafaxine (Effexor)	
Pharmacology class: Tricyclic antidepressants	**Indications:**[c] Depression, OCD, anxiety disorders **Adverse effects:** Anticholinergic effects
Medications: Generic names (trade names)	
Amitriptyline (Elavil) Clomipramine (Anafranil) Desipramine (Norpramin) Doxepin (Silenor) Imipramine (Tofranil) Nortriptyline (Aventyl, Pamelor) Trimipramine (Surmontil)	

(*Continued*)

TABLE 2-50 • Drugs for Anxiety and Insomnia. (*Continued*)

Pharmacology class: Monoamine oxidase inhibitor (MAOI)	**Indications:**[d] Depression, OCD, anxiety disorders **Adverse effects:** Orthostatic hypotension, headache, insomnia, diarrhea

Medications: Generic names (trade names)

Phenelzine (Nardil)
Tranylcypromine (Parnate)

Pharmacology class: Benzodiazepines	**Indications:**[e] Anxiety, phobias, panic, and insomnia **Adverse Effects:** Drowsiness, sedation, amnesia, weakness, disorientation, ataxia, sleep disturbance, blood pressure changes, blurred vision, nausea, vomiting

Medications: Generic names (trade names)

Alprazolam (Xanax)
Chlordiazepoxide (Librium)
Clonazepam (Klonopin)
Clorazepate (Tranxene)
Diazepam (Valium)
Lorazepam (Ativan)
Oxazepam (Serax)
Estazolam (Prosom)
Flurazepam (Dalmane)
Quazepam (Doral)
Temazepam (Restoril)
Triazolam (Halcion)

Pharmacology class: Sedative–hypnotic barbiturates	**Indications:**[e] Anxiety, phobias, panic, and insomnia **Adverse effects:** Drowsiness, sedation, amnesia, weakness, disorientation, ataxia, sleep disturbance, blood pressure changes, blurred vision, nausea, vomiting

Medications: Generic names (trade names)

Pentobarbital (Nembutal)
Secobarbital (Seconal)
Butabarbital (Butisol)
Phenobarbital (Luminal)

Pharmacology class: Nonbenzodiazepines, nonbarbiturate drugs for anxiety and insomnia	**Indications:**[e] Anxiety, phobias, panic, and insomnia **Adverse effects:** Drowsiness, daytime sedation, dizziness, amnesia, depression, nausea, confusion and vomiting, GI effects

Medications: Generic names (trade names)

Buspirone (BuSpar) sedative
Dexmedetomidine (Precedex) sedative
Valproate/valproic acid (Depakene, Depakote) antiseizure
Atenolol (Tenormin) beta-blocker
Propranolol (Inderal, InnoPran XL) beta-blocker
Eszopiclone (Lunesta) nonbenzodiazepine
Zaleplon (Sonata) nonbenzodiazepine
Zolpidem (Ambien, Edular, others) nonbenzodiazepine
Ramelteon (Rozerem) melatonin receptor drug
Tasimelteon (Hetlioz) melatonin receptor drug
Suvorexant (Belsomra) orexin receptor blocker
Diphenhydramine (Nytol and Sominex) antihistamine
Doxylamine (Unisom) antihistamine

[a]*SSRI prescribed varies by diagnosis;*
[b]*atypical antidepressants prescribed varies by diagnosis;*
[c]*X prescribed varies by diagnosis;*
[d]*MAOIs prescribed varies by diagnosis;*
[e]*benzodiazepines prescribed varies by diagnosis.*

TABLE 2-51 • Drugs for Depression.

Therapeutic class: Antidepressant

Pharmacology Class:	Indications:[a] Depression, anxiety disorders, obsessive-compulsive disorder (OCD), panic disorders, posttraumatic stress
Selective serotonin reuptake inhibitors (SSRIs)	**Adverse effects:** Serious reactions include dizziness, nausea, insomnia, somnolence, confusion, seizure, serotonin syndrome

Medications: Generic names (trade names)

Citalopram (Celexa)
Escitalopram (Lexapro)
Fluoxetine (Prozac)
Fluvoxamine (Luvox)
Paroxetine (Paxil)
Sertraline (Zoloft)
Vilazodone (Viibryd)

Pharmacology class:	Indications:[b] Depression, anxiety disorders, neuropathic pain, fibromyalgia
Atypical antidepressants	**Adverse effects:** Headache, insomnia, nervousness, dry mouth, dizziness, weight gain, sexual dysfunction, and chills

Medications: Generic names (trade names)

Bupropion (Wellbutrin)
Duloxetine (Cymbalta)
Mirtazapine (Remeron)
Nefazodone (Serzone)
Trazodone (Oleptro)
Venlafaxine (Effexor)
Vortioxetine (Trintellix)

Pharmacology class:	Indications:[c] Depression, OCD, anxiety disorders
Tricyclic antidepressants	**Adverse effects:** Anticholinergic effects

Medications: Generic names (trade names)

Amitriptyline (Elavil)
Amoxapine (Asendin)
Clomipramine (Anafranil)
Desipramine (Norpramin)
Doxepin (Sinequan)
Imipramine (Tofranil)
Maprotiline (Ludiomil)
Nortriptyline (Aventyl, Pamelor)
Trimipramine (Surmontil)

Pharmacology class:	Indications:[d] Depression, obsessive-compulsive disorder, anxiety disorders
Monoamine oxidase inhibitors (MAOIs)	**Adverse effects:** Orthostatic hypotension, headache, insomnia, diarrhea

Medications: Generic names (trade names)

Isocarboxazid (Marplan)
Phenelzine (Nardil)
Selegiline (Emsam)
Tranylcypromine (Parnate)

[a]*SSRI prescribed varies by diagnosis;*

[b]*atypical antidepressants prescribed varies by diagnosis;*

[c]*X prescribed varies by diagnosis;*

[d]*MAOIs prescribed varies by diagnosis.*

CHECKLIST

When you complete this chapter, you should be able to:

❏ Outline neuroanatomy and neurophysiology principles for clinical practice.

❏ Outline various neurologic pathologies.

❏ Compare neurologic interventions across different pathologies.

❏ Describe the various vestibular disorders and their assessment tests.

❏ Outline standardized outcome measures for various neurologic pathologies across practice settings.

❏ List developmental milestones with the appropriate age range of acquisition.

❏ Identify time course and presentation of primitive reflexes.

❏ Compare techniques to determine gestational age.

❏ Outline signs, symptoms, and clinical presentation of various pediatric pathologies.

❏ Compare developmental outcome measures and determine the population for use.

❏ Identify common pediatric durable medical equipment and their use.

❏ Compare seizure disorders.

▮ APPENDICES

ACADEMY OF NEUROLOGIC PHYSICAL THERAPY CLINICAL PRACTICE GUIDELINES

Clinical practice guidelines (CPGs) are recommendations based on the systematic review and evaluation of research evidence used to guide best practices for a specific condition. CPGs are essential to bridge the gap between research evidence and clinical practice. CPGs are a dynamic and growing resource.

For further details, please visit the ANPT website and access the professional resources: ANPT Clinical Practice Guidelines (http://neuropt.org/professional-resources/clinical-practice-guidelines and http://neuropt.org/professional-resources/clinical-practice-guidelines/vestibular-hypofunction-cpg).

RESOURCES FOR OUTCOME MEASURES

An outcome measure is one type of test and measure used in the patient management process. Outcome measures are used to assist in the diagnosis and prognosis of patient care and track changes in human performance and health status. Unlike measurement tools such as posture and manual muscle testing, many outcome measures have research evidence that provides psychometric properties for specific patient populations. Understanding the psychometric properties assists in patient-specific clinical decision-making and the application of evidence-based practice (EBP).

Two of the most widely used resources are the rehabilitation measures database (RMD) and the ANPT's EDGE documents. Using the RMD, one can search for a specific outcome measure and obtain useful clinically applicable information, such as a copy of the outcome measure itself, the ICF category, and a wealth of psychometrics. For further details, please visit https://www.sralab.org/rehabilitation-measures.

The ANPT has created EDGE documents for the following diagnoses: stroke, MS, TBI, SCI, PD, and vestibular disorders. In addition, the EDGE documents within each diagnosis are further categorized for recommended outcome measures in entry-level DPT education, research, and various clinical practice settings. For further details, please visit http://neuropt.org/professional-resources/neurology-section-outcome-measures-recommendations.

TABLE A-1 • Measures of Recovery in TBI.

Glasgow Coma Scale Score	JFK Coma Recovery Scale—Revised (Score)	Ranchos Los Amigos Cognitive Scale[a]	Braintree Scale	Disability Rating Scale[b]
3	Unarousable (0); none responsive on all scales (0); may have abnormal posturing (1); total = 0-1	Stage I: Unresponsive	1. Coma—unresponsive	No response on any scale and totally dependent; total score = 29
4-8	Startles to auditory and visual stimuli (1 each); flexor withdrawal to noxious stimulus (2); reflexive oral responses (1); opens eyes to stimulation (1); no communication; total = 6	Stage II: Generalized response—whole limb or body response to touch, requires complete assistance	2. Vegetative state—begins sleep-wake cycle	Opens eye to pain (2); incomprehensible speech—groans/moans (3); extends (4) or flexes (3) limb to pain or withdraws (2); no awareness for feeding, toileting, grooming (3 each); totally dependent (5) and nonemployable (3); total = 24-26
9-10	Localizes sound (1); object fixation—visual pursuit (2-3); localized response to noxious stimulus (3); vocalization/oral movement (2); intentional vocalizing (1); eye opening with or without stimulation (1-2); total = 10-12	Stage III: Localized response—moves part specific to site of touch/pinch, still requires total assistance	3. Minimally conscious—responds inconsistently, no speech	Opens eyes to speech (1) or spontaneously (0); incomprehensible speech (3); localized movement to stimulation (1); no feeding, toileting, or grooming (3 each); totally dependent (5); nonemployable (3); total = 21-22
12-14	Moves to command inconsistently/consistently (3-4); reaches to object or recognizes object (4-5); object manipulation or automatic movement or functional object use (4-6); verbalizations understood (3); communication is functional (2); some attention to situation (3); total = 19-23	Stage IV: Confused and agitated, can be abusive and easily provoked, maximal assistance required Stage V: Confused with less agitation but still inappropriate behavior, requires maximal supervision	4. Posttraumatic amnesia	Spontaneous eye opening (0); obeying commands to move (0); some awareness of feeding (2); some awareness of toileting needs (2); primitive ability to groom self (2); marked (4) assistance required; not employable (3); total = 17 Eye opening (0); confused speech (1); moving to commands (0); partial awareness of how to feed self, toileting and grooming (1 each); marked assistance all of the time (4); not employable (3); total = 10
15		Stage VI: Confused but more appropriate behavior; requires moderate supervision Stage VII: Automatic appropriate—can complete ADLs and routine activities if physically able with minimal supervision/assistance, but still have memory problems and difficulty with problem-solving Stave VIII: Purposeful, appropriate—independent in many tasks, understands limitations, still some behavioral problems, requires standby assistance	5. PTA resolution, increased independence 6. Increasing independence and social skills with return to community activity, work, etc	Eye opening (0); oriented speech (0); obeying movement commands (0); full awareness of feeding, toileting, grooming needs (0 each); moderately dependent—needs supervision in the home (3); not employable (3) or able to work in sheltered workshop (2); total = 5 or 6 Same as above but with increasing ability to perform independently with some supervision (1) and likely can work either in a sheltered workshop (2) or selected jobs (1); total = 2 or 3

[a]The Ranchos Scale actually has two more levels: IX, which is associated with increasing ability to maintain focus and switch focus from one task to another but continued mild emotional/behavioral challenges that may require caregiver assistance to refocus, and X, which is associated with good goal-directed function, the ability to multitask, but still with some attentional challenges and the need for more time to complete some activities. Therapists rarely see patients who are at levels VIII to X.

[b]The Disability Rating Scale has a final category of functioning = independent in all skills (0) and work = unrestricted work ability (0).

TABLE A-2 • ASIA Motor Scores.

ASIA Key Muscles	Right	Left
C5 elbow flexors	0/5	2/5
C6 wrist extensors	0/5	1/5
C7 elbow extensors	0/5	2/5
C8 finger flexors	0/5	0/5
T1 finger abduction	0/5	0/5
L2 hip flexors	0/5	2/5
L3 knee extensors	1/5	2/5
L4 ankle dorsiflexors	0/5	0/5
L5 long toe extensors	0/5	0/5
S1 ankle plantar flexor	1/5	2/5

Reproduced with permission from Nichols-Larsen DS, Kegelmeyer DA, Buford JA, et al., eds. *Neurologic Rehabilitation: Neuroscience and Neuroplasticity in Physical Therapy Practice*, 2016. Copyright © McGraw Hill LLC. All rights reserved. https://accessphysiotherapy.mhmedical.com.

TABLE A-3 • Neurology Terms to Know.

The following is a list of common terminology associated with the various neurologic diagnoses.

Asthenia Debility; loss of strength and energy; weakness.	**Dystonia** Impairment of muscular tonus; abnormal muscle tone.
Ataxia Failure of muscular coordination; irregular and incoordination of movements.	**Fasciculation** Visible, small, involuntary muscular contraction under the skin; seen lower motor neuron disease.
Athetosis Involuntary repetitive, slow, writhing movements.	**Graphesthesia** Tactile ability to recognize writing on the skin.
Barognosis Conscious perception of weight; able to differentiate the weight of objects.	**Hemiballismus** Violent motor restlessness of half of the body, most marked in the upper extremities.
Clasp-knife rigidity Seen in Parkinson disease; increased tension in the extensor of the joint when passively flexed, giving way suddenly on exertion of further pressure; seen in upper motor neuron disease.	**Lead-pipe rigidity** A smooth, rigidity in flexion and extension that continues through the entire range of motion of a stretched muscle; seen in Parkinson disease.
Clonus Involuntary muscular contraction and relaxation in rapid succession, initiated by the spinal cord below an area of spinal cord injury. Set in motion by reflexive movements.	**Stereognosis** The sense of being able to identify objects through means of touch without seeing the objects.
Dysdiadochokinesia Impairment of the ability to perform *rapid* alternating movements.	**Tremor** Involuntary, oscillatory movements, trembling of hands and nodding of the head. Secondary to basal ganglia lesion. Specific to etiology.
Dysmetria An aspect of ataxia, in which the ability to control distance, power, and speed of an act is impaired.	**Two-point discrimination** The ability to localize two points of pressure on the surface of the skin as discrete sensations.

ANPT diagnosis EDGE documents are as follows:

- Stroke (http://www.neuropt.org/professional-resources/neurology-section-outcome-measures-recommendations/stroke).
- Multiple sclerosis (http://www.neuropt.org/professional-resources/neurology-section-outcome-measures-recommendations/multiple-sclerosis).
- Spinal cord injury (http://www.neuropt.org/professional-resources/neurology-section-outcome-measures-recommendations/spinal-cord-injury).
- Traumatic brain injury (http://www.neuropt.org/professional-resources/neurology-section-outcome-measures-recommendations/traumatic-brain-injury).
- Parkinson disease (http://www.neuropt.org/professional-resources/neurology-section-outcome-measures-recommendations/parkinson-disease).
- Vestibular disorders (http://www.neuropt.org/professional-resources/neurology-section-outcome-measures-recommendations/vestibular-disorders).

RESOURCES FOR CODING AND REIMBURSEMENT

In clinical practice, coding and reimbursement are highly connected to the use of outcome measures, and when tied to Medicare, involve knowledge of G code information. The ANPT has organized support for G codes by diagnosis: stroke, MS, TBI, SCI, PD, and vestibular disorders. For further details, please visit the ANPT's website and access the professional resources for coding and reimbursement at http://neuropt.org/professional-resources/medicare-g-code-information.

■ NEUROSCIENCE/NEUROANATOMY QUESTIONS

1. **A 65-year-old man demonstrates ataxic movements during reaching and gait activities. Which region of the brain was most likely affected by the CVA?**
   A. Brainstem
   B. Cerebellum
   C. Frontal lobe
   D. Parietal lobe

2. **Damage to the basal ganglia is likely to result in what clinical signs and symptoms?**
   A. Unilateral sensory and motor loss
   B. Bilateral sensory and motor loss
   C. Rigidity, bradykinesia, postural instability, and tremor
   D. Spasticity, hyperkinesia, postural instability, and tremor

3. **A PTA tests a patient's ability to move the eye medially during cranial nerve testing. Which cranial nerve is the therapist testing?**
   A. Abducens nerve
   B. Optic nerve
   C. Oculomotor nerve
   D. Trochlear nerve

4. **A 68-year-old woman presents to the emergency room (ER) with signs and symptoms of a CVA. She has complaints of a left frontal headache and right foot drag. Muscle tone and reflexes were slightly hyperreflexive upon testing. She has a history of hypertension (HTN) and diabetes. Which is the MOST likely location of the lesion?**
   A. L Middle cerebral artery
   B. L Anterior cerebral artery
   C. R Anterior cerebral artery
   D. R Middle cerebral artery

5. **A patient with ALS presents to physical therapy. Cranial nerve testing reveals motor impairments of the tongue, including wasting and deviation on protrusion. Which cranial nerve is likely damaged based on these results?**
   A. IX
   B. X

   C. XI

   D. XII

6. **Which of the following is a clinical manifestation of an upper motor neuron lesion?**

   A. Spasticity

   B. Flaccidity

   C. Hypotonicity

   D. Areflexia

STROKE

7. **A patient presents to physical therapy following a CVA. During the treatment session, the PTA asks the patient to reach for a glass of water, and the patient is unable to do so. However, later during the treatment session the patient reaches for the glass and takes a drink of water. What impairment is the patient likely exhibiting?**

   A. Ideomotor apraxia

   B. Ideational apraxia

   C. Unilateral neglect

   D. Visual agnosia

8. **A patient presents to outpatient physical therapy 2 weeks following a left CVA. When attempting to reach for an item using the right upper extremity the patient can initiate the movement voluntarily, however, is unable to move out of an abnormal synergistic pattern. Muscle tone testing reveals spasticity in the flexor muscles of the upper extremity. According to Brunnstrom stages of motor recovery, which stage of recovery is this patient in?**

   A. Stage 1

   B. Stage 2

   C. Stage 3

   D. Stage 4

SPINAL CORD INJURY

9. **An individual with a complete SCI presents with sensory and motor loss affecting all four extremities. Which area of the spinal cord was likely damaged?**

   A. Cervical

   B. Thoracic

   C. Lumbar

   D. Sacral

10. **Autonomic dysreflexia typically occurs in SCI at what levels?**

   A. T6 and above

   B. T12 and above

   C. L1 and above

   D. L5 and above

11. **A patient sustained an incomplete T12 SCI from a stabbing injury. The patient has absent proprioception and motor function below T12 on the ipsilateral side and absent pain and temperature on the contralateral side below T12. These examination findings describe which syndrome?**

   A. Brown-Sequard syndrome

   B. Anterior cord syndrome

   C. Central cord syndrome

   D. Cauda equina syndrome

12. **A patient with an incomplete SCI presents to inpatient rehabilitation with paralysis and sensory loss to the upper extremities with normal sensory and motor function in the lower extremities. Which of the following syndromes is the most likely to have been diagnosed?**

   A. Brown-Sequard syndrome

   B. Anterior cord syndrome

C. Central cord syndrome

D. Cauda equina syndrome

PARKINSON DISEASE

13. **A patient with Parkinson disease presents with complaints of dizziness and light-headedness immediately after standing. What is the most likely cause of these symptoms?**
    A. BPPV
    B. Vestibulopathy
    C. Decreased proprioception in the lower extremities
    D. Orthostatic hypotension

14. **Which of the following is a cardinal sign of Parkinson disease?**
    A. Intention tremor
    B. Hypophonia
    C. Postural instability
    D. Decreased cognition

15. **How is the tremor in early Parkinson disease?**
    A. Typically bilateral
    B. Increased with activity
    C. Present at rest
    D. Usually improved with levodopa

16. **A PTA is working with a patient with advanced Parkinson disease. The patient has lost weight and his family is concerned with his ability to swallow. Which of the following would be the appropriate referral for additional services?**
    A. Speech therapy
    B. Social work
    C. Occupational therapy
    D. Dietitian

OUTCOME MEASURES

17. **Which of the following outcome measures would be the most appropriate to test a patient's ability to shift and adapt between the three sensory systems important for postural control?**
    A. Berg balance test
    B. Tinetti balance and gait test
    C. Clinical test of sensory integration of balance (CTSIB)
    D. Romberg test

18. **Which of the following assessment tools would be the most appropriate to measure the participation restrictions in an individual with Parkinson disease?**
    A. Berg Balance Scale (BBS)
    B. Six-minute walk test (6MWT)
    C. Medical Outcomes Study 36-Item Short-Form Health Survey (SF-36)
    D. Functional Reach Test (FRT)

INTERVENTION

19. **A patient is having difficulty with maintaining upright sitting posture following a CVA. The patient sits forward-flexed and leaning to the nonhemiplegic side. Which body segment should the PTA align *first*?**
    A. Scapula and ribcage
    B. Thoracic spine
    C. Pelvis
    D. Lower extremities

20. **Which of the following PNF bilateral upper extremity (UE) patterns is the *best* to improve upright posture for a patient with Parkinson disease who has an increase in thoracic kyphosis in sitting and standing?**
    A. Bilateral symmetrical UE Flex/Add/ER pattern
    B. Bilateral symmetrical reciprocal UE Flex/Add/ER and UE Ext/Abd/IR UE pattern
    C. Bilateral symmetrical reciprocal UE Flex/Abd/ER and UE Ext/Add/IR UE pattern
    D. Performing bilateral symmetrical UE Flex/Abd/ER pattern

21. **A patient with a diagnosis of multiple sclerosis requires moderate assist with sit to stand due to bilateral quad weakness. Which of the following is the *best* intervention to improve this patient's independent performance of sit to stand?**
    A. Partial squats performed against the wall
    B. Partial lunges bilaterally
    C. Repetitive sit to stand from a raised treatment table
    D. Long arc quads with cuff weights seated edge of mat

22. **A patient with a traumatic brain injury has difficulty ascending stairs due to weak lower extremity extensors. Which of the following would be the *best* treatment strategy to address the patient's deficit?**
    A. Alternating high-knee marching exercises with unilateral UE support
    B. Alternating 4-in step-ups with unilateral UE support
    C. Alternating quadruped hip extension exercises
    D. Alternating prone hip extension exercises

23. **Which of the following statements is *true* regarding compensatory and restorative approaches to rehabilitation?**
    A. A compensatory approach focuses on regaining strength and resuming the performance of functional abilities.
    B. A restorative strategy focuses on restoring the individual's ability to perform a task with the use of adaptive equipment using different movement strategies than the individual used before his/her injury.
    C. A restorative approach is always the most appropriate approach.
    D. A compensatory approach uses a variety of substitution movement strategies and/or adaptive equipment to accomplish desired tasks.

ICF

24. **Following a traumatic brain injury, which of the following would be an example of a restriction in the participation domain of the ICF model?**
    A. Inability to walk on the beach with a spouse
    B. Inability to stand from her couch without assistance
    C. Inability to load the step out of the shower without assistance
    D. Inability to walk without an assistive device

ASSISTIVE DEVICE AND WHEELCHAIR PRESCRIPTION

25. **An individual has a complete spinal cord injury C3 (ASIA A) from a motor vehicle accident. Which wheelchair will be most appropriate for this patient?**
    A. Power tilt and recline, joystick-controlled wheelchair and a universal cuff
    B. Power tilt and recline, joystick-controlled wheelchair and a mechanical ventilator
    C. Power tilt and recline, breath-controlled wheelchair and a universal cuff
    D. Power tilt and recline, breath-controlled wheelchair and a mechanical ventilator

26. **A PTA is working with a patient with Parkinson disease. The patient and his caregivers report the patient has begun falling and they would like to know what is the best assistive device for this patient. During the treatment session, the PTA notes the patient requires moderate assistance for losses of balance and demonstrates**

freezing of gait. The patient does not demonstrate festinating gait. Which assistive device would be the *most* appropriate for this patient?
A. Front-wheeled walker
B. Single-point cane
C. Standard four-point walker
D. Inverted cane

GAIT

27. A patient with multiple sclerosis is referred to physical therapy for difficulty walking. During initial contact to loading response, the patient's foot "slaps" the floor. Which is the most likely cause of this gait deviation?
A. Flaccid plantar flexors
B. Tight plantar flexors
C. Spastic dorsiflexors
D. Weak dorsiflexors

MULTIPLE SCLEROSIS

28. A patient with multiple sclerosis presents to physical therapy with reports of a sudden worsening in her symptoms since her move from New York to Miami. What could this change be attributed to?
A. Fatigue
B. Natural disease progression
C. CNS plaque formation
D. Uthoff phenomenon

DISEASE AND CONDITIONS

29. A patient reports difficulty picking up small items and writing with the left hand, but denies difficulty when using the right hand. The patient exhibits fasciculations and a positive Babinski sign in the left upper extremity. Which of the following is the *most* likely diagnosis?
A. Amyotrophic lateral sclerosis
B. Guillain–Barré syndrome
C. Multiple sclerosis
D. Stroke

30. A patient presents with a rapid onset of extreme fatigue and bilateral, symmetrical flaccid paralysis. The onset of muscle weakness occurred in a distal-to-proximal pattern. Patient reports an upper respiratory disorder approximately 2 weeks prior to symptom onset. What is the most likely diagnosis?
A. Multiple sclerosis
B. Amyotrophic lateral sclerosis
C. Guillain–Barré syndrome
D. Poliomyelitis

31. A PTA is working with a patient who has difficulty with sit-to-stand transfers. The therapist decides to teach the patient the skill by breaking it down into smaller components, having the patient practice these components, then putting the components together in one complete movement. What is this type of practice called?
A. Distributed practice
B. Part-to-whole task practice
C. Random practice
D. Massed practice

32. **The use of sit-to-stand practice as a method of strengthening the lower extremities is an example of what type of intervention?**
    A. Knowledge of performance
    B. Results-based
    C. Task-oriented
    D. Impairment-based

33. **A PT is evaluating a patient with suspected BPPV involving the posterior semi-circular canal. Which is the maneuver with the best diagnostic accuracy for this condition?**
    A. Dix-Hallpike maneuver
    B. Supine roll test
    C. Epley maneuver
    D. Semont liberatory maneuver

34. **A PT is evaluating a patient with suspected BPPV involving the lateral semicircular canal. Which is the maneuver with the best diagnostic accuracy for this condition?**
    A. Dix-Hallpike maneuver
    B. Supine roll test
    C. Epley maneuver
    D. Semont liberatory maneuver

35. **Current evidence-based practice indicates which maneuver is best in treating lateral semicircular canal BPPV?**
    A. Barbecue roll
    B. Dix-Hallpike maneuver
    C. Epley maneuver
    D. Semont liberatory maneuver

36. **Which standardized outcome measures is the most comprehensive and sensitive to change when assessing gait and balance dysfunction in a community-dwelling older adult with a vestibular pathology?**
    A. Functional gait assessment (FGA)
    B. Dynamic gait index
    C. Berg Balance Scale (BBS)
    D. Performance-oriented mobility assessment

37. **Which of the following descriptions of nystagmus is most consistent with an acute (4 days) left unilateral peripheral vestibular disorder?**
    A. Nystagmus that is purely vertical, observable in room light and with fixation blocked, and increases with upward gaze
    B. Nystagmus that is mixed right horizontal and torsional, not observable in room light, observable with fixation blocked, and increases with right gaze
    C. Nystagmus that is mixed left horizontal and torsional, not observable in room light, observable with fixation blocked, and increases with left gaze
    D. Nystagmus that is mixed left horizontal and torsional, observable in room light and with fixation blocked, and does not increase with gaze in any direction

38. **Habituation exercises are a component of vestibular rehabilitation. Which of the following is the premise behind these exercises?**
    A. Avoid head movement until the symptoms are alleviated.
    B. Perform rapid and repeated head motions to induce severe symptoms until the symptoms are alleviated.
    C. Gradually perform head and body movements that induce mild-to-moderate symptoms until the symptoms are alleviated.
    D. Take vestibular suppressants to desensitize the nervous system over time until the symptoms are alleviated.

39. **A PTA is working with a patient diagnosed with Guillain–Barré syndrome at an acute care hospital. The patient was diagnosed 3 days ago and is currently**

experiencing a gradual loss of strength and sensation. **What is the most appropriate treatment plan for this patient at this time?**
- A. Initiate an exercise program of supine therapeutic exercise including straight leg raises, gluteal squeezes, hip abduction, and ankle pumps to improve strength.
- B. Defer treatment now and educate the patient to limit all movement in bed and out of bed.
- C. Educate the patient and family on proper positioning in bed and gentle passive range of motion for ankles, knees, and hips to decrease risk of skin breakdown and development of joint contractures.
- D. Gradually progress the patient daily from sitting at the edge of the bed to eventually ambulating with appropriate assistive device to decrease his or her potential for losing functional mobility.

40. **A PTA is treating a patient with Guillain–Barré syndrome in an outpatient clinic three times per week. On arrival for his or her second treatment session the patient reports that he or she felt weaker and less stable when ambulating. What is the most appropriate course of action for this scheduled therapy session?**
- A. Hold the therapy session for the day and recommend the patient to visit his or her physician for an assessment and blood work.
- B. Perform fewer repetitions and lower intensity of the already established exercises.
- C. Educate the patient that this is a normal part of muscle strengthening and continue the current treatment plan.
- D. Eliminate any eccentric exercises and train muscles only concentrically for the remainder of rehabilitation.

■ ANSWERS AND RATIONALES

1. **The answer is B.** The cerebellum has a major role in the coordination of voluntary movement. Damage to the cerebellum often results in ataxia.

2. **The answer is C.** Damage to the basal ganglia is implicated in Parkinson disease; the four cardinal features of Parkinson disease are rigidity, bradykinesia, postural instability, and tremor.

3. **The answer is C.** The oculomotor nerve (CN III) is responsible for up, down, and medial eye movements. The oculomotor nerve is also responsible for pupillary constriction.

4. **The answer is B.** The left anterior cerebral artery is the most likely location of the lesion based on area of headache (left) and the contralateral hemiparesis involving the right lower extremity. The middle cerebral artery provides circulation to the area of the brain controlling contralateral upper extremity motor function, and the anterior cerebral artery provides circulation to the area of the brain controlling the contralateral lower extremity.

5. **The answer is D.** Cranial nerve XII is the hypoglossal nerve that innervates the muscles of the tongue.

6. **The answer is A.** Upper motor neuron signs include hypertonicity, including spasticity and hyperreflexia.

7. **The answer is A.** Ideomotor apraxia is a neurologic deficit represented by the inability to perform a motor function on request or imitate a motor activity while the ability to spontaneously perform the motor task remains intact.

8. **The answer is C.** Brunnstrom stages of motor recovery describe typical recovery of motor function following a stroke. There are six stages, from flaccidity and no voluntary movement immediately after a stroke (Stage 1) to full voluntary movement and minimal to no spasticity (Stage 6). The patient in this case has spasticity and voluntary limb control but is unable to move out of an abnormal muscle synergy pattern, which represents Stage 3 of Brunnstrom motor recovery scale.

9. **The answer is A.** The cervical spinal cord controls sensory and motor function for the upper extremities. A spinal cord injury at the cervical level will disrupt communication to all levels of the spinal cord caudal to the area of injury, which will result in sensory and motor loss affecting all four extremities and the trunk.

10. **The answer is A.** Autonomic dysreflexia is a phenomenon typically occurring in SCI above the T6 level. Signs and symptoms of autonomic dysreflexia include a sudden increase in blood pressure, pounding headache, flushing, and profuse sweating above the level of the SCI. It is due to disruption in the connection between the brain and the sympathetic neurons in the thoracolumbar spine.

11. **The answer is A.** The incomplete SCI clinical syndrome represented by proprioception and motor loss below the level of injury ipsilaterally and absent pain and temperature contralaterally below the level of injury is Brown-Sequard syndrome.

12. **The answer is C.** The incomplete SCI clinical syndrome represented by greater upper extremity motor and sensory loss than lower extremity motor and sensory loss is the central cord syndrome.

13. **The answer is D.** Orthostatic hypotension is a common side effect of the medication carbidopa-levodopa (Sinemet) used to treat Parkinson disease. It is characterized by a drop in blood pressure that occurs when changing positions causing dizziness, light-headedness, and syncope.

14. **The answer is C.** The cardinal signs of Parkinson disease include the direct impairments of tremor, bradykinesia, postural instability, and rigidity.

15. **The answer is C.** Unilateral tremor is often an early sign of PD. Tremor associated with PD is usually present at rest and is diminished with activity. Levodopa is more effective at improving bradykinesia and rigidity and less effective in reducing tremor and postural instability.

16. **The answer is A.** A referral to speech therapy to evaluate this patient's swallowing abilities is appropriate. Speech therapy can address the possibility of dysphagia, which could be potentially life-threatening, as it can lead to aspiration pneumonia. The speech therapist can also evaluate the patient's ability to speak clearly. Patients with Parkinson's disease frequently have difficulty related to speech production related to hypophonia and/or dysarthria.

17. **The answer is C.** The Clinical Test of Sensory Integration of Balance (CTSIB) is commonly referred to as the foam and dome test. This assessment measures the effectiveness of the three sensory systems for postural control with the ability to stand with eyes open and closed, on and off a compliant surface, and with inadequate visual cues with the use of a dome. The modified CTSIB does not use the dome.

18. **The answer is C.** The tool that measures participation restrictions is the Medical Outcomes Study 36-Item Short-Form Health Survey (SF-36), which assesses quality of life (including physical and mental domains) from the patient's point of view. The BBS, 6MWT, and FRT measure the direct impairments common in patients with PD: functional mobility, gait, balance, and postural stability.

19. **The answer is C.** In sitting, the pelvis should always be aligned first to provide a stable base from which to build.

20. **The answer is D.** To improve thoracic kyphosis the bilateral UE PNF pattern that promotes the most thoracic extension is bilateral symmetrical UE Flex/Abd/ER.

21. **The answer is C.** Task-specific functional mobility training to improve sit-to-stand can be done with repetitive sit-to-stand training.

22. **The answer is B.** Alternating 4-in step-ups with unilateral UE support are the most task-specific activities of the provided choices to improve ascending stairs.

23. **The answer is D.** Rehabilitation approaches may include teaching the individual compensatory strategies to allow them to perform tasks using substitution strategies and/or adaptive equipment to accomplish desired tasks. A restorative approach to rehabilitation is typically used in rehabilitation with the goal of recovery of normal movement and minimal compensations.

24. **The answer is A.** The inability to walk on the beach with a spouse is a participation restriction because it represents a social activity or an activity that is meaningful to the individual's life satisfaction. All other options represent activity limitations.

25. **The answer is D.** An individual with a complete spinal cord injury at the C3 level will require mechanical assistance with ventilation due to the lack of innervation at the diaphragm and accessory breathing musculature. The breath-controlled (also referred to as a sip-and-puff) power tilt and recline wheelchair will allow the individual to be independent with wheelchair locomotion and pressure reliefs.

26. **The answer is A.** A single-point cane will likely be insufficient to prevent falls in a patient with balance impairments requiring moderate assistance for recovery of balance. An inverted cane is used to provide a visual cue for a patient with freezing gait, but will likely also be insufficient to prevent a fall for this patient. A standard walker can worsen freezing episodes and will not help with retropulsion related falls. A front-wheeled walker can be used in patients with freezing of gait effectively to prevent falls but may be unsafe for patients with festinating gait, which this patient does not have.

27. **The answer is D.** In initial contact to loading response, the dorsiflexors work eccentrically to slow the progression of the foot from a dorsiflexed position to a plantarflexed position. Weak dorsiflexors cause this change in position to happen with less control, causing the foot to slap on the floor.

28. **The answer is D.** Uthoff phenomenon is characterized by a decline in neurologic symptoms caused by overheating of the body for individuals with MS. This overheating may be due to hot weather, exercise, body fever, saunas, hot tubs, or other heat-inducing environments. The patient in this case recently moved from a cooler to warmer climate, which may explain the sudden worsening of his or her symptoms.

29. **The answer is A.** ALS is a degenerative neurologic condition, which causes both upper and lower motor nerve degeneration. Muscle twitching, called fasciculation, is commonly seen in individuals with ALS and is a lower motor neuron sign. Babinski sign is an abnormal response of the foot to extend, typically seen in the great toe in response to stimulation on the plantar surface of the foot. A normal response to this is for the foot to plantarflex. An abnormal response in adults may be a sign of an upper motor neuron disfunction.

30. **The answer is C.** Guillain–Barré syndrome presents with bilateral, symmetrical flaccid paralysis progressing in a distal-to-proximal pattern.

31. **The answer is B.** Part-to-whole task practice was used in this example. The patient practiced the component tasks first, then practiced the entire task.

32. **The answer is C.** Using a functional task that is specific, both in regard to the task and the context, is the hallmark of the task-oriented approach.

33. **The answer is A.** The Dix-Hallpike maneuver should be used to diagnose posterior canal BPPV. The Epley maneuver is used to treat posterior canal BPPV once this is determined with a positive Dix-Hallpike maneuver. The roll test should be used to diagnose lateral canal BPPV, and the Semon liberatory is used to treat lateral canal BPPV.

34. **The answer is B.** The supine roll test should be used to diagnose lateral canal BPPV.

35. **The answer is A.** The barbecue roll maneuver is an effective maneuver to treat lateral canal BPPV. Forced prolonged positioning can also be used to treat lateral canal BPPV.

36. **The answer is A.** Although moderate correlations exist between all the options listed, the FGA is the most comprehensive and sensitive to change when assessing gait and balance dysfunction in community-dwelling elderly and in individuals with vestibular dysfunction. An FGA score of less than or equal to 22/30 is predictive of increased fall risk.

37. **The answer is B.** With a unilateral peripheral vestibular disorder, the patient may be able to suppress the nystagmus in room light after 3 days following symptom onset. Nystagmus is less likely to be suppressed with fixation blocked using Frenzel goggles. The direction of nystagmus will be mixed horizonal and torsional in the direction of the intact ear. According to Alexander's law, nystagmus will also increase when the patient looks toward the fast phase.

38. **The answer is B.** Habituation exercises involve repeated, gradual, and graded performance of exercises or activities that induce dizziness, with the goal of getting the nervous system accustomed to the stimuli without symptom provocation.

39. **The answer is C.** The patient has recently been diagnosed and is in a phase of decline, with progressive muscular weakness and sensation loss. It is important to educate the patient and family on proper positioning techniques and gentle range of motion to decrease risks of skin breakdown and joint contractures. This will reduce additional complications in his or her recovery once he or she is cleared for mobilization.

40. **The answer is A.** The patient may be experiencing overwork weakness, which is a serious contraindication to therapy. The patient needs to be evaluated by the physician and have laboratory work done to check for increased serum levels of creatine kinase. He must be cleared by his or her physician to resume exercise.

■ PEDIATRIC NEUROLOGY QUESTIONS

1. A physical therapist assistant initiates the treatment of an infant. The infant is observed sitting alone without support, reaching with one hand, and waving "bye-bye." The infant is demonstrating typical development for which of the following ages?
   A. 1 to 2 months
   B. 3 to 5 months
   C. 6 to 8 months
   D. 9 to 11 months

2. Your neighbor has discussed concern that their 4-month-old infant daughter has not been able to demonstrate the same gross motor activities as the same age cousin. You start by asking the neighbor if the infant can perform which of the milestones consistent with 4 months of age:
   A. Transitions sitting to crawling
   B. Stands with assistance
   C. Raises self to sit
   D. Pivots in prone position

3. Determination of pain is a key aspect of child examination. An appropriate pain assessment for a 13-month-old includes which of the following?
   A. Parents should determine pain levels.
   B. Faces pain scale.
   C. Visual analog scale.
   D. Face, legs, activity, cry, consolability behavioral scale.

4. Which is the best measure to determine the quantity of movement in children with cerebral palsy or Down syndrome?
   A. Gross motor function measure
   B. Denver Developmental Screening Test
   C. Peabody Developmental Motor Scales
   D. Test of gross motor development

5. The physical therapist assistant is observing a child limping while walking on a firm surface. The child demonstrates a shortened stance phase but has level hips.

Physical examination reveals range of motion limitation a tenderness at the hip only. Which gait type has the therapist identified?

A. Abductor lurch
B. Antalgic
C. Equines
D. Circumduction

6. A 5-year-old child presents to the clinic with joint inflammation involving many joints. Physical examination by the physical therapist reveals limitations in range of motion of the same joints, weakness, and significant pain. The parents report the child requires assistance with self-care and that handwriting has been difficult. Imaging reveals joint space narrowing. This description is most likely indicative of which of the following pediatric diseases affecting connective tissue?

A. Ehlers-Danlos syndrome
B. Juvenile idiopathic arthritis
C. Pediatric lupus erythematous
D. Hemophilia

7. During a school screening, a 10-year-old girl presents with a rib hump during the Adams Forward Bend test. Further testing with a sociometer was performed. Which of the following results should be referred to the physician?

A. 1- to 4-degree scoliometer trunk rotation angle
B. 5- to 9-degree scoliometer trunk rotation angle
C. 10-degree scoliometer trunk rotation angle
D. > 15-degree scoliometer trunk rotation angle

8. A 3-year-old child with developmental hip dysplasia presents to the clinic with gross motor delay. During treatment, the unstable hip joint should avoid which end-of-range hip positions?

A. Extension
B. Flexion
C. External rotation
D. Abduction

9. Gowers sign used by children with muscular dystrophy compensates for which of the following?

A. Distal weakness
B. Proximal weakness
C. Distal contractures
D. Proximal contractures

10. Congenital muscular torticollis is a nonprogressive unilateral contracture of the sternocleidomastoid muscle. Which of the following is true for typical neonatal cervical range of motion?

A. 25 degrees cervical rotation and 20 degrees of lateral flexion
B. 50 degrees cervical rotation and 35 degrees of lateral flexion
C. 90 degrees cervical rotation and 50 degrees of lateral flexion
D. 100 degrees or more cervical rotation and 65 degrees of lateral flexion

11. Brachial plexus injuries occur when nerve roots are damaged causing transient or permanent nerve damage. A teenager who spent the evening drinking fell from a height but was able to break the fall by holding on to a metal railing, stretching his neck and arm forcefully. He now presents with shoulder internal rotation and adduction, the wrist flexed, and the fingers extended. This position is characteristic of which of the following?

A. Total plexus palsy
B. Erb palsy
C. Klumpke palsy
D. Ulnar nerve palsy

12. **"W" sitting is used by children to assist with stability when sitting on the floor. Risks associated with prolonged use of "W" sitting include which of the following?**
    A. Limited unilateral use of the upper extremities
    B. Laxity of muscles at hips
    C. No hand preference
    D. Overstrengthening of core muscles

■ ANSWERS

1. **The answer is C.** Six to eight-month milestones include sitting alone, reaching with one hand, and waving goodbye.

2. **The answer is D.** Pivoting in prone is a customary developmental milestone between ages 4 and 5 months; the other answers are consistent with older infants.

3. **The answer is D.** Faces, legs, activity, cry, consolability behavioral scale is used for a child who is preverbal and cannot participate in a self-reporting scale. All other options require the child to report his or her pain.

4. **The answer is A.** Gross motor function measure was developed for use in children with cerebral palsy and Down syndrome. All other measures are norm-referenced test not specifically designed for cerebral palsy and Down syndrome.

5. **The answer is B.** Antalgic gait includes a shorted stance, tenderness, and reduced range on physical examination. Abductor lurch would present with a Trendelenburg sign, equinus would have heel cord contracture or limitations, and circumduction gait may be due to limb length discrepancy or weakness.

6. **The answer is B.** Juvenile idiopathic arthritis is believed to be an autoimmune dysfunction related to interleukin 1. Joint inflammation involving few or many joints with joint synovium proliferation causes overgrowth (pannus), which can erode the adjacent cartilage, causing joint narrowing and destruction. Significant pain is present. Ehlers-Danlos syndrome includes developmental delay, hyperextensibility of the skin and joints, scarring, hernias, easy bruising, and muscle hypotonia. The primary symptoms of pediatric lupus erythematous are inflammation, oral and nasal rash or ulcers, kidney dysfunction, headaches, cerebral vascular injury, and cognitive dysfunction. Pain, fatigue, and other discomfort may impact physical function. Hemophilia is a pathology associated with missing proteins required for blood clotting leading to chronic bleeding. Joint destruction leading to premature arthritis and chronic pain occurs. Muscle atrophy and range of motion limitations are noted.

7. **The answer is C.** Ten-degree or greater scoliometer trunk rotation angle should be referred to the physician.

8. **The answer is A.** Extreme or forceful extension should be avoided, as it may lead to dislocation. The most common intervention is the Pavlik harness, which maintains the hip in flexion, adduction, and slight external rotation.

9. **The answer is B.** Gowers sign used by children with muscular dystrophy compensates for proximal muscle weakness.

10. **The answer is D.** Typical neonates should have 100 degrees or more cervical rotation and 65 degrees of cervical lateral flexion.

11. **The answer is B.** Erb palsy presents with shoulder internal rotation and adduction, the wrist flexed and fingers extending. Klumpke palsy has motor deficits that affect muscles of the hand and lateral sensation of the medial arm. Total plexus palsy affects all the muscles of the arm and hand. Ulnar nerve palsy would present with a loss of sensation in the hand, especially the ring and little fingers, as well as loss of coordination in the fingers.

12. **The answer is C.** In a "W" sitting position, a child has too much trunk control and stability. It is very easy to use either hand to accomplish tasks, limiting the development of

hand preference. The wide sitting stance of the W position makes it easier to keep the body upright. Children sitting in a W position do not have to use their core muscles as much and will not develop them as they would in other sitting positions. The W position makes it difficult for children to rotate their upper bodies and reach across to either side with one or both arms, allowing them to use the upper extremity unilaterally with ease. If a child is prone to muscle tightness or hypertonia, sitting in a W position will increase tightness in hips, knees, and ankles.

REFERENCES

1. Connolly BH. Tests and assessment. In: Connolly BH, Montgomery PC, eds. *Therapeutic Exercise in Developmental Disabilities.* Thorofare, NJ: SLACK; 2001:15-33.

2. Grifka RG. Cyanotic congenital heart disease with increased pulmonary blood flow. *Pediatr Clin North Am.* 1999; 46:405-425.

Musculoskeletal System

MARK DUTTON

INTRODUCTION

The musculoskeletal system is designed to accommodate the stresses of everyday life. There-fore, understanding the composition of these structures and their stress response is essential for the evidence-based practitioner. Also, it is important to understand the mechanisms behind how energy is provided to the musculoskeletal structures for them to perform optimally.

▲ HIGH-YIELD TERMS

Collagen	The main structural protein found throughout the various connective tissues.
Elastin	A component of connective tissue that is very good at resisting tensile loads and determines the patterns of distension and recoil in most organs.
Stress-strain curve	A graphical representation of the relationship between the stress and strain that a specific material displays.
Crimp	The first line of response to stress by collagen tissue; occurs in the toe phase of the stress-strain curve. When a load is applied, the fibers line up in the direction of the applied force.
Creep	The gradual rearrangement of collagen fibers, proteoglycans, and water because of a continuously applied force after the initial lengthening caused by crimp has ceased.
Kinetics	The term applied to define the forces acting on the body.
Stress relaxation	A phenomenon in which stress or force within a deformed structure decreases with time while the deformation is constant.
Stiffness	The inelasticity of an object and the degree to which the object resists deformation in response to an applied force.
Plastic deformation	Occurs when a tissue remains deformed and does not recover its prestress length.
Stress response	The method by which a tissue responds to applied stress. Exercises may be used to change the physical properties of muscles/tendons and ligaments, as both have demonstrated adaptability to external loads with an increase in strength: weight ratios. The improved strength results from an increase in proteogly-can content and collagen cross-links.
Viscoelasticity	The time-dependent mechanical property of a material to stretch or compress over time and return to its original shape when the force is removed.
Open (loose)-packed position	The joint position that results in a slackening of the major ligaments of the joint, minimal surface congru-ity, minimal joint surface contact, maximum joint volume, and minimal stability of the joint.

Close-packed position	The joint position of maximal tautness of the major ligaments, maximal surface congruity, minimal joint volume, and maximum stability of the joint.
Capsular pattern	A capsular pattern of restriction is a limitation of pain and movement in a joint-specific ratio, which is usually present with osteoarthritis or following prolonged immobilization.
Neutral zone	The zone within a joint's motion in which the tissues offer little or no internal resistance to movement and the range in which the tissue's crimp is taken up.
Elastic zone	The zone in which the first barrier or restriction to movement occurs; takes place at the end of the neutral zone. After that, the elastic zone extends from the crimp area through the physiologic barrier (end of the active movement) and the anatomic barrier (end of the passive movement).
Plastic zone	The zone in which the tissue's deformation is extended beyond the tissue's elastic recoil and the tissue begins to deform; injury can occur if the deformation is sufficient in time or load.
Concave-convex rule	A concept used with joint mobilizations. If the joint surface is convex relative to the other surface, the slide (arthrokinematic motion) is opposite the osteokinematic motion. If, on the other hand, the joint surface is concave, the slide takes place in the same direction as the osteokinematic motion.

◼ ANATOMY AND BIOMECHANICS

Posture and movement are both governed by the body's ability to control these forces. A wide range of external and internal forces are either generated or resisted by the human body during daily activities. The inherent ability of a tissue to tolerate **load** can be observed experimentally.

STRUCTURES OF THE MUSCULOSKELETAL SYSTEM

Connective Tissue

Connective tissue (CT) is found throughout the body. It provides structural and metabolic support for the body's tissues and organs, including bone, cartilage, tendons, ligaments, and blood tissue. These connective tissues are made up of two proteins: collagen and elastin. Collagenous and elastic fibers are sparse and irregularly arranged in loose CT but are tightly packed in dense CT. The various types of connective tissue found within the musculoskeletal system are outlined in Table 3-1. The major ligaments of the upper and lower quadrants are described in Tables 3-2 and 3-3. Finally, the general structure of bone and associated conditions are depicted in Table 3-4.

Skeletal Muscle

The myofiber (single muscle cell), wrapped in a CT envelope called endomysium, comprises thousands of myofibrils (Figure 3-1). Bundles of myofibers, which form a whole muscle (fasciculus), are encased in the perimysium. A connective sheath called the epimysium surrounds groups of muscles. Myofibrils are composed of sarcomeres (the contractile machinery of a muscle) arranged in series.

The graded contractions of whole muscles occur because the number of fibers participating in the contraction varies. Thus, increasing the force of the movement is achieved by recruiting more cells into cooperative action. Myofilaments, which have a striated appearance, consist primarily of two components:

- Actin (thin). I bands containing tropomyosin and troponin function as the switch for muscle contraction and relaxation (Figure 3-2). In a relaxed state, the tropomyosin physically blocks the cross-bridges from binding to the actin. Therefore, the tropomyosin must be removed before a contraction can occur.
- Myosin (thick). A bands. Motor proteins that interact with the actin filaments.

Each muscle fiber is limited by a cell membrane called a **sarcolemma**. A somatic motor neuron innervates each myofiber. One neuron and the muscle fibers it innervates constitute a motor unit, or functional unit, of the muscle. A skeletal muscle is capable of producing different types of contraction:

- Isometric. Static contraction without a change in length.

TABLE 3-1 • Various Types of Connective Tissue Within the Musculoskeletal System.

Type	Description	Function
Fascia	Loose connective tissue.	Provides support and protection for the joint and acts as an interconnection between tendons, aponeuroses, ligaments, capsules, nerves, and muscle.
Tendon	Dense regular connective tissue with three distinct sections: • Bone-tendon junction—absorbs and distributes stress and is therefore vulnerable to injury. • Tendon midsubstance. • Musculotendinous junction (MTJ). Very susceptible to tensile failure. Common sites of failure include the MTJ of the biceps and triceps brachii, rotator cuff muscles, flexor pollicis longus, fibularis (peroneus) longus, medial head of the gastrocnemius, rectus femoris, adductor longus, iliopsoas, pectoralis major, semimembranosus, and the whole hamstrings group.	Produces joint motion, stores elastic energy that contributes to movement when stretched, and allows for the optimal distance between the muscle belly and the joint it is acting upon. The main function of tendons is to transmit the load from muscle to bone. Designed to resist strong tensile loads well but are not designed to resist shear or compressive forces.
Ligaments	Dense regular connective tissue (except for the ligamentum flavum and the nuchal ligament, a small amount of elastin is found in ligaments). The midportion of a ligament is avascular with a reduced nerve supply, whereas the end portion is highly vascular and more densely innervated.	Serve to connect bones across joints. Prevent excessive joint motion/provide stability. Provide proprioceptive input.
Cartilage	Exists in three primary forms: • Hyaline (articular)—the most abundant cartilage in the body. It is avascular and aneural, and its thickness is determined by the degree of peak pressures (the higher the pressure, the thicker the cartilage); the patella has the thickest cartilage in the body. • Elastic. Found in the outer ear and larynx. • Fibrocartilage. Avascular, aneural, and alymphatic. Examples include symphysis pubis, glenoid labrum, hip labrum, triangular fibrocartilage complex (TFCC) of the wrist, the intervertebral disk, and the menisci of the knee.	Hyaline: Functions to distribute and dissipate forces. Covers the ends of long bones. Permits frictionless motion between the articular surfaces of diarthrodial (synovial) joints. Elastic: Provides strength and elasticity to maintain the shape of certain structures. Fibrocartilage: Primarily functions as a shock absorber.
Bone	A dynamic tissue that undergoes constant metabolism and remodeling. Two types are recognized: • Cortical. Forms the outer shell of a bone. • Cancellous. Forms the epiphyseal and metaphyseal regions of long bones and the interior aspect of short bones.	Functions to provide support, enhance leverage, protect vital structures, provide attachments for both tendons and ligaments, and store minerals, particularly calcium. The strength of bone is directly related to its density. Skeletal structures develop by one of two methods: • Intramembranous ossification by mesenchymal stem cells (cranium, facial bones, ribs, clavicle, mandible). • Endochondral ossification (appendicular and axial bones).

- Isotonic. Tension within a muscle remains constant as the muscle shortens or lengthens, although, in most contractions, the tension varies based on the weight used, joint velocity, muscle length, and contraction type.
- Concentric. Produces a shortening of the muscle.
- Eccentric. Muscle lengthens, resulting in maximum lengthening muscle tension. Capable of generating more force than isometric or concentric and is primarily used with activities that require deceleration.
- Isokinetic. Muscle maximally contracts at the same speed throughout the range of its related lever.

Muscle contractions occur at the neuromuscular junction (NMJ), or motor endplate, which is the area of contact between a nerve and the muscle fiber. For example, a contraction occurs in the following manner:

STUDY PEARL (CONTINUED)
present with a history of progressive pain that is constant and not relieved with rest.

- Fibrosarcoma. This type has a mesenchymal stem cell (bone marrow) origin and may arise within the medullary canal or from the periosteum. Most lesions occur around the knee, the proximal femur and hip region, or the proximal upper extremity. Again, pain and swelling are the most common findings.

TABLE 3-2 • Major Ligaments of the Upper Quadrant.

Joint	Ligament	Function
Shoulder complex	Coracoclavicular Costoclavicular	Fixes the clavicle to the coracoid process Fixes the clavicle to the costal cartilage of the first rib
Glenohumeral	Coracohumeral Glenohumeral ("Z") Coracoacromial	Reinforces the upper portion of the joint capsule Reinforces the anterior and inferior aspect of the joint capsule Protects the superior aspect of the joint
Elbow	Annular Ulnar (medial) collateral Radial (lateral) collateral	Maintains the relationship between the head of the radius and the humerus and ulna Provides stability against valgus (medial) stress, particularly in the range of 20-130° of flexion and extension Provides stability against varus (lateral) stresses and functions to maintain the ulno-humeral and radiohumeral joints in a reduced position when the elbow is loaded in supination
Wrist	Extrinsic palmar Intrinsic Interosseous	Provides the majority of the wrist stability Serves as rotational restraints, binding the proximal carpal row into a unit of rotational stability Binds the carpal bones together
Fingers	Anterior and collateral interphalangeal	Prevent displacement of the interphalangeal joints

TABLE 3-3 • Major Ligaments of the Spine and Lower Quadrant.

Joint	Ligament	Function
Spine	Anterior longitudinal ligament Posterior longitudinal ligament Ligamentum flavum Interspinous Iliolumbar (lower lumbar)	Functions as a minor assistant in limiting anterior translation and vertical separation of the vertebral body Resists vertebral distraction of the vertebral body Resists posterior shearing of the vertebral body Acts to limit flexion over several segments Provides some protection against intervertebral disk protrusions Resists separation of the lamina during flexion Resists separation of the spinous processes during flexion Resists flexion, extension, axial rotation, and side-bending of L5 on S1
Sacroiliac	Sacrospinous Sacrotuberous Interosseous Dorsal sacroiliac (long)	Creates the greater sciatic foramen Resists forward tilting of the sacrum on the ilium during weight-bearing Creates the lesser sciatic foramen Resists forward tilting (nutation) of the sacrum on the ilium during weight-bearing Resists anterior and inferior movement of the sacrum Resists backward tilting (counternutation) of the sacrum on the ilium during weight-bearing
Hip	Ligamentum teres Iliofemoral Ischiofemoral Pubofemoral	Transports nutrient vessels to the femoral head Limits hip extension Limits anterior displacement of the femoral head Limits hip extension
Knee	Medial collateral Lateral collateral Anterior cruciate Posterior cruciate	Stabilizes the medial aspect of the tibiofemoral joint against valgus stress Stabilizes the lateral aspect of the tibiofemoral joint against varus stress Resists anterior translation of the tibia and posterior translation of the femur Resists posterior translation of the tibia and anterior translation of the femur
Ankle	Medial collaterals (deltoid) Lateral collaterals	Provides stability between the medial malleolus, navicular, talus, and calcaneus against eversion Static stabilizers of the lateral ankle, especially against inversion
Foot	Long plantar Bifurcate Calcaneocuboid	Provides indirect plantar support to the calcaneocuboid joint by limiting the amount of flattening of the lateral longitudinal arch of the foot Supports the medial and lateral aspects of the foot when weight-bearing in a plantarflexed position Provides plantar support to the calcaneocuboid joint and possibly helps to limit flattening of the lateral longitudinal arch

TABLE 3-4 • General Structure of Bone.

Site	Comment	Conditions	Result
Epiphysis	Mainly develops under pressure Apophysis forms under traction Forms bone ends Supports articular surface	Epiphyseal dysplasias Joint surface trauma Overuse injury Damaged blood supply	Distorted joints Degenerative changes Fragmented development Avascular necrosis
Physis	Epiphyseal or growth plate Responsive to growth and sex hormones Vulnerable before growth spurt occurs Mechanically weak	Physeal dysplasia Trauma Slipped epiphysis	Short stature Deformed or angulated growth or growth arrest
Metaphysis	Remodeling expanded bone end Cancellous bone heals rapidly Vulnerable to osteomyelitis Affords ligament attachment	Osteomyelitis Tumors Metaphyseal dysplasia	Sequestrum formation Altered bone shape Distorted growth
Diaphysis	Forms shaft of the bone Large surface for muscle origin Significant compact cortical bone Strong in compression	Fractures Diaphyseal dysplasias Healing slower than at metaphysis	Able to remodel angulation Cannot remodel rotation Involucrum with infection Dysplasia gives altered density and shape

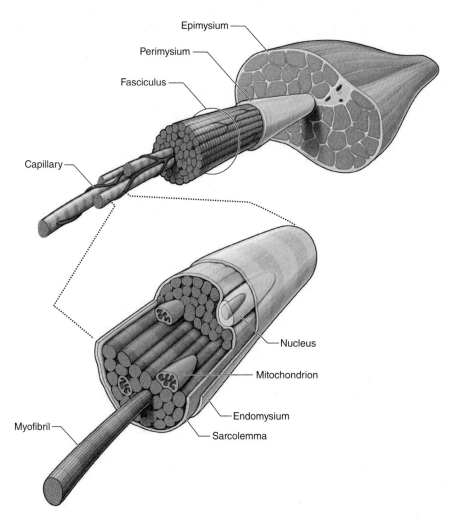

Figure 3-1. Microscopic structure of the muscle. (Reproduced with permission from Dutton M. *Dutton's Orthopaedic Examination, Evaluation and Intervention*, 4th ed. 2017. Copyright © McGraw Hill LLC. All rights reserved. https://accessphysiotherapy.mhmedical.com.)

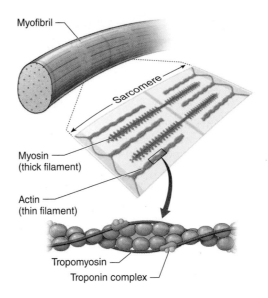

Figure 3-2. Troponin and tropomyosin action during a muscle contraction. (Reproduced with permission from Dutton M. *Dutton's Orthopaedic Examination, Evaluation and Intervention*, 4th ed. 2017. Copyright © McGraw Hill LLC. All rights reserved. https://accessphysiotherapy.mhmedical.com.)

STUDY PEARL (CONTINUED)
The most common time cancer is detected in physical therapy is during discussions with the patient. The physical therapist assistant (PTA) must be alert to any mention of pain unrelated to movement, especially at night, any unexplained growth or mass, or sudden weight loss.

STOP RED FLAG

The PTA needs to be aware of the more common bone tumors and their clinical manifestations and report any suspicions to the supervising PT immediately.

- Acetylcholine (ACh) is released at the NMJ.
- Calcium (Ca^{2+}) is released from the sarcoplasmic reticulum (SR). SR forms a network around the myofibrils, storing and providing Ca^{2+} required for a muscle contraction. As SR is associated with both contraction and relaxation, any change in its ability to release or sequester Ca^{2+} markedly affects both the time course and magnitude of force output by the muscle fiber.
- The Ca^{2+} diffuses into the sarcomeres, binds to troponin, and displaces the tropomyosin, thereby allowing the actin to bind with the myosin cross-bridges. Thus, whenever a somatic motor neuron is activated, all the muscle fibers it innervates are stimulated and contract with *all-or-none* twitches.

At the end of the contraction, the SR accumulates Ca^{2+} through active transport, requiring degradation of adenosine triphosphate (ATP) to adenosine diphosphate.

Several muscle fiber types exist (Tables 3-5 and 3-6):

- Type I. Tonic, slow-twitch. Used for endurance (aerobic) and stabilization activities—for example, postural, back, and trunk muscles.
- Type II. Phasic fast-twitch. Used for quick, explosive (anaerobic), and dynamic activities.

TABLE 3-5 • Comparison of Muscle Fiber Types.			
Characteristics	Type I	Type II A	Type IIx
Size (diameter)	Small	Intermediate	Very large
Resistance to fatigue	High	Fairly high	Low
Capillary density	High	High	Low
Glycogen content	Low	Intermediate	High
Twitch rate	Slow	Fast	Fast
Energy system	Aerobic	Aerobic	Anaerobic
Maximum muscle shortening velocity	Slow	Fast	Fast
Major storage fuel	Triglycerides	Creatine phosphate glycogen	Creatine phosphate glycogen

TABLE 3-6 • Functional Division of Muscle Groups.	
Movement Group	**Stabilization Group**
Primarily type II A	Primarily type I
Prone to adaptive shortening	Prone to develop weakness
Prone to develop hypertonicity	Prone to muscle inhibition
Dominate in fatigue and new movement situations	Fatigue easily
Generally cross two joints	Primarily cross one joint
Examples	*Examples*
Gastrocnemius/soleus	Fibularis (peronei)
Tibialis posterior	Tibialis anterior
Short hip adductors	Vastus medialis and lateralis
Hamstrings	Gluteus maximus, medius, and minimus
Rectus femoris	Serratus anterior
Tensor fascia lata	Rhomboids
Erector spinae	Lower portion of the trapezius
Quadratus lumborum	Short/deep cervical flexors
Pectoralis major	Upper limb extensors
Upper portion of the trapezius	Rectus abdominis
Levator scapulae	
Sternocleidomastoid	
Scalenes	
Upper limb flexors	

Data from Twomey LT, Taylor JR, eds. *Physical Therapy of the Low Back: Clinics in Physical Therapy. 1987.*
Copyright © Churchill Livingstone. All rights reserved.

Depending on the type and structure, skeletal muscle can serve many roles:

- Prime mover (agonist). Directly responsible for the desired movement.
- Antagonist. Produces an action directly opposite the agonist.
- Synergist (supporter). Provides cooperative muscle function relative to the agonist.

The effects of velocity can impact the quality of a muscle contraction:

- Concentric contractions. Inverse relationship (increased speed leads to a decreased force).
- Eccentric. Direct relationship (increased speeds lead to an increased force initially); during slow eccentric muscle actions, the work produced approximates an isometric contraction.

Muscle length can also impact the quality of a muscle contraction:

- Active insufficiency. A muscle in a shortened or excessively lengthened position places the actin/myosin cross-bridges at a disadvantage such that the muscle cannot fully shorten to produce a full range of motion (ROM). For example, the hamstrings may limit hip flexion when the knee is in full extension.
- Passive insufficiency. Occurs when a two-joint muscle cannot stretch to the extent required for full ROM in the opposite direction at all joints crossed. For example, when making a fist with the wrist fully flexed, the active shortening of the finger and wrist flexors results in a passive lengthening of the finger extensors.

CT disorders include systemic lupus erythematosus (SLE), rheumatoid arthritis (RA), spondyloarthropathies (eg, ankylosing spondylitis, reactive arthritis), polymyalgia rheumatica, polymyositis and dermatomyositis, scleroderma, Sjögren syndrome, crystal-induced arthropathies (eg, gout), and juvenile RA.

Joints
Several major joint types exist:

Synarthrosis

There are two types of synarthrosis:

- Fibrous joints. Formed from dense fibrous CT. Examples include suture (eg, skull), gomphosis (eg, tooth, maxilla, mandible), and syndesmosis (eg, tibiofibular joint, radioulnar joint).
- Cartilaginous. Generally stable joints with little movement (eg, symphysis pubis).

Diarthrosis (Synovial)

Provides greater mobility, unites long bones, the joint capsule contains synovial fluid. Several types exist:

- Simple (uniaxial) or hinge joint. An example is the humeroulnar joint.
- Compound (biaxial), or condyloid. Examples include the metacarpophalangeal (MCP) joint of the finger and the saddle joint of the thumb-carpometacarpal (CMC).
- Complex (multiaxial). These joints allow movement in and around three planes. In addition, they have an intra-articular inclusion within the joint, like a meniscus or disk, which increases the number of joint surfaces. An example is the ball-and-socket joint of the hip.
- Synovial. Synovial joints have some distinguishing characteristics:
  - A joint cavity enclosed by a capsule and which is composed of two layers.
  - Hyaline cartilage that covers the surfaces of the enclosed bones.
  - Synovial fluid provides joint lubrication, viscoelastic properties, and anti-inflammatory and antinociceptive properties. In addition to being found within joints, synovial fluid is also found in bursae (enclosed, round, flattened sacs lined with synovium and which function to separate exposed areas of bone from overlapping muscles [deep bursae], or skin and tendons [superficial bursae]).
  - A synovial membrane that lines the inner surface of the capsule.

MOVEMENTS OF THE BODY SEGMENTS

Movements of the body segments are described using a series of planes and axes. The more common planes of the body include (Figure 3-3):

- Sagittal (anterior-posterior, or median plane). Divides the body vertically into left and right halves of equal size.
- Frontal (coronal or lateral plane). Divides the body equally into front and back.
- Transverse (horizontal). Divides the body equally into top and bottom halves.

The axes of the body, around which movement occurs, are always perpendicular to the plane in which they occur. As with the planes of the body, there are three common types:

- Mediolateral or coronal axis: Perpendicular to the sagittal plane.
- Vertical or longitudinal axis: Perpendicular to the frontal plane.
- Anteroposterior (AP) axis: Perpendicular to the transverse plane.

Some familiar directional terms describe the relationship of body parts or an external object's location to the body. The following are commonly used directional terms:

- Superior or cranial: Closer to the head.
- Inferior or caudal: Closer to the feet.
- Anterior or ventral: Toward the front of the body.
- Posterior or dorsal: Toward the back of the body.
- Medial: Toward the midline of the body.
- Lateral: Away from the midline of the body.
- Proximal: Closer to the trunk.
- Distal: Away from the trunk.
- Superficial: Toward the surface of the body.
- Deep: Away from the surface of the body in the direction of the inside of the body.

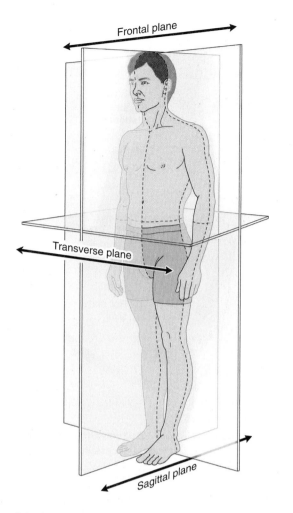

Figure 3-3. Planes of the body. (Reproduced with permission from Dutton M. *Dutton's Orthopaedic Examination, Evaluation and Intervention*, 4th ed. 2017. Copyright © McGraw Hill LLC. All rights reserved. https://accessphysiotherapy.mhmedical.com.)

The center of gravity (COG), or center of mass (COM), of the body, is the point at which all the mass of the object or segment is concentrated; the point at which the line of gravity balances the body (located at the S2 level in a rigid human body).

The body's base of support (BOS) includes the body part in contact with the supporting surface and the prevailing area. During static standing, the body's line of gravity is between the individual's feet, which serve as the BOS.

Joint Kinematics

Kinematics is the study of motion and describes how something is moving. Within the study of joint kinematics, two significant types of motion are commonly described: (1) osteokinematic and (2) arthrokinematic.

- Osteokinematic (bone movement). This includes physiologic movements that can be performed voluntarily, for example, flexion of the shoulder.
- Arthrokinematic (joint movement). This includes the motion of the bone surfaces within a joint. These movements cannot be performed voluntarily and can only occur when resistance to active motion is applied or when the patient's muscles are completely relaxed. The more common types of joint plane motion include the following:
  - Roll: The joint motion occurs in the same direction as the swinging bone, and compression of the joint surfaces occurs in the direction of the roll.
  - Slide: Translation of joint surfaces, also referred to as *translatory* motion. The shape of the articulating surface determines the direction of the slide. This concept is often

STUDY PEARL
Both the COG and BOS are important factors of balance and stability.

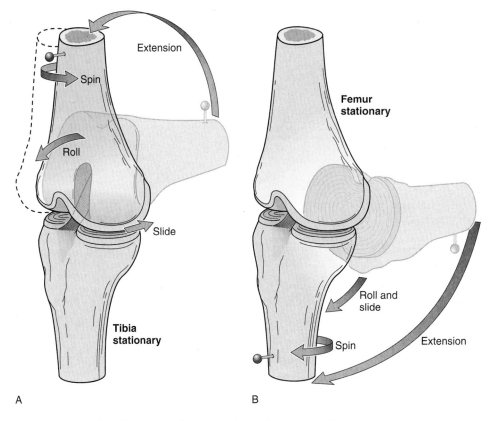

A   B

Figure 3-4. Arthrokinematics of motion. (Reproduced with permission from Dutton M. *Dutton's Orthopaedic Examination, Evaluation and Intervention*, 4th ed. 2017. Copyright © McGraw Hill LLC. All rights reserved. https://accessphysiotherapy.mhmedical.com.)

referred to as the *concave-convex rule* and is used when applying joint mobilizations (see **Appendix A**):

- If the joint surface is convex relative to the other surface, the slide occurs in the opposite direction to the osteokinematic motion (Figure 3-4).
- If the joint surface is concave, the slide takes place in the same direction as the osteokinematic motion (Figure 3-5).
- Spin: Involves a rotation of one surface on an opposing surface around a vertical axis, for example, rotation of the radial head during forearm pronation and supination.

A wide range of external and internal forces are either generated or resisted by the human body during daily activities. Examples of these external forces include ground reaction forces, gravity, and applied forces through contact. Examples of internal forces include muscle contraction, joint contact, and joint forces, including shear, compression, and tension (Figure 3-6).

The terms *strain* and *stress* have specific mechanical meanings. Strain is defined as the change in length of a material due to an imposed load, divided by the original length. Stress, or load, is given in units of force per area and is used to describe the type of force applied. As a clinical example, tendons display more elasticity at lower strain rates and more stiffness at higher tensile loading rates and deform less than ligaments.

The load-deformation curve, or stress-strain curve, of a structure (Figure 3-7) depicts the relationship between the amount of force applied to a structure and the structure's response regarding deformation or acceleration. The horizontal axis (deformation or strain) represents the ratio of the tissue's deformed length to its original length. The graph's vertical axis (load or stress) denotes the internal resistance generated as a tissue resists deformation, divided by its cross-sectional area. The load-deformation curve is split into four regions, with each region representing a biomechanical property of the tissue (Figure 3-7).

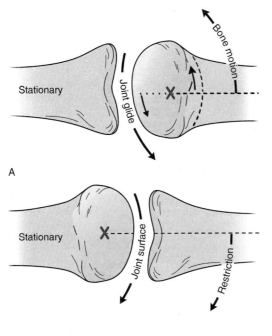

Figure 3-5. **Gliding motions according to joint surfaces.** (Reproduced with permission from Dutton M. *Dutton's Orthopaedic Examination, Evaluation and Intervention*, 4th ed. 2017. Copyright © McGraw Hill LLC. All rights reserved. https://accessphysiotherapy.mhmedical.com.)

The body uses different types of levers to reduce stress and strain by manipulating the mechanical advantage (MA) (Figure 3-8):

- First class. The fulcrum is located between two forces (eg, cervical flexion/extension). Therefore, the MA varies depending on the location of the axis of rotation.
- Second class (MA > 1). The load (resistance) is located between the fulcrum and the effort, so it takes less force to move the resistance (eg, heel raises).

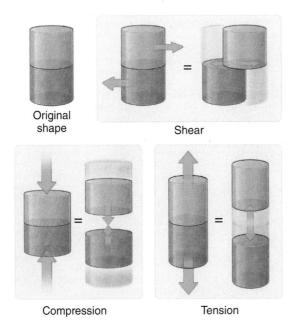

Figure 3-6. **Internal forces acting on the body.** (Reproduced with permission from Dutton M. *Dutton's Orthopaedic Examination, Evaluation and Intervention*, 4th ed. 2017. Copyright © McGraw Hill LLC. All rights reserved. https://accessphysiotherapy.mhmedical.com.)

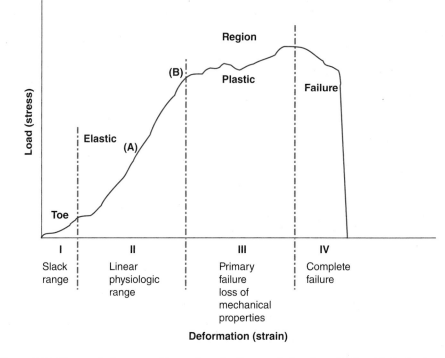

Figure 3-7. **Stress-strain curve.** (Reproduced with permission from Dutton M. *Dutton's Orthopaedic Examination, Evaluation and Intervention*, 4th ed. 2017. Copyright © McGraw Hill LLC. All rights reserved. https://accessphysiotherapy.mhmedical.com.)

- Third class (MA < 1). The load is located between the fulcrum and the load at the end of the lever and effort. Thus, the effort expended is greater than the load, but the load is moved a greater distance. Most moveable joints in the body use third-class levers (eg, flexion of the elbow).

The term *kinematic chain* is used in rehabilitation to describe an extremity or trunk's function or activity regarding a series of linked chains. The efficiency of an activity can be dependent on how well these chain links work together. Two types of kinematic chain

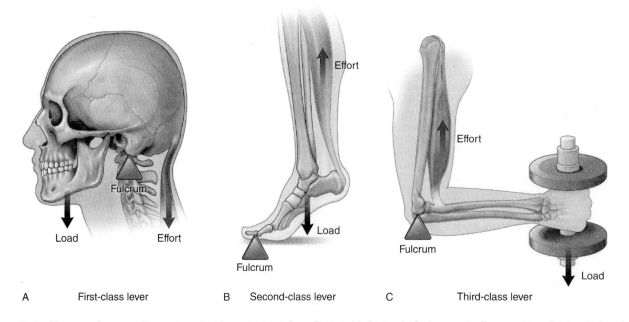

Figure 3-8. **Classes of levers.** (Reproduced with permission from Dutton M. *Dutton's Orthopaedic Examination, Evaluation and Intervention*, 4th ed. 2017. Copyright © McGraw Hill LLC. All rights reserved. https://accessphysiotherapy.mhmedical.com.)

TABLE 3-7 • Differential Features of OKC and CKC Exercises.

Exercise Mode	Characteristics	Advantages	Disadvantages
Open kinematic chain	1. Single muscle group 2. Single axis and plane 3. Emphasizes concentric contraction 4. Non–weight-bearing	1. Isolated recruitment 2. Simple movement pattern 3. Minimal joint compression	1. Limited function 2. Limited eccentrics 3. Less proprioception and joint stability with increased joint shear forces
Closed kinematic chain	1. Multiple muscle groups 2. Multiple axes and planes 3. Balance of concentric and eccentric contractions 4. Weight-bearing exercises	1. Functional recruitment 2. Functional movement patterns 3. Functional contractions 4. Increased proprioception and joint stability	1. Difficult to isolate 2. More complex 3. Loss of control of target joint 4. Compressive forces on articular surfaces

Data from Greenfield BH, Tovin BJ. The application of open and closed kinematic chain exercises in rehabilitation of the lower extremity. *J Back Musculoskel Rehabil.* 1992;2:38-51.

systems are recognized: *closed kinematic chain* (CKC) and *open kinematic chain* (OKC) systems (Table 3-7).

When referring to a joint's stability, the two terms, close-packed and open-packed, are commonly used.

Close-packed position (Table 3-8). A joint is said to be in its close-packed position when there is:

- Maximum congruity of joint surfaces.
- Maximum tautness of major ligaments.

TABLE 3-8 • Close-Packed Position of the Joints.

Joint	Position
Zygapophyseal (spine)	Extension
Temporomandibular	Teeth clenched
Glenohumeral	Abduction and external rotation
Acromioclavicular	Arm abducted to 90°
Sternoclavicular	Maximum shoulder elevation
Ulnohumeral	Extension
Radiohumeral	Elbow flexed 90°; forearm supinated 5°
Proximal radioulnar	5° of supination
Distal radioulnar	5° of supination
Radiocarpal (wrist)	Extension with radial deviation
Metacarpophalangeal	Full flexion
Carpometacarpal	Full opposition
Interphalangeal	Full extension
Hip	Full extension, internal rotation, and abduction
Tibiofemoral	Full extension and external rotation of the tibia
Talocrural (ankle)	Maximum dorsiflexion
Subtalar	Supination
Midtarsal	Supination
Tarsometatarsal	Supination
Metatarsophalangeal	Full extension
Interphalangeal	Full extension

TABLE 3-9 • Open-Packed (Resting) Position of the Joints.

Joint	Position
Zygapophyseal (spine)	Midway between flexion and extension
Temporomandibular	Mouth slightly open (freeway space)
Glenohumeral	55° of abduction, 30° of horizontal adduction
Acromioclavicular	Arm resting by the side
Sternoclavicular	Arm resting by the side
Ulnohumeral	70° of flexion, 10° of supination
Radiohumeral	Full extension, full supination
Proximal radioulnar	70° of flexion, 35° of supination
Distal radioulnar	10° of supination
Radiocarpal (wrist)	Neutral with slight ulnar deviation
Carpometacarpal	Midway between abduction-adduction and flexion-extension
Metacarpophalangeal	Slight flexion
Interphalangeal	Slight flexion
Hip	30° of flexion, 30° of abduction, slight lateral rotation
Tibiofemoral	25° of flexion
Talocrural (ankle)	10° of plantarflexion, midway between maximum inversion and eversion
Subtalar	Midway between the extremes of the range of movement
Midtarsal	Midway between the extremes of the range of movement
Tarsometatarsal	Midway between the extremes of the range of movement
Metatarsophalangeal	Neutral
Interphalangeal	Slight flexion

- Minimum joint volume.
- Maximum stability.

STUDY PEARL
The close-packed position is often associated with a fall on an outstretched hand (FOOSH) injury.

Open-packed position (Table 3-9). A joint is said to be in its open-packed position when there is:

- Slackening of the major ligaments.
- Minimal joint surface congruity and contact.
- Maximum joint volume.
- Minimal stability.

STUDY PEARL
The open-packed position of the joint is often associated with capsular and ligamentous injuries. Because this position places the joint in its most relaxed position, the open-packed position is commonly used in joint mobilization interventions.

A **capsular pattern of restriction** (Table 3-10) is a limitation of pain and movement in a joint-specific ratio, which is usually present with arthritis or following prolonged immobilization. Thus, the passive range of motion (PROM) for that joint will be limited in a capsular pattern, and there will be decreased joint play movement. However, it is worth remembering that a consistent capsular pattern for a particular joint might not exist and that these patterns are based on empirical findings and tradition rather than on research.

The quality of resistance encountered by the clinician at the end range of passive motion is referred to as the **end feel**. The end feel is evaluated for quality and tenderness, as it can indicate to the clinician the cause of the motion restriction (Tables 3-11 and 3-12).

TABLE 3-10 • Capsular Patterns of Restriction.	
Joint	**Limitation of Motion (Passive Angular Motion)**
Glenohumeral	External rotation > abduction > internal rotation (3:2:1)
Acromioclavicular	No true capsular pattern; possible loss of horizontal adduction and pain (and sometimes slight loss of end range) with each motion
Sternoclavicular	See acromioclavicular joint
Humeroulnar	Flexion > extension (±4:1)
Humeroradial	No true capsular pattern; possible equal limitation of pronation and supination
Superior radioulnar	No true capsular pattern; possible equal limitation of pronation and supination with pain at end ranges
Inferior radioulnar	No true capsular pattern; possible equal limitation of pronation and supination with pain at end ranges
Wrist (carpus)	Flexion = extension
Radiocarpal	See wrist (carpus)
Carpometacarpal	Flexion = extension
Midcarpal	Flexion = extension
Carpometacarpal 1	Retroposition
Carpometacarpals 2-5	Fan > fold
Metacarpophalangeal 2-5	Flexion > extension (±2:1)

Interphalangeal 2-5
  Proximal (PIP)
  Distal (DIP)
	Flexion > extension (±2:1)
	Flexion > extension (±2:1)

Hip	Internal rotation > flexion > abduction = extension > other motions
Tibiofemoral	Flexion > extension (±5:1)
Superior tibiofibular	No capsular pattern; pain at the end range of translatory movements
Talocrural	Plantarflexion > dorsiflexion
Talocalcaneal (subtalar)	Varus > valgus
Midtarsal	Inversion (plantarflexion, adduction, and supination)
Talonavicular calcaneocuboid	> Dorsiflexion
Metatarsophalangeal 1	Extension > flexion (±2:1)
Metatarsophalangeals 2-5	Flexion ≥ extension

Interphalangeals 2-5
  Proximal
  Distal
	Flexion ≥ extension
	Flexion ≥ extension

DIP, distal interphalangeal; PIP, proximal interphalangeal.
Data from Cyriax J. *Textbook of Orthopaedic Medicine, Diagnosis of Soft Tissue Lesions*, 8th ed. 1982. Copyright © Bailliere Tindall. All rights reserved.

The term **arc of pain** describes temporary pain that occurs during active or passive motion but disappears before the end of the movement. The presence of a painful arc indicates that some structure is being compressed:

- A painful arc associated with a positive resistive test (for pain) usually indicates a contractile lesion.
- A painful arc associated with a negative resistive test (for pain) usually indicates an inert lesion.

A joint can be described as being normal, **hypomobile**, **hypermobile**, or **unstable**.

- *Hypomobile.* A joint that moves less than normal when compared to the same joint on the opposite extremity. A contracture of CT may cause hypomobility. The presence of

TABLE 3-11 • Normal End Feels.		
Type	**Cause**	**Characteristics and Examples**

Bony	Produced by bone-to-bone approximation	Abrupt and unyielding; it gives the impression that further forcing will break something
		Examples:
		  Normal: elbow extension
		  Abnormal: cervical rotation (may indicate osteophyte)

Elastic	Produced by the muscle-tendon unit; may occur with adaptive shortening	Stretches with elastic recoil and exhibits constant-length phenomenon; further forcing feels as if it will snap something
		Examples:
		  Normal: wrist flexion with finger flexion, the straight leg raise, and ankle dorsiflexion with the knee extended
		  Abnormal: decreased dorsiflexion of the ankle with the knee flexed

Soft tissue approximation	Produced by contact of two muscle bulks on either side of a flexing joint where joint range exceeds other restraints	Very forgiving end feel that gives the impression that further normal motion is possible if enough force could be applied
		Examples:
		  Normal: knee flexion and elbow flexion in extremely muscular subjects
		  Abnormal: elbow flexion with obese subject

Capsular	Produced by capsule or ligaments	Various degrees of stretch without elasticity; the ability to stretch is dependent on the thickness of the tissue
		Strong capsular or extracapsular ligaments produce a hard capsular end feel, whereas a thin capsule produces a softer one
		The impression given to the clinician is that if further force is applied, something will tear
		Examples:
		  Normal: wrist flexion (soft), elbow flexion in supination (medium), and knee extension (hard)
		  Abnormal: inappropriate stretchability for a specific joint; if too hard, may indicate hypomobility due to arthrosis; and if too soft, hypermobility

Data from Meadows JTS. *Manual Therapy: Biomechanical Assessment and Treatment, Advanced Technique.* 1995. Copyright © Swodeam Consulting. All rights reserved.

TABLE 3-12 • Abnormal End Feels.		
Type	**Causes**	**Characteristics and Examples**

Springy	Produced by articular surface rebounding from intra-articular meniscus or disk; the impression is that if forced further, something will give way	Rebound sensation as if pushing off from a rubber pad
		Examples:
		  Normal: axial compression of cervical spine
		  Abnormal: knee flexion or extension with displaced meniscus

Boggy	Produced by viscous fluid (blood) within joint	"Squishy" sensation as joint is moved toward its end range; further forcing feels as if it will burst joint
		Examples:
		  Normal: none
		  Abnormal: hemarthrosis at the knee

(Continued)

TABLE 3-12 • Abnormal End Feels. (*Continued*)

Type	Causes	Characteristics and Examples
Spasm	Produced by reflex and reactive muscle contraction in response to irritation of nociceptor, predominantly in articular structures and muscle; forcing it further feels as if nothing will give	Abrupt and "twangy" end to the movement that is unyielding while the structure is being threatened but disappears when threat is removed (kicks back) With joint inflammation, it occurs early in range, especially toward a close-packed position, to prevent further stress With irritable joint hypermobility, it occurs at the end of what should be the normal range, as it prevents excessive motion from further stimulating the nociceptor Spasm in grade II muscle tears becomes apparent as muscle is passively lengthened and is accompanied by a painful weakness of that muscle *Note:* Muscle guarding is not a true end feel, as it involves cocontraction *Examples:* Normal: none Abnormal: significant traumatic arthritis, recent traumatic hypermobility, and grade II muscle tears
Empty	Produced solely by pain; frequently caused by serious and severe pathologic changes that do not affect joint or muscle and so do not produce spasm; demonstration of this end feel is, except for acute subdeltoid bursitis, de facto evidence of serious pathology; further forcing just increases pain to unacceptable levels	Limitation of motion has no tissue resistance component, and resistance is from the patient being unable to tolerate further motion due to severe pain; it is not the same feeling as voluntary guarding, but rather it feels as if the patient is both resisting and trying to allow movement simultaneously *Examples:* Normal: none Abnormal: acute subdeltoid bursitis and sign of the buttock
Facilitation	Not truly an end feel, as facilitated hypertonicity does not restrict motion; it can, however, be perceived near end range	Light resistance as from constant light muscle contraction throughout the latter half of range that does not prevent the end of the range from being reached; resistance is unaffected by the rate of movement *Examples:* Normal: none Abnormal: spinal facilitation at any level

hypomobility in the absence of contraindications indicates joint mobilizations as the intervention of choice.

- *Hypermobile.* A joint that moves more than normal is considered normal compared to the same joint on the opposite extremity. May occur as a generalized phenomenon or be localized to just one direction of movement—the result of damaged CT. The presence of hypermobility is a contraindication to joint mobilizations.

- *Unstable.* An unstable joint disrupts joint's bony and ligamentous structures, resulting in function loss. Joint instability is a factor of joint integrity, elastic energy, passive stiffness, and muscle activation.

■ QUESTIONS

1. **Which of the following best describes the characteristics of hyaline cartilage?**
   A. Distributes forces, is avascular and aneural, and is located in diarthrosis joints.
   B. Distributes forces, is highly vascular, contains free-nerve endings, and is located in fibrocartilaginous joints.
   C. Resists compressive forces, is highly vascular and aneural, and is located within synovial joints.
   D. Resists compressive forces, is avascular, contains free-nerve endings, and is located in synarthrodial joints.

2. **Which type of connective tissue (CT) in the musculoskeletal system is made up of dense CT and provides joint stability and proprioceptive input?**
   A. Fascia
   B. Tendons
   C. Ligaments
   D. Cartilage

3. **Which of the following joint categories best describes the classification of the intermetatarsal joint?**
   A. Spheroid
   B. Trochoid
   C. Planar
   D. Saddle

4. **A patient performing a bicep curl with a 10-lb weight in his/her hand is an example of which type of lever?**
   A. First-class lever
   B. Second-class lever
   C. Third-class lever
   D. Fourth-class lever

5. **After the initial lengthening caused by crimp, what is the term that describes the gradual rearrangement of collagen fibers, proteoglycans, and water due to a continuously applied force?**
   A. Creep
   B. Tension
   C. Stress-strain curve
   D. Elasticity

6. **What is the protein that fibroblasts produce?**
   A. Albumin
   B. Collagen
   C. Actin
   D. Myosin

7. **The heel raise exercise (rising on the toes) is an example of which type of lever?**
   A. First-class lever
   B. Second-class lever
   C. Third-class lever
   D. Fourth-class lever

■ ANSWERS WITH RATIONALES

1. **The answer is A.** Hyaline cartilage contains no nerves or blood vessels and is found on the anterior ends of ribs, in the larynx, trachea, and bronchi, and on the articulating surfaces of bones.

2. **The answer is C.** Ligaments function as check-reins to joint motion.

3. **The answer is C.** The intermetatarsal joints, which are a good example of a planar joint, are the articulations between the base of metatarsal bones.

4. **The answer is C.** The third-class lever has the input force between the output force and the fulcrum. So the elbow joint is the fulcrum, the 10-lb weight is the resistance/load, and the force is the biceps muscle when the elbow is flexed.

5. **The answer is A.** Creep is the time-dependent elongation of tissue when subjected to constant stress.

6. **The answer is B.** Fibroblasts are cells within connective tissue that synthesize the extracellular matrix and form collagen.

7. **The answer is B.** A second-class lever has the fulcrum at one end, the effort (which is always less than the load) on the opposite end, and the load in the middle.

■ TISSUE RESPONSE TO INJURY

Maintaining the health of the various tissues is a delicate balance because insufficient, excessive, or repetitive stresses can prove harmful. Fortunately, most tissues have an inherent ability to self-heal—a process that is an intricate phenomenon.

▲ HIGH-YIELD TERMS TO LEARN

Macrotrauma	Typically, a severity of force sufficient to cause an immediate injury.
Microtrauma	Typically lacks enough force to cause an immediate injury.
Injury classifications	Acute, subacute, chronic, and acute on chronic.
Stages of healing	Coagulation and inflammation (acute), migratory and proliferative (subacute), and remodeling (chronic).
Osteoarthritis	A disease process resulting from the failure of chondrocytes to repair damaged articular cartilage in synovial joints.
Osteoporosis	A disease process in which new bone creation does not keep up with old bone removal.
Sarcopenia	Refers specifically to the universal, involuntary decline in lean body mass that can occur with age, primarily due to the loss of skeletal muscle volume.

TISSUE INJURY

The two major types of tissue injury are as follows:

- Macrotrauma (primary). Acute stress (loading) of a single force large enough to cause injury to biological tissues. It can be self-inflicted, caused by another individual or entity, or caused by the environment. The acute stress/load is sufficient to cause injury to biological tissues.
- Microtrauma (secondary). This type of injury occurs when repeated or chronic stress over some time causes an injury. Microtraumatic injuries, which include tendinopathy, tenosynovitis, and bursitis, can be intrinsic or extrinsic:
  - Intrinsic factors: Physical characteristics that predispose an individual to microtrauma injuries, for example, muscle imbalances, leg length discrepancies, anatomic anomalies.
  - Extrinsic factors: The most common cause of microtrauma. Related to external conditions by which the activity is performed, for example, training errors, type of terrain, environmental temperature, or incorrect use of equipment.

An injury to the musculoskeletal system can be classified as follows:

- Acute. Acute injuries are usually caused by macrotrauma or refer to the early phase of injury and healing, the latter of which typically lasts 4 to 6 days. An acute injury is characterized by:
  - Swelling (due to an increase in the permeability of the venules, plasma proteins, and leukocytes, which leak into the site of injury).
  - Redness.
  - Heat.
  - Impairment or loss of function.
- Subacute. A subacute injury typically lasts 10 to 17 days after the acute phase has ended, but it can last for weeks in tissues with limited circulation (eg, tendons). From a clinical perspective, the "active" swelling and local erythema of the inflammatory stage is usually no longer present. However, residual swelling may still be present at this time and resist reabsorption.
- Chronic. The chronic stage of healing has several definitions but usually refers to the final stage of healing, which occurs 26 to 34 days after injury but can last up to 1 year depending on the amount of damage and the type of tissue involved. Because this phase may last

STUDY PEARL
There is typically pain at rest or with active motion in the presence of an acute injury or when specific stress is applied to the injured structure.

several months or even years, it is extremely important to continue applying controlled stresses to the tissue long after healing appears to have occurred.

- Acute on chronic. This is not a normal stage of healing but an acute exacerbation of a chronic condition.

TISSUE HEALING

Some of the factors that can impact healing include the following:

- The extent of the injury. Large tears cause more tissue having to be repaired.
- Age. The ability to heal decreases with age.
- Drugs. Nonsteroidal anti-inflammatory drugs (NSAIDs) and corticosteroids reduce inflammation and swelling, but the latter must be used judiciously.
- Edema. Increased pressure can impede nutrition and inhibit neuromuscular control.
- Obesity. Oxygen pressure is lower.
- Absorbent dressings. The epithelium regenerates twice as quickly in a moist environment.
- Hemorrhage. Similar negative effects to edema.
- Malnutrition. Need protein and vitamins essential for healing.
- Temperature. Hypothermia adversely affects healing.
- Poor vascular supply. Inadequate nutrition to the healing tissues.
- Hormone levels. Affect composition and structure of tissues.
- Infection. Inhibits healing processes.
- Muscle spasm. Causes tension in already torn tissue; impedes approximation.
- Comorbidities. Preexisting conditions such as diabetes, obesity, congestive heart failure can hinder tissue healing.
- Excessive scarring. Can reduce blood flow.

Three major stages of healing are recognized in Table 3-13.

SPECIFIC TISSUE BEHAVIOR, INJURY, HEALING, AND TREATMENT

The various musculoskeletal tissues respond and heal based on morphology.

Muscle

Behavior. Muscle behaves in a variety of ways in response to stress/injury, each of which depends on the following:

- Age. There is decreased cross-sectional area of muscle, with decreased type II fibers being the most impacted. This loss can be minimized or reversed with exercise. A particular muscle fiber atrophy can occur with aging (senescence sarcopenia), resulting in a 20% to 25% loss of skeletal mass and a reduced power output from the muscles.
- Temperature. There is an inverse temperature-elastic modulus relationship whereby increased temperature results in increased elasticity and decreased stiffness.

TABLE 3-13 • Stages of Wound Healing.	
Stage	**General Characteristics**
Coagulation and inflammation (acute)	The area is red, warm, swollen, and painful Pain is present without any motion of the involved area Usually lasts 48-72 hours but can last as long as 7-10 days
Migratory and proliferative (subacute)	The pain usually occurs with activity or motion of the involved area Usually lasts 10 days to 6 weeks
Remodeling (chronic)	The pain usually occurs after activity Usually lasts 6 weeks to 12 months

TABLE 3-14 • Classification of Muscle Injury.	
Type	**Related Factors**
Exercise-induced muscle injury (delayed muscle soreness)	Increased activity Unaccustomed activity Excessive eccentric work Viral infections Secondary to muscle cell damage
Strains	
First degree (mild): minimal structural damage; minimal hemorrhage; early resolution Second degree (moderate): partial tear; a large spectrum of injury; significant early functional loss Third degree (severe): complete tear; may require aspiration; may require surgery	Onset at 24-48 hours after exercise Sudden overstretch Sudden contraction Decelerating limb Insufficient warm-up Lack of flexibility Increasing severity of strain associated with greater muscle fiber death, more hemorrhage, and more eventual scarring Steroid use or abuse Previous muscle injury Collagen disease
Contusions Mild, moderate, severe Intramuscular vs intermuscular	A direct blow, associated with increasing muscle trauma and tearing of fiber proportionate to the severity

- Immobilization or disuse. If a muscle is immobilized in a shortened position, it becomes less capable of producing force, and its shorter length makes it more susceptible to a stretching injury. In contrast, if a muscle is immobilized in its lengthened position, it can produce greater force requiring a more significant change in length to cause a tear than in a nonimmobilized muscle.

Injury. Muscle strains are the most common injury in sports. A muscle injury can be classified in several ways based on severity (Table 3-14). Some factors that contribute to muscle injury include the following:

- Inadequate flexibility.
- Inadequate strength or endurance.
- Dyssynergistic muscle contraction.
- Insufficient warm-up.
- Inadequate rehabilitation from a previous injury.

Healing. A muscle tends to heal in three phases:

- Destruction phase. This phase is associated with muscle atrophy, with the amount of atrophy dependent on the usage before the injury and the muscle's original function. For example, antigravity muscles (eg, quadriceps) are more prone to atrophy than their antagonists (eg, hamstrings). Research has demonstrated that a single bout of exercise can protect against muscle damage, with the effects lasting between 6 and 9 months.
- Repair phase. This phase typically involves three steps: hematoma formation, matrix formation, and collagen formation.
- Remodeling phase. During this phase, the application of controlled mobility and stress is necessary for proper healing.

Treatment. The type of treatment to use for a muscle injury depends on the stage of healing. All or some of the following can be used:

- Prevention and patient education.
- Controlled mobility and activity.

- Medications (pain and anti-inflammatory) and modalities.
- Exercise progression initiated with PROM, then active-assisted range of motion (AAROM), then active range of motion (AROM), then submaximal isometrics within the protective range, then throughout the whole range, then maximum isometrics in multiple angles, then throughout the whole range, then progressive resisted exercises (PREs).

Tendon

Behavior. Because the collagen fibers are more parallel in tendons than in ligaments, the toe region of the stress-strain curve is smaller in tendons than ligaments since less realignment occurs. The muscle-tendon junction (MTJ) is the weakest point in the muscle-tendon unit; therefore, strain injuries are common here.

Injury. Several terms were traditionally used for tendon injuries, including tendinosis and tendinitis. However, these terms have recently been encompassed into the umbrella term of tendinopathy:

- Tendinopathy. A clinical syndrome characterized by pain, swelling, and impaired performance, often implying overuse of a tendon. The most common tendinopathies occur at the patellar and Achilles tendons in the lower extremity and the supraspinatus tendon and extensor carpi radialis brevis (ECRB) tendons in the upper extremity.

Stages of Healing. A tendon heals during several stages.

- Inflammatory response (but only if the acute tendon injury disrupts vascular tissues within the tendon). During this phase, a hematoma forms within erythrocytes and platelets, and there is an infiltration of inflammatory cells.
- Repair. Deposition of collagen and tendon matrix components.
- Remodeling. Collagen structure and organization. It is worth noting that an injured tendon never achieves its original histologic or mechanical features.

Treatment. The treatment approach for tendons has changed over the years. There is no longer an emphasis on anti-inflammatory strategies since studies have consistently shown an absence of inflammatory infiltrates with tendinopathy. Instead, the following approach is currently recommended:

- Eccentric exercises. This type of exercise produces about 20% more load on the tendon than concentric training.
- Pain control—modalities and isometric exercises.
- Addressing the entire kinetic chain.
- Identification and removal of all negative internal and external forces/factors.

Ligament

Behavior. A ligament loses mass, stiffness, structural strength, and viscosity with age. Also, loss of ligament strength and stiffness occurs with low deprivation. In contrast, movement/exercise can maintain and enhance ligament strength and stiffness.

Injury (Sprains). Ligament injuries typically occur when an applied load is sufficient to deform a taut ligament beyond its elastic (recovery) limit. A ligament injury is characterized by the following:

- Point tenderness.
- Joint effusion.
- History of trauma.

If sufficient, damage to the ligament can result in loss of joint stability. The classification of ligament injuries is outlined in Table 3-15.

TABLE 3-15 • Ligament Injuries.			
Grade	Description	Signs and Symptoms	Implications
I (mild)	Some stretching or tearing of the ligamentous fibers	Mild pain Little or no swelling Some joint stiffness Minimal loss of structural integrity No abnormal motion Minimal bruising	Minimal functional loss Early return to training—some protection may be necessary
II (moderate)	Some tearing and separation of the ligamentous fibers	Moderate-to-severe pain Joint stiffness Significant structural weakening with abnormal motion Often associated hemarthrosis and effusion	Tendency to recurrence Need protection from the risk of further injury May need modifying immobilization May stretch out further with time
III (complete)	Total rupture of the ligament	Severe pain initially followed by little or no pain (total disruption of nerve fibers) Profuse swelling and bruising Loss of structural integrity with marked abnormal motion	Needs prolonged protection Surgery may be considered Often permanent functional instability

Stages of Healing. The process of healing for ligaments is essentially the same as for other vascular tissues. Normal healing occurs in four phases: hemorrhagic (hematoma fills the tissue gap), inflammatory (influx of macrophages and growth factors), proliferation (fibroblasts to produce collagen and the initial matrix), and remodeling/maturation (organization of matrix). Although the healing tissue matures, it never regains preinjury/normal quality. Total healing can take as long as 3 years—a ligament may reach 50% of its normal tensile strength by 6 months and 80% after 1 year.

Treatment. The treatment of a ligament injury depends on the location and severity but generally follows these guidelines:

- Minimization of immobilization time. A prolonged period of immobilization dramatically compromises the properties of ligaments.
- Controlled mobility. Very low cyclical loads make ligaments stronger and structurally stiffer.
- Transverse friction massage (TFM).

More invasive techniques include the following:

- Surgical repair.
- Growth factors.
- Gene therapy.

Articular Cartilage

Behavior. In general, articular cartilage demonstrates low metabolic activity and poor regenerative capacity. In addition, with increasing age, there is increased cartilage stiffness, resulting in increased stresses to subchondral bone. Also, immobilization results in degenerative changes similar to those found in osteoarthritis (OA).

Injury. Degradation of articular cartilage occurs because of an imbalance between extracellular matrix (ECM) synthesis and degradation (eg, OA). Stress deprivation (eg, immobilization or bed rest) can have a similar effect. Other causes of articular cartilage damage include the following factors:

STUDY PEARL
Intra-articular ligaments (ie, the anterior cruciate ligament [ACL]) do not heal as well as extra-articular ligaments due to the limited blood supply and the presence of synovial fluid, which can hinder the inflammatory process.

- Developmental etiologies leading to an abnormal force transmission (eg, hip dysplasia, coxa valgus, genu valgum).
- Joint surface incongruity and instability.
- Disease (eg, rheumatoid arthritis [RA]).

Three major types of injury are typically cited:

- Type I: Superficial. Characterized by microscopic damage to chondrocytes and ECM (cell injury).
- Type II: Partial thickness. Characterized by microscopic disruption of the chondral surface (chondral fractures or fissuring). This type has a poorer prognosis due to the lack of penetration of the subchondral bone and therefore no inflammatory response.
- Type III: Full thickness. Characterized by disruption of the articular cartilage with infiltration of the subchondral bone and significant inflammatory response.

Healing

- Limited capacity, dependent on the depth of injury.
- Type I and II tissues become necrotic and do not repair; progress to degeneration.
- Type III tissues undergo repair as a result of access to bone-blood supply.
  - Repaired tissue is different than normal hyaline cartilage; 50% result in fibrillation, fissuring, and extensive degenerative changes.
  - Degenerated cartilage in OA does not usually undergo repair but instead progressively degenerates.

> **STUDY PEARL**
> As the articular cartilage is avascular, there is no inflammatory phase of healing.

Treatment. The treatment approach for articular cartilage varies but typically includes a combination of the following:

- Exhaustion of conservative measures to avoid significant reconstructive surgery. Typical conservative measures include attempts to decrease joint pain and improve function through modalities, patient education, low-impact aerobic exercise, and ROM and strengthening exercises.
- Pharmacologic pain control (NSAIDs, opioid analgesics, intra-articular corticosteroid injections).
- Unloading braces to decrease joint stress.
- Intra-articular viscosupplementation.
- Mesenchymal stem cells.
- Surgical management.

Bone

Behavior. Bone tissue reacts well to compression but not to tension. The health of the bone matrix, which is an organic mineral, and fluid is influenced by diet, hormone levels, and biomechanics. In particular, exercise has been shown to result in increased cortical thickness and mineral content.

Injury. In general, injury to bone tissue involves some form of fracture. The most commonly encountered fracture for the physical therapist is the stress fracture, a fatigue fracture of the bone caused by repeated submaximal stress.

The diagnostic indicators for stress fractures include the following:

- X-rays; however, a fracture is often not apparent if x-rays are taken too early in the course.
- Bone scan.
- Magnetic resonance imaging (MRI).

> **STUDY PEARL**
> Eighty percent to 90% of stress fractures occur in the lower limb, with the tibia being the most common site (50%).

Some diseases, including osteoarthritis and osteoporosis, can cause bone (pathological) fractures.

Healing. The healing of bone occurs through the repair of the original tissue and not by scar tissue. Two types of bone healing are recognized:

- Primary (cortical). Cortical healing unites the cortex.
- Secondary (callus). Responses occur in the periosteum and external soft tissues with subsequent formation of callus. The majority of fractures heal by secondary fracture healing.

The stages of bone healing include the following:

- Hematoma formation (inflammatory) phase.
- Soft callus formation (reparative or revascularization) phase.
- Hard callus formation (modeling) phase.
- Remodeling phase.

The determinants of fracture healing include the following:

- Angiogenesis.
- The amount of movement at the fracture ends. Small degrees of micromotion aid in healing due to stimulation of blood flow, but excessive motion prevents the establishment of intramedullary blood vessel bridging.
- Environment.
- Hormones impact osteoblastic and osteoclastic activities.

The following techniques are occasionally required to augment healing:

- Pulsed electromagnetic fields (PEMF); stimulates cellular repair.
- Pulsed ultrasound.
- Direct current.
- Demineralized bone matrix (DBM).

Treatment. The treatment for a bone fracture depends on the location and level of severity but typically includes some or all of the following:

- Stabilization of the fracture site through casting. During this period, submaximal isometrics are introduced and progressed to ROM exercises once a clinical union is confirmed.
- Surgery, if indicated. Postsurgical complications can include the following:
- Infection.
- Deep vein thrombosis (DVT).
- Pulmonary embolism (PE).
- Poor wound healing.
- Scars and adhesions.

■ QUESTIONS

1. **Which of the following primary cells are involved in the proliferation phase of healing?**
   A. Fibroblasts
   B. Macrophages
   C. Leukocytes
   D. Osteoclasts

2. **If a patient sustained an injury 18 days ago and progressed appropriately through the phases of healing, what is the expected stage of healing?**
   A. Coagulation
   B. Inflammatory
   C. Proliferative
   D. Remodeling

3. **Which of the following tissues requires satellite cells to proliferate for proper healing to occur?**
   A. Tendon
   B. Ligament
   C. Bone
   D. Muscle

4. **Which of the following is an age-associated change in a tissue?**
   A. Decreased muscle power
   B. Increased number of sarcomeres in series
   C. Increased crimp in a tendon
   D. Decreased stiffness of tendinous tissue

5. **Which of the following tissues respond best to very low cyclic loading to promote scar proliferation and material remodeling?**
   A. Muscle
   B. Tendon
   C. Ligament
   D. Bone

■ ANSWERS WITH RATIONALES

1. **The answer is A.** Fibroblasts produce the structural framework for tissues during wound healing.

2. **The answer is C.** The proliferative phase of wound healing, which occurs approximately after 3 days and lasts for 21 days, involves the rebuilding of the wound with new tissue made up of collagen and extracellular matrix.

3. **The answer is D.** Satellite cells are precursors to skeletal muscle cells.

4. **The answer is A.** Decreased muscle power is the only one that occurs from the choices given. The decrease in muscle power can be reduced with strengthening exercises.

5. **The answer is C.** Ligaments require controlled motion to heal effectively.

■ ENERGY SYSTEMS

When a person undertakes work or exercise, some of the body systems adapt to the demands of the required tasks, particularly the cardiorespiratory and neuromuscular systems.

▲ HIGH-YIELD TERMS TO LEARN

Aerobic	Relating to or denoting exercise that improves or is intended to improve the body's cardiovascular system's efficiency in absorbing and transporting oxygen. Refers to the use of oxygen to adequately meet energy demands during exercise via aerobic metabolism.
Anaerobic	A metabolism that does not depend on oxygen. Anaerobic exercise is powered primarily by metabolic pathways that do not use oxygen. Such pathways produce lactic acid, resulting in metabolic acidosis. Examples of anaerobic exercise include sprinting and heavy weight lifting.
Adenosine triphosphate (ATP)	ATP is the energy currency of life. ATP is a high-energy molecule found in every cell. Its job is to store and supply the cell with the needed energy.
Phosphocreatine (PCr)	Phosphocreatine, also known as creatine phosphate, is an energy source for muscle contraction naturally present in the skeletal muscle tissue of humans and other vertebrates. It enables the expression of explosive power in the muscles, lasting no longer than 8 to 12 seconds.

TYPES OF ENERGY

Several systems provide energy for the body, including the following:

- Phosphagen (ATP-PCr) system. Used during anaerobic, ATP-PCr, short-term, high-energy activities; primary energy source first 10 seconds of short, intense activities; active at the start of all exercise; small maximum capacity.
- Glycolytic system. Glycolysis is the metabolic pathway by which glucose is converted into two pyruvates. The pathway involves an anaerobic carbohydrate breakdown (glycogen in muscle or glucose in the blood) into pyruvate to produce ATP through glycolysis, then transformed into lactic acid through anaerobic glycolysis. This system is slower to become fully active than the ATP-PCr system but has a greater capacity to provide energy, so it supplements the ATP-PCr system during maximum exercise.
- Oxidative system. An aerobic system requiring O_2, glycogens, fats, and proteins. This is the primary energy source at rest and low-intensity activities. The relative contributions to ATP production for this system are as follows:
  - 0 to 10 seconds: ATP-PCr (phosphagen) system.
  - 10 to 30 seconds: ATP-PCr plus anaerobic glycolysis.
  - 30 seconds to 2 minutes: Anaerobic glycolysis.
  - 2 to 3 minutes: Anaerobic glycolysis plus oxidative.
  - > 3 minutes: Oxidative.

SKILL KEEPER QUESTIONS

1. A patient is training for a track meet, and begins to run. Which energy system is predominantly used in the first 10 seconds of his run? Which is used in the next 30 seconds?

2. Should a patient increase or decrease speed with an eccentrically biased exercise or a concentrically biased exercise to increase force production?

3. If you are developing an exercise program for a marathon runner with back pain, would you want to bias your program toward type I or type II muscle fibers? What about a sprinter with a quadriceps injury?

SKILL KEEPER ANSWERS

1. First 10 seconds: ATP-PCr; next 30 seconds: ATP-PCr + anaerobic glycolysis.

2. Increased speed produces more force with an eccentric exercise provided the patient maintains control of the lengthening (ie, they do not allow gravity to lower the weight). With a concentric-biased exercise, the opposite is true; more force production is achieved with slower speeds, partly due to the tendency to use momentum with faster concentric exercises (Figure 3-9). Therefore, eccentric activities will increase force production with increasing speed, and concentric activities will increase force production with slower speeds.

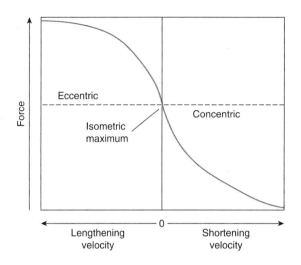

Figure 3-9. The force–velocity relationship for muscle tissue. When the resistance (force) is negligible, muscle contracts with maximal velocity. As the load progressively increases, concentric contraction velocity slows to zero at isometric maximum. As the load increases further, the muscle lengthens eccentrically. (Reproduced with permission from Hall S, ed. *Basic Biomechanics*, 7th ed. 2015. Copyright © McGraw Hill LLC. All rights reserved. https://accessphysiotherapy.mhmedical.com.)

3. Marathon runner: Type I muscle fibers need to be recruited for the endurance muscles (postural trunk muscles), so the aerobic energy system has to be stimulated. Sprinter: Type II because now training the quadriceps muscles, which are dynamic, phasic, will need to work more on the anaerobic energy system required for sprinting.

■ FUNCTIONAL ANATOMY AND BIOMECHANICS OF SPECIFIC JOINTS

Understanding the functional anatomy and biomechanics of the various joint complexes is essential for every intervention.

SHOULDER COMPLEX

The shoulder complex (Figure 3-10) is composed of four articulations:

- The glenohumeral (G-H) joint.
- The acromioclavicular (A-C) joint.

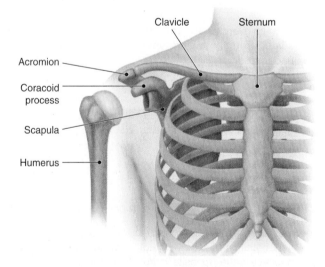

Figure 3-10. Skeletal structures of the shoulder complex. (Reproduced with permission from Burke-Doe A, Dutton M, eds. *National Physical Therapy Examination and Board Review*. 2019. Copyright © McGraw Hill LLC. All rights reserved. https://accessphysiotherapy.mhmedical.com.)

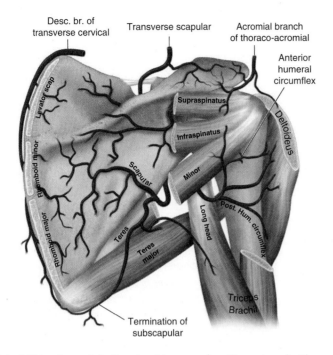

Figure 3-11. Arterial blood supply to the shoulder complex. (Reproduced with permission from Burke-Doe A, Dutton M, eds. *National Physical Therapy Examination and Board Review*. 2019. Copyright © McGraw Hill LLC. All rights reserved. https://accessphysiotherapy.mhmedical.com.)

- The sternoclavicular (S-C) joint.
- The scapulothoracic pseudoarticulation.

The blood supply to the shoulder complex comes from several arteries (Figure 3-11), but primarily from the anterior and posterior circumflex humeral arteries and the suprascapular artery.

▲ HIGH-YIELD TERMS TO LEARN

Open and closed kinetic chain	The expression *kinematic chain* is used in rehabilitation to describe an extremity or trunk's function or activity as a series of linked chains.
Scaption	The forward elevation of the arm in the scapular plane.
Scapulohumeral rhythm	During elevation of the arm overhead, approximately one-third of the motion occurs at the scapulothoracic joint, and two-thirds occur at the glenohumeral joint. Thus, the scapula rotates upwardly, externally, and tilts posteriorly.
Scapular dyskinesia	Also referred to as an abnormal scapulohumeral rhythm, scapular winging, and scapular dysrhythmia that describes abnormal or atypical scapular movement during normal active motion tasks. The finding is common in patients with an unstable glenohumeral joint and patients with impingement syndrome. Scapular dyskinesia may occur primary or secondary to shoulder impingement and instability.
Snapping scapula	Attributed to friction between the mobile scapula and its attached soft tissues and the relatively stable thoracic wall. Anatomic explanations for snapping scapula include thickened bursa, bone spurs on the scapula or a rib, and osteochondroma.
Hill-Sachs lesion	A compression fracture of the humeral head's posterolateral aspect during an anterior dislocation of the shoulder causes an impact on the anteroinferior rim of the glenoid.

Reverse Hill-Sachs lesion	Also referred to as a McLaughlin lesion. It is defined as an impaction fracture of the humeral head's anteromedial aspect following a posterior dislocation of the humerus.
Bankart lesion	An avulsion or detachment of the anterior portion of the inferior glenohumeral ligament complex and glenoid labrum of the glenoid's anterior rim. Bankart lesions can contribute to recurrent instability.
Superior labrum anterior and posterior (SLAP)	An injury to the glenoid labrum associated with overhead and throwing activities.
Myotome	A muscle or group of muscles served by a single nerve root. *Key muscle* is a better, more accurate term, as the muscles tested are the most representative of the supply from a particular segment.
Cubital tunnel	A fibro-osseous canal through which the ulnar nerve passes. The cubital tunnel volume is greatest with the elbow held in extension and the least in full elbow flexion.
The triangular space	Formed by the long head of the triceps laterally, the teres minor superiorly, and the teres major inferiorly. Through it passes the circumflex scapular artery, a branch of the scapular artery.
The quadrangular space	Formed by the shaft of the humerus laterally, the long head of the triceps medially, the teres minor muscle superiorly, and the teres major muscle inferiorly. Through it pass the axillary nerve and the posterior humeral circumflex artery.

GLENOHUMERAL JOINT

- The convex humeral head articulates with the concave glenoid fossa of the scapula. The humeral head is retroverted 20 to 30 degrees. The longitudinal axis of the head is 135 degrees from the axis of the neck.
- The glenoid is retroverted approximately 7 degrees. It faces anteriorly at an angle of approximately 45 degrees to the coronal plane as it sits on the chest wall. The glenoid fossa's depth is enhanced by the glenoid labrum, contributing up to 50% of the fossa's depth.
- The scapula is a flat triangular bone situated over the second through seventh ribs. The glenoid fossa is located on the scapula's lateral angle and faces anteriorly, laterally, and superiorly. This orientation places true abduction at 30 degrees anterior to the frontal plane.
- An important bony landmark in the shoulder is the coracoid process, medial and lateral to which run the major blood vessels and brachial plexus. In addition, the coracoid serves as a muscular attachment for the pectoralis minor, the short head of the biceps, and the coracobrachialis.
- The shoulder complex's ligaments (Table 3-16) function as static stabilizers during arm motion to reciprocally tighten and loosen, thereby limiting translation and rotation of the joint surfaces in a load-sharing fashion.
- The bursae (small fluid-filled sacs) of the shoulder (Table 3-17) decrease friction and aid mobility.

Several common dysfunctions are associated with the shoulder complex (Table 3-18).

The G-H joint is relatively unstable:

- Static stability for the joint is provided by the previously mentioned labrum and various ligaments (Table 3-16). In addition, the joint capsule is reinforced by the G-H ligaments, which are distinct capsular thickenings that limit excessive rotation and translation of the humeral head by reinforcing the connection between the glenoid fossa and the humerus.

Joint	Ligament	Function
Shoulder complex	Coracoclavicular Costoclavicular	Fixes the clavicle to the coracoid process. Fixes the clavicle to the costal cartilage of the first rib.
Glenohumeral	Coracohumeral Glenohumeral ("Z")	Reinforces the upper portion of the joint capsule. Reinforces the anterior and inferior aspects of the joint capsule. • Inferior glenohumeral ligament (IGHL): A complex—parts include the anterior band, axillary pouch, and posterior band. The IGHL provides anterior stabilization, especially during abduction of the arm. • Middle glenohumeral ligament: Strongest of the glenohumeral ligaments and provides anterior stabilization during the combined motion of external rotation and 45° abduction. • Superior glenohumeral ligament: Runs from glenoid rim to anatomic neck and works in conjunction with the coracohumeral ligament to provide inferior stabilization during adduction.
	Coracoacromial	Protects the superior aspect of the joint.

TABLE 3-16 • Major Ligaments of the Shoulder.

- Dynamic stability for the joint is afforded by the dynamic stabilizers, particularly the rotator cuff, the biceps tendon, and the muscles of scapular motion (Table 3-19). Normal strength ratios for the shoulder are as follows:
- Internal and external rotation 3:2.
- Adduction and abduction 2:1.
- Extension and flexion 5:4.

Available ranges of motion of the shoulder complex, the end feels, and potential causes of pain are listed in Table 3-20.

Sternoclavicular Joint

The S-C joint, a saddle joint, is the only joint that directly attaches the upper extremity to the thorax. This saddle joint allows elevation and depression, protraction and retraction, and rotation. The biomechanics of the S-C and A-C joints are discussed in Table 3-21.

Acromioclavicular Joints

A plane joint, but also described as diarthrodial, with fibrocartilage surfaces—a convex clavicle and a concave acromion. The joint contains an intra-articular fibrocartilaginous disk, which degenerates during the third and fourth decades of life.

TABLE 3-17 • Major Bursae of the Shoulder.

Bursa	Location
Subacromial-subdeltoid	Located between the rotator cuff muscles and the deltoid muscle. As the humerus elevates, this bursa permits the rotator cuff to slide easily beneath the deltoid muscle.
Subcoracoid	Located between the joint capsule and the coracoid process of the scapula.
Subscapular (subtendinous bursa of the scapularis)	Located between the capsule and the tendon of the subscapularis muscle.
Coracobrachial	Located between the subscapularis muscle and the tendon of the coracobrachialis muscle.

TABLE 3-18 • Differential Diagnosis for Common Causes of Shoulder Pain.

Condition	Patient's Age (Approximate)	Mechanism of Injury	Area of Symptoms	Symptoms Aggravated by	Observation	AROM	PROM	End Feel	Pain with Resisted	Tenderness Palpation
Rotator cuff tendinitis										
Acute	20-40	Microtrauma/macrotrauma	Anterior and lateral shoulder	Overhead motions	Swelling—anterior shoulder	Limited abduction	Limited abduction	ER	Abduction	Pain below the anterior acromial rim
Chronic	30-70	Microtrauma/macrotrauma	Anterior and lateral shoulder	Overhead motions Atrophy of shoulder area	Atrophy of scapular area	Limited abduction and flexion	Pain on IR and ER at 90° abduction	ER IR	Abduction Pain below the anterior acromial rim	Anterior shoulder
Bicipital tendinitis	20-45	Microtrauma	Anterior shoulder	Overhead motions / May see signs of concomitant rotator cuff pathology	Possible swelling—anterior shoulder / Pain on full flexion from full extension	Limited ER when arm at 90° abduction / Biceps stability test may be abnormal (if tendon unstable)	Pain on the combined extension of shoulder and elbow	Speed test painful, Yergason test occasionally painful	Elbow flexion	Of biceps tendon over the bicipital groove
Rotator cuff rupture	40+	Macrotrauma	Posterior/superior shoulder	Arm elevation	Atrophy of scapular area	Limited abduction Pain with or without restriction	Full and pain-free	ER	Abduction	Pain below the antero-lateral acromial rim
Adhesive capsulitis	35-70	Microtrauma/macrotrauma	Shoulder and upper arm—poorly localized	All motions	Atrophy of shoulder area	All motions limited, especially ER and abduction	All motions limited, especially ER and abduction	Capsular	Most/all	Varies
A-C joint sprain	Varies	Macrotrauma	Point of shoulder	Horizontal adduction	Step/bump at point of shoulder	Limited abduction / Limited horizontal adduction	Limited abduction / Pain with horizontal adduction	Flexion / Flexion	ER / Soft tissue thickening at point of shoulder	Point of shoulder

Condition	Age	Onset / Mechanism	Location of symptoms	Aggravating factors	Observation	ROM	Pain on IR at 90° abduction	End feel	Resistive / Strength	Palpation
Subacromial bursitis	Varies	Microtrauma	Anterior and lateral shoulder	Overhead motions	Often unremarkable	Limited abduction and IR / May have full range, but the pain is in the midrange of flexion/abduction	Pain on IR at 90° abduction / The pain only in the midrange of abduction and flexion		Most/all	Pain below the anterolateral acromial rim
Glenohumeral arthritis	50+	Gradual onset but can be traumatic	Poorly localized	Arm activity	Possible posterior positioning of the humeral head	Capsular pattern (ER > abduction > IR)	Pain	Capsular	Weakness of the rotator cuff, rather than pain	Poorly localized
SICK scapula	20-40	Microtrauma	Anterior/superior shoulder; Posterosuperior scapular; Arm, forearm, hand	Overhead activities	Scapular malposition; Inferior medial border prominence; Dyskinesia of Scapular movement	Decreased forward flexion which diminishes when clinician manually repositions the scapula into retraction and posterior tilt	Normal		Weakness rather than pain	Medial coracoid; Superomedial angle of scapula
Cervical radiculopathy	Varies	Typically none but can be traumatic	Upper back, below shoulder	Cervical extension, cervical side-bending and rotation to the ipsilateral side, full arm elevation	May have a lateral deviation of the head away from the painful side	Decreased cervical flexion, cervical side-bending, and rotation to ipsilateral side; decreased arm elevation on the involved side	Painful into the restricted active range of motions; Positive Spurling test	Empty	Weakness rather than pain; Other neurologic changes	Varies; may have numbness over dermatomal area

ER, external rotation; IR, internal rotation.

173

TABLE 3-19 • Muscles of the Shoulder Complex According to Their Actions on the Scapula and at the Glenohumeral Joint.

Action	Nerve Supply	Blood Supply
Scapular Abductors Trapezius Serratus anterior (upper fibers)	Accessory nerve (motor), cervical spinal nerves C3 and C4 (motor and sensation) Long thoracic nerve (C5-C7)	*Shoulder complex*: Primarily provided by branches of the axillary artery, a continuation of the subclavian artery. The axillary artery meets the brachial plexus in the neck, and here they are encased in the axillary sheath, together with the axillary vein.
Scapular Adductors Levator scapulae Rhomboids	Posterior (dorsal) scapular nerve (C3-C5) Posterior (dorsal) scapular nerve (C4-C5)	*G-H joint*: Receives its blood supply from the anterior and posterior circumflex humeral (Figure 2-9) as well as the
Scapular Flexors Serratus anterior (lower fibers)	Long thoracic nerve (C5-C7)	suprascapular and circumflex scapular vessels.
Scapular Extensors Pectoralis minor	Medial pectoral nerve (C6-C8)	*Labrum*: Vascular supply arises mostly from its peripheral attachment to the capsule and is from a combination of
Scapular External Rotators Trapezius Rhomboids	Accessory nerve (motor), cervical spinal nerves C3 and C4 (motor and sensation) Posterior (dorsal) scapular nerve (C4-C5)	the suprascapular circumflex scapular branch of the subscapular and posterior humeral circumflex arteries.
Shoulder Flexors Coracobrachialis Short and long head of biceps Pectoralis major Anterior deltoid	Musculocutaneous nerve (C5-C7) Musculocutaneous nerve (C5-C7) Medial (lower fibers) pectoral nerves (C8-T1); Lateral (upper fibers) pectoral nerves (C5-C7) Axillary (C5-C6)	*Rotator cuff*: Consists of three main sources: the thoracoacromial, suprahumeral, and subscapular arteries. *Brachial artery*: Provides the dominant arterial supply to each of the two heads of the biceps brachii. The artery travels in the medial intermuscular
Shoulder Extensors Triceps Posterior deltoid Teres minor Teres major Latissimus dorsi	Radial (C6-C8) and axillary nerve Axillary (C5-C6) Axillary (C5-C6) Lower subscapular nerve (C5-C6) Lower subscapular nerve (C5-C6)	septum and is bordered by the biceps muscle anteriorly, the brachialis muscle medially, and the medial head of the triceps muscle posteriorly.
Shoulder Abductors Supraspinatus Deltoid	Suprascapular nerve (C5-C6) Axillary (C5-C6)	
Shoulder Adductors Subscapularis Pectoralis major Latissimus dorsi Teres major Teres minor	Upper and lower subscapular nerve (C5-C6) Medial (lower fibers) pectoral nerves (C8-T1) Lateral (upper fibers) pectoral nerves (C5-C7) Lower subscapular nerve (C5-C6) Lower subscapular nerve (C5-C6) Axillary (C5-C6)	
Shoulder Internal Rotators Pectoralis major and minor Serratus anterior Subscapularis Pectoralis major Latissimus dorsi Teres major	(See above) Long thoracic nerve (C5-C7) Upper and lower subscapular nerve (C5-C6) Medial (lower fibers) pectoral nerves (C8-T1); Lateral (upper fibers) pectoral nerves (C5-C7) Lower subscapular nerve (C5-C6) Lower subscapular nerve (C5-C6)	
Shoulder External Rotators Infraspinatus Supraspinatus Deltoid Teres minor	Suprascapular nerve (C5-C6) Suprascapular nerve (C5-C6) Axillary (C5-C6) Axillary (C5-C6)	

TABLE 3-20 • Movements of the Shoulder Complex, Normal Ranges, End Feels, and Potential Causes of Pain.

Motion	Range Norms (Degrees)	End Feel	Potential Source of Pain
Elevation-flexion (sagittal plane—spin) Muscles performing motion: Pectoralis major (clavicular portion), deltoid (anterior fibers), coracobrachialis, biceps brachii Peripheral nerves involved: Lateral and medial pectoral, axillary, musculocutaneous	0-180	Tissue stretch Motion limited by: Posterior band of the coracohumeral ligament, inferoposterior joint capsule	Suprahumeral impingement Stretching of glenohumeral, acromioclavicular, sterno-clavicular joint capsule Triceps tendon if elbow flexed
Extension (sagittal plane—spin) Muscles performing motion: Deltoid (posterior fibers), teres major, latissimus dorsi, pectoralis major (sternocostal portion) Peripheral nerves involved: Axillary, lower subscapularis, thoracodorsal, lateral and medial pectoral	0-60	Tissue stretch Motion limited by: Coracohumeral ligament, anterior joint capsule.	Stretching of the glenohumeral joint capsule Severe suprahumeral impingement Biceps tendon if elbow extended
Elevation-abduction (frontal plane—humerus rolls superiorly, glides inferiorly) Muscles performing motion: Deltoid, supraspinatus Peripheral nerves involved: Axillary, suprascapular	0-180	Tissue stretch Motion limited by: Inferior joint capsule, glenohumeral ligament, an approximation of the greater tuberosity and glenoid labrum	Suprahumeral impingement Acromioclavicular arthritis at terminal abduction
External rotation (transverse plane—humerus rolls posteriorly, glides anteriorly) Muscles performing motion: Infraspinatus, deltoid (posterior fibers), teres minor Peripheral nerves involved: Lateral and medial pectoral, axillary, thoracodorsal, lower subscapularis, upper and lower subscapularis	0-85	Tissue stretch Motion limited by: Anterior capsule, glenohumeral ligament	Anterior glenohumeral instability
Internal rotation (transverse plane—humerus rolls anteriorly, glides posteriorly) Muscles performing motion: Pectoralis major, deltoid (anterior fibers), teres major, subscapularis Peripheral nerves involved: Suprascapular, axillary	0-95	Tissue stretch Motion limited by: Posterior capsule	Suprahumeral impingement Posterior glenohumeral instability

ELBOW COMPLEX

The elbow complex (Figure 3-12) is composed of four articulations:

- The humeroulnar joint.
- The humeroradial joint.
- The proximal radioulnar joint.
- The distal radioulnar joint (DRUJ).

The elbow is a very congruous joint, and hence inherently very stable. However, much of this stability is due to several ligaments (Figure 3-13) (Tables 3-22 and 3-23).

The elbow's dynamic stability and motion are also afforded by numerous muscles (Table 3-24).

The bursae of the elbow (Table 3-25) serve to decrease friction and aid mobility.

The cubital fossa represents the triangular space, or depression, located over the elbow joint's anterior surface, which serves as an "entrance" to the forearm or antebrachium. The boundaries of the fossa are described below:

TABLE 3-21 • Movements of the Acromioclavicular and Sternoclavicular Complex.

Motion of the Proximal Clavicle at the A-C Joint	Range of Motion	Motion Limited By
Protraction: The concave surface of the proximal clavicle moves on the convex sternum, producing an anterior glide of the clavicle and an anterior rotation of the distal clavicle *Muscles performing motion*: Serratus anterior, pectoralis minor *Peripheral nerves involved*: Long thoracic, lateral and medial pectoral	The distal clavicle (at the S-C joint) moves approximately 10 cm	Anterior S-C ligament, costoclavicular ligament (posterior portion), anterior capsule of the S-C joint
Retraction: The proximal clavicle articulates with a flat surface and tilts or swings, causing an anterolateral gapping, and a posterior rotation at the distal end *Muscles performing motion*: Trapezius, rhomboids *Peripheral nerves involved*: Spinal accessory, dorsal scapular	The distal clavicle (at the S-C joint) moves approximately 3 cm	Posterior S-C ligament, costoclavicular ligament (anterior portion), posterior capsule of the S-C joint
Elevation: The clavicle rotates upward on the manubrium and produces an inferior glide to maintain joint contact; only slight angular motion of the clavicle *Muscles performing motion*: Upper trapezius, levator scapulae *Peripheral nerves involved*: Spinal accessory, directly via C3-C4 and dorsal scapular	The distal clavicle (at the S-C joint) moves approximately 10 cm	Costoclavicular ligament, inferior capsule of the S-C joint
Depression: The clavicle rotates downward on the manubrium and produces a superior glide to maintain joint contact; only slight angular motion of the clavicle *Muscles performing motion*: Serratus anterior (lower portion), pectoralis minor *Peripheral nerves involved*: Long thoracic, lateral and medial pectoral	The distal clavicle (at the S-C joint) moves approximately 3 cm	Interclavicular ligament, S-C ligament, articular disk of S-C joint, superior capsule of S-C joint
Rotation: The clavicle rotates passively as the scapula rotates *Muscles performing motion*: Upper trapezius, serratus anterior (lower portion) *Peripheral nerves involved*: Spinal accessory, long thoracic	30° occurs at A-C joint, then 30° at the S-C joint	S-C: Anterior and posterior sternoclavicular ligament, interclavicular ligament, costoclavicular ligament A-C: A-C ligament, coracoclavicular ligament (conoid [limits backward rotation], trapezoid [limits forward rotation])

- Lateral—brachioradialis and extensor carpi radialis longus (ECRL) muscles.
- Medial—pronator teres muscle.
- Proximal—an imaginary line that passes through the humeral condyles.
- Floor—brachialis muscle.

The contents of the fossa are as follows:

- The tendon of the biceps brachii lies as the central structure in the fossa.
- The median nerve runs along the lateral edge of the pronator teres muscle.
- The brachial artery enters the fossa just lateral to the median nerve, medial to the biceps brachii tendon.
- The radial nerve runs along the medial edge of the brachioradialis and ECRL muscles and is vulnerable to injury here.
- The median cubital or intermediate cubital cutaneous vein crosses the surface of the fossa.
- The elbow complex receives its blood supply from the brachial artery, anterior ulnar recurrent artery, posterior ulnar recurrent artery, radial recurrent artery, and the middle collateral branch of the arteria profunda brachii.

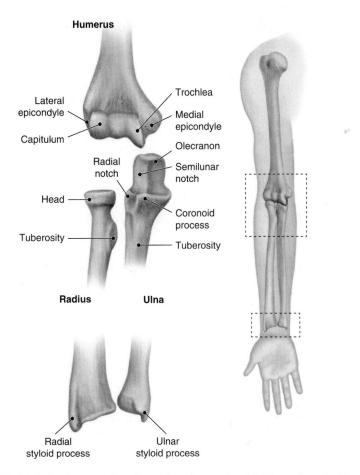

Figure 3-12. **Skeletal structures of the elbow, forearm, and wrist.** (Reproduced with permission from Burke-Doe A, Dutton M, eds. *National Physical Therapy Examination and Board Review*. 2019. Copyright © McGraw Hill LLC. All rights reserved. https://accessphysiotherapy.mhmedical.com.)

Humeroulnar Joint

The motions that occur at the humeroulnar joint involve impure flexion and extension, which are primarily the result of the rotation of the ulna about the trochlea. The range of flexion-extension is from 0 to 150 degrees, with about 10 degrees hyperextension being available. Full active extension in the normal elbow is 5 to 10 degrees short of that obtainable by forced extension due to passive muscular restraints (biceps, brachialis, and supinator).

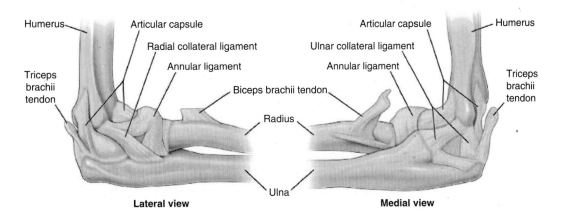

Figure 3-13. **Ligaments of the lateral and medial aspects of the elbow.** (Reproduced with permission from Burke-Doe A, Dutton M, eds. *National Physical Therapy Examination and Board Review*. 2019. Copyright © McGraw Hill LLC. All rights reserved. https://accessphysiotherapy.mhmedical.com.)

TABLE 3-22 • Major Ligaments of the Elbow.

	Function
Annular	Maintains the relationship between the head of the radius and the humerus and ulna
Ulnar (medial) collateral	Primary stabilizer against valgus (medial) stress, particularly in the range of 20°-130° of flexion and extension
Radial (lateral) collateral	Provides stability against varus (lateral) stress and functions to maintain the ulnohumeral and radiohumeral joints in a reduced position when the elbow is loaded in supination

TABLE 3-23 • Articular and Ligamentous Contributions to Elbow Stability.

Stabilization	Elbow Extended	Elbow Flexed 90°

Valgus stability	Anterior capsule
	UCL and bony articular (proximal half of sigmoid notch)
	  equally divided
		UCL provides 55%
		0% anterior capsule and bony articulation
		  (proximal half of sigmoid notch)

Varus stability	Anterior capsule (32%) Joint articulation (55%) RCL (14%)	Joint articulation (75%) Anterior capsule (13%) RCL (9%)
Anterior displacement	Anterior oblique ligament Anterior joint capsule Trochlea-olecranon articulation (minimal)	
Posterior displacement	Anterior capsule Radial head against the capitellum Coracoid against the trochlea	
Distraction	Anterior capsule (85%) RCL (5%) UCL (5%) Triceps, biceps, brachialis, brachioradialis, and forearm muscles	RCL (10%) UCL (78%) Capsule (8%)

RCL, radial collateral ligament; UCL, ulnar collateral ligament.

Data from Zachazewski JE, Magee DJ, Quillen WS, eds. *Athletic Injuries and Rehabilitation.* 1996. Copyright © WB Saunders. All rights reserved.

TABLE 3-24 • Muscles of the Elbow and Forearm: Their Actions, Nerve Supply, and Nerve Root Derivation.

Action	Muscles Acting	Peripheral Nerve Supply	Nerve Root Deviation	Blood Supply
Elbow flexion	Brachialis Biceps brachii Brachioradialis Pronator teres Flexor carpi ulnaris	Musculocutaneous Musculocutaneous Radial Median Ulnar	C5-C6 (C7) C5-C6 C5-C6, (C7) C6-C7 C7-C8	The vascular supply to the elbow includes the brachial artery, the radial and ulnar arteries, the middle and radial collateral arteries laterally, and the superior and inferior ulnar collateral arteries.
Elbow extension	Triceps Anconeus	Radial Radial	C7-C8 C7-C8, (T1)	
Forearm supination	Supinator Biceps brachii	Posterior interosseous (radial) Musculocutaneous	C5-C6 C5-C6	
Forearm pronation	Pronator quadratus Pronator teres Flexor carpi radialis	Anterior interosseous (median) Median Median	C8, T1 C6-C7 C6-C7	

TABLE 3-25 • Major Bursae of the Elbow.	
Bursa	**Location**
Olecranon	Located posteriorly between the skin and the olecranon process; the main bursa of the elbow joint complex
Deep intratendinous and deep subtendinous	Located between the triceps tendon and olecranon
Bicipitoradial	Separates the biceps tendon from the radial tuberosity
Coracobrachial	Located between the subscapularis muscle and the tendon of the coracobrachialis muscle

- Passive extension is limited by the impact of the olecranon process on the olecranon fossa and tension on the ulnar collateral ligament and anterior capsule.
- Passive flexion is limited by bony structures (the head of the radius against the radial fossa and the coronoid process against the coronoid fossa), tension of the posterior capsular ligament, and passive tension in the triceps.
- The elbow's normal carrying angle varies with flexion and extension, ranging from 6 degree varus with full flexion to 11 degrees valgus in full extension. Women tend to have a larger carrying angle.

Humeroradial Joint

The motions occurring at this joint include flexion and extension of the elbow. Some supination and pronation also occur at this joint due to a spinning of the radial head.

Proximal Radioulnar Joint

At the proximal radioulnar joint, pronation and supination occur. Pronation and supination involve the articulations at the elbow as well as the DRUJ and the radiocarpal articulation.

Motion at the elbow is primarily gliding for both flexion and extension. Rolling occurs in the final 5 to 10 degrees of ROM for both flexion and extension.

FOREARM, WRIST, AND HAND

The wrist and hand joint complex (Figure 3-14) comprises the following:

- The DRUJ.
- Eight carpal bones.
- The bases of five metacarpals.
- More than 20 radiocarpal, intercarpal, and CMC joints.

While these structures can be differentiated anatomically, they are functionally interrelated, with movement in one joint affecting the motion of neighboring joints. The major ligaments of the wrist and hand are described in Table 3-26.

The forearm muscle compartments are described in Table 3-27, and the wrist and hand muscles are described in Table 3-28. The AROM norms for the forearm, wrist, and hand are described in Table 3-29.

Distal Radioulnar Joint

The DRUJ is a double-pivot joint that unites the distal radius and ulna and an articular disk. The articular disk, known as the triangular fibrocartilaginous complex (TFCC), helps bind the distal radius and is the main stabilizer of the DRUJ, as it improves joint congruency and cushions against compressive forces.

Supination tightens the anterior capsule, while pronation tightens the posterior part, adding to the wrist's overall stability.

STUDY PEARL
The proximal and distal radial ulnar joints are intimately related biomechanically, with the function and stability of both dependent on the configuration and the distance between the two bones.

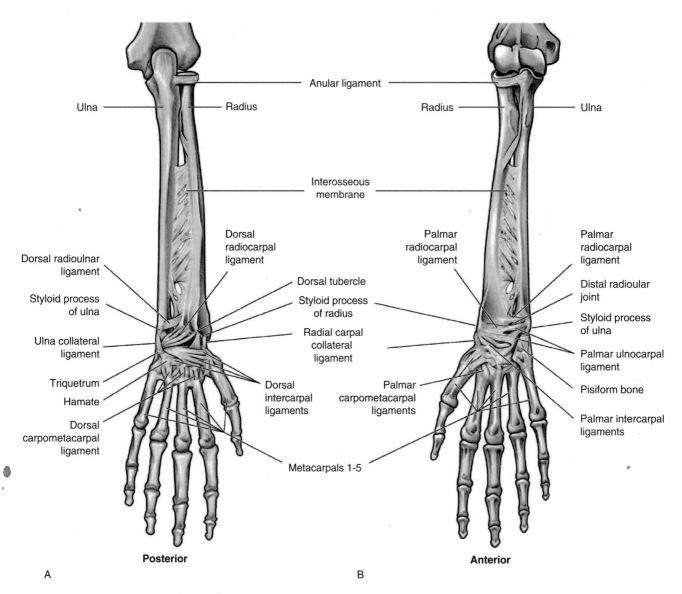

Figure 3-14. Ligaments of the forearm, wrist, and hand. (Reproduced with permission from Burke-Doe A, Dutton M, eds. *National Physical Therapy Examination and Board Review*. 2019. Copyright © McGraw Hill LLC. All rights reserved. https://accessphysiotherapy.mhmedical.com.)

THE WRIST

The Carpals

The carpal bones lie in two transverse rows (Figure 3-15).

The proximal row contains (from radial to ulnar) the scaphoid (navicular), lunate, triquetrum, and pisiform. The distal row holds (radial to ulnar) the trapezium, trapezoid, capitate, and hamate. Various instabilities can occur in the carpal joints (Table 3-30).

TABLE 3-26 • Major Ligaments of the Wrist and Hand.		
Wrist	Extrinsic palmar	Provides the majority of the wrist stability
	Intrinsic	Serves as rotational restraint, binding the proximal carpal row into a unit of rotational stability
	Interosseous	Binds the carpal bones together
Fingers	Anterior and collateral interphalangeal	Prevent displacement of the interphalangeal joints

TABLE 3-27 • Muscle Compartments of the Forearm.	
Compartment	**Principal Muscles**
Anterior	Pronator teres Flexor carpi radialis Palmaris longus Flexor digitorum superficialis Flexor digitorum profundus Flexor pollicis longus Flexor carpi ulnaris Pronator quadrates
Posterior	Abductor pollicis longus Extensor pollicis brevis Extensor pollicis longus Extensor digitorum communis Extensor digitorum proprius Extensor digiti quinti Extensor carpi ulnaris
Mobile wad	Brachioradialis Extensor carpi radialis longus Extensor carpi radialis brevis

Midcarpal Joints

The midcarpal joint lies between the two rows of carpals. Due to the wrist's morphology, movement at this joint complex involves a coordinated interaction between several articulations, including the radiocarpal joint, the proximal row of carpals, and the distal row of the carpals. The wrist's flexion and extension movements are shared between the radiocarpal articulation and the intercarpal articulation in varying proportions.

Wrist flexion, extension, and radial deviation are mainly midcarpal joint motions. Each carpal in the proximal row is convex on its lateral surface and concave on its medial surface. At their distal aspect:

- The scaphoid and lunate present with a concave surface to the distal row of carpals.
- The triquetrum presents with a convex surface to the distal row of carpals.

The wrist also allows relatively extensive traction and gliding accessory movements. A physiologic ulnar deviation exists at rest—approximately 40 degrees of ulnar deviation and 15 degrees of radial deviation.

Carpal Ligaments. Migration of the carpal bones is prevented by strong ligaments and the ulnar support provided by the TFCC. The wrist's major ligaments include the anterior and posterior extrinsic and intrinsic ligaments.

Radiocarpal Joint

The radiocarpal joint is formed by the large articular concave surface of the distal end of the radius, the scaphoid and lunate of the proximal carpal row, and the TFCC.

Antebrachial Fascia

The antebrachial fascia is a dense connective tissue "bracelet" that encases the forearm and maintains the tendon relationships that cross the wrist.

Extensor Retinaculum

At the point where the tendons cross the wrist, a retinaculum serves to prevent the tendons from "bow-stringing" when the tendons turn a corner at the wrist. The tunnel-like structures formed by the retinaculum and the underlying bones are called fibro-osseous compartments. There are six fibro-osseous compartments, or tunnels, on the dorsum of

STUDY PEARL

The wrist position in flexion or extension influences the tension of the long, or "extrinsic," muscles of the digits because the finger flexors or extensors are not long enough to allow maximal ROM at the wrist and the fingers simultaneously.

TABLE 3-28 • Muscles of the Wrist and Hand.

Action	Muscles	Nerve Supply
Wrist extension	Extensor carpi radialis longus Extensor carpi radialis brevis Extensor carpi ulnaris	Radial C6, C7 Posterior interosseous C6, C7 Posterior interosseous C7, C8
Wrist flexion	Flexor carpi radialis Flexor carpi ulnaris	Median C6, C7 Ulnar C8, T1
Ulnar deviation of the wrist	Flexor carpi ulnaris Extensor carpi ulnaris	Ulnar C8, T1 Posterior interosseous C7, C8
Radial deviation of the wrist	Flexor carpi radialis Extensor carpi radialis longus Abductor pollicis longus Extensor pollicis brevis	Median C6, C7 Radial C6, C7 Posterior interosseous C7, C8 Posterior interosseous C7, C8
Finger extension	Extensor digitorum communis Extensor indicis Extensor digiti minimi	Posterior interosseous C6-C8 Posterior interosseous C7, C8 Posterior interosseous C7, C8
Finger flexion	Flexor digitorum profundus Flexor digitorum superficialis Lumbricals Interossei Flexor digiti minimi	Anterior interosseous, lateral two digits C8, T1 Ulnar, medial two digits C8, T1 Median C7, C8, T1 First and second: median C8, T1 Third and fourth: ulnar C8, T1 Ulnar C8, T1 Ulnar C8, T1
Abduction of fingers	Posterior interossei Abductor digiti minimi	Ulnar C8, T1 Ulnar C8, T1
Adduction of fingers	Palmar interossei	Ulnar C8, T1
Thumb extension	Extensor pollicis longus Extensor pollicis brevis Abductor pollicis longus	Posterior interosseous C7, C8 Posterior interosseous C7, C8 Posterior interosseous C7, C8
Thumb flexion	Flexor pollicis brevis Flexor pollicis longus Opponens pollicis	Superficial head: median C8, T1 Deep head: ulnar C8, T1 Anterior interosseous C8, T1 Median C8, T1
Abduction of thumb	Abductor pollicis longus Abductor pollicis brevis	Posterior interosseous C7, C8 Median C8, T1
Adduction of thumb	Adductor pollicis	Ulnar C8, T1
Opposition of the thumb and little finger	Opponens pollicis Flexor pollicis brevis Abductor pollicis brevis Opponens digiti minimi	Median C8, T1 Superficial head: median C8, T1 Median C8, T1 Ulnar C8, T1

the wrist. The compartments, from lateral to medial, contain the tendons of the following muscles:

1. Abductor pollicis longus (APL) and extensor pollicis brevis (EPB).
2. ECRL and ECRB.
3. Extensor pollicis longus (EPL).
4. Extensor digitorum and indicis.
5. Extensor digiti minimi.
6. Extensor carpi ulnaris.

STUDY PEARL

The mnemonic 2 2 1 2 1 1 helps remember the number of tendons in each compartment.

Flexor Retinaculum

The flexor retinaculum (transverse carpal ligament) spans the pisiform, hamate, scaphoid, and trapezium. It transforms the carpal arch into a tunnel, through which passes the median

TABLE 3-29 • Active Range of Motion Norms for the Forearm, Wrist, and Hand.

Motion	Degrees
Forearm pronation	85-90
Forearm supination	85-90
Radial deviation	15
Ulnar deviation	30-45
Wrist flexion	80-90
Wrist extension	70-90
Finger flexion	MCP: 85-90; PIP: 100-115; DIP: 80-90
Finger extension	MCP: 30-45; PIP: 0; DIP: 20
Finger abduction	20-30
Finger adduction	0
Thumb flexion	CMC: 45-50; MCP: 50-55; IP: 85-90
Thumb extension	MCP: 0; IP: 0-5
Thumb adduction	30
Thumb abduction	60-70

CMC, carpometacarpal; DIP, distal interphalangeal; IP, interphalangeal; MCP, metacarpophalangeal; PIP, proximal interphalangeal.

nerve and some of the hand tendons. Proximally, the retinaculum attaches to the tubercle of the scaphoid and the pisiform. Distally, it attaches to the hook of the hamate and the tubercle of the trapezium. The tendons that pass *deep* to the flexor retinaculum include the following:

- Flexor digitorum superficialis (FDS).
- Flexor digitorum profundus (FDP).

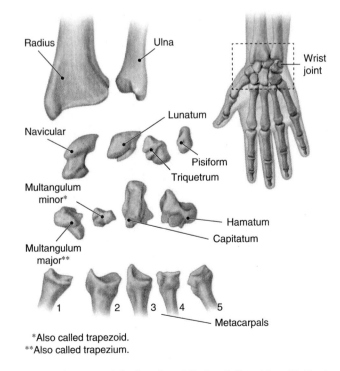

*Also called trapezoid.
**Also called trapezium.

Figure 3-15. The carpal bones of the hand and their relationship with the bones of the wrist and fingers. (Reproduced with permission from Burke-Doe A, Dutton M, eds. *National Physical Therapy Examination and Board Review.* 2019. Copyright © McGraw Hill LLC. All rights reserved. https://accessphysiotherapy.mhmedical.com.)

TABLE 3-30 • Common Wrist Dysfunctions.	
Dysfunction	**Cause**
Dorsal intercalated segment instability (DISI)	Results from disruption between the scaphoid and lunate, allowing the scaphoid to rotate into anterior flexion. The remaining components of the proximal row rotate into dorsiflexion because of loss of connection to the scaphoid.
Volar intercalated segment instability (VISI)	Results from disruption of the ligamentous support to the triquetrum and lunate and leads to anterior rotation of the lunate and extension of the triquetrum.
Scapholunate dissociation	A complete tear of the scapholunate ligaments may result from a hyperextension injury. The lunate and triquetrum extend abnormally, supinate, and deviate radially, while the scaphoid tilts into flexion, pronation, and ulnar deviation (see Watson test).
Triangular fibrocartilaginous complex (TFCC) tear	This injury typically occurs following a fall on the supinated outstretched wrist or as the result of chronic repetitive rotational loading. Patients complain of medial wrist pain just distal to the ulna, which is increased with end-range forearm pronation/supination and with forceful gripping. TFCC tears can be a cause of distal radioulnar joint/wrist instability.

- Flexor pollicis longus (FPL).
- Flexor carpi radialis (FCR).

Structures that pass *superficial* to the flexor retinaculum include the following:

- Ulnar nerve and artery.
- Tendon of the palmaris longus.
- Sensory branch (anterior branch) of the median nerve.

Carpal Tunnel

The carpal tunnel serves as a conduit for the median nerve and nine flexor tendons (the eight tendons of the FDS and FDP, and the FPL).

- The anterior radiocarpal ligament and the anterior ligament complex form the floor of the canal.
- The roof of the tunnel is formed by the flexor retinaculum (transverse carpal ligament).
- The ulnar and radial borders are formed by carpal bones (hook of hamate and trapezium, respectively).

STUDY PEARL

Most hand surgeons refer to the hand area represented by the distal crease in the palm and the middle crease in the finger as "no man's land," or zone II (Figure 3-16). This is because the area is one complex anatomy and has demonstrated a poor healing level due to an increased chance of adhesion formation.

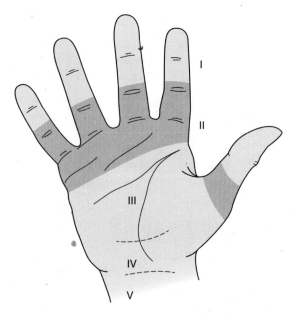

Figure 3-16. Zone II of the flexor tendon zones—the surgical no man's land of the hand. (Reproduced with permission from Burke-Doe A, Dutton M, eds. *National Physical Therapy Examination and Board Review*. 2019. Copyright © McGraw Hill LLC. All rights reserved. https://accessphysiotherapy.mhmedical.com.)

Within the tunnel, the median nerve divides into a motor branch and distal sensory branches.

Tunnel of Guyon

The tunnel of Guyon is a depression superficial to the flexor retinaculum, located between the hook of the hamate and the pisiform bones. From radial to ulnar, the ulnar artery and ulnar nerve pass through the canal. The flexor carpi ulnaris tendon is most ulnar but lies outside the tunnel.

Phalanges

The 14 phalanges each consist of a base, shaft, and head. Two shallow depressions, which correspond to the pulley-shaped heads of the adjacent phalanges, mark the concave proximal bases. The phalangeal motion thus follows the concave-convex rule.

Metacarpophalangeal Joints of the Second to Fifth Fingers

The second to fifth metacarpals articulate with the respective proximal phalanges in biaxial joints. The MCP joints allow flexion-extension and medial-lateral deviation associated with a slight degree of axial rotation. Motions at these joints follow the concave-convex rule.

- Approximately 90 degree flexion is available at the second MCP. The amount of available flexion progressively increases toward the fifth MCP.
- Active extension at these joints is 25 to 30 degrees, while 90 degree is obtainable passively.
- Approximately 20 degrees abduction/adduction can occur in either direction, with more available in extension than flexion.
- Abduction-adduction movements of the MCP joints are restricted in flexion and freer in extension.

The joint capsule of these joints is relatively lax and redundant, endowed with collateral ligaments. Although lax in extension, these collateral ligaments become taut in approximately 70 to 90 degrees flexion of the MCP joint.

Carpometacarpal Joints

The distal borders of the distal carpal row bones articulate with the metacarpal bases, thereby forming the CMC joints. The CMC joints progress in mobility from the second to the fifth.

The anterior and posterior CMC and intermetacarpal ligaments provide stability for the CMC joints. While the trapezoid articulates with only one metacarpal, the distal carpal row's remaining members combine one carpal bone with two or more metacarpals.

First Carpometacarpal Joint

The thumb is the most important digit of the hand, and the sellar (saddle-shaped) CMC joint is the most important joint of the thumb. Motions that can occur at this joint include flexion/extension, adduction/abduction, and opposition (varying flexion, internal rotation, and anterior adduction motions). At the first CMC joint, the following biomechanics are involved:

- Flexion/extension of metacarpal occurs around an anterior-posterior axis in the frontal plane perpendicular to the sagittal plane of finger flexion and extension: The metacarpal surface is concave, and the trapezium surface is convex.
  - The swing of the bone occurs in an anteromedial/posterolateral direction.
  - The base glides and rolls in an anteromedial/posterolateral direction.
  - Flexion occurs with a conjunct rotation of internal rotation of the metacarpal. Extension occurs with a conjunct rotation of external rotation of the metacarpal.
- Abduction/adduction of the metacarpal occurs around a medial-lateral axis in the sagittal plane, which is perpendicular to the frontal plane of finger abduction and adduction: The convex metacarpal surface moves on the concave trapezium.
  - The swing of the bone occurs in an anterolateral/posteromedial direction.

- The base glides in the opposite direction of the swing and rolls in the same direction as the swing.
- Abduction occurs with a conjunct rotation of internal rotation. Adduction occurs with a conjunct rotation of external rotation.
- Thumb opposition involves a wide arc of motion from the anatomic position, comprises sequential anterior adduction and flexion accompanied by internal rotation of the thumb. Retroposition of the thumb returns the thumb to the anatomic position, a motion that incorporates elements of abduction with extension and external rotation of the metacarpal.

Metacarpophalangeal Joint of the Thumb

The MCP joint of the thumb is a hinge joint. Its bony configuration, which resembles the interphalangeal (IP) joints, provides some inherent stability. Also, anterior and collateral ligaments provide support for the joint. Approximately 75 to 80 degrees of flexion is available at this joint. The extension movements, as well as the abduction and adduction motions, are negligible. Traction, gliding, and rotatory accessory movement are also present. Motions follow the concave-convex rule.

Interphalangeal Joints

Adjacent phalanges articulate in hinge joints that allow movement in only one plane. The congruency of the interphalangeal (IP) joint surfaces contributes greatly to finger joint stability. The motions follow the concave-convex rule.

Proximal Interphalangeal Joint. The proximal interphalangeal (PIP) joint is a hinged joint capable of flexion and extension and is stable in all positions. The supporting ligaments and tendons provide the bulk of the static and dynamic stability of this joint. The motions available at these joints consist of approximately 110 degrees flexion at the PIP joints and 90 degrees at the thumb IP joint. Extension reaches 0 degree at the PIP joints and 25 degrees at the thumb IP joint. Traction, gliding, and accessory movement also occur at the IP joints.

Distal Interphalangeal Joints. The distal interphalangeal (DIP) joint has similar structures but less stability and allows slight hyperextension. The motions available at these joints consist of approximately 80 degrees active flexion and 25 degrees passive extension. Traction, gliding, and accessory movements also occur at the DIP joints.

Anterior Aponeurosis

The anterior aponeurosis, a dense fibrous structure continuous with the palmaris longus tendon and fascia, is located just deep to the subcutaneous tissue. It is covering the thenar and hypothenar muscles.

Extensor Hood

At the MCP joint level, the tendon of the extensor digitorum (ED) fans out to cover the posterior aspect of the joint in a hood-like structure. A complex tendon that covers the posterior aspect of each digit is formed from a combination of the tendons of insertion of the ED, extensor indicis, and extensor digiti minimi. The distal portion of the hood receives the tendons of the lumbricals and interossei over the proximal phalanx. The tendons of the intrinsic muscles pass anterior to the MCP joint axes but posterior to the PIP and DIP joint axes. Between the MCP and PIP joints, the complete, complex ED tendon (after all contributions have been received) splits into three parts—a central slip and two lateral bands:

- Central slip. This band inserts into the proximal posterior edge of the middle phalanx.
- Lateral bands. The lateral bands rejoin over the middle phalanx into a terminal tendon that inserts into the distal phalanx's proximal posterior edge. Rupture of the tendon insertion into the distal phalanx produces a "mallet" finger (see Common Orthopedic Conditions section, later)
- The arrangement of the muscles and tendons in this expansion hood creates a "cable" system that provides a mechanism for *extending* the MCP and IP joints and allows the

lumbrical and possibly the interosseous muscles to assist in the *flexion* of the MCP joints and extension of the IP joints.

Synovial Sheaths

Synovial sheaths can be thought of as long narrow balloons filled with synovial fluid, which wrap around a tendon. During wrist motions, the sheaths move longitudinally, reducing friction.

At the wrist, the tendons of both the FDS and FDP are essentially covered by a synovial sheath and pass deep to the flexor retinaculum. As a result, the FDP tendons are deeper than those of the FDS.

The FDS and FDP tendons are covered for a variable distance by a synovial sheath in the palm.

At the digit base, both sets of tendons enter a "fibro-osseous tunnel" formed by the bones of the digit (head of the metatarsals and phalanges) and a fibrous digital tendon sheath on the anterior surface of the digits.

Flexor Pulleys

Annular (A) and cruciate (C) pulleys restrain the flexor tendons to the metacarpals and phalanges and contribute to fibro-osseous tunnels through which the tendons travel, allowing the muscles to move the wrist and hand.

Anatomic Snuffbox

The anatomic snuffbox is represented by a depression on the hand's posterior surface at the thumb base, just distal to the radius. The tendons of the APL and EPB form the radial border of the snuffbox, while the tendon of the EPL forms the ulnar border. Along the snuffbox floor are the deep branch of the radial artery and the tendinous insertion of the ECRL. Underneath these structures, the scaphoid and trapezium bones are found.

Nerve Supply

The three peripheral nerves that supply the skin and muscles of the wrist and hand include the median, ulnar, and radial nerve. The following areas of the hand typically have autonomous innervation:

- The posterior thumb-index webspace (radial nerve).
- The distal tip of the little finger (ulnar nerve).
- The volar tip of the index finger (median nerve).

Blood Supply

The brachial artery bifurcates at the elbow into radial and ulnar branches, which are the main arterial branches to the hand. Kienböck disease is in avascular necrosis of the lunate, usually as a result of distant trauma. It has also been associated with relative shortening of the ulna (negative ulnar variance) compared with the radius bone. The four stages of the disease are sclerosis, fragmentation, collapse, and arthritis.

HIP JOINT

Anatomy

The hip joint is classified as an unmodified ovoid (ball and socket) joint. The acetabulum comprises three bones: the ilium, ischium, and pubis (Figure 3-17).

The acetabular labrum deepens the acetabulum and increases articular congruence. Many muscles act across the hip (Table 3-31).

The femur is largely held in the acetabulum by three ligaments (Figure 3-18) (Table 3-32).

STUDY PEARL
Tenderness with palpation in the anatomic snuffbox suggests a scaphoid fracture but can also present in minor wrist injuries or other conditions.

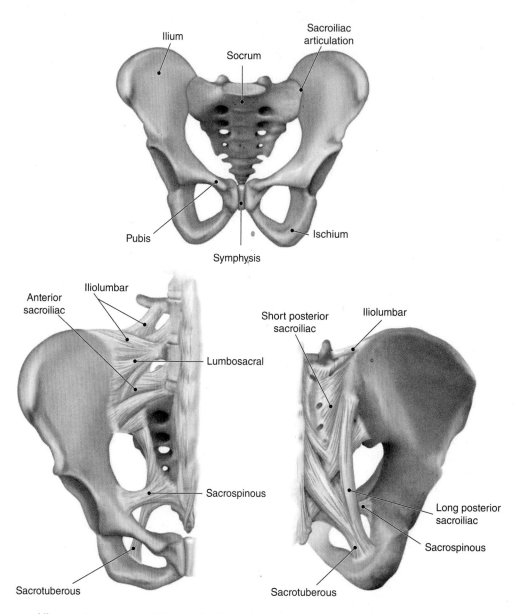

Figure 3-17. Bony and ligament structures of the pelvis. (Reproduced with permission from Burke-Doe A, Dutton M, eds. *National Physical Therapy Examination and Board Review*. 2019. Copyright © McGraw Hill LLC. All rights reserved. https://accessphysiotherapy .mhmedical.com.)

Vascular Supply

The femur's proximal shaft and the femoral neck have a plentiful blood supply from the medial circumflex femoral artery and its branches. On the other hand, the femoral head has an extremely tenuous blood supply from a small branch of the obturator artery that passes within the femoral ligament.

Biomechanics

Motion at the hip occurs in three planes: sagittal (flexion and extension around a transverse axis), frontal (abduction and adduction around an anterior-posterior axis), and transverse (internal and external rotation around a vertical axis).

The angle between the femoral shaft and the neck is called the **collum/inclination** angle. The collum angle has an important influence on the hips. This angle is approximately 125 to 135 degrees (according to source) but can vary with body types. For example, in a tall person, the collum *angle* is larger. The opposite is true with a shorter individual. An increase in the collum angle, known as **coxa valga**, causes the femoral head to be directed more

TABLE 3-31 • Muscles Acting Across the Hip Joint and Major Actions.

Muscle	Origin	Insertion	Innervation
Adductors			
Adductor brevis	External aspect of the body and inferior ramus of the pubis	By an aponeurosis to the line from the greater trochanter of the linea aspera of the femur	Obturator nerve, L3
Adductor longus	Pubic crest and symphysis	By an aponeurosis to the middle third of the linea aspera of the femur	Obturator nerve, L3
Adductor magnus	Inferior ramus of pubis, ramus of ischium, and inferolateral aspect of the ischial tuberosity	By an aponeurosis to the linea aspera and adductor tubercle of the femur	Obturator nerve and the tibial portion of the sciatic nerve, L2-L4
Pectineus	Pecten pubis	Along a line leading from the lesser trochanter to the linea aspera	Femoral or obturator or accessory obturator nerves, L2
Gracilis	The body and inferior ramus of the pubis	The anterior-medial aspect of the shaft of the proximal tibia, just proximal to the tendon of the semitendinosus	Obturator nerve, L2
Hip Extensors			
Biceps femoris (long head)	Arises from the sacrotuberous ligament and posterior aspect of the ischial tuberosity	By way of a tendon, on the lateral aspect of the head of the fibula, the lateral condyle of the tibial tuberosity, the lateral collateral ligament, and the deep fascia of the leg	The tibial portion of the sciatic nerve, S1
Semimembranosus	Ischial tuberosity	The posterior-medial aspect of the medial condyle of the tibia	Tibial nerve, L5-S1
Semitendinosus	Ischial tuberosity	The upper part of the medial surface of the tibia behind the attachment of the sartorius and below that of the gracilis	Tibial nerve, L5-S1
Gluteus maximus	Posterior gluteal line of the ilium, iliac crest, aponeurosis of the erector spinae, posterior surface of the lower part of the sacrum, side of the coccyx, sacrotuberous ligament, and intermuscular fascia	Iliotibial tract of the fascia lata, gluteal tuberosity of the femur	Inferior gluteal nerve, S1-S2
Hip Abductors			
Gluteus medius	The outer surface of the ilium between the iliac crest and the posterior gluteal line, anterior gluteal line, and fascia	The lateral surface of the greater trochanter	Superior gluteal nerve, L5
Tensor fasciae latae	The outer lip of the iliac crest and the lateral surface of the anterior superior iliac spine	Iliotibial tract	Superior gluteal nerve, L4-L5
Gluteus minimus	The outer surface of the ilium between the anterior and inferior gluteal lines and the margin of the greater sciatic notch	A ridge laterally situated on the anterior surface of the greater trochanter	Superior gluteal nerve, L5
Hip Flexors			
Iliacus	Super two-thirds of the iliac fossa, the upper surface of the lateral part of the sacrum	Fibers converge with the tendon of the psoas major to the lesser trochanter	Femoral nerve, L2
Psoas major	Transverse processes of all the lumbar vertebrae, bodies, and intervertebral disks of the lumbar vertebrae	Lesser trochanter of the femur	Lumbar plexus, L2-L3
Rectus femoris	By two heads, from the anterior inferior iliac spine and a reflected head from the groove above the acetabulum	The base of the patella	Femoral nerve, L3-L4
Sartorius	Anterior superior iliac spine and notch below it	The upper part of the medial surface of the tibia in front of the gracilis	Femoral nerve, L2-L3

(Continued)

Muscle	Origin	Insertion	Innervation
TABLE 3-31 • Muscles Acting Across the Hip Joint and Major Actions. (*Continued*)			
External Rotators			
Gemelli (superior and inferior)	The superior-posterior surface of the spine of the ischium, inferior-upper part of the tuberosity of the ischium	The superior and inferior-medial surface of the greater trochanter	Sacral plexus, L5-S1
Quadratus femoris	Ischial body next to the ischial tuberosity	Quadrate tubercle on femur	Nerve to quadratus femoris
Obturator internus	Internal surface of the anterolateral wall of the pelvis and obturator membrane	Medial surface of the greater trochanter	Sacral plexus, S1
Piriformis	Front of the sacrum, the gluteal surface of the ilium, the capsule of the sacroiliac joint, and sacro-tuberous ligament	The upper border of the greater trochanter of the femur	Sacral plexus, S1
Obturator externus	Rami of the pubis, ramus of the ischium, medial two-thirds of the outer surface of the obturator membrane	Trochanteric fossa of the femur	Obturator nerve, L4

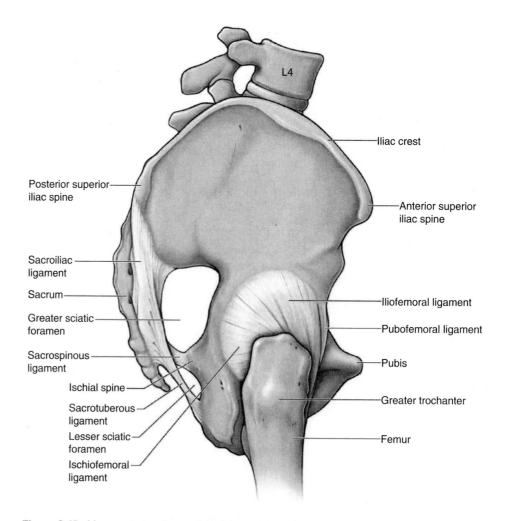

Figure 3-18. Ligament structures of the hip and the relationship of the hip joint to the lateral pelvis. (Reproduced with permission from Burke-Doe A, Dutton M, eds. *National Physical Therapy Examination and Board Review*. 2019. Copyright © McGraw Hill LLC. All rights reserved. https://accessphysiotherapy.mhmedical.com.)

TABLE 3-32 • Ligaments of the Hip.

Ligament	Origin	Insertion	Action
Iliofemoral (Y ligament of Bigelow) Consists of two parts: an inferior (medial) portion and a superior (lateral) portion, making it resemble an inverted Y	The anterior inferior iliac spine at its apex	The medial portion inserts into the inferior aspect of the trochanteric line, while the lateral portion inserts onto the superior aspect of the trochanteric line	Exhibits the greater stiffness and prevents anterior translation during extension and external rotation, in both flexion and extension Hip adduction tightens the superior portion of the iliofemoral ligament
Pubofemoral	Blends with the inferior band of the iliofemoral and with the pectineus muscle	Attaches medially to the iliopectineal eminence, the superior pubic ramus, and the obturator crest and membrane, and laterally to the anterior surface of the trochanteric line	Its fibers tighten in extension and also tighten in external rotation
Ischiofemoral	Posterior thickening of the joint capsule	The anterior aspect of the femur	Tightens with internal rotation of the hip in flexion and extension, as well as adduction of the flexed hip More commonly injured than the other hip ligaments

superiorly in the acetabulum. If the collum angle is reduced, it is known as **coxa vara** and is associated with genu valgum.

Femoral alignment in the transverse plane also influences the mechanics of the hip joint.

Anteversion is defined as the anterior position of the axis through the femoral condyles. **Retroversion** is defined as a femoral neck axis that is parallel or posterior to the condylar axis. The normal range for femoral alignment in the transverse plane in adults is 12 to 15 degrees of anteversion. Subjects with excessive anteversion usually have more hip internal rotation ROM than external rotation and gravitate to the typical "frog-sitting" posture as a position of comfort. There is also associated in-toeing while weight-bearing.

The degree of pelvic tilt, known as the angle of inclination, is measured as the angle between the horizontal plane and a line connecting the anterior superior iliac spine (ASIS) with the posterior superior iliac spine (PSIS), varying from 5 to 12 degrees in normal individuals. Angles less than this can be associated with posterior pelvic tilt, and angles greater than this may be associated with anterior pelvic tilt.

KNEE JOINT COMPLEX

The knee joint complex includes three articulating surfaces, which form two distinct joints within a single joint capsule: the patellofemoral and tibiofemoral joint (Figure 3-19).

Despite its proximity to the tibiofemoral joint, the patellofemoral joint can be considered its own entity in much the same way as the craniovertebral joints are when compared to the rest of the cervical spine. The muscles that impact the knee joint complex are described in Table 3-33.

Tibiofemoral Joint

The tibiofemoral joint, or knee joint, is a ginglymoid or modified hinge joint. Joint stability depends on the static restraints of the joint capsule, ligaments, and menisci (Figure 3-19) and (Table 3-34), and the dynamic restraints of the quadriceps, hamstrings, and gastrocnemius.

STUDY PEARL
The most stable position of the hip is the normal standing position: hip extension, slight abduction, and slight internal rotation.

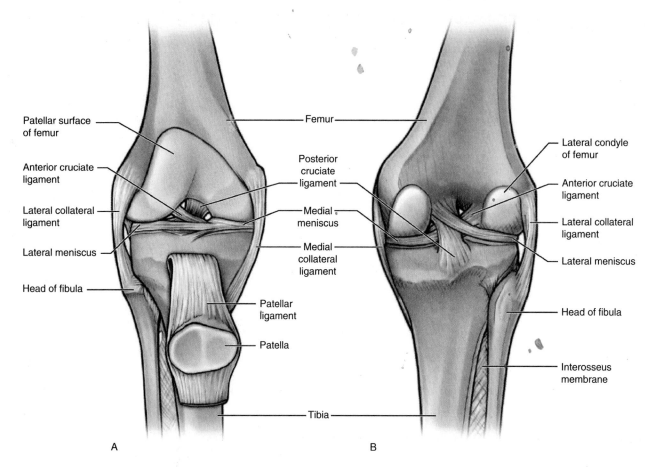

Figure 3-19. Ligaments and menisci of the (A) anterior and (B) posterior knee. (Reproduced with permission from Burke-Doe A, Dutton M, eds. *National Physical Therapy Examination and Board Review.* 2019. Copyright © McGraw Hill LLC. All rights reserved. https://accessphysiotherapy.mhmedical.com.)

TABLE 3-33 • Muscles of the Knee: Actions, Nerve Supply, and Nerve Root Derivation.			
Action	**Primary Muscles**	**Peripheral Nerve Supply**	**Nerve Root Derivation**
Flexion of the knee	Biceps femoris	Sciatic	L5, S1-S2
	Semimembranosus	Sciatic	L5, S2-S2
	Semitendinosus	Sciatic	L5, S1-S2
	Gracilis	Obturator	L2-L3
	Sartorius	Femoral	L2-L3
	Popliteus	Tibial	L4-L5, S1
	Gastrocnemius	Tibial	S1-S2
	Tensor fascia latae	Superior gluteal	L4-L5
Extension of the knee	Rectus femoris	Femoral	L2-L4
	Vastus medialis	Femoral	L2-L4
	Vastus intermedius	Femoral	L2-L4
	Vastus lateralis	Femoral	L2-L4
	Tensor fascia latae	Superior gluteal	L4-L5
Internal rotation of the flexed leg (non–weight-bearing)	Popliteus	Tibial	L4-L5
	Semimembranosus	Sciatic	L5, S1-S2
	Semitendinosus	Sciatic	L5, S1-S2
	Sartorius	Femoral	L2-L3
	Gracilis	Obturator	L2-L3
External rotation of flexed leg (non–weight-bearing)	Biceps femoris	Sciatic	L5, S1-S2

Data from Magee DJ. *Orthopaedic Physical Assessment*, 7th ed. 2020. Copyright © WB Saunders. All rights reserved.

TABLE 3-34 • Common Ligamentous and Meniscal Injuries.		
	Mechanism of Injury	**Subjective Complaints**
MCL	Most commonly involves external valgus or rotational force while the leg is firmly planted; often associated with an ACL injury	Localized swelling and tenderness over the injured area
ACL	Commonly involves noncontact pivoting/twisting mechanism while the foot is planted; non-contact hyperextension; sudden deceleration; forced internal rotation; sudden valgus impact	Reports of being unable to continue activity; hearing "pop" in the knee; extreme pain at the time of injury; acute knee swelling (within 1-2 hours of injury)
Meniscus	Usually caused by noncontact injury; rotational/torsional force applied to a flexed knee with the foot firmly planted	Reports of swelling developing within 12 hours of injury; localized swelling and tenderness over the injured area, history of popping, clicking, or locking with knee motions

Patellofemoral Joint

The quadriceps tendon (extensor mechanism) represents the confluence of four muscle-tendon units (rectus femoris, vastus lateralis, vastus intermedius, and vastus medialis) and inserts on the superior pole of the patella.

- Laterally, the iliotibial band (ITB) supports the extensor mechanism and is an important lateral stabilizer of the patellofemoral joint. It originates above the hip joint as a wide fascial band, originating from the gluteal muscles, tensor fascia lata, and vastus lateralis.
- Distally, the ITB consists of two tracts. The iliotibial tract inserts on the Gerdy tubercle of the lateral tibial plateau.

The patellar retinaculum is an important soft tissue stabilizer of the patellofemoral joint. The thicker lateral retinaculum comprises a distinct thick, deep layer and a thin superficial layer.

The patella, the largest sesamoid bone in the body, possesses the thickest articular cartilage. The articular surface, which can have a variable contour, articulates with the femur's trochlear groove.

The patellar tendon, occasionally termed the patellar ligament, originates at the patella's inferior pole and inserts onto the tibial tuberosity.

Biomechanics

The biomechanics of the knee complex are the most complex in the body.

Tibiofemoral Joint

The tibiofemoral joint motions consist of rolling, gliding, and rotation between the femoral condyles and the tibial plateaus. This rolling, gliding, and rotation occur almost simultaneously, albeit in different directions.

The femur rolls posteriorly and glides anteriorly during the knee flexion, with the opposite occurring with knee extension. This arrangement resembles a twin wheel rolling on a central rail. In the last 30 to 5 degrees of weight-bearing knee extension, the femur's lateral condyle and the lateral meniscus (LM) become congruent, moving the axis of movement more laterally. The tibial glide now becomes much greater on the medial side, which produces the femur's internal rotation, and the ligaments, both extrinsic and intrinsic, start to tighten near terminal extension. At this point, the cruciates become crossed and are tightened.

STUDY PEARL
For knee flexion to be initiated from a full extension position, the knee joint must first be "unlocked." The service of a locksmith is provided by the popliteus muscle, which acts to internally rotate the tibia on the femur, enabling the flexion to occur.

In the last 5 degrees of extension, rotation is the only movement accompanying the extension. This rotation is referred to as the *screw home mechanism* and is a characteristic motion in the normal knee in which the tibia externally rotates and the femur internally rotates as the knee approaches extension. Zero to 15 degrees of knee hyperextension is usually available. During knee hyperextension, the femur does not continue to roll anteriorly but instead tilts forward. In the normal knee, hyperextension is checked by the soft tissue structures.

Patellofemoral Joint

The patella is a passive component of the knee extensor mechanism, where the static and dynamic relationships of the underlying tibia and femur determine the patellar-tracking pattern. There are several static and dynamic restraints to assist in controlling the forces around the patellofemoral joint. The static restraints include the following:

- The medial retinaculum.
- Bony configuration of the trochlea.
- The medial patellomeniscal ligament and the lateral retinaculum.

The passive restraints to a medial translation of the patella are provided by the structures that form the superficial and deep lateral retinaculum.

The primary dynamic restraints to patellar motion are the quadriceps muscles, particularly the vastus medialis oblique (VMO). VMO contraction timings relative to the other quadriceps muscles, especially the vastus lateralis, are associated with patellar malalignment, and the VMO is vulnerable to inhibition when swelling is present.

The Quadriceps Angle

The quadriceps ("Q") angle can be described as the angle formed by the bisection of two lines, one line drawn from the ASIS to the center of the patella and the other from the center of the patella to the tibial tubercle. Various normal values for the Q-angle have been reported in the literature. However, the most common ranges cited are 8 to 14 degrees for males and 15 to 17 degrees for females. The discrepancy between males and females is supposedly due to the female's wider pelvis, although this has yet to be proven.

STUDY PEARL
Q-angle measurements can vary significantly with foot pronation and supination compared with measurements made in the supine position.

Patella-Femur Contact and Loading

The amount of contact between the patella and the femur appears to vary according to several factors, including (1) the angle of knee flexion, (2) the location of the contact, (3) the surface area of contact, and (4) the patellofemoral joint reaction force.

Patellar Tracking

The patella glides in a curved path inferiorly and superiorly in the normal knee during flexion and extension, respectively.

Open and Closed Kinetic Chain Activities

A closed-chain motion at the knee joint complex occurs when the knee bends or straightens, while the lower extremity is weight-bearing, or when the foot is in contact with any firm surface. An open-chain motion occurs when the knee bends or straightens when the foot is not in contact with any stable surface.

Whether the motion occurring at the knee joint complex occurs as a closed or open kinetic chain has implications on the biomechanics and the joint compressive forces induced.

Closed-Chain Motion

Tibiofemoral Joint. During closed-chain knee flexion, the femoral condyles roll backward and glide forward on the tibia. When the femur rolls posteriorly, the distance between the tibial and femoral insertions of the ACL increases. Since the ACL cannot lengthen, it guides the femoral condyles anteriorly. In contrast, during closed-chain extension of the knee, the distance between the femoral and tibial insertions of the posterior cruciate ligament (PCL) increases. Since the PCL cannot lengthen, the ligament guides the femoral condyles posteriorly as the knee extends.

Patellofemoral Joint. During closed kinetic exercises, the flexion moment arm increases as the angle of knee flexion increases. From 90 to 120 degrees of flexion, the articular pressure remains essentially unchanged because the quadriceps tendon is in contact with the trochlea, which effectively increases the contact area. Due to the effect of joint reaction forces, CKC exercises involving the patellofemoral joint are performed in the 0 to 45 degrees range of flexion, with caution used when exercising between 90 and 50 degrees of knee flexion as the patellofemoral joint reaction forces can be significantly greater.

Open-Chain Motion

Tibiofemoral Joint. During open-chain flexion, the tibia rolls and glides posteriorly on the femur, while during extension, the opposite occurs. Open-chain knee extension involves a conjunct external rotation of the tibia, while open-chain knee flexion involves a conjunct internal rotation of the tibia.

Open-chain activities produce shear forces at the tibiofemoral joint in the direction of tibial movement.

Open-chain knee flexion, resulting from an isolated contraction of the hamstrings, reduces ACL strain throughout the ROM but increases the PCL strain as flexion increases from 30 to 90 degrees.

Patellofemoral Joint. In an open-chain activity, the forces across the patella are their lowest at 90 degrees of flexion. Due to the effect of joint reaction forces, OKC exercises for the patellofemoral joint should be performed from 25 to 90 degrees of flexion (60-90 degrees if there are distal patellar lesions) or at 0 degree of extension (or hyperextension) from the point of view of cartilage stress. OKC exercises are not recommended for the patellofemoral joint between 0 and 45 degrees of knee flexion, especially if there are proximal patellar lesions, as the patellar joint reaction forces (PJRFs) are significantly greater.

ANKLE AND FOOT JOINT COMPLEX

The majority of the support provided to the ankle and foot joints comes by way of the ankle mortise and the numerous ligaments found here (Table 3-35).

Further stabilization is afforded by an abundant number of short and long tendons that cross this joint complex (Tables 3-36 and 3-37). These tendons are also involved in producing foot and ankle movements and are held in place by the retinacula.

Even with this remarkable protection level, the foot and ankle complex is at the mercy of truly impressive forces that act upon it during normal and athletic activities. Thus, as elsewhere, injuries to this area can be either microtraumatic or macrotraumatic.

Biomechanics

Terminology. Motions of the leg, foot, and ankle consist of single-plane and multiplane movements.

The single-plane motions include the following:

- The frontal plane motions of inversion and eversion.
- The sagittal plane motions of dorsiflexion and plantarflexion.
- The horizontal plane motions of adduction and abduction.

Triplanar motions occur at the talocrural, subtalar, and midtarsal joints and the first and fifth rays. Pronation and supination are considered triplanar motions.

TABLE 3-35 • Ankle and Foot Joints and Associated Ligaments.

Joint	Associated Ligament	Fiber Direction	Motions Limited
Distal tibiofibular	Anterior tibiofibular Posterior tibiofibular Interosseous	Distolateral Distolateral	Distal glide of the fibula Plantarflexion Distal glide of the fibula Plantarflexion Separation of tibia and fibula

Ankle	Deltoid (medial collateral)
	Superficial
	  Tibionavicular
	  Tibiocalcaneal
	  Posterior tibiotalar
	Deep
	  Anterior tibiotalar
	Lateral or fibular collateral
	  Anterior talofibular
	  Calcaneofibular
	  Posterior talofibular
	Lateral talocalcaneal
	Anterior capsule
	Posterior capsule
		
		Plantar-anterior
		Plantar, plantar-posterior
		Plantar-posterior
		
		Anterior
		Anterior-medial
		Posterior-medial
		Horizontal (lateral)
		Posterior-medial
			
			Plantarflexion, abduction
			Eversion, abduction
			Dorsiflexion, abduction
			Eversion, abduction, plantarflexion
			Plantarflexion
			
			Inversion
			Anterior displacement of the foot
			Inversion
			Dorsiflexion
			Dorsiflexion
			Posterior displacement of the foot
			Inversion
			Dorsiflexion
			Plantarflexion
			Dorsiflexion

Subtalar	Interosseous talocalcaneal
	  Anterior band
	  Posterior band
	Lateral talocalcaneal
	Deltoid
	Lateral collateral
	Posterior talocalcaneal
	Medial talocalcaneal
	Anterior talocalcaneal (cervical ligaments)
		
		Proximal-anterior-lateral
		Proximal-posterior-lateral
		(See ankle)
		(See ankle)
		(See ankle)
		Vertical
		Plantar-anterior
		Plantar-posterior-lateral
			
			Inversion
			Joint separation
			Inversion
			Joint separation
			Dorsiflexion
			Eversion
			
			Inversion

Main ligamentous support of longitudinal arches	Long plantar Short plantar Plantar calcaneonavicular Plantar aponeurosis	Anterior, slightly medial Anterior Posterior-anterior-medial Anterior	Eversion Eversion Eversion Eversion

Midtarsal or transverse	Bifurcated
	  Medial band
	  Lateral band
	Posterior talonavicular
	Posterior calcaneocuboid ligaments supporting the arches
		
		Longitudinal
		Horizontal
		Longitudinal
		Longitudinal
			
			Joint separation
			Plantarflexion
			Inversion
			Plantarflexion of talus on navicular
			Inversion, plantarflexion

Intertarsal	Numerous ligaments named by two interconnected bones (posterior and plantar ligaments) Interosseous ligaments connecting cuneiforms, cuboid, and navicular ligaments supporting arches		Joint motion in a direction causing ligament tightening Flattening of the transverse arch
Tarsometatarsal	Posterior, plantar, and interosseous		Joint separation
Intermetatarsal	Posterior, plantar, and interosseous Deep transverse metatarsal		Joint separation Joint separation Flattening of the transverse arch
Metatarsophalangeal	Fibrous capsule Dorsally, thin—separated from extensor tendons by bursae Inseparable from the deep surface of the plantar and collateral ligaments Collateral Plantar, grooved for flexor tendons	 Plantar-anterior	Flexion Extension Flexion, abduction, or adduction in flexion Extension
Interphalangeal	Collateral Plantar Extensor hood replaces posterior ligaments		Flexion, abduction, or adduction in flexion Extension Flexion

TABLE 3-36 • Intrinsic Muscles of the Foot.			
Muscle	**Attachments**	**Action**	**Innervation**
Extensor digitorum brevis	Proximal: Superior surface of the calcaneus Distal: Posterior surface of second through fourth toes, the base of proximal phalanx	Extends digits 2 through 4	Deep peroneal S1 and S2
Abductor hallucis	Proximal: Tuberosity of calcaneus and plantar aponeurosis Distal: Base of the proximal phalanx, medial side	Abducts hallux	Medial plantar L5 and S1 (L4)
Adductor hallucis	Proximal: Base of second, third, and fourth metatarsals and deep plantar ligaments Distal: Proximal phalanx of first digit lateral side	Adducts hallux	Medial and lateral plantar S1 and S2
Lumbricals	Proximal: Medial and adjacent sides of flexor digitorum longus tendon to each lateral digit Distal: Medial side of the proximal phalanx and extensor hood	Flex metatarso-phalangeal joints; extend interphalangeal joints	Medial and lateral plantar L5, S1, and S2 (L4)
Plantar interossei First Second Third	Proximal: Base and medial side of the third metatarsal Distal: Base of the proximal phalanx and extensor hood of the third digit Proximal: Base and medial side of the fourth metatarsal Distal: Base of the proximal phalanx and extensor hood of the fourth digit Proximal: Base and medial side of the fifth metatarsal Distal: Base of the proximal phalanx and extensor hood of the fifth digit	Adduct toes	Medial and lateral plantar S1 and S2
Posterior interossei First Second Third Fourth	Proximal: First and second metatarsal bones Distal: Proximal phalanx and extensor hood of the second digit medially Proximal: Second and third metatarsal bones Distal: Proximal phalanx and extensor hood of the second digit laterally Proximal: Third and fourth metatarsal bones Distal: Proximal phalanx and extensor hood of the third digit laterally Proximal: Fourth and fifth metatarsal bones Distal: Proximal phalanx and extensor hood of the fourth digit laterally	Abduct toes	Medial and lateral plantar S1 and S2
Abductor digiti minimi	Proximal: Lateral side of the fifth metatarsal bone Distal: Proximal phalanx of the fifth digit	Flexion and abduction of the fifth toe	Lateral plantar S1 and S2

- The body plane motions during pronation are abduction in the transverse plane, dorsiflexion in the sagittal plane, and eversion in the frontal plane.
- The plane motions during supination are a combined movement of adduction, plantarflexion, and inversion.

In pronation, the forefoot is rotated big toe downward and little toe upward, whereas in supination, the reverse occurs.

Distal Tibiofibular Joint

The two tibiofibular joints (proximal and distal) are described as individual articulations, but they function as a pair. Thus, the movements that occur at these joints are primarily a result of the ankle's influence.

The ligaments of the distal tibiofibular joint are more commonly injured than the anterior talofibular ligament. Ankle syndesmosis injuries most often occur with forced external rotation of the foot or during internal rotation of the tibia on a planted foot. Hyperdorsiflexion may also be a contributing mechanism.

TABLE 3-37 · Extrinsic Muscle Attachments and Innervation.

Muscle	Attachments	Action	Innervation
Gastrocnemius	Proximal: Medial and lateral condyle of the femur Distal: Posterior surface of calcaneus through Achilles tendon	Plantarflexes foot flexes knee	Tibial S2 (S1)
Plantaris	Proximal: Lateral supracondylar line of femur Distal: Posterior surface of calcaneus through Achilles tendon	Plantarflexes foot and flexes knee	Tibial S2 (S1)
Soleus	Proximal: Head of the fibula, the proximal third of shaft, soleal line, and midshaft of the posterior tibia Distal: Posterior surface of calcaneus through Achilles tendon	Plantarflexes foot	Tibial S2 (S1)
Tibialis anterior	Proximal: Distal to the lateral tibial condyle, proximal half of lateral tibial shaft, and interosseous membrane Distal: First cuneiform bone, medial and plantar surfaces, and base of the first metatarsal	Dorsiflexion and inversion of the foot	Deep fibular (peroneal) L4 (L5)
Tibialis posterior	Proximal: Posterior surface of the tibia, proximal two-thirds posterior of the fibula, and interosseous membrane Distal: Tuberosity of navicular bone, tendinous expansion to other tarsals and metatarsals	Plantarflexion and inversion of the foot	Tibial L4 and L5
Fibularis (peroneus) longus	Proximal: Lateral condyle of tibia, head, and proximal two-thirds of the fibula Distal: Base of the first metatarsal and first cuneiform, lateral side	Plantarflexion, eversion of the foot	Superficial fibular (peroneal) L5 and S1 (S2)
Fibularis (peroneus) brevis	Proximal: Distal two-thirds of the lateral fibular shaft Distal: Tuberosity of the fifth metatarsal	Plantarflexion, eversion of the foot	Superficial fibular (peroneal) L5 and S1 (S2)
Fibularis (peroneus) tertius	Proximal: Lateral slip from extensor digitorum longus Distal: Tuberosity of the fifth metatarsal	Dorsiflexion and eversion of the foot	Deep fibular (peroneal) L5 and S1
Flexor hallucis brevis	Proximal: Plantar surface of cuboid and third cuneiform bones Distal: Base of proximal phalanx of the great toe	Flexion of the hallux	Medial plantar S3 (S2)
Flexor hallucis longus	Proximal: Posterior distal two-thirds of the fibula Distal: Base of distal phalanx of the great toe	Flexion of all joints of the big toe; plantarflexion of the ankle joint	Tibial S2 (S3)
Flexor digitorum brevis	Proximal: Tuberosity of calcaneus Distal: One tendon slips into the base of the middle phalanx of each of the lateral four toes	Flexion of the lateral four digits	Medial and lateral plantar S3 (S2)
Flexor digitorum longus	Proximal: Middle three-fifths of the posterior tibia Distal: Base of distal phalanx of lateral four toes	Flexion of the four smaller digits	Tibial S2 (S3)
Extensor hallucis longus	Proximal: Middle half of anterior shaft of fibula Distal: Base of distal phalanx of the great toe	Extension of the big toe and assists in dorsiflexion of the foot at the ankle Also, a weak evertor/invertor	Deep fibular (peroneal) L5 and S1
Extensor hallucis brevis	Proximal: Distal superior and lateral surfaces of calcaneus Distal: Posterior surface of proximal phalanx	Extends the hallux	Deep fibular (peroneal) S1 and S2
Extensor digitorum longus	Proximal: Lateral condyle of tibia proximal anterior surface of shaft of fibula Distal: One tendon to each lateral four toes, to middle phalanx and extending to distal phalanges	Extension of toes and dorsiflexion of the ankle	Deep fibular (peroneal) L5 and S1

Talocrural Joint

The primary motions at this joint are dorsiflexion and plantarflexion, with a total range of 70 to 80 degrees. The talocrural joint axis is 20 to 30 degrees posterior to the frontal plane as it passes posteriorly from the medial malleolus to the lateral malleolus. Although talocrural motion occurs primarily in the sagittal plane, appreciable horizontal motion appears to occur in the horizontal plane, especially during internal rotation of the tibia or pronation of the foot.

Stability for this joint in weight-bearing is provided by the articular surfaces, while in non–weight-bearing, the ligaments appear to provide the majority of stability.

Subtalar Joint

The subtalar joint is responsible for the inversion and eversion of the hindfoot (Figure 3-20). Approximately 50% of apparent ankle inversion observed comes from the subtalar joint. The axis of motion for the subtalar joint is approximately 45 degrees from horizontal and 20 degrees medial to the midsagittal plane.

This axis, which moves during subtalar joint motion, allows the subtalar joint to produce a triplanar (pronation/supination) and varies according to whether the joint is weight-bearing (close chain) or non–weight-bearing (open chain).

- During weight-bearing activities, pronation involves calcaneal eversion, adduction and plantarflexion of the talus, and internal rotation of the tibia, whereas supination involves a combination of calcaneal inversion, abduction and dorsiflexion of the talus, and external rotation of the tibia.
- During non–weight-bearing activities, pronation involves calcaneal eversion and abduction and dorsiflexion of the talus, whereas supination involves a combination of calcaneal inversion and adduction and plantarflexion of the talus.

> **STUDY PEARL**
> The tibia internally rotates during pronation and externally rotates during supination.

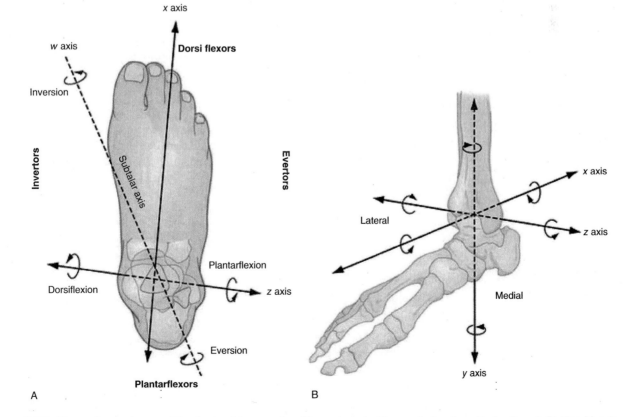

Figure 3-20. Biomechanical axes of the foot-ankle complex. (Reproduced with permission from Burke-Doe A, Dutton M, eds. *National Physical Therapy Examination and Board Review.* 2019. Copyright © McGraw Hill LLC. All rights reserved. https://accessphysiotherapy.mhmedical.com.)

Joint	Degrees of Freedom	Motions Available
Talocalcaneal	2	Plantar-/dorsiflexion, inversion/eversion
Cuneonavicular	2	Plantar-/dorsiflexion, inversion/eversion
Intercuneiform and cuneocuboid	1	Inversion/eversion
Metatarsophalangeal	2	Flexion/extension, abduction/adduction
First metatarsophalangeal	2	Flexion/extension, abduction/adduction
Interphalangeal (IP)	1	Flexion/extension

TABLE 3-38 • Motion Available for the Ankle and Foot Joints.

STUDY PEARL

In normal individuals, there is an eversion to inversion ratio of 2:3 to 1:3, which amounts to approximately 20 degrees inversion and 10 degrees eversion. Therefore, a minimum of 4 to 6 degrees of eversion and 8 to 12 degrees of inversion is required for normal gait.

The subtalar joint controls supination and pronation with help from the transverse tarsal joints of the midfoot.

Stability for the subtalar joint is provided by the calcaneofibular ligament (CFL), the cervical ligament, the interosseous ligament, the lateral talocalcaneal ligament, the fibulotalocalcaneal ligament (ligament of Rouviere), and the extensor retinaculum.

Midtarsal (Transverse Tarsal) Joint Complex

The midtarsal joint complex's function is to provide the foot with an additional mechanism for raising and lowering the arch and absorbing some of the horizontal plane tibial motion transmitted to the foot during stance. The joints of the foot and ankle have varying amounts of motion (Table 3-38).

The great toe's function is to provide stability to the medial aspect of the foot and provide for normal propulsion during gait. Normal alignment of the first metatarsophalangeal (MTP) joint varies between 5 degrees varus and 15 degrees valgus.

The great toe is characterized by having a remarkable discrepancy between active and passive motion. Approximately 30 degrees active plantarflexion is present and at least 50 degrees active extension, the latter of which can be frequently increased passively to between 70 and 90 degrees.

CRANIOVERTEBRAL JOINTS

The craniovertebral (CV) junction is a collective term that refers to the region of the cervical spine where the skull and vertebral column articulate. It comprises the foramen magnum, occiput, atlas, and axis, and their supporting ligaments. The posterior portion of the foramen magnum houses the brainstem-spinal cord junction.

Occipito-Atlantal Joint

The occipito-atlantal (O-A) joint is formed between the occipital condyles and the superior articular facets of the atlas (C1). The paired occipital condyles are ovoid structures with their long axis situated in a posterolateral-to-anteromedial orientation.

Atlantoaxial Joint

The atlantoaxial (A-A) joint is a relatively complex articulation, which consists of the following:

- Two lateral synovial zygapophyseal joints between the articular surfaces of the inferior articular processes of the atlas and the superior processes of the axis.
- Two medial synovial joints: One between the anterior surface of the dens of the axis and the anterior surface of the atlas, and the other between the posterior surface of the dens and the anterior hyalinated surface of the transverse ligament.

Craniovertebral Ligaments

The craniovertebral ligaments (Figure 3-21) are outlined in Table 3-39.

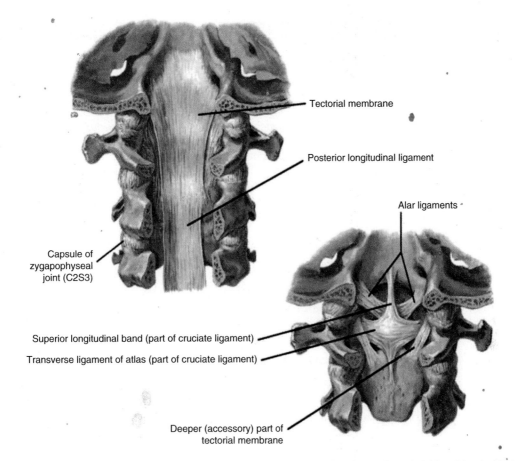

Figure 3-21. **Ligaments of the upper cervical spine.** (Reproduced with permission from Burke-Doe A, Dutton M, eds. *National Physical Therapy Examination and Board Review*. 2019. Copyright © McGraw Hill LLC. All rights reserved. https://accessphysiotherapy. mhmedical.com.)

TABLE 3-39 • Craniovertebral Ligaments.	
Ligament	**Description**
Capsule and accessory capsular	These ligaments are quite lax to permit maximal motion, so they provide only moderate support to the joints during contralateral head rotation.
Apical	Extends from the apex of the dens to the anterior rim of the foramen magnum. The ligament appears to be only a moderate stabilizer against a posterior translation of the dens relative to both the atlas and the occipital bone.
Vertical and transverse bands of the cruciform	The transverse portion stretches between tubercles on the medial aspects of the lateral masses of the atlas. The transverse portion's major responsibility is to counteract an anterior translation of the atlas relative to the axis, thereby maintaining the position of the dens relative to the anterior arch of the atlas. The transverse ligament also limits the amount of flexion between the atlas and axis. These limiting functions are of extreme importance because the excessive movement of either type could result in the dens compressing the spinal cord, epipharynx, vertebral artery, or superior cervical ganglion.
Alar and accessory alar	Connect the superior part of the dens to fossae on the medial aspect of the occipital condyles, although they can also attach to the lateral masses of the atlas. The function of the ligament is to resist flexion, contralateral side-bending, and rotation. Due to the ligament connections, side-bending of the head produces a contralateral rotation of the C2 vertebra.
Anterior occipito-atlantal membrane	Thought to be the superior continuation of the anterior longitudinal ligament. It extends from the anterior arch of vertebra C1 to the anterior aspect of the foramen magnum.
Posterior occipito-atlantal membrane	A continuation of the ligamentum flavum. This ligament interconnects the posterior arch of the atlas and the posterior aspect of the foramen magnum.
Tectorial membrane	Interconnects the occipital bone and the axis. This ligament is the superior continuation of the posterior longitudinal ligament and connects the body of vertebra C2 to the anterior rim of the foramen magnum. This bridging ligament is an important limiter of upper cervical flexion.

Region	Specific Muscle	Function	Nerve Supply
Anterior suboccipital	Rectus capitis anterior	Aids in neck/head flexion.	C1, C2
	Rectus capitis lateralis	Aids in side flexion. Also stabilizes the occipito-atlantal joint.	C1, C2
Posterior suboccipital	Rectus capitis posterior major Rectus capitis posterior minor Obliquus capitis superior Obliquus capitis inferior	These muscles function in controlling segmental sliding between C1 and C2, and may have an important role in proprioception, having more muscle spindles than any other muscle for their size. All of the posterior suboccipital muscles are innervated by the posterior ramus of C1 and are strongly linked with the trigeminal nerve. The suboccipitals receive their blood supply from the vertebral artery.	Suboccipital nerve

TABLE 3-40 • Muscles of the Craniovertebral Region.

Craniovertebral Muscles

The muscles of the craniovertebral region are outlined in Table 3-40.

Biomechanics

The upper cervical spine is responsible for approximately 50% of the motion in the entire cervical spine. Motion at the A-A joint occurs relatively independently, while below C2, normal motion is a combination of motion occurring at other levels.

Occipito-Atlantal Joint

The primary motion at this joint is flexion and extension, although side-bending and rotation also occur. It is generally agreed that rotation and side-bending at this joint occur to opposite sides when they are combined.

Occipital rotation, and to some degree anterior-posterior translation of the occiput on C1, is thought to be limited by the alar ligaments.

Atlantoaxial Joint

The major motion at all three of the A-A articulations is axial rotation, totaling approximately 40 to 47 degrees to each side.

A-A joint flexion and extension movements amount to a combined range of 10 to 15 degrees: 10 degrees flexion and 5 degrees extension.

CERVICAL SPINE

The cervical spine is made up of seven vertebrae, C1 to C7. Eight pairs of cervical spinal nerves exit bilaterally through the intervertebral foramina. Each spinal nerve is named for the vertebra above which it exits; for example, the C6 nerve exits above the C6 vertebra. This naming changes at the C7-T1 segment. The C8 nerve exits at the C7-T1 segment. All of the spinal nerves inferior to this segment are named for the vertebra beneath; for example, the T1 nerve exits at the T1-T2 segment.

With stability being sacrificed for mobility, the cervical spine is more vulnerable to direct and indirect trauma. The cervical spine can be the source of many pain syndromes, including neck, upper thoracic periscapular syndromes, cervical radiculopathy, and shoulder and elbow syndromes.

Biomechanics

At the zygapophyseal joints, significant flexion occurs at C5-C6 and extension around C6-C7. The only significant arthrokinematic motion available to the zygapophyseal joint is an inferior, medial glide of the inferior articular process of the superior facet during extension and a superior, lateral glide during flexion. Segmental side-bending is, therefore, an extension of the ipsilateral joint and flexion of the contralateral joint. Rotation, coupled with ipsilateral side-bending, involves an extension of the ipsilateral joint and flexion of the contralateral.

Muscle Control

The cervical region's muscle groups may be divided into those producing global movements and those local muscles that sustain postures or stabilize the segments.

- The neck's global muscles are the sternocleidomastoid (anteriorly) and the semispinalis capitis and splenius capitis (posteriorly).
- The local system comprises the longus capitis and longus colli and semispinalis cervicis, and multifidus.

TEMPOROMANDIBULAR JOINT

The temporomandibular joint (TMJ) is a synovial, compound modified ovoid bicondylar joint formed between the articular eminence of the temporal bone, the intra-articular disk, and the head of the mandible. The maxilla and the mandible, which support the teeth, and the temporal bone, which supports the mandible's articulation with the skull, make up the masticatory system. The TMJ is unique in that, even though the joint is synovial, the articulating surfaces are covered, not by hyaline cartilage but by fibrocartilage. The development of fibrocartilage over the load-bearing surface of the TMJ indicates that the joint is designed to withstand large and repeated stresses and that this area of the joint surface has a greater capacity to repair itself than would hyaline cartilage.

Located between the articulating surface of the temporal bone and the mandibular condyle is a fibrocartilaginous disk (sometimes incorrectly referred to as "meniscus"). The shape of the condyle and the articulating fossa determines the biconcave shape of the disk. The disk effectively divides the TMJ into a lower and upper joint cavity.

Muscles of the TMJ Region

The muscles of this region are described in Table 3-41.

The muscles of the TMJ, working in various combinations, are involved as follows:

- Mouth opening—bilateral action of the lateral pterygoid and digastric muscles.
- Mouth closing—bilateral action of the temporalis, masseter, and medial pterygoid muscles.
- Lateral deviation—the action of the ipsilateral masseter and contralateral medial pterygoid muscles.
- Protrusion—bilateral action of the lateral pterygoid, medial pterygoid, and anterior fibers of the temporalis muscles.
- Retrusion—bilateral action of the posterior fibers of the temporalis muscle and the digastric, stylohyoid, geniohyoid, and mylohyoid muscles.

Supporting Structures

The supporting structures of the TMJ are outlined in Table 3-42.

Nerve Supply

The TMJ is primarily supplied from three nerves that are part of the mandibular division of the fifth cranial (trigeminal) nerve.

Biomechanics

Two primary arthrokinematic movements (rotation and anterior translation) occur at this joint around three planes: sagittal, horizontal, and frontal.

- Mouth opening, contralateral deviation, and protrusion all involve an anterior osteokinematic rotation of the mandible and an anterior, inferior, and lateral glide of the mandibular head and disk.
- Mouth closing, ipsilateral deviation, and retrusion all involve a posterior osteokinematic rotation of the mandible and a posterior, inferior, and lateral glide of the mandibular head and disk.

TABLE 3-41 · Muscles of the Face, Mouth, and Pharynx.

	Anatomy	Action	Innervation
Muscles of the Face			
Levator anguli oris	Arises from the canine fossa of the maxilla and inserts into the upper and lower lips	Contraction results in drawing the corner of the mouth up and medially	Superior buccal branches of CN VII
Zygomatic major (zygomaticus)	Arises lateral to the zygomatic minor on the zygomatic bone Courses obliquely and inserts into the corner of the orbicularis oris	Elevates and retracts the angle of the mouth (smiling)	
Depressor labii inferioris	Originates from the mandible and courses up and in to insert into the lower lip	Dilation of the orifice of the mouth; pulls the lips down and out; counterpart to the levator triad	Mandibular marginal branches of VII
Depressor anguli oris (triangularis)	Originates along the lateral margins of the mandible Fanlike fibers converge on the orbicularis oris and upper lip at the corner	Depresses the corners of the mouth and compresses the upper lip against the lower lip	
Mentalis	Arises from the region of the incisive fossa of the mandible and inserts into the skin of the chin	Contraction elevates and wrinkles the chin and pulls the lower lip out	Innervated by the mandibular marginal branch of the facial nerve
Platysma (also considered a neck muscle)	Arises from the fascia overlying the pectoralis major and deltoid Courses superiorly and inserts into the corner of the mouth below the symphysis mente, the lower margin of the mandible, and then into the skin near the masseter	Appears to assist in depression of the mandible	The cervical branch of CN VII
Muscles of the Mouth			
Orbicularis oris	Considered a single muscle encircling the mouth opening as well as paired upper and lower muscles (obicularis oris superior, obicularis oris inferior)	Serves as a point of insertion for other muscles	Branches of the VII facial nerve
Risorius	Superficial to the buccinators, it originates from the posterior region of the face along the fascia of the masseter muscle; courses forward, and inserts into the corners of the mouth	Retracts the lips at the corners (smiling)	Cranial nerve VII (facial nerve)
Buccinator	Deep to the risorius; originates on the pterygomandibular ligament and the posterior alveolar portion of the mandible and maxillae; courses forward to insert into the upper and lower orbicularis oris	Involved in mastication; also constricts the oropharynx	Cranial nerve VII (facial nerve)
Levator triad (a group of three muscles)	1. Levator labii superioris alaeque nasi (most medial)—courses vertically along the lateral margin of the nose, arising from the frontal process of maxilla; inserts into the wing of the nostril and UL (flares the nares) 2. Levator labii superioris (intermediate)—originates from the infraorbital margin of the maxilla; courses down and into the upper lip 3. Zygomatic minor (lateral)—originates at the facial surface of the zygomatic bone and courses downward into the upper lip	Dominant muscles for lip elevation and also dilate the oral opening	Buccal branches of CN VII

(Continued)

TABLE 3-41 • Muscles of the Face, Mouth, and Pharynx. (Continued)			
	Anatomy	**Action**	**Innervation**
Intrinsic Muscles of the Tongue			
Median fibrous septum	Divides right and left halves of the tongue—originates on the body of the hyoid bone via the hyoglossal membrane; courses the length of the tongue	Serves as the point of origin for the transverse muscle of the tongue Forms tongue attachment with the hyoid	
Longitudinal muscle (superior lingualis)	A thin layer of oblique and longitudinal muscle fibers lying just deep to the mucous membrane of the dorsum Fibers arise from the submucous fibrous tissue near the epiglottis, hyoid, and the median fibrous septum Fibers fan forward and outward, then insert into the lateral margins of the tongue	A bilateral contraction will elevate the tongue tip A unilateral contraction will pull the tongue toward the side of the contraction	
Inferior longitudinal muscle (inferior lingualis)	A bundle of muscle fibers located on the undersurface of the tongue (absent in the medial tongue base) Originates at the root of the tongue and corpus hyoid Courses between the genioglossus and hyoglossus muscles and to the apex of the tongue Longitudinal muscle fibers interdigitate with them	A bilateral contraction will pull the tip of the tongue downward and assist in retraction of the tongue if cocontracted with the superior longitudinal A unilateral contraction will cause the tongue to turn toward the contracted side and downward	
Transverse muscle (transverse lingualis)	Fibers originate at the median fibrous septum Courses laterally to insert into the submucous tissue at the lateral margins of the tongue Some fibers continue as the palatopharyngeus muscle	Contraction pulls the edges of the tongue toward the midline, narrowing and elongating the tongue	
Vertical muscles (vertical lingualis)	Originate from the mucous membrane of the dorsum Course vertically downward and somewhat laterally Fibers of the transverse and vertical muscles interweave Insert into the sides and inferior surface of the tongue	Contraction flattens the tongue	
Extrinsic Tongue Muscles			
Genioglossus	A flat, triangular muscle located close to the median plane Arises from the inner mandibular surface at the symphysis Lower fibers course to the hyoid bone and attach by a thin aponeurosis to the upper part of the body The remainder of the fibers radiate fanlike to the dorsum of the tongue, inserting into the submucous fibrous tissues	The prime mover of the tongue (strongest and largest of the extrinsic muscles) Contraction of the anterior fibers results in retraction of the tongue Contraction of the posterior fibers draws the tongue forward to aid protrusion of the apex Contraction of both anterior and posterior fibers will draw the middle portion of the tongue down into the floor of the mouth (cupping the tongue)	
Hyoglossus	Arises from the length of the greater cornu and lateral body of the hyoid Courses upward and inserts into the lateral portions of the tongue	Contraction pulls the sides of the tongue down The antagonist to the palatoglossus	

	Anatomy	Action	Innervation
TABLE 3-41 • Muscles of the Face, Mouth, and Pharynx. (*Continued*)			
Extrinsic Tongue Muscles (Cont.)			
Styloglossus	Originates from the anterolateral margin of the styloid process Courses forward and down to insert into the inferior sides of the tongue Divides into two portions: One interdigitates with the inferior longitudinal muscle and the other with the hyoglossus	Bilateral contraction draws the tongue back and up	
Chondroglossus	Also considered to be a part of the hyoglossus Arises from the lesser cornu of the hyoid Courses up to interdigitate with the intrinsic muscles of the tongue medial to the point of insertion of the hyoglossus	Contraction depresses the tongue	
Palatoglossus	Can be considered a muscle of the tongue or the velum	Serves a dual purpose—depresses the soft palate, and elevates the back of the tongue	
Mandibular Elevators			
Masseter	The most superficial of the mastication muscles Originates on the lateral, inferior, and medial surfaces of the zygomatic arch External fibers insert into the ramus Internal (deep) fibers terminate on the coronoid process	Places maximum force on the molars Contraction elevates the mandible, closing the jaw Clenching the teeth will make the muscular belly visible	Innervated by CN V—trigeminal nerve
Temporalis	Deep to the masseter Arises from the temporal fossa (a region of the temporal and parietal bones) The broad, thin, fan-shaped muscle converges as it courses down and forward The terminal tendon passes through the zygomatic arch and inserts in the coronoid process and ramus	Contraction elevates the mandible and draws it back if protruded	Innervated by CN V—trigeminal
Medial ptery-goid (internal pterygoid mus-cle, internal masseter)	Originates primarily in the vertically directed pterygoid fossa and from the medial surface of the lateral pterygoid plate Fibers course down and back inserting into the ramus	Contraction elevates the mandible in conjunction with the masseter	Innervated by CN V
Mandibular Protrusors			
Lateral pterygoid	Arises from the sphenoid bone Two heads—lateral pterygoid plate; the greater wing of the sphenoid bone Fibers course back to insert into the pterygoid fossa (fovea) of the mandible (a depression on the anterior neck of the condyle of the mandible) and to the anterior margin of the articular disk of the temporomandibular articulation	Contraction protrudes the mandible, causing the condyle to slide down and forward on the articular eminence Unilateral contraction moves the jaw in a grinding motion	

(Continued)

TABLE 3-41 • Muscles of the Face, Mouth, and Pharynx. (*Continued*)			
	Anatomy	**Action**	**Innervation**
Mandibular Depressors			
Digastricus	Anterior and posterior	When infrahyoid musculature is fixed, contraction of the anterior digastricus will depress the mandible Bilaterally, the digastrics assist in forced mouth opening by stabilizing the hyoid The posterior bellies are especially active during coughing and swallowing	
Mylohyoid	Forms floor of the mouth	When the hyoid is in a fixed position, the contraction will depress the mandible Stabilizes or elevates the tongue during swallowing and elevates the floor of the mouth in the first stage of deglutition	
Geniohyoid	A narrow muscle situated under the mylohyoid muscle	Contraction depresses the mandible if the hyoid is fixed; elevates the hyoid bone if the mandible is fixed	
Platysma	Also considered a muscle of the face	Contraction depresses the mandible	
Hyoid Muscles			
Sternohyoid Omohyoid Sternothyroid and thyrohyoid Stylohyoid	A strap-like muscle Situated lateral to the sternohyoid; consists of two bellies Located deep to the sternohyoid muscle	Functions to depress the hyoid as well as assist in speech and mastication Functions to depress the hyoid The sternothyroid muscle is involved in drawing the larynx downward, while the thyrohyoid depresses the hyoid and elevates the larynx Elevates the hyoid and base of the tongue and has an undetermined role in speech, mastication, and swallowing	C1-C3 by a branch of ansa cervicalis (cervical loop)
Pharyngeal Constrictors			
Superior pharyngeal constrictor Middle pharyngeal constrictor Inferior pharyngeal constrictor Cricopharyngeus muscle Thyropharyngeus muscle	The constrictors, innervated by the vagus nerve, work to convey a food bolus downward into the esophagus. The superior pharyngeal constrictor is a quadrilateral muscle in the pharynx that is the most superior muscle of the three constrictors. The middle pharyngeal constrictor is a fan-shaped muscle, which is the smallest of the three constrictors. Inferior pharyngeal constrictor is the thickest of the three constrictors. The upper esophageal sphincter (UES) is a musculoskeletal valve composed of the cricopharyngeus muscle, the lower part of the inferior pharyngeal constrictor, and the cricoid cartilage, to which these muscles attach.		

TABLE 3-42 • Supporting Structures of TMJ.	
Structure	**Description**
Joint capsule or capsular ligament	Surrounds the entire joint; is thought to provide proprioceptive feedback regarding joint position and movement.
Temporomandibular (or lateral) ligament	The temporomandibular joint capsule is reinforced laterally by an outer, oblique portion and an inner horizontal portion of the temporomandibular ligament, which function as a suspensory mechanism for the mandible during moderate opening movements. The ligament also functions to resist rotation and posterior displacement of the mandible.
Stylomandibular ligament	This ligament becomes taut and acts as a guiding mechanism for the mandible, keeping the condyle, disk, and temporal bone firmly opposed.
Sphenomandibular ligament	This ligament acts to check the mandible angle from sliding as far forward as the condyles during the translatory cycle and serves as a mandible suspensory ligament during wide mouth opening.

Resting Position

The resting position, or "freeway space," of the TMJ corresponds to the position where the residual tension of the muscles is at rest, and no contact occurs between maxillary and mandibular teeth. In this position, the tongue is against the palate of the mouth with its most anterior-superior tip in the area against the palate, just posterior to the rear of the upper central incisors.

THORACIC SPINE AND RIB CAGE

In the thoracic spine, protection and function of the thoracic viscera take precedence over segmental spinal mobility. Each thoracic segment includes 12 articulations, 10 of which are synovial. The posterior thoracic muscles, spinous processes, anterior and posterior longitudinal ligaments, vertebral bodies, zygapophyseal and costotransverse joints, inferior and superior articular processes, pars interarticularis, intervertebral disk (IVD), nerve root, joint meniscus, and dura mater are all capable of producing pain in this region.

Biomechanics

There is very little agreement in the literature concerning the biomechanics of the thoracic spine.

Respiration

During inspiration, in the upper ribs, an anterior elevation (pump handle) occurs, and in the middle and lower ribs (excluding the free ribs), a lateral elevation (bucket handle) occurs (Figure 3-22).

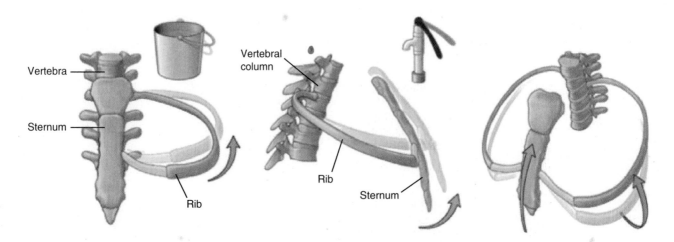

Figure 3-22. Artistic impression of the two main rib motions during breathing—bucket handle (right) and pump handle (left). (Reproduced with permission from Burke-Doe A, Dutton M, eds. *National Physical Therapy Examination and Board Review*. 2019. Copyright © McGraw Hill LLC. All rights reserved. https://accessphysiotherapy.mhmedical.com.)

The former movement increases the thoracic cavity's anterior-posterior diameter, and the latter increases the transverse diameter. The reverse occurs with expiration.

The action of the diaphragm produces both kinds of rib motion. The seventh through tenth ribs act to increase the abdominal cavity to afford space for the descending diaphragm.

LUMBAR SPINE

The spinous process is primarily horizontal in orientation. The region between the superior articular process and the lamina is the pars interarticularis.

The lumbar spine's primary ligamentous support includes the anterior longitudinal ligament, the posterior longitudinal ligament, the attachments of the annulus fibrosis, the facet joints, and the interosseous ligaments between the spinous processes.

Biomechanics

Motions at the lumbar spine joints can occur in three cardinal planes: sagittal (flexion and extension), frontal (side-bending), and transverse (rotation).

The amount of segmental motion at each vertebral level varies. Most of the lumbar spine's flexion and extension occurs in the lower segmental levels, whereas most of the lumbar spine's side-bending occurs in the midlumbar area. Rotation, which occurs with side-bending as a coupled motion, is minimal and occurs most at the lumbosacral junction. The amount of range available in the lumbar spine decreases with age.

SACROILIAC JOINT

Substitutions by other muscle groupsthan motion. However, studies have documented that motion does occur at the joint; therefore, slightly subluxed and even locked positions can occur.

▲ HIGH-YIELD TERMS TO LEARN

Referred pain	Used to describe symptoms that have their origin at a site other than where the patient feels the pain.
Patient history	The information gained by a clinician by asking specific questions, either of the patient or other people who know the patient.
Systems review	A questioning technique to elicit those aspects of the medical history from a patient that could preclude the patient from receiving physical therapy.
Special test	A clinical test designed to help confirm a working hypothesis/diagnosis.
Accessory joint motion	A motion that occurs at joint surfaces to allow movement to occur. Accessory motion is assessed using joint mobility testing.
Differential diagnosis	A process by which a particular disease or condition is differentiated from others that present with similar clinical features.

Stability at the SIJ is provided not just by the ridges present in the joint but also by the presence of generously sized ligaments. The ligamentous structures offer resistance to shear and loading. In addition, many large and small muscles have relationships with these ligaments and the SIJ. These include the piriformis, biceps femoris, gluteus maximus and minimus, erector spinae, latissimus dorsi, thoracolumbar fascia, and iliacus.

Biomechanics

There is very little agreement among disciplines or within disciplines about the pelvic complex's biomechanics. However, the numerous studies on SIJ mobility have led to various hypotheses about pelvic mechanics over the years.

■ EXAMINATION OF THE MUSCULOSKELETAL SYSTEM

ACTIVE RANGE OF MOTION

The expected active range of motion for all major joints is outlined in Table 3-43. The measurement of range of motion using goniometry is outlined in **Appendix B**.

TABLE 3-43 • Active Ranges of the Major Joints.

Joint	Action	Degrees of Motion
Shoulder	Flexion Extension Abduction Internal rotation External rotation	0-180 0-40 0-180 0-80 0-90
Elbow	Flexion	0-150
Forearm	Pronation Supination	0-80 0-80
Wrist	Flexion Extension Radial deviation Ulnar deviation	0-60 0-60 0-20 0-30
Finger flexion	Flexion	MCP: 85-90 PIP: 100-115 DIP: 80-90
Hip	Flexion Extension Abduction Adduction Internal rotation External rotation	0-100 0-30 0-40 0-20 0-40 0-50
Knee	Flexion	0-150
Ankle	Plantarflexion Dorsiflexion	0-40 0-20
Foot	Inversion Eversion	0-30 0-20

Toe	Flexion
	
	Extension
		Great toe:
		  MTP, 45
		  IP, 90
		Lateral four toes:
		  MTP, 40
		  PIP, 35
		  DIP, 60
		Great toe:
		  MTP, 70
		  IP, 0
		Lateral four toes:
		  MTP, 40
		  PIP, 0
		  DIP, 30

TABLE 3-44 • Findings from Muscle Testing.

Finding	Possible Explanation
Strong and painless contraction	Normal finding
Strong and painful contraction	Grade I contractile lesion
Weak and painless contraction	Palsy (nerve compression, neuropathy) Complete rupture of the muscle-tendon unit/avulsion
Weak and painful contraction	Serious pathology such as significant muscle tear, fracture, tumor, etc

MANUAL MUSCLE TESTING

The Guide to Physical Therapist Practice[1] lists manual muscle testing (MMT) and dynamometry as appropriate muscle strength measures.

- MMT is a procedure for the evaluation of the function and strength of individual muscles and muscle groups
- Dynamometry is a strength testing method using sophisticated strength measuring devices (eg, hand-grip, handheld, fixed, and isokinetic dynamometry).

Valuable information can be gleaned from these tests, including the following:

- The amount of force the muscle can produce and the amount of force produced varies with the joint angle.
- The endurance of the muscle and how much substitution occurs during the test.
- Whether any pain or weakness is produced with the contraction (Table 3-44).

Examples of common grading scales used with MMT are depicted in Table 3-45.

To be a valid test, strength testing must elicit a maximum contraction of the muscle being tested. Five strategies ensure this:

- Placing the joint that the muscle to be tested crosses in or close to its open-packed position.
- Placing the muscle to be tested in a shortened position. This puts the muscle in an ineffective physiologic position and has the effect of increasing motor neuron activity.
- Having the patient perform an eccentric muscle contraction using the command "Don't let me move you." As the tension at each cross-bridge and the number of active cross-bridges are greater during an eccentric contraction, the maximum eccentric muscle tension developed is greater with an eccentric contraction than a concentric one.
- Breaking the contraction. It is important to break the patient's muscle contraction to ensure that the patient is making a maximal effort and that its full power is being tested.
- Holding the contraction for at least 5 seconds. Weakness due to nerve palsy has a distinct fatigability. Therefore, if a muscle appears to be weaker than normal, further investigation is required.

The test is repeated three times. Muscle weakness resulting from disuse will be consistently weak and should not get weaker with several repeated contractions.

Another muscle that shares the same innervation (spinal nerve or peripheral nerve) is tested. Knowledge of both spinal nerve and peripheral nerve innervation will help the clinician determine which muscle to select (Tables 3-46 through 3-48).

NEUROLOGIC TESTING

The evaluation of the transmission capability of the nervous system by the physical therapist is performed to detect the presence of either an upper motor neuron (UMN) lesion or a lower motor neuron (LMN) lesion (Table 3-49). Also, the neurologic examination can often help the physical therapist determine the exact site of the lesion.

STUDY PEARL
Substitutions by other muscle groups during testing indicate the presence of weakness. It does not, however, tell the clinician the cause of the weakness. Therefore, the same muscle is tested on the opposite side whenever possible, using the same testing procedure, and a comparison is made.

TABLE 3-45 • Comparison of MMT Grades.

Medical Research Council	Daniels and Worthingham	Kendall and McCreary	Explanation
5	Normal (N)	100%	Holds test position against maximal resistance
4+	Good + (G+)		Holds test position against moderate to strong pressure
4	Good (G)	80%	Holds test position against moderate resistance
4−	Good − (G−)		Holds test position against slight to moderate pressure
3+	Fair + (F+)		Holds test position against slight resistance
3	Fair (F)	50%	Holds test position against gravity
3−	Fair − (F−)		Gradual release from the test position
2+	Poor + (P+)		Moves through partial ROM against gravity OR Moves through complete ROM gravity eliminated and holds against pressure
2	Poor (P)	20%	Able to move through full ROM gravity eliminated
2−	Poor − (P−)		Moves through partial ROM gravity eliminated
1	Trace (T)	5%	No visible movement; palpable or observable tendon prominence/flicker contraction
0	0	0%	No palpable or observable muscle contraction
Grades of 0, 1, and 2 are tested in the gravity-minimized position (contraction is perpendicular to the gravitational force) All other grades are tested in the anti-gravity position	The more functional of the three grading systems because it tests a motion that utilizes all of the agonists and synergists involved in the motion	Designed to test a specific muscle rather than the motion, and requires both selective recruitment of a muscle by the patient and sound knowledge of anatomy and kinesiology on the part of the clinician to determine the correct alignment of the muscle fibers	

SPECIAL TESTS

This list of special tests is provided for reference as the PTA can see mention of these tests in the patient's medical record and should therefore know the rationale behind each test and the possible implications based on the results.

SPECIAL TESTS OF THE UPPER EXTREMITY

Special Tests of the Shoulder Complex

The special tests for the shoulder are divided into diagnostic categories. Selection for their use is at the clinician's discretion and is based on a complete patient history.

Subacromial Impingement Tests. Patients with subacromial impingement syndrome usually perceive pain when a compressing force is applied to the greater tuberosity and

TABLE 3-46 • Peripheral Nerves of the Upper Quadrant.

Nerves	Nerve Root	Muscles	Action
Musculocutaneous	C5-C6	Biceps, brachialis Coracobrachialis	Flexion of elbow Shoulder flexion
Lateral brachial cutaneous nerve of the arm	C5-C6	Sensory only	
Median	C5-T1	Flexor carpi radialis Flexor digitorum sublimis Flexor digitorum profundus (lateral half) Pronator teres, pronator quadratus Abductor pollicis brevis Opponens pollicis brevis Flexor pollicis longus Flexor pollicis brevis	Radial flexion of the wrist Flexion of middle phalanges (digiti II-V) Flexion of distal phalanges (digiti II, III) Pronation of forearm Abduction of thumb Opposition of thumb Flexion of distal phalanx of thumb Flexion of proximal phalanx of thumb
Axillary	C5-C6	Deltoid Teres minor	Shoulder abduction
Radial	C5-T1	Triceps Brachioradialis Extensor carpi radialis/ulnaris Supinator Extensor pollicis brevis Extensor pollicis longus Extensor indicis proprius Extensor digiti proprius Extensor digiti communis	Extension at elbow Flexion of forearm Extension at the wrist with radial/ulnar deviation Supination of forearm Extension of thumb (proximal) Extension of thumb (distal) Extension of the index (proximal) Extension of the little finger (proximal) Extension of digits (II-V, proximal)
Medial (posterior) cutaneous (antebrachial) nerve of the forearm	C6-T1	Sensory only	
Lateral cutaneous (antebrachial) nerve of the forearm	C5-C6	Sensory only	
Ulnar	C8-T1	Flexor carpi ulnaris Flexor digitorum profundus (medial half) Abductor digiti minimi All other intrinsics of hand	Ulnar flexion of the wrist Flexion of distal phalanges (digiti IV, V) Abduction of digiti V Finger abduction/adduction

rotator cuff region. Pain may also be elicited with shoulder abduction in internal or external rotation.

- Neer impingement test
- Hawkins-Kennedy impingement test
- Yocum test

Rotator cuff rupture tests

Drop Arm Test. If the patient's arm drops at any point in the descent, this indicates a full-thickness tear.

Biceps and Superior Labral Tear Tests
- Clunk test
- Crank test
- Speed test
- Yergason test
- O'Brien test
- Anterior slide test

TABLE 3-47 • Peripheral Nerves of the Lumbar Plexus.

Nerves	Nerve Root	Muscles	Action
The iliohypogastric nerve	T12, L1	Sensory	The lateral (iliac) branch supplies the skin of the upper lateral part of the thigh The anterior (hypogastric) branch supplies the skin over the symphysis
The ilioinguinal nerve	L1	Sensory	Supplies the skin of the upper medial part of the thigh and the root of the penis and scrotum or mons pubis and labium majores
The genitofemoral nerve	L1, L2	Sensory	The genital branch supplies the cremasteric muscle and the skin of the scrotum or labia The femoral branch supplies the skin of the middle-upper part of the thigh and the femoral artery
Femoral	L2-L4	Iliopsoas Quadriceps	Flexion of hip Extension of knee
Saphenous	L3-L4		
Obturator	L2-L4	Adductor longus, adductor brevis, adductor magnus	Adduction of hip
Lateral cutaneous (femoral) nerve of the thigh	L2-L3	Sensory	
Posterior cutaneous nerve of the thigh	L2-L3	Sensory	
Anterior cutaneous (femoral) nerve of the thigh	L2-L3	Sensory	

TABLE 3-48 • Nerves of the Sacral Plexus.

Nerves	Nerve Root	Muscles	Action
Superior gluteal	L4, L5, S1	Gluteus medius Gluteus minimus Tensor of the fascia latae	Abduction of hip
Inferior gluteal	L5-S2	Gluteus maximus	Extension of the hip
Sciatic	L4-S3	Biceps femoris, semitendinosus, semimembranosus	Flexion of the leg at the knee
Sciatic branches: Deep fibular (peroneal)	L4-S2	Tibialis anterior Extensor digitorum longus Extensor hallucis longus	Dorsiflexion of foot Extension of toes Extension of the great toe
Sciatic branches: Superficial fibular (peroneal)	L4-S1	Fibularis (peroneus) muscles	Eversion of foot
Sciatic branches: Tibial	L4-S3	Gastrocnemius, soleus Flexor digitorum longus Flexor hallucis longus Flexor digitorum brevis Flexor hallucis brevis	Plantar flexion of foot Flexion of distal phalanges (II-IV) Flexion of distal phalanges (I) Flexion of middle phalanges (II-V) Flexion of middle phalanges (I)
Lateral cutaneous nerve of the leg	L4-S2	Sensory	
Medial plantar	L4-L5		
Sural	S1-S2		
Lateral plantar	S1-S2		

TABLE 3-49 • Major Differences Between UMN and LMN Lesion Signs and Symptoms.

	Upper Motor Neuron Lesion	Lower Motor Neuron Lesion
Location/structures	Central nervous system—cortex, brainstem, corticospinal tracts, spinal cord	Cranial nerve nuclei/nerves and anterior horn cell, spinal roots, peripheral nerve
Pathology	Cerebrovascular accident (CVA), traumatic brain injury (TBI), spinal cord injury (SCI), myelopathy	Peripheral nerve neuropathy, radiculopathy, polio, Guillain–Barré syndrome
Tone	Increased: Hypertonia, velocity-dependent	Decreased or absent: Hypotonia, flaccidity, non–velocity-dependent
Reflexes	Increased: Hyperreflexia, clonus, exaggerated cutaneous and autonomic reflexes, + pathologic reflexes (Babinski, Hoffman, inverted supinator)	Decreased or absent: Hyporeflexia, cutaneous reflexes decreased/absent
Involuntary movements	Muscle spasms: Flexor or extensor	Fasciculations: With denervation
Voluntary movements	Impaired or absent: Dyssynergic patterns, mass synergies	Weak or absent (if nerve integrity interrupted)
Strength	Weakness or paralysis: Ipsilateral (stroke) or bilateral (SCI) Corticospinal: Contralateral if above decussation in the medulla; ipsilateral if below Distribution: Never focal	Ipsilateral weakness or paralysis in limited distribution: Segmental/focal/root pattern
Muscle appearance	Disuse atrophy: Variable, widespread distribution, especially of anti-gravity muscles	Neurogenic atrophy

The remaining tests are reserved for when the clinician needs to differentiate the structure causing the symptoms, when the provocation of symptoms during the examination has been minimal, or to rule out the possibility of instability.

Acromioclavicular Tests
- Acromioclavicular shear test
- Stability testing
- Glenohumeral—load and shift test
- Apprehension test
- Jobe subluxation/relocation test
- Anterior release test
- Sulcus sign for inferior instability
- Rockwood test for anterior instability

Special Tests of the Elbow Complex

Tennis Elbow (Lateral Elbow Tendinopathy) Tests
- Cozen
- Mill

Cubital Tunnel Syndrome
- Elbow flexion test
- Pressure provocation test
- Tinel sign (at the elbow)

Special Tests of the Wrist and Hand
Several tests can be used to document the neurovascular status of the wrist and hand.

Neurologic and Autonomic Tests
- Tinel sign at carpal tunnel
- Phalen (wrist flexion) test

- Reverse Phalen (prayer test)
- Carpal compression test
- Froment sign
- Egawa sign
- Wrinkle (shrivel) test
- Weber (Moberg) two-point discrimination test

Vascular Tests

- Allen test

Ligament, Capsule, and Joint Instability Tests

- Ligamentous instability tests for the fingers
- MP collateral ligament test
- PIP collateral ligament test
- DIP collateral ligament test
- Test for tight retinacular ligaments (retinacular or Bunnel-Littler test)
- Lunotriquetral ballottement (Reagan) test
- Murphy sign
- Watson (scaphoid shift) test
- Scaphoid stress test
- "Piano keys" test
- Axial load test
- Pivot shift test of the midcarpal joint
- Grind test
- Tabletop test

Tests for Tendons and Muscles

- Finkelstein test
- Flexor digitorum profundus
- Flexor digitorum superficialis test
- Test for extensor hood rupture
- Linburg sign
- Mallet finger test

SPECIAL TESTS OF THE LOWER EXTREMITY

Special Tests of the Hip

- Quadrant
- Faber (Patrick)
- Trendelenburg
- Pelvic drop test
- Sign of the buttock

Muscle Length Tests

- Thomas test and modified Thomas test
- Ely test
- Ober test
- Straight leg raise test for hamstring length
- 90-90 straight leg raise
- Piriformis

- Hip adductors
- Leg length discrepancy

Special Tests of the Knee Complex

Stress Tests

- Abduction valgus stress
- The stable Lachman test
- Anterior drawer test
- Gravity (Godfrey) sign
- Posterior drawer
- Active posterolateral drawer test
- Hughston posterior-lateral drawer test
- Hughston external rotational recurvatum test
- Hughston posterior-medial drawer test
- Pivot shift test
- MacIntosh (true pivot shift)
- Slocum test

Meniscal Lesion Tests

- Modified McMurray test
- Apley test
- O'Donahue test
- Boehler test
- Thessaly test

Special Tests for Specific Diagnoses

- Plical irritation
- Supra-/infrapatellar tendinopathy
- *McConnell test*
- *Zohler (patellar grind) test*
- *Clarke test*
- *Waldron test*
- Fairbanks apprehension test for patellar instability
- Wilson test for osteochondritis dissecans
- Hamstring flexibility
- Iliotibial band flexibility
- *Renne creak test*
- *Noble compression test*

Special Tests of the Ankle and Foot

Ligamentous Stress Tests

- Mortise/syndesmosis
- *Clunk (cotton) test*
- *Posterior drawer test*
- *Squeeze (distal tibiofibular compression) test*
- *Lateral collaterals*
- *Anterior talofibular ligament (ATFL)*
- *Anterior drawer test*
- *Dimple sign*
- *Calcaneofibular ligament*
- *Posterior talofibular*

- Medial collaterals (deltoid complex)
- *Kleiger (external rotation) test*
- Thompson test for Achilles tendon rupture
- Arc sign for Achilles tendinopathy
- The Royal London Hospital test for Achilles tendinopathy
- Patla test for tibialis posterior length
- Feiss line test
- "Too many toes" sign

Articular Stability Tests
- Navicular drop test
- Talar rock

Neurovascular Status
- Homan sign
- Buerger test
- Morton test
- Duchenne test
- Tinel sign
- Dorsal pedis pulse

Special Tests of the Upper Cervical Spine
Cervical Arterial Dysfunction Tests
- Vertebral artery tests
- *Muscle compression test*
- *Barre test*
- *Hautard (Hautant, Hautart, or Hautarth) test*
- *Cervical quadrant test*

Cervical Ligamentous Integrity Tests
- Modified Sharp-Purser test

Special Tests of the Cervical Spine and Temporomandibular Joint
- Temporomandibular joint screen
- Lhermitte Symptom

Thoracic Outlet Tests
- Adson vascular test
- Allen pectoralis minor test
- Costoclavicular test
- Hallstead maneuver
- Roos test
- Overhead test
- Hyperabduction maneuver (Wright test)
- Passive shoulder shrug

Special Tests of the Lumbar Spine and SIJ
Neurodynamic Mobility Testing
- *Straight leg raise test*
- Pheasant test

Stress Testing

- Anterior SI joint stress (gapping) test
- Posterior sacroiliac joint stress (anterior compression) test
- FADE positional test
- Posterior-anterior pressures
- Bicycle test of van Gelderen

■ COMMON ORTHOPEDIC CONDITIONS

Frequently encountered orthopedic conditions are described here. The intervention strategies for many of these conditions are described in the Intervention Principles for Musculoskeletal Injuries section. In addition, treatments specific to certain conditions are included in the descriptions.

OSTEOARTHRITIS

OA, or degenerative joint disease, occurs when the joint cartilage deteriorates to a point when pain and/or dysfunction occur.

▲ HIGH-YIELD TERMS TO LEARN

Osteoarthritis	Degeneration of joint cartilage and the underlying bone, most common from middle age onward. It causes pain and stiffness, especially in the hip, knee, and thumb joints.
Osteoporosis	A medical condition in which the bones become brittle and fragile from loss of tissue, typically due to hormonal changes or deficiency of calcium or vitamin D.
Autoimmune disease	A disease in which the body produces antibodies that attack its own tissues, leading to the deterioration and, in some cases, the destruction of such tissue.
Red flags	Signs or symptoms indicating a more serious problem.
Neurogenic claudication	Group of symptoms commonly associated with spinal stenosis, which is the narrowing of the spinal canal. This condition commonly develops in the lumbar (lower) region with the symptoms of pain, numbness, and tingling.
Vascular claudication	Sometimes called intermittent claudication, this condition generally affects the blood vessels in the legs, but claudication can also affect the arms. Pain is caused by too little blood flow, usually during exercise.
Sprain	Stretch or tearing of ligaments.
Strain	Stretch or tearing of muscle or tendon.

Clinical Significance

Primary OA is an idiopathic phenomenon occurring in previously intact joints related to the aging process and typically occurs in older individuals. Primary OA occurs most commonly in the hands, particularly in the DIP, PIP, and first CMC joints. Secondary OA is a degenerative disease of the synovial joints that results from some predisposing condition, usually trauma that has adversely altered the articular cartilage and/or subchondral bone of the affected joints. Secondary OA often occurs in relatively young individuals.

Tests and Measures and Response

Signs and symptoms include the following:

- Swelling: Variable from minimum to severe.
- Warmth.
- Pain with weight-bearing activities and potentially at rest.

- Capsular pattern of motion limitation common.
- Diagnosis confirmed through radiograph/diagnostic tests.

Clinical Findings, Secondary Effects, or Complications

Impaired mobility, impaired muscle performance, impaired balance, and activity limitations, and participation restrictions. Deep, achy joint pain exacerbated by extensive use is the primary symptom. Also, reduced ROM and crepitus are frequently present. In addition, joint malalignment may be visible. Heberden nodes, representing palpable osteophytes in the DIP joints, are characteristic in women but not men. (Heberden nodes are OA features, not rheumatoid arthritis, and they have no known association with G-H disease or inguinal lymphadenopathy.) Inflammatory changes are typically absent or at least not pronounced.

Comorbidities such as obesity and cardiovascular disease can negatively impact the clinical course.

Diagnostic Tests

The diagnostic tests used to confirm OA include joint aspiration, x-rays, or MRI (in the early stages of the disease).

Common findings on radiograph with OA:

- Joint space narrowing.
- Sclerosis.
- Osteophytes.
- Lucent cysts.
- Swelling.

Interventions/Treatment

Medical—The extent of the medical intervention depends on the severity of the disease and can range from a conservative course to various surgical procedures. A typical medical intervention includes the following:

- NSAIDs.
- Corticosteroid injections.
- Topical analgesics.

Surgical procedures that can be used in advanced cases of OA include the following:

- Total or partial joint replacement.
- Osteotomy to change a bony alignment.

Pharmacologic—NSAIDs and acetaminophen (Tylenol).
Physical therapy—The goals of a physical therapy intervention include the following:

- Reduction of pain and muscle spasm through the use of modalities and relaxation training.
- Improvement of balance and ambulation.
- Maintenance or improvement of ROM.
- Correction of muscle imbalances in both strength and flexibility.

Physical therapy interventions to meet these goals are as follows:

- Strengthening exercises.
- Flexibility exercises.
- Balance and neuromuscular training.
- Functional training.
- Assistive devices as needed (canes, walkers, orthotics, reachers, etc).

- Aerobic conditioning using low- to nonimpact exercises (walking program, pool exercises).
- Patient education and empowerment:
  - Joint protection strategies.
  - Energy conservation techniques.
  - Activities to avoid.
  - Promotion of healthy lifestyle, for example, weight reduction.

BURSITIS

Bursitis is defined as inflammation of a bursa and occurs when the synovial fluid becomes infected by bacteria or irritated because of too much friction. When inflamed, the synovial cells increase in thickness and may show villous hyperplasia.

Clinical Significance

Common forms of bursitis include the following:

- Subacromial (subdeltoid) bursitis. Repetitive activities with an elevated arm most frequently cause inflammation of this bursa. As a result, difficulty in G-H abduction may occur, specifically from 70 to 100 degrees.
- Olecranon bursitis. Because of its superficial location, this bursa is easily traumatized from acute blows or chronic stress. Trauma of the skin and surrounding tissues makes the olecranon a frequent location for infectious bursitis.
- Iliopsoas bursitis. This type of bursitis is often associated with hip pathology (eg, RA, OA) or recreational injury (eg, running). Pain from iliopsoas bursitis radiates down the thigh's anteromedial side to the knee and increases with hip extension, adduction, and internal rotation.
- Trochanteric bursitis. Although the trochanteric bursa can become inflamed, it is now thought that the more common cause for lateral hip pain is gluteal tendinopathy. The bursae can become inflamed through either friction or direct trauma, such as a fall on the side of the hip. Palpable tenderness and the reproduction of the pain when the ITB is stretched across the trochanter with hip adduction, or the extremes of internal or external hip rotation, indicate either gluteal tendinopathy or trochanteric bursitis. Resisted abduction, extension, or external rotation of the hip are also painful.
- Ischial bursitis. Inflammation of this bursa commonly arises due to trauma, prolonged sitting on a hard surface (weaver's bottom), or prolonged sitting in the same position (spinal cord injury).
- Prepatellar bursitis. The inflammation arises from trauma or constant friction between the skin and the patella, most commonly when frequent forward kneeling is performed.
- Infrapatellar bursitis. The symptoms from this bursitis, often caused by frequent kneeling in an upright position, are located more distally than those of prepatellar bursitis.
- Pes anserine bursitis. This type of bursitis can result from an abnormal pull of any of the three tendons (sartorius, gracilis, and semitendinosus) or can be due to repetitive friction from a dysfunctional gait. Patients with pes anserine bursitis are commonly obese, older females with a history of OA of the knees.

Tests and Measures and Response

There are no specific clinical tests to diagnose bursitis. Instead, the diagnosis is made through the patient's history (complaints of aching muscle stiffness, pain with pressure on the affected area), presenting signs (red and swollen area), and tenderness on palpation.

Clinical Findings, Secondary Effects, or Complications

- Inflammation/edema.
- Localized tenderness.

- Warmth.
- Erythema.
- Loss of function.

Diagnostic Tests

Although not commonly used, the physician may prescribe a series of x-rays to rule out bone spurs/arthritis or aspiration of the bursa to examine the fluid and rule out such conditions as gout or infection.

Interventions/Treatment

Pharmacologic—NSAIDs to help control pain and inflammation.
Physical therapy

- Modalities to reduce swelling and pain.
- Patient education on activity modification.
- Therapeutic exercise to progress back to full ROM and strength.
- Functional training.

RHEUMATIC DISEASES

There are more than 100 rheumatic diseases. Rheumatic diseases are a series of pathologies that affect joints and muscles, which can also be classified as autoimmune diseases. Some of the more common ones are presented here.

Rheumatoid Arthritis

Rheumatoid arthritis (RA) is a disease that affects the entire body and the whole person. It is a systemic autoimmune disease in which the immune system attacks the synovium. The cycle of stretching, healing, and scarring resulting from the inflammatory process seen in RA causes significant damage to the soft tissues, periarticular structures, joint destruction, and laxity.

Clinical Significance. RA is the most common type of autoimmune arthritis. It is now well accepted that early treatment of RA helps prevent joint damage, increases muscle strength, and provides better long-term results.

Tests and Measures and Response. The diagnosis of RA is made radiographically, through bloodwork or joint aspiration.

Clinical Findings, Secondary Effects, or Complications

- Systemic manifestations: Morning stiffness lasting for more than 30 minutes, anorexia, weight loss, and fatigue.
- Arthritis of three or more joint areas: The 14 more commonly involved joints include the right or left PIP, MCP, wrists, elbow, knee, ankle, and MTP joints. On the one hand, many common deformities can be seen, such as ulnar deviation of the MCP joints, radial deviation of the CMC block, boutonnière deformity, and swan-neck deformities of the digits.
- Muscle atrophy and myositis.
- Tenosynovitis.
- Positive laboratory tests: Elevated erythrocyte sedimentation rate (ESR) or C-reactive protein; synovial fluid analysis.
- Radiographic findings.

Interventions/Treatment

Medical—The medical interventions for RA, usually by a rheumatologist, depend on the acuity and severity, but almost all interventions include some form of drug therapy.

Pharmacologic—While there is no cure for RA, disease-modifying antirheumatic drugs (DMARDs) help relieve symptoms and slow the progression of joint damage. In addition, patients with more advanced cases of the disease may be prescribed biological response modifiers.

Physical therapy—The following concepts form the foundation of any intervention to manage RA based on the pathomechanics of the rheumatoid process:

- Decrease pain.
- Control the inflammation.
- Increase or maintain the ROM of all joints sufficient for functional activities.
- Increase or maintain muscle strength sufficient for functional activities.
- Increase joint stability and decrease mechanical stress on all affected joints.
- Increase endurance for or functional activities.
- Promote independence in all activities of daily living (ADLs), including bed mobility and transfers.
- Improve efficiency and safety of gait pattern.
- Establish adequate physical activity or exercise patterns to maintain or improve musculoskeletal and cardiovascular fitness and general health.
- Educate the patient, family, and other personnel to promote the individual's capacity for self-management.

Gout

Gout (known as podagra when it involves the big toe) is caused by an altered purine metabolism that leads to hyperuricemia and the accumulation of uric acid crystals in synovial joints.

Clinical Significance. The rising prevalence of gout stems from dietary changes, environmental factors, increasing longevity, subclinical renal impairment, and the increased use of drugs, particularly diuretics.

Tests and Measures and Response. There are no specific physical therapy tests to diagnose gout, but the following signs and symptoms usually highlight its presence: sudden attacks of pain, erythema, and swelling of one or a few joints in the lower extremities.

Clinical Findings, Secondary Effects, or Complications. Gout can present in several ways, although the most usual is a gouty arthritis attack of acute inflammatory arthritis (red, tender, hot, swollen) of the involved joint.

Diagnostic Tests. Diagnosis is confirmed clinically by the visualization of the characteristic crystals in joint fluid.

Interventions/Treatment

Medical—Modifiable risk factors (eg, diuretic therapy, high-purine diet, alcohol use, and obesity) are typically addressed.

Pharmacologic—NSAIDs or corticosteroids are usually the first drugs to be used, depending on comorbidities. Colchicine is prescribed in the more recalcitrant cases.

Physical therapy—During an acute exacerbation, physical therapy is focused on pain management and splinting, orthotics, or other assistive devices to protect the affected joint(s). During periods of nonacute exacerbation, the intervention is focused on maintenance of ROM, strength, and function, a suitable home exercise program, and patient education about weight control.

Ankylosing Spondylitis

Ankylosing spondylitis (AS, also known as Bekhterev or Marie-Strümpell disease) is an autoimmune systemic inflammatory disease that impacts the enthesitis (the attachment sites of tendons and ligaments to bone).

Clinical Significance. The patient is usually between 15 and 40 years of age, and although males are affected more frequently than females, mild courses of AS are more common in the latter. The disease includes the involvement of the anterior longitudinal ligament and ossification of the disk, thoracic zygapophyseal joint joints, costovertebral joints, manubriosternal joint, and the SIJ. This multijoint involvement makes the checking of chest expansion measurements a required test in this region. In time, AS progresses to involve the whole spine and results in spinal deformities, including flattening of the lumbar lordosis, kyphosis of the thoracic spine, and hyperextension of the cervical spine.

Tests and Measures and Response. The inspection usually reveals a flat lumbar spine and gross limitation of side bending in both directions. Mobility loss tends to be bilateral and symmetric. There is a loss of spinal elongation on flexion (Schober test), although this can also occur in patients with chronic low back pain or spinal tumors. The patient may relate a history of costochondritis, and upon examination, rib springing may give a hard end feel. Basal rib expansion often is decreased. The glides of the costotransverse joints and distraction of the sternoclavicular joints are decreased, and the lumbar spine exhibits a capsular pattern.

As the disease progresses, the pain and stiffness can spread up the entire spine, pulling it into flexion so that the patient adopts the typical stooped-over position. The patient gazes downward, the entire back is rounded, the hips and knees are semiflexed, and the arms cannot be raised beyond a limited amount at the shoulders.

Exercise is particularly important for these patients to maintain mobility of the spine and involved joints for as long as possible and prevent the spine from stiffening in an unacceptable kyphotic position.

Clinical Findings, Secondary Effects, or Complications. The most characteristic feature of the back pain associated with AS is pain at night. Patients often awaken in the early morning (between 2:00 and 5:00 am) with back pain and stiffness. Backache during the day is typically intermittent. Although not as common, AS can also cause peripheral joint pain, particularly in the hips, knees, ankles, shoulders, and neck.

Diagnostic Tests. The AS diagnosis is generally confirmed with radiographs, which typically show the characteristic finding of a "bamboo spine."

Interventions/Treatment
Physical therapy—Much of the physical therapy intervention involves patient education and instruction. The patient is taught a strict regimen of daily exercises, including positioning spinal extension and breathing exercises. Several times a day, patients should lie prone for 5 minutes, and they should be encouraged to sleep on a hard mattress and avoid the sidelying position. Swimming is the best routine sport.

Systemic Lupus Erythematosus

SLE, sometimes referred to as lupus, is a chronic inflammatory autoimmune disorder that can affect any organ or body system. More than 90% of cases of SLE occur in women, often starting at childbearing age.

Clinical Significance. The seronegative arthropathies include ankylosing spondylitis, Reiter syndrome (the classic triad of arthritis, conjunctivitis, and urethritis), psoriatic arthritis, and arthritis associated with inflammatory bowel disease.

Tests and Measures and Response. SLE can affect almost any organ system; thus, its presentation and course are highly variable. Nevertheless, the classic triad of fever, joint pain, and rash in a woman of childbearing age should prompt exploration into SLE diagnosis.

Clinical Findings, Secondary Effects, or Complications. Clinical manifestations for the physical therapist to note include the following:

- Musculoskeletal involvement: Arthralgias and arthritis constitute the most common presenting manifestations of SLE.
- Cardiopulmonary signs: Pleuritis, pericarditis, and dyspnea.
- Neurologic involvement: Headaches, depression, seizures, peripheral neuropathy (Raynaud phenomenon).
- Kidney dysfunction or failure.

Physical therapy goals include the following:

- Patient education on how to control and restrict activities—energy conservation.
- Careful observation for signs of renal failure such as weight gain, edema, or hypertension.
- If Raynaud phenomenon is present, patient education on how to warm and protect the hands and feet.

Diagnostic Tests. The diagnosis of SLE is based on a combination of clinical findings and laboratory results. According to the American College of Rheumatology (ACR), a person is considered to have SLE if 4 of the following 11 criteria, conveniently put into a mnemonic of SOAP BRAIN MD, are present:

- Serositis.
- Oral ulcers.
- Arthritis—nonerosive arthritis of two or more peripheral joints characterized by tenderness, swelling, or effusion.
- Photosensitivity.
- Blood disorders—hemolytic anemia, leukopenia, leukopenia, or thrombocytopenia.
- Renal involvement.
- Antinuclear antibodies—abnormal titer.
- Immunologic phenomena (eg, double-stranded DNA [dsDNA]; anti-Smith [Sm] antibodies).
- Neurologic disorder.
- Malar rash.
- Discoid rash.

Interventions/Treatment

Medical—The medical management of SLE typically depends on the individual's disease severity and manifestations.

Pharmacologic—Medications used to treat SLE manifestations include antimalarials (eg, hydroxychloroquine), short-term use of corticosteroids, nonbiological and biological DMARDs, and NSAIDs.

Physical therapy—Physical therapy interventions focus on addressing the musculoskeletal manifestations of the disease and concentrating on improving the decreased level of aerobic physical fitness often found in this population. Each patient is examined and then provided with an individualized and effective plan of care to help reduce pain, stiffness, and inflammation and improve joint ROM and functional mobility.

Psoriatic Arthritis

Psoriatic arthritis is an inflammatory arthritis associated with psoriasis, which affects men and women with equal frequency. Its peak onset is in the fourth decade of life, although it may occur in children and older adults.

Clinical Significance. Psoriatic arthritis can manifest in one of several patterns, including distal joint disease (affecting the DIP joints of the hands and feet), arthritis mutilans (a severe destructive form of arthritis), asymmetric oligoarthritis, polyarthritis (which tends to be asymmetric in half the cases), and spondyloarthropathy.

Tests and Measures and Response. There are no specific physical therapy tests to diagnose psoriatic arthritis.

Clinical Findings, Secondary Effects, or Complications. The spondyloarthropathy of psoriatic arthritis may be distinguished from AS by the sacroiliitis pattern—the sacroiliitis in AS tends to be symmetric, affecting both SIJs to the same degree, whereas it tends to be asymmetric in psoriatic arthritis.

The most telling signs are the skin and nail (occur in > 80% of patients) changes. The nail changes include discolorations and "pitting"—forming depressions in the fingernails or toenails. Another feature of psoriatic arthritis is dactylitis, tenosynovitis (often digital, flexor and extensor tendons, and Achilles tendons), and enthesitis.

Diagnostic Tests. The diagnosis is typically made based on the signs and symptoms, the physical examination, the patient's medical and family history, imaging studies, bone density tests, and a series of blood tests (rheumatoid factor [RF] and anti-CCP antibody tests can rule out RA).

Interventions/Treatment

Medical—Psoriatic arthritis is treated similarly to RA. The main goal of treatment is to control joint inflammation through medications.

Pharmacologic—The most commonly prescribed medications include NSAIDs initially and then nonbiological and/or biological DMARDs as needed.

Physical therapy—The physical therapy intervention focuses on using ultraviolet (UV) therapy, hydrotherapy, and thermal modalities to decrease pain. In addition, cryotherapy can be used to reduce joint swelling and tenderness.

OSTEOMYELITIS

Osteomyelitis is an infectious process of the bone and its marrow. The term can refer to infections caused by pyogenic microorganisms but can also be used to describe other sources of infection such as tuberculosis, viral infections, syphilitic infections (Charcot arthropathy), specific fungal infections (mycotic osteomyelitis), and parasitic infections (hydatid disease).

Clinical Significance. Certain conditions can weaken the immune system, increasing the risk of developing osteomyelitis, including the following:

- Diabetes (a common cause).
- RA.
- HIV or AIDS.
- Sickle cell disease.
- Intravenous drug use.
- Alcoholism.
- Long-term use of steroids.
- Hemodialysis.

Tests and Measures and Response. There are no specific physical therapy clinical tests that can diagnose osteomyelitis.

Clinical Findings, Secondary Effects, or Complications. Findings at the physical examination may include the following:

- Fever or no fever.
- Edema.

- Warmth.
- Tenderness to palpation.
- Reduction in the use of the extremity.

Diagnostic Tests. Diagnosis of osteomyelitis is often based on radiologic results showing a lytic center with a sclerosis ring, but a culture of material taken from a bone biopsy is needed to identify the specific pathogen.

Interventions/Treatment

Medical—Osteomyelitis may require surgical debridement. Severe cases may lead to the loss of a limb.

Pharmacologic—Osteomyelitis often requires prolonged antibiotic therapy, with a course lasting a matter of weeks or months.

Physical therapy—The major physical therapy role in osteomyelitis is one of early detection. In general, rehabilitation aims to restore normal ROM, flexibility, strength, and endurance to maintain function and enhance mobility.

OSTEOPOROSIS

Osteoporosis is a systemic skeletal disorder characterized by decreased bone mass and deterioration of bony microarchitecture. Osteoporosis results from genetic and environmental factors that affect both peak bone mass and the rate of bone loss.

Clinical Significance

Skeletal demineralization, caused by an imbalance between bone formation and bone resorption, can be a primary or secondary disorder to various other diseases or disorders such as hyperparathyroidism. The term *skeletal demineralization* refers to a loss of mass and calcium content from the bones. Skeletal demineralization can vary in severity:

- Less severe bone loss: Osteopenia. Osteopenia may be apparent as radiographic lucency (measured as a T-score—see Tests and Measures and Response) but is not always noticeable until approximately 30% of bone mineral is lost.
- More severe bone loss: Osteoporosis. Osteoporosis accounts for the largest number of fractures among the elderly.

Risk factors for skeletal demineralization include those that are modifiable and those that are nonmodifiable. The modifiable risk factors include the following:

- Gender (female > male).
- Race.
- Age.
- Family history.
- Body size.
- Early menopause.

The nonmodifiable risk factors include the following:

- Use of specific medications.
- Low calcium intake.
- Low vitamin D levels.
- Estrogen deficiency.
- Excessive alcohol intake.
- Cigarette smoking.
- Physical inactivity.
- Prolonged overuse of thyroid hormone.

Tests and Measures and Response

- The lower a person's T-score, the lower the bone density.
- A T-score of −1.0 or above is normal bone density. Examples are 0.9, 0, and −0.9.
- A T-score between −1.0 and −2.5 indicates low bone density or osteopenia.
- A T-score of −2.5 or below is a diagnosis of osteoporosis.

Clinical Findings, Secondary Effects, or Complications

Osteoporosis may be either primary or secondary.

- Primary. Primary osteoporosis is subdivided into types I and II.
  - Type I, or postmenopausal osteoporosis, is thought to result from gonadal (ie, estrogen, testosterone) deficiency, resulting in accelerated bone loss. Increased recruitment and responsiveness of osteoclast precursors and increased bone resorption, which outpace bone formation, occur. After menopause, women experience an accelerated bone loss for the first 5 to 7 years. The result is a decrease in trabecular bone and an increased risk of Colles and vertebral fractures.
  - Type II, or senile, osteoporosis occurs in women and men because of decreased formation of bone and decreased renal production of $1,25(OH)_2 D_3$ occurring late in life. The consequence is a loss of cortical and trabecular bone and an increased risk for fractures of the hip, long bones, and vertebrae.
- Secondary. Secondary osteoporosis, also called type III, occurs secondary to medications, especially glucocorticoids, or other conditions that cause increased bone loss by various mechanisms.

Osteoporosis can occur in either a generalized or a regional form. The cardinal feature is a fracture, and the clinical picture depends on the fracture site. Most fractures occur in the mid-to-lower thoracic or upper lumbar spine. The pain is described variably as sharp, nagging, or dull; movement may exacerbate pain, and sometimes pain radiates to the abdomen.

Acute pain usually resolves after 4 to 6 weeks. However, in multiple fractures with severe kyphosis or dowager hump, the pain may become chronic. When kyphosis becomes severe, the patient may develop a restrictive pattern of respiratory impairment.

Diagnostic Tests

To definitively diagnose osteoporosis, one must perform some type of quantitative imaging study on the bone in question. Medical and screening tests of bone mineral density are available:

- Screening tests include finger densitometry and heel (calcaneal) ultrasonography.
- Medical tests include single-photon absorptiometry (SPA) and dual-energy x-ray absorptiometry (DXA). Radiographs may show fractures or other conditions, such as OA, disk disease, or spondylolisthesis.

Bone mineral density (BMD) testing is the best predictor of fracture risk. Although measurement at any site can assess overall fracture risk, measurement at a particular site is the best predictor of fracture risk at that site. BMD is reported as a T-score, which compares the patient's BMD to a healthy young adult (see Tests and Measures and Response).

Interventions/Treatment

Medical—Effective medical therapy helps prevent and treat osteoporosis, including drug therapy and gonadal hormone replacement.

Pharmacologic—Several pharmaceutical agents are used to treat osteoporosis calcitonin, selective estrogen receptor modulators, and bisphosphonates, although these agents reduce bone resorption with little, if any, effect on bone formation.

STUDY PEARL
Vertebral fracture often manifests as acute back pain after bending, lifting, coughing, or asymptomatic progressive kyphosis with loss of height.

STUDY PEARL
Forearm, hip, and proximal femoral fractures usually occur after falls, with falling forward often resulting in Colles fractures and backward falls resulting in hip fractures. Rib fractures are most often associated with osteoporosis secondary to corticosteroid use or Cushing syndrome, but they can also be observed with other etiologies.

Physical therapy—The physical therapy intervention for osteoporosis includes the following factors:

- Weight-bearing and aerobic exercise, which have been shown to have a positive effect on BMD, although the exact mechanism is not known. Regular exercise should be encouraged in all patients, including children and adolescents, to strengthen the skeleton during the maturation process. Also, exercise improves agility and balance, thereby reducing the risk of falls.
- Postural correction and training—should address walking, standing, and sitting.
- Pain control methods—adjunctive interventions including thermal and nonthermal modalities and transcutaneous electrical nerve stimulation (TENS).

GLENOHUMERAL INSTABILITY

Laxity is the physiologic motion and a necessary attribute of the G-H joint that allows normal ROM in an asymptomatic shoulder. Instability is the abnormal and symptomatic motion of the G-H joint that affects normal joint kinematics and results in pain, subluxation, or dislocation of the shoulder.

Clinical Significance

G-H instability is typically associated with reports of "slipping" or "popping out" of the shoulder during overhead activities. Instability of the shoulder can be classified by direction, frequency (acute or chronic), magnitude, and origin. Acute traumatic instability with shoulder dislocation is the most dramatic variety and often requires manipulative reduction. Shoulder instability may also be classified according to the subluxation direction as either unidirectional (anterior, posterior, or inferior), bidirectional, or multidirectional. Posterior instability, which results either from avulsion of the posterior glenoid labrum from the posterior glenoid or stretching of the posterior capsuloligamentous structures, is often difficult to diagnose, with no single test having high sensitivity and specificity.

Tests and Measures and Response

Several physical therapy special tests exist to help confirm a diagnosis of G-H instability (see Special Tests of the Shoulder Complex).

Clinical Findings, Secondary Effects, or Complications

Most patients presenting with hypermobility or instability of the anterior G-H joint are athletic adolescents or young adults with joint laxity. The most common presenting complaint is pain. Anterior instability occurs when the abducted shoulder is repetitively placed in the anterior apprehension position of external rotation (ER) and horizontal abduction. Such individuals may have pain with overhead movements due to an inability to control the laxity through muscle support. In addition, they may develop enough instability in a superior direction with impingement-like symptoms (instability–impingement overlap), especially in abduction and ER positions. In general, the patients have had normal asymptomatic shoulder function until some event precipitates symptoms. The event usually involves only relatively minor trauma than the traumatic causes of unidirectional instability, or repetitive microtrauma.

Diagnostic Tests

Diagnosis of G-H instability is through a thorough history, radiology, and physical therapy special tests.

Interventions/Treatment

Medical—Two acronyms are commonly used to describe shoulder instability, TUBS (*T*raumatic, *U*nidirectional instability with *B*ankart lesion requiring *S*urgery) and AMBRII (*A*traumatic onset of *M*ultidirectional instability accompanied by *B*ilateral laxity or hypermobility. *R*ehabilitation is the primary course of intervention to restore G-H stability. However, if an operation is necessary, a procedure such as a capsulorrhaphy is performed to tighten the *I*nferior capsule and the rotator *I*nterval).

Pharmacologic—The use of medications for G-H instability varies according to severity but may include NSAIDs and pain relief medications.

Physical therapy—Intervention goals for G-H instability are to restore dynamic stability and control to the shoulder using the dynamic scapular and G-H stabilizers to contain the humeral head within the glenoid and correct any scapular dyskinesis.

SUBACROMIAL IMPINGEMENT SYNDROME

Subacromial impingement syndrome (SIS) is a recurrent condition closely related to rotator cuff (RC) disease. The RC problems occur because of trauma, attrition, and the anatomic structure of the subacromial space.

Clinical Significance

In the presence of a normal RC, normal scapular pivoters, and no capsular contractures, the humeral head translates less than 3 mm superiorly during the midranges of active elevation, whereas at the end ranges, A-P and superoinferior translations of 4 to 10 mm do occur, all of which are coupled with the specific motions of IR or ER. An increase in superior translation with active elevation may result in the encroachment of the coracoacromial arch. This encroachment produces a compression of the suprahumeral structures against the anteroinferior aspect of the acromion and coracoacromial ligament. Repetitive compression of these structures, coupled with other predisposing factors, results in a condition called SIS.

Tests and Measures and Response

Several physical therapy special tests exist to help confirm a diagnosis of SIS (see Special Tests of the Shoulder Complex)

Clinical Findings, Secondary Effects, or Complications

Both intrinsic and extrinsic factors have been implicated as etiologies of the impingement process, and several impingement types have evolved.

The most common symptoms associated with SIS include the following:

- Age 40 to 60.
- Painful arc (90-120 degrees with forward flexion or abduction).
- Anterior and lateral shoulder pain during arm elevation, but no pain radiating below the elbow.
- Increased pain with overhead activities.
- Weakness.
- Positive impingement tests.

Diagnostic Tests

An SIS diagnosis can usually be made based on the patient's history, physical examination, radiographs (A-P view, outlet Y view, axillary view), and MRI.

Interventions/Treatment

Medical—The extent of the medical intervention depends on the severity and can range between conservative and surgical. The indications for a surgical repair are persistent pain that interferes with ADLs, work, or sports; patients who are unresponsive to a 4- to 6-month period of conservative care; or acute full-thickness RC tear in an active young patient (< 50 years of age).

Pharmacologic—NSAIDs.

Physical therapy—Physical therapy typically involves a gradual progression of ROM and strengthening exercises for the rotator cuff muscles and the scapular stabilizers.

ACROMIOCLAVICULAR JOINT INJURIES

An A-C joint injury, commonly referred to as a shoulder separation, can be caused by direct trauma or overuse.

Clinical Significance

A-C joint injuries typically occur in active or athletic young individuals. The injury's clinical significance depends on the severity (see Clinical Findings, Secondary Effects, or Complications).

Tests and Measures and Response

The A-C shear test (See Special Tests of the Shoulder Complex) may or may not provide useful information.

Clinical Findings, Secondary Effects, or Complications

Six types (I-VI) of A-C injury have been categorized based on the direction and amount of displacement.

- Types I, II, III, and V all involve inferior displacement of the acromion to the clavicle. However, they differ in the severity of injury to the ligaments and the amount of resultant displacement.
- Types I and II usually result from a fall or a blow to the point on the lateral aspect of the shoulder, or a FOOSH, producing a sprain.
- Types III and IV usually involve a dislocation (commonly called A-C separations) and a distal clavicle fracture, both of which commonly disrupt the coracoclavicular ligaments. Type V injuries are characterized by posterior displacement of the clavicle.
- Type VI injuries have a clavicle inferiorly displaced into either a subacromial or subcoracoid position. These types (IV-VI) also have a complete rupture of all the ligament complexes and are rarer injuries than types I through III.

Diagnostic Tests

Typically, an A-C joint injury is diagnosed radiographically.

Interventions/Treatment

The intervention for A-C joint injuries has long been the subject of debate.
Medical—Types I and II injuries are typically treated nonoperatively. Types IV to VI generally require surgical repair. However, no real consensus exists regarding the optimal management of acute type III injuries.
Pharmacologic—Medications may be prescribed for pain relief.
Physical therapy—Physical therapy intervention usually only occurs in types I to III (Table 3-50).

TABLE 3-50 • Physical Therapy Intervention for A-C Joint Injuries.	
Injury Type	**Intervention**
Type I	Does not require immobilization Ice is recommended for pain If return to sport involves contact or impact forces, a donut pad placed over the shoulder helps to protect the joint
Type II	Patients are typically prescribed a sling as necessary ROM exercises are initiated as tolerated, often beginning with PROM to minimize muscle activation of the trapezius and deltoid; however, because the deltoid and trapezius fibers reinforce the A-C joint capsule, specific strengthening exercises for these muscles are part of the long-term rehabilitation program Return to function usually occurs within 2-3 weeks after injury
Type III	The most appropriate intervention is somewhat controversial and can be either surgical or conservative The most commonly used device for reduction is the Kenny–Howard harness

A-C, acromioclavicular; PROM, passive range of motion.

ADHESIVE CAPSULITIS

Adhesive capsulitis often termed *frozen shoulder*, is associated with female gender, age older than 40 years, posttrauma, diabetes, prolonged immobilization, thyroid disease, poststroke or myocardial infarction, certain psychiatric conditions, and certain autoimmune diseases.

Tests and Measures and Response

The six ROM measurements that should be taken include flexion, external rotation at the side, external rotation in abduction, internal rotation in abduction, horizontal abduction, and functional internal rotation up the back.

Clinical Findings, Secondary Effects, or Complications

The three classic stages of adhesive capsulitis include the following:

- The early painful stage (freezing). Lasts between 2 and 9 months. Patients have diffuse pain, difficulty sleeping on the affected side, and restricted movement secondary to pain.
- The stiffening stage (freezing). Lasts between 4 and 12 months. Characterized by progressive loss of ROM and decreased function.
- Recovery stage (thawing). Lasts between 5 and 24 months. Characterized by gradual increases in ROM and decreased pain.

Diagnostic Tests

Adhesive capsulitis is diagnosed primarily by physical examination—patients demonstrate limited active and passive ROM with a capsular restriction pattern. The shoulder's capsular pattern is a motion restriction of external rotation > abduction > internal rotation, often noted in frozen shoulders. The shoulder's reverse capsular pattern, often noted in impingement syndrome, is internal rotation > elevation (abduction/flexion).

Interventions/Treatment

Medical—Surgical intervention (manipulation) is reserved for those who do not respond to conservative intervention.
Pharmacologic—Most patients with adhesive capsulitis are prescribed NSAIDs or oral glucocorticoids in cases of severe refractory conditions.
Physical therapy—The primary goal of physical therapy is to restore ROM and focus on applying controlled tensile stresses using stretching and joint mobilizations to produce elongation of the restricting tissues.

- The patient with capsular restriction and low irritability may require aggressive soft tissue and joint mobilization.
- The patient with high irritability may require pain-easing manual therapy techniques.
- Treatment for the patient with limited ROM due to nonstructural changes aims to address the cause of the pain.

LATERAL ELBOW TENDINOPATHY (TENNIS ELBOW)

Lateral elbow tendinopathy (LET) represents a pathologic condition of the tendons that control wrist extension and radial deviation, resulting in pain on the elbow's lateral side. This pain is aggravated with the wrist movements, by palpation of the lateral side of the elbow, or by contraction of the wrist's extensor muscles.

Clinical Significance

Two types of elbow tendinopathy are commonly described: lateral (tennis elbow) and medial (golfer's elbow). The lateral type is far more common than the medial. LET is usually the result of overuse but can be traumatic in origin. Individuals who perform repetitive wrist extension against resistance are particularly at risk, such as those who participate in tennis, baseball, javelin, golf, squash, racquetball, swimming, and weightlifting.

STUDY PEARL
While the terms *epicondylitis* and *tendinitis* have been commonly used to describe tennis elbow and golfer's elbow, histopathologic studies have demonstrated that these conditions are often not inflammatory conditions; rather, they are degenerative conditions. Therefore, tendinopathy better describes the condition.

Tests and Measures and Response

Several physical therapy special tests have been designed to confirm a LET diagnosis (see Special Tests of the Elbow Complex).

Clinical Findings, Secondary Effects, or Complications

A thorough but focused history and physical examination are critical to a timely and accurate diagnosis. Pain is the primary symptom of LET. The pain is often activity-related. Diffuse achiness and morning stiffness are also common complaints. Occasionally, the pain is experienced at night, and the patient may report frequent dropping of objects, especially if they are carried with the palm facing down. Tenderness is usually found over the ECRB and ECRL, especially at the lateral epicondyle. The site of maximum tenderness is most commonly over the anterior aspect of the lateral epicondyle.

Diagnostic Tests

In most cases, a LET diagnosis can be made on the strength of the patient's history and physical examination.

Interventions/Treatment

Medical—Lateral epicondylosis is a self-limiting complaint; without intervention, the symptoms will usually resolve within 8 to 12 months. Surgery is indicated if the symptoms do not resolve despite properly performed nonoperative treatments lasting 6 months.

Pharmacologic—NSAIDs.

Physical therapy—To date, there is no consensus on the optimal treatment approach for LET, which is largely due to its unclear underlying etiology. Poor technique, particularly with racket sports, is the cause of many elbow problems. Emphasis should be placed on recruiting the whole of the shoulder and trunk when hitting the ball to dissipate the forces as widely as possible. In addition to correcting poor technique, patient education should address racket size, grip size, and string tension.

An exercise regimen consisting of progressive resistance exercise to the wrist extensors, with the elbow flexed to 90 degrees, and the elbow straight is recommended, performed as a 10-repetition maximum, morning and night. Gradually, the weight must be increased so that the 10-repetition maximum is always maintained. Contrary to popular belief, tennis elbow braces have been shown to have little effect on vibrational dampening.

MEDIAL ELBOW TENDINOPATHY (GOLFER'S ELBOW)

Medial elbow tendinopathy (MET) is only one-third as common as LET and primarily involves tendinopathy of the common flexor origin, specifically the flexor carpi radialis and the humeral head of the pronator teres. To a lesser extent, the palmaris longus, flexor carpi ulnaris, and FDS may also be involved.

Clinical Significance

The mechanism for medial epicondylosis is not usually related to direct trauma but rather to overuse, commonly for three reasons:

- The flexor-pronator tissues fatigue in response to repeated stress.
- There is a sudden change in stress level that predisposes the elbow to medial ligamentous injury.
- The ulnar collateral ligament fails to stabilize the valgus forces sufficiently.

Chronic symptoms result from a loss of tissue extensibility, leaving the tendon unable to attenuate tensile loads.

Tests and Measures and Response

See Special Tests of the Elbow Complex.

Clinical Findings, Secondary Effects, or Complications

The typical clinical presentation for MET is pain and tenderness over the flexor-pronator origin, slightly distal and anterior to the medial epicondyle, in an aggressive advanced-level athlete. The symptoms are typically exacerbated with either resisted wrist flexion and pronation or passive wrist extension and supination.

Diagnostic Tests

In the vast majority of cases, a MET diagnosis can be made on the strength of the patient's history and physical examination.

Interventions/Treatment

Medical—A self-limiting complaint; within 8 to 12 months. Surgery is indicated if the symptoms do not resolve despite properly performed nonoperative treatments lasting 6 months.

Pharmacologic—NSAIDs.

Physical therapy—The physical therapy intervention for this condition initially involves rest, activity modification, and local modalities. Once the acute phase has passed, the focus is to restore the ROM and correct flexibility and strength imbalances. The strengthening program is progressed to include concentric and eccentric exercises of the flexor-pronator muscles. Splinting or the use of a counterforce brace may be a useful adjunct.

LITTLE LEAGUE ELBOW

Little league elbow is a common term for an avulsion lesion to the medial apophysis.

Clinical Significance

Repetitive throwing results in muscular and bony hypertrophic changes about the elbow and can also result in ligament damage, reflected by an increase in the number of medial ulnar collateral ligament reconstruction ("Tommy John") procedures performed on injured throwers. The repetitive motions involved in the various phases of throwing place enormous valgus strains on the immature elbow, particularly during the late cocking and acceleration phases, which can result in inflammation, scar formation, loose bodies, ligament sprains or ruptures, and the more serious conditions of osteochondritis, or an avulsion fracture.

Tests and Measures and Response

In an adolescent-aged pitcher (typically aged between 9 and 14), complaints of medial elbow pain occur with throwing and worsen when they throw more innings.

Clinical Findings, Secondary Effects, or Complications

Little league elbow may start insidiously or suddenly. Usually, a sudden onset of pain is secondary to fracture at the site of the lesion. Clinical findings include a history of pain on the elbow's medial side, with and without throwing. Physical findings relate to the specific lesion but are commonly a persistent elbow discomfort or stiffness due to the injury's aggravation. A locking or "catching" sensation indicates a loose body.

Diagnostic Tests

Radiographs: An MRI may be required for a closer examination of the growth plates and to evaluate for ligament injury when the radiographic findings are unclear.

Interventions/Treatment

Medical—In most cases, a conservative approach is recommended, which typically includes a period of complete rest from throwing for a minimum of 4 to 6 weeks. Surgical intervention is reserved for those patients with symptoms of a loose body, osteochondritis, or who fail to respond to conservative therapy.

Pharmacologic—NSAIDs.

Physical therapy—Physical therapy management involves rest and eliminating the offending activity for 3 to 6 weeks. If osteochondritis dissecans is present, the joint is protected for several months. The patient cannot return to pitching until full and pain-free motion has returned. To prevent elbow disorders, young athletes should adhere to little league rules, limiting the number of pitches per game, per week, and season, and the number of days of rest between pitching. The pitch count is the most important of these statistics.

CARPAL TUNNEL SYNDROME

Carpal tunnel syndrome (CTS) results from the entrapment of the median nerve in the carpal tunnel's relatively unyielding space, resulting in numbness, pain, or paresthesia of the thumb, index, and middle fingers. Compression of the nerve in the carpal tunnel is compounded by an increase in synovial fluid pressure and tendon tension, which decreases the available volume.

Clinical Significance

CTS results from an ischemic compression of the median nerve at the wrist as it passes through the carpal tunnel. CTS more commonly occurs between the fourth and sixth decades. CTS is the most common compression neuropathy. The compression of the median nerve may result from a wide variety of factors, several of which can easily be remembered using the pneumonic PRAGMATIC:

- **P**regnancy secondary to fluid retention.
- **R**enal dysfunction.
- **A**cromegaly.
- **G**out and pseudogout.
- **M**yxedema or mass.
- **A**myotrophy. Neuralgic amyotrophy is the most likely diagnosis in patients who suddenly develop arm pain followed within a few days by arm paralysis in the distribution of single or multiple nerves or extending over multiple myotomes.
- **T**rauma (repetitive or direct). About half of the CTS cases are related to repetitive and cumulative trauma in the workplace, making it the occupational epidemic syndrome of our time.
- **I**nfection.
- **C**ollagen disorders. The incidence of carpal tunnel syndrome in patients with polyarthritis is high.

Other causes include rheumatoid arthritis, diabetes, hypothyroidism, and hemodialysis. Less common causes include incursion of the lumbrical muscles within the tunnel during finger movements and hypertrophy of the lumbricals, lunate laxity, or malposition.

Tests and Measures and Response

Physical therapy special tests include the Phalen test and Tinel sign; the upper limb tension test (ULTT) for the median nerve, which examines the effect of upper extremity position on median nerve tension, is specific.

Clinical Findings, Secondary Effects, or Complications

The physical assessment focuses on examining the motor and sensory functions of the hand compared to the uninvolved hand.

Diagnostic Tests

An experienced clinician most reliably makes a CTS diagnosis after reviewing the patient's history and a physical examination. This syndrome's clinical features include intermittent pain and paresthesias in the hand's median nerve distribution, which can become persistent as the condition progresses. The symptoms are typically worse at night, exacerbated by strenuous wrist movements, and can be associated with morning stiffness. The pain may radiate proximally into the forearm and arm.

Interventions/Treatment

Medical—These include the median nerve conduction study (NCS) and electromyography (EMG) study. A carpal tunnel view radiograph may be the only view that shows abnormalities within the carpal tunnel. Evaluation for surgical management is necessary for patients with atrophy of the thenar muscles, decreased sensation, and persistent symptoms that are intolerable despite conservative therapy.

Pharmacologic—NSAIDs and/or diuretics.

Physical therapy—The conservative intervention for mild cases typically includes splints, activity, ergonomic modification, and isolated tendon excursion exercises. Patient education is also important to avoid sustained pinching or gripping, repetitive wrist motions, and sustained positions of full wrist flexion.

DE QUERVAIN DISEASE

de Quervain disease is a progressive stenosing tenosynovitis, which affects the tendon sheaths of the first posterior compartment of the wrist, resulting in a thickening of the extensor retinaculum, a narrowing of the fibro-osseous canal, and an eventual entrapment and compression of the tendons, especially during radial deviation.

Clinical Significance

Overuse, repetitive tasks that involve overexertion of the thumb or radial and ulnar deviation of the wrist, and arthritis are the most common predisposing factors, as they cause the greatest stresses on the structures of the first posterior compartment. Such activities include golfing, fly-fishing, typing, sewing, knitting, and cutting.

Tests and Measures and Response

The Finkelstein test is commonly used to confirm the diagnosis (see Special Tests of the Wrist and Hand).

Clinical Findings, Secondary Effects, or Complications

Frequently, patients report a gradual and insidious onset of a dull ache over the radial aspect of the wrist made worse by turning doorknobs or keys. Examination of the wrist may reveal the following:

- A localized swelling with tenderness in the region of the radial styloid process and wrist pain radiating proximally into the forearm and distally into the thumb.
- Severe pain with wrist ulnar deviation and thumb flexion and adduction. A reproduction of the pain can also be reported with thumb extension and abduction.
- Crepitus of the tendons moving through the extensor sheath.
- Palpable thickening of the extensor sheath and the tendons distal to the extensor tunnel.
- A loss of abduction of the CMC joint of the thumb.

Diagnostic Tests

de Quervain tenosynovitis is diagnosed based on the typical appearance, location of pain, and tenderness of the involved wrist.

Interventions/Treatment

Medical—Although the diagnosis is mostly clinical, posterior-anterior and lateral radiographs of the wrist can be obtained to rule out any bony pathology, such as a scaphoid fracture, radioscaphoid, or triscaphoid arthritis, and Kienböck disease. If a conservative approach does not give relief, surgical tendon sheath release is an option.

Pharmacologic—NSAIDs and possibly cortisone injections.

Physical therapy—Physical therapy includes rest, continuous immobilization through splinting with a thumb spica for 3 weeks, and anti-inflammatory medication. Following removal of the splint, ROM exercises are prescribed, with a gradual progression to strengthening.

DUPUYTREN CONTRACTURE

Dupuytren contracture is a fibrotic condition of the palmar aponeurosis that results in nodule formation in the palmar and digital fascia or scarring of the aponeurosis, which may ultimately cause finger flexion contractures.

Clinical Significance

The nodules that are associated with this condition occur in specific locations along longitudinal tension lines. The appearance of the nodules is followed by the formation of tendon-like cords, which are due to the pathologic change in the normal fascia. The contractures form at the MCP joint, the PIP joint, and occasionally the DIP joint.

Tests and Measures and Response

The tabletop test can be used to help confirm the diagnosis (see Special Tests of the Wrist and Hand).

Clinical Findings, Secondary Effects, or Complications

The diagnosis of Dupuytren disease in its early stages may be difficult and is based on the palpable nodule, characteristic skin changes, changes in the fascia, and progressive joint contracture. The skin changes are caused by a retraction of the skin, resulting in dimples or pits. The disease is usually bilateral, with one hand being more severely involved. However, there appears to be no association with hand dominance. The patient may have one, two, or three rays involved in the more severely affected hand. The most commonly involved digit is the ring finger.

Diagnostic Tests

In most cases, the diagnosis can be made from the physical examination. Other tests are rarely necessary.

Interventions/Treatment

Medical—Needling has been used to break down the tissue cords, although the cords often reappear. Enzyme injections have also been used to help soften the fascia. However, these somewhat conservative interventions have not yet proven clinically useful or of any long-term value in the treatment of established contractures. Therefore, surgery is the intervention of choice when the MCP joint contracts approximately 30 degrees and the deformity becomes a functional problem.

Pharmacologic—Medications are not typically prescribed for this condition.

Physical therapy—Scar management and splinting are important parts of postoperative management. Active, active-assisted, and passive exercises are usually initiated at the first treatment session.

SLIPPED CAPITAL FEMORAL EPIPHYSIS

Slipped capital femoral epiphysis (SCFE) is characterized by a sudden or gradual anterior displacement of the femoral neck from the capital femoral epiphysis while the head remains in the acetabulum.[2,3] The initiating traumatic episode may be as minimal as turning over in bed. Approximately 45% will have knee or lower thigh pain as their initial symptom.[3] If the patient can walk, it is with difficulty and with a limp, often with ER of the involved foot.

Clinical Significance

SCFE is one of the most common hip pathologies that occur during adolescence. The natural history of SCFE is that the capital femoral epiphysis eventually will fuse with the femoral neck at the end of adolescence. Patients with chronic SCFE generally have a history of groin or medial thigh pain for months to years.

Tests and Measures and Response

The hip will often show decreased ROM, particularly of internal rotation, abduction, and flexion. On passive flexion of the hip, the patient will frequently externally rotate the leg (Drehmann sign).

Clinical Findings, Secondary Effects, or Complications

In the stable hip, weight-bearing is possible with or without crutches. However, the patient presents with fracture-like symptoms in the unstable hip, with pain so severe that weight-bearing is impossible.

Three complications that can adversely affect the outcome are avascular necrosis (osteonecrosis), femoroacetabular impingement, and chondrolysis.[2] These complications are uncommon sequelae in the untreated slip but are serious complications in the operative and nonoperative management of SCFE.

Diagnostic Tests

Diagnosis is confirmed by bilateral hip radiography, which should include anteroposterior and frog-leg views in patients with stable SCFE, and anteroposterior and cross-table lateral views in unstable SCFE.[4]

Interventions/Treatment

Medical—Patient placed on non–weight-bearing crutches or in a wheelchair and urgently referred to an orthopedic surgeon. The current method of choice is in situ surgical fixations to maintain the sphericity of the femoral head. Prophylactic pinning may be indicated in high-risk patients, such as younger patients and those with obesity or an endocrine disorder.[4]

Pharmacologic—Medications, if any, include NSAIDs.

Physical therapy—Conservative intervention includes traction for the relief of symptoms, at home or in the hospital, for periods ranging from 1 or 2 days to several weeks. Postoperative rehabilitation protocols for SCFE are poorly described in the literature. Gait training postsurgery is initiated as soon as LE strength and ROM are adequate for ambulation skills. The weight-bearing status can vary but is usually non–weight-bearing or touch-down weight-bearing. Full weight-bearing is permitted when the growth plate has fused (within approximately 3-4 months). ROM exercises for the hip should be performed in all planes, emphasizing hip flexion, internal rotation, and abduction. Strengthening of the affected extremity is introduced when sufficient healing has occurred.

LEGG-CALVE-PERTHES DISEASE

Legg-Calvé-Perthes disease (LCPD) is osteonecrosis of the capital femoral epiphysis of the femoral head in young children, the definitive cause of which remains unknown. However, there is considerable epidemiologic, histologic, and radiographic evidence to support the theory that LCPD is probably a localized manifestation of a generalized disorder of epiphyseal cartilage manifested in the proximal femur because of its unusual and precarious blood supply.[5,6] The young patient complains of a vague ache in the groin that radiates to the medial thigh and inner aspect of the knee. Muscle spasm is another common complaint in the early stages of the disease.

Clinical Significance

At the hip, the proximal femur grows in three areas: the apophyseal growth of the greater trochanter, the femoral neck isthmus, and the physial plate. Although the hip joint is fully formed by the 11th week of gestation, the acetabulum continues to evolve throughout gestation and into childhood, making the watershed age for the prognosis of pediatric hip conditions to be 8 years old, as this is the age when most acetabular development is complete.[5,6]

Tests and Measures and Response

A positive Trendelenburg sign is often seen, and there may be some out-toeing of the involved extremity.

Clinical Findings, Secondary Effects, or Complications

The child may be small for his/her age. On observation, there is usually decreased abduction and internal rotation. The ROM examination may show contracture in hip flexion and adduction. There may also be a slight dragging of the leg and slight atrophy of the thigh muscles.

Diagnostic Tests

Children under 6 years of age (possibly 5 years in girls) and those with minimal capital femoral epiphysis involvement and normal ROM are often followed with intermittent physical examinations and radiographs approximately every 2 months.

Interventions/Treatment

Medical—In the more severe cases, there is a lack of agreement regarding whether operative or nonoperative intervention is beneficial as most patients (70%-90%) are active and pain-free regardless of intervention.[5,6]

Pharmacologic—Medications, if any, include NSAIDs.

Physical therapy—An awareness of this disease and its manifestations will facilitate early recognition and referral by the PTA to the supervising physical therapist. Treatment methods include the following:

- Observation only.
- ROM exercises in all planes of hip motion (especially IR and abduction).
- Bracing.
- Casting.

ACETABULAR LABRAL TEAR

Mechanical impingement and/or instability of the femoroacetabular joint are common causes of labral chondral pathology. Direct trauma, sporting activities, and certain hip movements, including torsional or twisting movements, have been cited for causing labral tears.

Clinical Significance

Labral tears of the hip are more common than previously thought. In patients with mechanical hip pain, the prevalence of labral tears has been reported to be high. However, many labral tears are not associated with any known specific event or cause and may occur insidiously. Two common types of scenarios have been recognized:

1. A young person with a twisting injury to the hip, usually an external rotation force in a hyperextended position.
2. An older person with a history of hip and/or acetabular dysplasia, or the result of repeated pivoting and twisting.

Tests and Measures and Response

ROM of the hip may or may not be limited, but there may be pain at the extremes in those cases where it is not limited. There is little information regarding the sensitivity, specificity, or likelihood ratios associated with a single clinical test or a cluster of tests in diagnosing a labral tear. Generally speaking, the combined movement of flexion and rotation causes pain in the groin.

Clinical Findings, Secondary Effects, or Complications

Labral tears of the hip are often misdiagnosed as common groin strains, and it is not uncommon for the diagnosis to be missed for many months. Therefore, in young, active patients with a predominant complaint of groin pain with or without a history of trauma, the diagnosis of a labral tear should be suspected.[7]

Diagnostic Tests

Diagnosis can often be made based on the history and physical examination, although labral tears can have various clinical presentations associated with a wide degree of clinical findings.

Interventions/Treatment

Medical—Conservative intervention has traditionally included bed rest with or without traction, followed by a period of protected weight-bearing. Operative treatment consists of arthrotomy or arthroscopy with resection of the entire labrum or the portion of the torn labrum.

Pharmacologic—Medications typically include NSAIDs.

Physical therapy—The appropriate physical therapy intervention for a patient with an acetabular labral tear has yet to be established. A common approach, based on clinical findings, typically includes progressive resisted strengthening and closed-chain exercises with emphasis on hip and lumbopelvic stabilization, correction of hip muscular imbalance, and biomechanical control.

ILIOTIBIAL BAND FRICTION SYNDROME

As its name suggests, iliotibial band friction syndrome (ITBFS) is a repetitive stress injury common in runners and cyclists, caused by friction of the ITB as it slides over the prominent lateral femoral epicondyle at approximately 30 degrees of knee flexion. The friction has been found to occur at the band's posterior edge, which is tighter against the lateral femoral condyle than the anterior fibers.

Clinical Significance

ITB syndrome can cause significant morbidity and lead to the cessation of exercise. At the hip, an ITB contracture can lead to gluteal tendinopathy by increasing compression and friction of the subgluteus maximus bursa between the ITB and the greater trochanter. Pelvic and trunk motion in the coronal plane will usually be increased in this population, and given the potential for proximal compensations, pelvic and trunk motion should be assessed for abnormal movements during the dynamic examination of this group of patients.

Tests and Measures and Response

The classic test for ITB contracture is the Ober test (see Special Tests of the Hip). Three commonly used physical therapy special tests for ITBFS include Noble compression and the Renne (creak) test (see Special Tests of the Knee Complex).

Clinical Findings, Secondary Effects, or Complications

Subjectively, the patient reports pain with repetitive motions of the knee. The lateral knee pain is described as diffuse and hard to localize. Although walking on level surfaces does not generally reproduce symptoms, especially if a stiff-legged gait is used, climbing or descending stairs often aggravates the pain. Patients do not complain of pain during sprinting, squatting, or during such stop-and-go activities as tennis or racquetball. The progression of symptoms is often associated with a change in training surface, increased mileage, or training on crowned roads.

Objectively, there is localized tenderness to palpation at the lateral femoral condyle and/or Gerdy tubercle on the anterior-lateral portion of the proximal tibia. The resisted tests are likely to be negative for pain. The special tests for the ITB (Ober test, prone lying test, and retinacular test) should be positive for pain, crepitus, or both, especially at 30 degrees of weight-bearing knee flexion. In addition to the finding of a tight ITB, a cavus foot (calcaneal varus) structure, leg length difference (with the syndrome developing on the shorter side), fatigue, internal tibial torsion (increased lateral retinaculum tension), an anatomically prominent lateral femoral epicondyle, and genu varum, have all been associated with ITB friction problems, although they have yet to be substantiated.

Diagnostic Tests

The diagnosis for ITBFS is usually based on the history and physical examination. An MRI may be ordered if another joint pathology is suspected or if surgery is being considered. The MRI will show a thickened ITB over the lateral femoral epicondyle in cases of ITBFS and often detects a fluid collection deep to the ITB in the same region.

Interventions/Treatment

Medical—Surgical intervention, consisting of resection of the posterior half of the ITB at the level that passes over the lateral femoral condyle, is reserved for the more recalcitrant cases.

Pharmacologic—NSAIDs.

Physical therapy—Activity modification to reduce the irritating stress (decreasing mileage, changing the bike seat position, changing the training surfaces), using new running shoes, heat or ice applications, strengthening the hip abductors, and ITB stretching.

ANTERIOR CRUCIATE LIGAMENT TEAR

When the outer aspect of the knee receives a direct blow that causes valgus stress, the MCL often is torn first, followed by the ACL, which becomes the second component of a sports-related ACL injury.

Clinical Significance

Almost all ACL tears are complete midsubstance tears. ACL injury rates are two to eight times higher in women than in men participating in the same sports. Young athletes may sustain growth plate injuries (eg, avulsion fractures) rather than midsubstance tears because the epiphyseal cartilage in their growth plates is structurally weaker than their ligaments, collagen, or bones.

Symptomatic ACL deficiencies in young athletes' knee joints are subject to the same long-term detrimental effects that occur in adult athletes. Young athletes may also be more pre-disposed to more long-term degenerative knee conditions due to more years of chronic rotary knee instabilities from ACL deficiencies.

Tests and Measures and Response

Numerous physical therapy special tests exist to aid in confirming an ACL tear (see Special Tests of the Knee Complex).

Clinical Findings, Secondary Effects, or Complications

All ACL tears (ie, sprains) are categorized as grade I, II, or III injuries. Ligament tears are classified according to the degree of injury, ranging from overstretched ligament fibers (ie, partial or moderate tears) to ligament ruptures (ie, complete tears or disruptions). Patients commonly describe the sensation of their knee "popping" or "giving out" as the tibia sub-luxes anteriorly. Other signs and symptoms of ACL injuries include pain, immediate dys-function, instability in the involved knee, and the inability to walk without assistance. A classic sign of ACL injuries is acute hemarthrosis (ie, extravasation of blood into a joint or synovial cavity). Atrophy of the quadriceps is an almost constant finding with patients who have a torn ACL.

Diagnostic Tests

Thorough patient histories and physical examinations are essential for accurate diagnoses of ACL injuries. An arthrometer, such as a KT-1000, is a mechanical testing device for measuring anterior-posterior knee ligament instability. This noninvasive device assesses the amount of displacement between the femur and the tibia at a given force in millime-ters. Although most patients who have a complete tear of the ACL have increased tibial translation on instrumented testing, it is unknown how many of these patients will have "giving-way" of the knee or how many knees will have overt or latent damage of the carti-lage within a few years.

MRI scans are useful for diagnosing ACL injuries, although their use in discriminating between complete and partial ACL tears is limited. Diagnostic MRI scans, however, can detect associated meniscal tears that routine radiographs cannot show.

Interventions/Treatment

Medical—The primary healing potential of the ACL has been reported to be extremely poor in both clinical and experimental studies due to its minimal blood supply and the presence of joint fluid, both of which contribute to a reduced healing potential. Patients with either partial (grades I and II) ACL tears (negative pivot shifts) or "isolated" ACL tears, who lead a less active lifestyle and participate in linear, nondeceleration activities, are considered to be candidates for conservative intervention. However, to return to normal preinjury activity levels, patients must be thoroughly rehabilitated, and protective measures (eg, knee bracing and activity restrictions) must be taken to prevent further knee injuries. ACL reconstruction is one of the most commonly performed orthopedic surgeries in the United States. Surgical treatment of the torn ACL includes direct repair, repair with augmentation, and reconstruction with autografts or allografts (single-bundle or double-bundle). The clinical evidence for double-bundle ACL reconstruction is mounting but is still inconclusive. Currently, arthroscopic reconstruction remains the treatment of choice.

Pharmacologic—Analgesics both preoperatively and postoperatively.

Physical therapy—Numerous lower extremity rehabilitation protocols following injury or surgery have been reported in the literature. Emphasis on regaining extension and closed-chain 0 to 45 degrees strengthening exercises are consistent among most ACL rehab protocols. For the middle-aged and older athlete, physical therapy often is the treatment of choice unless the patient plans to participate in sports activities that expose the knees to vigorous twisting forces. However, certain sports activities must be avoided, especially those involving jumping, quick starts and stops, and abrupt lateral movements (eg, soccer, basketball). Identifying the nonoperative patient population who return to an active lifestyle (copers) and those who modify activity level (adapters) from surgical candidates (noncopers) should use an ACL screening examination. The best criterion for this screening examination is an area of ongoing study. Current recommendations include the KOS-Sport, Global Knee Function Rating, hop tests, and Quadriceps Index.

MENISCAL INJURIES

Meniscal injuries are a common sports-related problem and the most frequent injury to the knee joint. Such injuries are especially prevalent among competitive athletes, particularly those who play soccer, football, and basketball.

Clinical Significance

The outer 25% to 30% of the menisci is known to be vascular.[8] Tears in the vascular region are repairable, as are tears extending into the avascular midsubstance if vascularity is stimulated through abrasion of the perimeniscal synovium and/or implantation of a fibrin clot. Next to an adequate blood supply, the most important factor influencing the meniscus repair's prognosis is ACL stability.

Tests and Measures and Response

Common clinical findings include a twisting mechanism of injury, delayed effusion, and mechanical complaints such as catching or locking. Numerous physical therapy special tests exist to aid in confirming a meniscal injury (see Special Tests of the Knee Complex).

Clinical Findings, Secondary Effects, or Complications

Meniscal tears can be classified into two types, traumatic and degenerative:

- Traumatic tears: Most commonly found in young, athletically active individuals, not necessarily associated with contact injuries; frequently associated with ACL tears, and less commonly with PCL tears. Vertical longitudinal tears are the most common; transverse or radial tears are also common. Injuries to the healthy meniscus are usually produced by combining compressive forces coupled with rotation of the flexed knee as it starts to move into extension. The final type and location of the tear are determined by the direction and magnitude of the force acting on the knee and the position of the knee when injured.
- Degenerative tears: Tend to occur in patients older than 40 years. No history of a traumatic event is present. These tears have minimal or no healing capacity, and horizontal cleavage tears, flap tears, and complex tears are most common.

The most common report following meniscal injury is one of joint-line pain. The patient may also report joint clicking or locking and the knee giving way. Tests to evaluate the menisci are outlined in the Special Tests of the Knee section.

Severe damage or loss or removal of the menisci frequently leads to joint instability and later accelerated DJD, resulting in further disability and joint replacement.

Diagnostic Tests

A torn meniscus can often be diagnosed based on the physical examination alone. An MRI is the best imaging study to detect and confirm a torn meniscus.

Interventions/Treatment

Medical—Depending on the type, size, and location of the tear, the initial approach is conservative. If the conservative approach fails or there is repetitive locking of the knee, a surgical repair of the meniscus is typically recommended.

Pharmacologic—Analgesics both preoperatively and postoperatively.

Physical therapy—The rehabilitation process is based on the healing phases: initial protection and joint activation phase, followed by a progressive joint loading and functional restoration phase, and finally an activity restoration phase. Patients may progress through the rehabilitation process at different rates, depending on individual characteristics, lesion features, and concomitant pathology.

OSGOOD-SCHLATTER DISEASE

Osgood-Schlatter disease is a self-limiting traction apophysis that is one of the most common causes of adolescent knee pain. Repeated stress from the quadriceps contracting during rapid growth periods may result in a partial avulsion fracture through the ossification center of a small portion of the partially developed tibial tuberosity. The condition occurs in active boys and girls aged 11 to 18 years, coinciding with periods of growth spurts, and occurs more frequently in boys than in girls.[9]

Clinical Significance

Two factors that impact epiphyseal plate injury are (1) the ability of the growth plate to resist failure and (2) the forces applied to the bone or the stresses induced in the growth plate. The majority of epiphyseal fractures are due to high-velocity injuries.

Tests and Measures and Response

No specific physical therapy special tests exist to confirm a diagnosis. The diagnosis is typically made based on the patient's age, history, and palpable tenderness at the tibial tuberosity.

Clinical Findings, Secondary Effects, or Complications

Symptoms are typically unilateral, although 20% to 30% of cases can be bilateral.[10] In the acute phase, the pain is severe and continuous. The pain occurs during running, jumping, squatting, especially during kneeling, acute knee impact, and ascending or descending stairs. There is often a visible lump over the site. The pain can be reproduced by extending the knee against resistance or stressing the quadriceps.

Diagnostic Tests

These are usually unnecessary, but x-rays will show soft tissue swelling with loss of the patellar tendon's sharp margins in the acute phase, and bone fragmentation at the tibial tuberosity may be evident 3 to 4 weeks after the onset.

Interventions/Treatment

Medical—This is usually a self-limiting condition. Surgical intervention is only usually required if complications arise.

Pharmacologic—NSAIDs or analgesics, depending on the severity.

Physical therapy—Avoidance of the offending activity and judicious stretching of the quadriceps and hamstrings (adaptively shortened hamstrings require increased quadriceps force to overcome the tight posterior structures).

PATELLAR TENDINOPATHY

Patellar tendinopathy (jumper's knee) and quadriceps tendinopathy are overuse conditions frequently associated with eccentric overloading during deceleration activities (repeated jumping and landing, downhill running, etc). The high stresses placed upon these areas during closed kinetic chain functioning place them at high risk for overuse injuries.

STUDY PEARL
Orthopedic injuries commonly seen in the pediatric population include Osgood-Schlatter disease, spondylolysis, stress fractures, little league elbow, and growth plate disorders.

Clinical Significance

Chronic tendinopathy.

Tests and Measures and Response

No specific physical therapy special tests exist to confirm a diagnosis.

Clinical Findings, Secondary Effects, or Complications

Patellar tendinopathy is one of many potential diagnoses for a patient presenting with anterior knee pain. Pain upon palpation near the patellar insertion is present in both patellar and quadriceps tendinopathy.

Diagnostic Tests

A comprehensive examination of the complete lower extremity is necessary to identify any relevant deficits at the hip, knee, and ankle/foot regions.

Interventions/Treatment

Medical—These are usually self-limiting conditions. Surgical intervention is only usually required if significant tendinosis develops and is successful in most patients.
Pharmacologic—NSAIDs or analgesics, depending on the severity.
Physical therapy—Patellar tendinopathies typically respond well to rest, stretching, eccentric strengthening, bracing, and other conservative techniques.
Several protocols have been advocated for the conservative intervention of patellar tendinopathy based on symptoms. Lesions characterized by no undue functional impairment and pain only after the activity are addressed with localized heating of the area, an adequate warm-up before training and ice massage after a detailed flexibility assessment, and evaluation of athletic techniques. Also, a concentric-eccentric program for the anterior tibialis muscle is prescribed, which progresses into a purely eccentric program as the pain decreases.

PATELLOFEMORAL PAIN SYNDROME

Anterior knee pain, or patellofemoral pain syndrome (PFS), is characterized by pain in the vicinity of the patella, worsened by sitting and during activities that require knee flexion and forceful contraction of the quadriceps (eg, during squats, ascending/descending stairs). The pain, characteristically located behind the kneecap (ie, retropatellar) and/or along the patella's borders at the medial or lateral retinaculum attachment sites, may worsen in intensity and duration and rapidity of onset if the aggravating activity is performed repeatedly.

Clinical Significance

Although PFS can occur in anyone—particularly athletes—women who are not athletic appear to be more prone to this problem than men who are not athletic. The impairments resulting from patellofemoral dysfunction have been related to problems that cannot be improved by physical therapy and those that can. The former includes anatomic variance (femoral trochlear dysplasia, patellar morphology and the amount of patellofemoral joint congruency, the natural positioning of the patella (alta/baja) joint, and gender (females are more predisposed).

Tests and Measures and Response

Several physical therapy special tests exist to assess the patella's mobility (see Special Tests of the Knee Complex).

Clinical Findings, Secondary Effects, or Complications

The usual physical findings are localized around the knee.

- Tenderness often is present along the facets of the patella. The facets are most accessible to palpation while the knee is fully extended and the quadriceps muscle is relaxed.
- Tenderness with palpation to medial or lateral retinaculum.
- An apprehension sign may be elicited by manually fixing the patella's position against the femur and having the patient contract the ipsilateral quadriceps.

- Crepitus may be present, but crepitus alone does not allow for a definitive diagnosis.
- An alteration in the Q-angle.
- Movement analysis may demonstrate excessive foot pronation, excessive knee valgus, excessive hip internal rotation, an antalgic gait pattern, and excessive hip adduction and internal rotation with squatting, stairs, and landing from a jump.
- Repetitive squatting may reproduce knee pain.
- Genu recurvatum and hamstring weakness.

Diagnostic Tests

PFS is primarily a clinical diagnosis based on a thorough physical examination.

Interventions/Treatment

Medical—PFS is generally treated conservatively. Surgery may be considered for those patients in whom other causes of anterior knee pain have been excluded and whose symptoms persist despite completing at least 6 to 12 months of a thorough rehabilitation program.

Pharmacologic—The physician may prescribe analgesics, depending on the severity.

Physical therapy—The focus of physical therapy intervention is to find the cause of the PFS (eg, muscle imbalance, leg length discrepancy, or other structural problems). Ice, electrical stimulation, and biofeedback may be used. The basic exercise principles for the management of PFS are as follows:

- Restoration of muscle balance within the quadriceps group. Quadriceps strengthening is traditionally performed while the knee is flexed 0 to 30 degrees. Controversy remains as to the extent that the individual muscle groups comprising the quadriceps can selectively be strengthened. Stretching of the quadriceps should be of long duration (20-30 seconds) and with low force. Also, restoration of hip muscle balance should be addressed, focusing on the hip abductors and external rotators and the gluteus maximus.
- Improving flexibility, including exercises to stretch the ITB, hip, hamstring, and gastrocnemius. Manual stretching of the lateral retinaculum may be used as a conservative approach, partially mimicking the effect of lateral retinacular release.
- Improving ROM.
- Restricting the offending physical activity.
- Home exercise programs that include both stretching and strengthening exercises.
- Patellar taping techniques (McConnell method) can be used to reduce the friction on the patella. If successful, the clinician can teach the patient self-taping techniques to use at home.
- Proper footwear also is important. The clinician can evaluate the patient's biomechanics and recommend proper shoes and/or orthotics.

ACHILLES TENDINOPATHY

Achilles tendinopathy is the most common overuse syndrome of the lower leg.

Clinical Significance

Achilles tendinopathy symptoms consist of a gradual onset of pain and swelling in the Achilles tendon 2 to 3 cm proximal to the tendon's insertion, exacerbated by activity. Some patients will present with pain and stiffness along the Achilles tendon when rising in the morning or pain at the start of activity that improves as the activity progresses.

Tests and Measures and Response

Several tests and measures have been designed specifically to detect Achilles tendinopathy. These can include passive stretching of the tendon to elicit pain, having the patient perform a unilateral heel raise while asking the patient to unilaterally hop on the affected side either in place or in various directions. Additional findings include the arc sign and the Royal London Hospital test (see Special Tests of the Ankle and Foot).

Several factors appear to contribute to the development of Achilles tendinopathy:

- Biomechanical factors: The rapid and repeated transitions from pronation to supination cause the Achilles tendon to undergo a "whipping" or "bowstring" action. Moreover, if the foot remains pronated after knee extension has begun, the external tibial rotation at the knee and the internal tibial rotation at the foot results in a "wringing" or twisting action of the tendon.
- Training variables: A lack of stretching programs, a faster training pace, and hill training have all been found to correlate with increased incidence.
- Overtraining has been found to correlate to calf muscle fatigue and microtears of the tendon.
- Muscular insufficiency has been cited as a significant factor in the inability to eccentrically restrain dorsiflexion during the beginning of the support phase of running.
- The compensatory overpronation resulting from the inflexibility of the cavus foot is a precursor to Achilles tendinitis.
- Shoe type. Spiked shoes lock the feet on the surface during a run's single support phase increasing the athlete's foot grip and transferring lateral and torque shear forces directly to the foot and ankle and through to the Achilles tendon.
- Sacroiliac joint dysfunction: Changes in sacroiliac joint mechanics as compared with the contralateral side.

Clinical Findings, Secondary Effects, or Complications

Upon observation, the patient will often be found to have pronated feet, and the presence of swelling is common. Observation during gait may reveal an antalgic gait, with the involved leg held in external rotation during both stance and swing phase.

- Localization of the tenderness with palpation is extremely important.
- Tenderness that is located 2 to 6 cm proximal to the insertion is indicative of noninsertional tendinopathy.
- Pain at the bone-tendon junction is more indicative of insertional tendinopathy.
- If there is an area in the tendon itself that is discrete and painful with side-to-side pressure of the fingers, this often indicates an area of mucoid degeneration or a small partial rupture of the tendon.
- If the tenderness is in the retrocalcaneal bursa area, noted by side-to-side pressure in that area, this is the primary area of involvement.

A lack of normal dorsiflexion in knee extension signifies adaptive gastrocnemius shortening, and the inability to perform a normal range of dorsiflexion in knee flexion implicates the soleus as well.

There is often pain with resisted testing of the gastrocnemius/soleus complex.

Diagnostic Tests

Achilles tendinopathy is typically diagnosed through the description of symptoms and an examination of the Achilles tendon. An ultrasound scan or MRI is used in cases where the diagnosis is not conclusive.

Interventions/Treatment

Medical—For most individuals, Achilles tendinopathy symptoms usually clear with 3 to 6 months of conservative treatment. In cases that do not respond to a conservative approach, surgery may become an option.

Pharmacologic—Short-term analgesics are used to help relieve the pain. However, corticosteroids in the treatment of Achilles tendinopathy have declined due to the adverse effects of these drugs on the tendon structure.

Physical therapy—The patient should temporarily discontinue any activity that seems to provoke the symptoms.

The intervention strategies for tendon injuries are outlined in Intervention Principles for Musculoskeletal Injuries section.

LATERAL ANKLE SPRAINS

The ankle is stable in the neutral position or dorsiflexion because the widest part of the talus is in the mortise. However, in plantarflexion, ankle stability is decreased, as the narrow posterior portion of the talus is in the mortise. Thus, the most common mechanism of an ankle sprain is one of inversion and plantarflexion.

Clinical Significance

Ankle sprains are the most common injuries in sports and recreational activities, and if left untreated, it can lead to chronic instability and impairment. Most acute ankle injuries occur in people 21 to 30 years old, although injuries in the younger and older groups tend to be more serious. Sprains of the lateral ligamentous complex represent the majority of ankle ligament sprains. Lateral ligament sprains are more common than medial ligament sprains for two major reasons:

- The lateral malleolus projects more distally than the medial malleolus, producing more bony obstruction to eversion than inversion.
- The deltoid ligament is much stronger than the lateral ligaments.

The high ankle sprain, or syndesmotic sprain, which involves disruption of the ligamentous structures between the distal fibula and tibia, just proximal to the ankle joint, occurs less frequently than the lateral ankle sprain.

Tests and Measures and Response

Several physical therapy special tests help diagnose a lateral ankle sprain (see Special Tests of the Ankle and Foot).

Clinical Findings, Secondary Effects, or Complications

Lateral ankle sprains can be graded according to severity:

- Grade I sprains are characterized by minimum to no swelling, no laxity, and localized tenderness over the ATFL.
- Grade II sprains are characterized by localized swelling and laxity and more diffuse lateral tenderness.
- Grade III sprains are characterized by significant swelling, laxity, pain, and ecchymosis and should be referred to a specialist. Grade III injuries may require greater than 6 weeks to return to full function.

Diagnostic Tests

No single symptom or test can provide a completely accurate diagnosis of a lateral ankle ligament rupture, but the collection of findings can be strongly indicative.

- The absence of swelling at the time of the delayed (after 4 days) physical examination suggests that there is no ligament rupture, whereas extensive swelling at this time is indicative of ligament rupture.
- Pain on palpation of the involved ligament suggests involvement.
- The presence of a hematoma suggests a rupture.
- Positive anterior drawer test suggests a rupture.
- Impairment of walking ability after injury suggests involvement.

X-rays are indicated to rule out a fracture of the ankle when there is bone tenderness in the posterior half of the lower 6 cm of the fibula or tibia and an inability to bear weight immediately after an injury. Similarly, if there is bone tenderness over the navicular and/or fifth metatarsal and an inability to bear weight immediately after injury, then radiographs of the foot are indicated.

Interventions/Treatment

Medical—Conservative intervention is consistently effective in treating grades I and II ankle sprains. However, surgical intervention may yield slightly better outcomes for function and instability for severe acute ankle sprains than conservative treatment.

Pharmacologic—Except for NSAIDs, pharmacologic intervention is typically not needed.

Physical therapy—Once pain and inflammation are under control (4-14 days), the patient begins dynamic balance and proprioceptive exercises, with or without a brace. Exercises that promote ankle dorsiflexion past the neutral position, enabling a closer to a normal walking pattern, are introduced. Open-chain (non–weight-bearing) progressive resistive exercises with rubber tubing resistance are performed (two sets of 30 reps each) for isolated plantarflexion, dorsiflexion, inversion, and eversion. Stationary cycling can also be performed (at a comfortable intensity for up to 30 minutes) to provide cardiovascular endurance training and controlled ankle ROM. Plyometric activities are introduced during the return-to-activity phase.

PLANTAR FASCIITIS

Plantar fasciitis is reported to be the most common cause of inferior heel pain. The role of the heel spur in plantar fasciitis is controversial.

Clinical Significance

Plantar heel pain is usually unilateral, although both feet can be affected. Although more common in active individuals, plantar heel pain can also affect the sedentary population, although the reasons for this remain elusive.

Tests and Measures and Response

Several special tests are available to help confirm the diagnosis of plantar fasciitis, of which the windlass test is considered the most reliable.

Clinical Findings, Secondary Effects, or Complications

Common findings include a history of pain and tenderness on the plantar medial aspect of the foot's heel and/or plantar surface, especially during initial weight-bearing in the morning. Interference with daily activities is common. Plantar fasciitis is usually unilateral, although both feet can be affected. The heel pain often decreases during the day but worsens with increased activity (such as jogging, climbing stairs, or going up on the toes) or after a period of sitting.

Upon physical examination, there will be localized pain on palpation along the medial edge of the fascia or its origin on the anterior edge of the calcaneus, although firm finger pressure is often necessary to localize the point of maximum tenderness. The tenderness is typically just over and distal to the medial calcaneal tubercle, and there is usually one small exquisitely painful area. Tenderness in the center of the heel's posterior part may be due to bruising or atrophy of the heel pad or subcalcaneal bursitis. Slight swelling in the area is common. The fascia needs to be stretched with a bowstring type test/windlass maneuver to test for plantar fasciitis. This maneuver can be performed by manually fixing the patient's heel in eversion, grasping the first metatarsal, and placing it in dorsiflexion before extending the big toe as far as possible. Pain should be elicited at the medial tubercle.

Diagnostic Tests

The clinical diagnosis for plantar fasciitis is normally based on the patient's history, evidence of risk factors (eg, pes cavus, excessive foot pronation, obesity, occupations involving prolonged standing/walking), and the physical examination. In the form of plain radiography, imaging is only ever used to rule out other heel pathology.

Interventions/Treatment

Medical—In the vast majority of cases, plantar fasciitis responds well to a conservative approach. However, in recalcitrant cases, plantar fascia release surgery may be required.

Pharmacologic—NSAIDs.

STUDY PEARL

The clinician should be suspicious of any insidious onset of bilateral plantar fasciitis (or Achilles tendinopathy) due to the possibility of a systemic inflammatory condition.

Physical therapy—Several physical therapy interventions have been suggested over the years for plantar fasciitis. These include the following:

- Night splinting.
- Orthotics.
- Taping.
- Heel cups.
- Stretching (gastrocnemius) and strengthening of the leg muscles and foot intrinsics.
- Progressive loading of the plantar fascia.
- Deep frictional massage.
- Dexamethasone iontophoresis.
- Shoe modifications.
- Casting.
- Extracorporeal shock wave lithotripsy.

CERVICOGENIC HEADACHES

A cervicogenic headache (CH) is defined as one that meets the following criteria: (1) pain localized to the neck and occipital region that may project to the forehead, orbital region, temples, vertex, or ears; (2) pain precipitated or aggravated by specific neck movements or sustained neck posture; and (3) resistance to or limitation of active or passive physiologic and accessory neck movements or abnormal tenderness of neck muscles, or both.

Clinical Significance

CHs are difficult to define and classify because of their variable distribution and character of symptoms.

Tests and Measures and Response

Jull et al.[11] provided a cluster of examination findings to discern CHs from primary headaches. The combination of reduced cervical ROM, painful upper cervical segmental manual palpation, and reduced strength in the cervical cranioflexor muscles delineated people with CHs from those with primary headaches with 100% sensitivity and 90% specificity.[11]

Clinical Findings, Secondary Effects, or Complications

The patient with a CH usually reports a dull, aching pain of moderate intensity, which begins in the neck or occipital region and then spreads to include a greater part of the cranium.

Diagnostic Tests

According to the International Headache Society (IHS), a radiologic examination must reveal at least one of the following: (1) movement abnormalities during flexion-extension, (2) abnormal posture, or (3) fractures, bone tumors, RA, congenital abnormalities, or other distinct pathology other than spondylosis or osteochondrosis.

Interventions/Treatment

Medical—The typical approach for a CH (once other causes have been ruled out) is conservative.

Pharmacologic—Analgesics may be prescribed.

Physical therapy—Several interventions have been recommended for CHs, including posture training, manual therapy, exercise, rest, and minor analgesics. Manual therapy studies have demonstrated positive effects on both the impairment (pain and muscle function) and the disability level, with most studies focusing on short-term outcomes. McKenzie[12] recommends a home program of cervical retraction exercises to decrease CH symptoms and maintain correct cervical alignment.

TEMPOROMANDIBULAR JOINT DYSFUNCTION

Temporomandibular joint internal derangement is one of the most common forms of temporomandibular joint dysfunction (TMD) and is associated with characteristic clinical findings such as pain, joint sounds, and irregular or deviating jaw function. When related to TMD, the term *internal derangement* denotes an abnormal positional relationship of the articular disk to the mandibular condyle and the articular eminence. This abnormal positional relationship may result in mechanical interference and restriction of the normal range of mandibular activity.

Clinical Significance

Approximately 50% to 75% of the general population has experienced unilateral TMD on a minimum of one occasion, and at least 33% have reported a minimum of one continuing persistent symptom.[13]

Tests and Measures and Response

The most common procedure used by physical therapists to detect a TMD is the TMJ screen (see Special Tests of the Cervical Spine and TMJ).

Clinical Findings, Secondary Effects, or Complications

Currently, clinical examination is the gold standard for diagnosing TMDs. Due to its proximity, the cervical spine must be thoroughly examined in conjunction with the TMJ.

Diagnostic Tests

MRI is currently the most accurate imaging modality for identifying disk positions of the TMJ and may be regarded as the gold standard for disk position identification purposes.[14]

Interventions/Treatment

Medical—There is a lack of a consistent method for identifying and diagnosing TMD. Complicating matter is that most of the symptoms associated with TMD are self-limiting and resolve without active intervention.

Pharmacologic—Medications may be prescribed for any psychosocial characteristics identified. Analgesics may be prescribed for pain management.

Physical therapy—The physical therapy intervention for this condition depends on the causative factors. Typically, the focus is on the following factors:

- Pain management techniques.
- Postural education.
- Elimination of any occlusal disharmony.
- Joint mobilizations to the TMJ and/or subcranial spine.
- Psychological stress reduction. Biofeedback can help the patient recognize periods of stress.
- Habit training to develop a path of mandibular movement that avoids any interference.
- Reduce or eliminate parafunctional habits (cheek biting, nail-biting, pencil chewing, teeth clenching, or bruxism).
- A reduction in chewing force while encouraging chewing on the affected side to decrease the interarticular pressure.
- Methods to prevent the disk-condyle complex from returning to the closed position by applying a permanent stabilization splint for a few months. When symptoms have been reduced, the patient should be weaned off the splint during the day, and eventually, at night.

IDIOPATHIC SCOLIOSIS

Scoliosis represents a progressive disturbance of a series of spinal segments that produces a three-dimensional deformity (lateral curvature and vertebral rotation) of the spine. Despite extensive research devoted to discovering the cause of idiopathic scoliosis, the mechanics and specific etiology are not clearly understood, hence the name. Scoliosis is generally described by the location of the curve or curves. One should also describe whether the convexity of the curve points to the right or left. If there is a double curve, each curve must be described and measured.

Clinical Significance

The following are the main factors that influence the probability of progression in the skeleton of the immature patient:

- The younger the patient at diagnosis, the greater the risk of progression.
- Double-curve patterns have a greater risk for progression than single-curve patterns.
- Curves with greater magnitude are at a greater risk to progress.
- The risk of progression in females is approximately 10 times that of males with curves of comparable magnitude.
- Greater risk of progression is present when curves develop before menarche.

Tests and Measures and Response

Visual observation is used during Adams forward bending test, which involves asking the patient to bend forward at the waist as though touching his or her toes while the clinician, who is standing behind the patient, looks along the line at the back and determines whether one side is higher than the other. If scoliosis is suspected, the magnitude of a rib hump is quantified by placing a scoliometer (an inclinometer) over the spinous process at the curve's apex during Adams forward bending test and measuring the angle of trunk rotation as the patient bends forward.

Clinical Findings, Secondary Effects, or Complications

During the physical examination by the patient's physician, a determination is made as to whether the deformity is structural (cannot be corrected with active or passive movement and there is rotation toward the convexity of the curve) or nonstructural (fully corrects clinically and radiographically with trunk side bending toward the apex of the curve and lacks vertebral rotation). Nonstructural scoliotic curves can result from leg length discrepancies, muscle disuse/overuse, habitual postures, and muscle guarding.

If scoliosis is neglected, the curves may progress dramatically, creating significant physical deformity and even cardiopulmonary problems with very severe curves.

Diagnostic Tests

Radiographs, which are usually only considered when a patient has a curve that might require treatment or could progress to a stage requiring treatment, can be used to determine the location, type, and magnitude of the curve (using the Cobb method), as well as skeletal age. Alternatively, a noninvasive (reduces radiation exposure) technique called Moiré topography can be used, in which light is projected through grids onto the back of the patient to assess topographical asymmetry.

Skeletal maturity is determined using the Risser sign, a measurement of the progressive ossification from anterolaterally to posteromedially in the iliac apophysis. Once a child reaches a grade 5 on the Risser scale, their scoliotic curve will stabilize.

Interventions/Treatment

Medical—Most curves can be treated nonoperatively with observation and periodic radiographs to check for curve progression. Orthoses are typically prescribed for children with idiopathic scoliosis who are skeletally immature (with a Risser sign of 0, 1, or 2) and have a curve from 25 to 45 degrees. The active theory of orthotics is that curve progression is prevented by muscle contractions responding to the brace wear.

Pharmacologic—Not usually prescribed except in rare cases for pain.

Physical therapy—Physical therapy interventions for scoliosis are based on the child's skeletal maturity, the child's growth potential, and the curve's magnitude. The primary benefits of exercise in a nonsurgical patient with scoliosis are as follows[15]:

- Help correct postural alignment and asymmetrical postural habits to prevent further development following the bracing program.
- Maintain proper respiration and chest mobility.
- Improve overall spinal mobility and help reduce back pain.
- Help the patient resume prebracing functional skills.
- Maintain muscle strength, particularly in the abdominals.
- Maintain or improve the correct length and strength relationships of the spinal and extremity musculature. The general rule is to strengthen the muscles on the convex side and stretch the muscles on the concave side.

LUMBAR HERNIATED NUCLEUS PULPOSUS

IVD herniation in the lumbar spine may occur from adolescence into old age. Degenerative changes are the body's attempts at self-healing as the body ages. The water-retaining ability of the nucleus pulposus progressively declines with age, resulting in a decrease in the disk's mechanical stiffness, allowing the annulus to bulge with a corresponding loss of disk and foramina height.

Clinical Significance

The clinical course of low back pain can be described as acute, subacute, recurrent, or chronic. Disk deterioration and loss of disk height may shift the balance of weight-bearing to the facet joint. Nuclear material that is displaced into the spinal canal is associated with a significant inflammatory response—macrophages respond to this displaced foreign material and seek to clear the spinal canal. Compression of a motor nerve results in weakness, and sensory nerve compression results in numbness. Radicular pain results from inflammation of the nerve. Furthermore, degeneration may result in radial tears and leakage from the nuclear material, which is toxic to the nerves. The resultant inflammatory response causes neural irritation with radiating pain without numbness, weakness, or loss of reflex, as neural compression is absent.

Tests and Measures and Response

One of the best ways to detect lumbar disk pathology is for the physical therapist to use the Cyriax lower quadrant examination.

Clinical Findings, Secondary Effects, or Complications

The pertinent historical information begins with an analysis of the chief complaint:

- The provocation of radiating pain down the leg is the most sensitive test for a lumbar disk herniation while assessing the pattern of pain regarding a dermatomal distribution or assessing the organicity of the complaints.
- It is important to specifically exclude red flags, such as nonmechanical pain—pain at night unrelated to activity or movement, which may indicate a tumor or infection.

The physical therapist's examination is essentially a neurologic assessment of weakness, dermatomal numbness, reflex change, or, most importantly, tension in the lumbar spine, sciatic or femoral nerve roots. For a higher lumbar lesion, reverse straight-leg raising or hip extension stretching the femoral nerve is analogous to a straight-leg raising sign.

Diagnostic Tests

Depending on the severity and complexity of the presenting symptoms, any of the following diagnostic tests may be used: x-rays, MRI, computed tomography (CT) scan, electrodiagnostics, bone scan, discography.

Interventions/Treatment

Medical—The natural history of radiculopathy and disk herniation is not quite as favorable as for simple low back pain, but it is still excellent. Surgery is often recommended after 4 to 6 weeks if the symptoms persist, following MRI and CT scan findings.

Pharmacologic—Analgesics, NSAIDs, and cortisone injections.

Physical therapy—With radiculopathy, the goal is to decrease radiating symptoms into the limb and centralize the pain using specific maneuvers or positions, such as the lateral shift correction. Once this centralizing position is identified, the patient can perform these maneuvers repetitively or sustain certain positions for specific periods throughout the day. Also, the patient is instructed in a lumbar stabilization program, in which neutral zone mechanics are practiced in various positions to decrease stress to the lumbosacral spine. It is theorized that these exercises may strengthen the stabilizer muscles, which control and limit the free movement of one vertebra on the other, thereby accelerating the herniated disk's recovery process.

SPINAL STENOSIS (DEGENERATIVE)

Degenerative spinal stenosis (DSS) is defined as a narrowing of the spinal canal, nerve root canal (lateral recess), or intervertebral foramina of the lumbar spine. It is predominantly a disorder of the elderly.

Clinical Significance

Spinal stenosis may be classified as central or lateral.

- Central stenosis is characterized by spinal canal narrowing around the thecal sac, which contains the cauda equina in the lumbar spine or the spinal cord in the cervical and thoracic regions. The causes for this type of stenosis include facet joint arthrosis and hypertrophy, thickening and bulging of the ligamentum flavum, bulging of the IVD, osteophytes, instability/spondylolisthesis, or tumor/space-occupying lesion.
- Lateral stenosis is characterized by an encroachment of the spinal nerve in the spinal canal's lateral recess or the intervertebral foramen. The causes for this type include facet joint hypertrophy, loss of IVD height, IVD bulging, or spondylolisthesis. In addition, nerve compression within the canal results in a limitation of the arterial supply or claudication due to venous return compression. Compression of the foraminal contents in the canal may occur more with certain movements or changes in posture:
  - The length of the canal is shorter in lumbar lordosis than in kyphosis.
  - Extension and, to a lesser degree, side-bending of the lumbar spine toward the involved side produces a narrowing of the canal.
  - Flexion of the lumbar spine reverses the process, returning both the venous capacity and blood flow to the nerve.

Tests and Measures and Response

Two commonly used tests in physical therapy to help diagnose degenerative spinal stenosis are the combination of the bicycle test of van Gelderen and treadmill walking. Both cycling and walking increase symptoms in vascular claudication due to the increased demand for blood supply. However, neurogenic claudication symptoms worsen with walking but are unaffected by cycling if the patient leans forward (lumbar spine flexed) due to the differing positions of the lumbar spine adopted in each of these activities. Patients with neurogenic claudication are far more comfortable leaning forward or sitting, which flexes the spine more than walking. The forward flexion position increases the anteroposterior diameter of the intervertebral canal, which allows a greater volume of the neural elements and improves the microcirculation.

Clinical Findings, Secondary Effects, or Complications

Both the history and the examination findings for DSS are very specific.

Patients with lumbar spinal stenosis who are symptomatic often relate a long history of low back pain. Unilateral or bilateral leg pain is usually a predominant symptom. Approximately half of the patients with lumbar spinal stenosis will present with neurogenic claudication (also referred to as pseudoclaudication). Subjectively, the patient reports an increase in symptoms with lumbar extension activities such as walking, prolonged standing, and to a lesser degree, side-bending. On observation, the patient presents with a flattened lumbar lordosis.

The physical examination usually reveals reduced flexibility or shortening of the hip flexors (iliopsoas and rectus femoris). The hip extensor muscles (gluteus maximus and hamstrings) are usually lengthened. This lengthening places them at a mechanical disadvantage, which leads to early recruitment of the lumbar extensor muscles and may lead to excessive lumbar extension.

Patients with cervical or thoracic central stenosis can experience UMN signs and symptoms (see Table 3-49) due to the spinal cord's compression. Myelopathy, disease, or compression of the spinal cord, which is the most common in females older than 45 years, can be caused by stenosis, tumor, osteophytes, congenital narrowing of the central canal, inflammatory process, tumor, encroachment of ligaments/membranes (ligamentum flavum, posterior longitudinal membranes, subcranial membranes), or instability. The signs and symptoms of myelopathy include bilateral or quadrilateral paresthesias in a nondermatomal pattern (glove/stocking distribution), weakness in a nonmyotomal pattern, ataxic gait, clumsiness, positive pathologic reflexes (Babinski, Hoffman, inverted supinator test), hyperreflexia, changes in bowel and bladder, and UMN signs and symptoms.

Diagnostic Tests
Radiographs or MRIs may be ordered to find the site and source of stenosis.

Interventions/Treatment
Medical—An initial conservative approach, including pain medication and physical therapy, is generally recommended for nerve root compression signs and symptoms. Failure to respond to a conservative approach is an indication of a nerve root and sinuvertebral nerve infiltration. Permanent relief in lateral recess stenosis has been reported with a local anesthetic injection around the nerve root. When nerve root infiltration fails, surgical decompression of the nerve root is indicated.

Pharmacologic—Analgesics, NSAIDs, and cortisone injections may also be implemented to help control inflammation.

Physical therapy—An MD referral is the first line of treatment in cases of suspected myelopathy. Once evaluated and cleared for therapy, common interventions for cervical spinal stenosis include a therapeutic exercise progression, including postural education, stretching of any tight musculature such as the pectorals and suboccipitals, and stabilization exercises targeting the deep neck flexors. For lumbar spine stenosis, the approach includes stretching of the hip flexors and rectus femoris and stabilization exercises targeting the lumbar paraspinals, transverse abdominals, multifidi, and gluteals, aerobic conditioning, and positioning such as a posterior pelvic tilt.

SPONDYLOLYSIS/SPONDYLOLISTHESIS

Spondylolysis is a defect of the pars interarticularis of the spine, which lies between the superior and inferior articular facets of the vertebral arch. The actual defect covers a broad range of etiologies, from a stress fracture to a traumatic bony fracture with separation.

Spondylolisthesis is a diagnostic term that identifies anterior slippage and inability to resist shear forces of a vertebral segment with the vertebral segment immediately below it. Spondylolisthesis usually occurs in the lumbar spine.

Clinical Significance
Newman[16] described five groups represented by this deformity based on etiology:

1. *Congenital* spondylolisthesis, due to dysplasia of the fifth lumbar and sacral arches and zygapophyseal joints.
2. *Isthmic* spondylolisthesis, caused by a defect in the pars interarticularis due to an acute fracture, a stress fracture, or an elongation of the pars.
3. *Degenerative* spondylolisthesis, due to disk and zygapophyseal joint degeneration. Degenerative spondylolisthesis usually affects older people and occurs most commonly at L4-L5. The slip occurs because of arthritis in the zygapophyseal joint with loss of their ligamentous support.
4. *Traumatic* spondylolisthesis. This fairly rare type occurs with a fracture or acute dislocation of the zygapophyseal joint.
5. *Pathologic* spondylolisthesis. This condition may result from a systemic disease causing a weakening of the pars, pedicle, zygapophyseal joint, or a local condition such as a tumor.

Spondylolisthesis acquisita, a sixth etiologic category, was added to represent the slip caused by the surgical disruption of ligaments, bone, and disk.

Tests and Measures and Response
Refer to Tests and Measures and Response in the spinal stenosis section (see Special Tests of the Lumbar Spine and SIJ).

Clinical Findings, Secondary Effects, or Complications

Clinically, these patients will complain of mechanical low back pain—worsened with activity and alleviated with rest. There may also be complaints of leg pain, which can either be of a radicular type pattern or, more commonly, be one of neurogenic claudication. If neurogenic claudication is present, the patient may complain of bilateral thigh and leg tiredness, aches, and fatigue. The questions regarding bicycle use versus walking can help differentiate neurogenic versus vascular claudication (see earlier). Vascular claudication occurs because not enough blood is flowing to a muscle. While there may be sufficient blood flow to the muscle car at rest, the narrowed artery may not supply enough blood during exercise. ROM of the lumbar spine flexion frequently is normal with both types of claudication. Some patients will be able to touch their toes without difficulty. Strength is usually intact in the lower extremities. Sensation also is usually intact. A check of distal pulses is important to rule out any coexisting vascular insufficiency. Findings such as hairless lower extremities, coldness of the feet, or absent pulses are signs of peripheral vascular disease. Sensory defects in a stocking-glove distribution are more suggestive of diabetic neuropathy. The deep tendon reflexes generally will be normal or diminished.

Diagnostic Tests

Radiography.

Interventions/Treatment

Medical—The recommended treatment program for an active spondylolysis is bracing to immobilize the spine for a short period (approximately 4 months).
Pharmacologic—Analgesics and/or NSAIDs prescribed as needed.
Physical therapy—The therapeutic exercise progression for this population includes postural education, hip flexor, rectus femoris and lumbar paraspinal stretching, lumbar (core) stabilization exercises targeting the abdominals and gluteals, aerobic conditioning, and positioning through a posterior pelvic tilt.

PELVIC FLOOR DYSFUNCTION

Pelvic floor dysfunction (PFD) may result in a group of clinical disorders that includes urinary incontinence (UI), anal incontinence, pelvic organ prolapse, sensory and emptying abnormalities of the lower urinary tract, defecatory dysfunction, sexual dysfunction, and several chronic pain syndromes.[17]

UI includes the various types of incontinence: stress incontinence, urge incontinence, or mixed incontinence (see Chapter 9).[18]

Clinical Significance

The contributing factors to UI can be a weakness or damage to numerous pelvic floor structures, including fascial structures, nerves, and the pelvic floor musculature.

Tests and Measures and Response

There are no specific tests and measures designed to diagnose PFD. Instead, the diagnosis is typically made based on patient or family reports of incontinence.

Clinical Findings, Secondary Effects, or Complications

The pelvic floor muscles demonstrate abnormalities of muscle activation and relaxation (either an elevated resting or involuntary relaxation of the pelvic floor muscles) associated with continence and evacuation.[17]

Diagnostic Tests

Several tests exist to help in the diagnosis of PFD, including the following:

- Cystoscopy.
- Urinalysis.
- Urodynamics.

Interventions/Treatment

Medical—Surgical intervention can include catheterization and surgically implanted artificial sphincters and bladder generators (sends impulses to the nerves to control the bladder function).

Pharmacologic—Medications prescribed to relieve urge incontinence: estrogen replacement therapy, anticholinergics, α-adrenergic blockers to increase bladder outlet/sphincteric tone, antispasmodics, and combination therapy using tricyclic antidepressant agents and antidiuretic hormone.[19-23]

Physical therapy—There is high-quality evidence for pelvic floor muscle training to manage urinary incontinence in women, for women who are antepartum and postpartum or who have pelvic organ prolapse, and for men.[24] The patients are initially educated in PFM awareness. Several teaching methods can be used, including verbal cues, visualization with an anatomic model, palpation, objective PFM contraction at the anus, or biofeedback with EMG recordings via a rectal probe.[25]

■ INTERVENTION PRINCIPLES FOR MUSCULOSKELETAL INJURIES

Several principles should guide the intervention through the various stages of musculoskeletal tissue healing. These include the following:

- Control pain, inflammation, and swelling (edema).
- Promote and progress healing.
- Instructions to the patient on a therapeutic exercise program that:
  - Corrects any imbalances between strength and flexibility.
  - Addresses postural and movement dysfunctions.
  - Integrates the open and closed kinetic chains.
  - Incorporates neuromuscular reeducation.
  - Maintains or improves overall strength and fitness.
  - Improves the functional outcome of the patient.

CONTROL OF PAIN AND INFLAMMATION

The clinician has many tools at his or her disposal to help control pain, inflammation, and swelling (edema). These include the application of electrotherapeutic and physical modalities, gentle ROM exercises, and graded manual techniques. During the acute stage of healing, the principles of POLICE (Protection, Optimal Loading, Ice, Compression, Elevation) are recommended. In addition, cryotherapy, electrical stimulation, pulsed ultrasound, and iontophoresis are used during the acute phase, and thermotherapy, phonophoresis, electrical stimulation, ultrasound (US), iontophoresis, and diathermy in the later healing stages. The applications of cold and heat are taught to the patient at the earliest opportunity.

▲ HIGH-YIELD TERMS TO LEARN

Primary joint replacement or arthroplasty	The first replacement surgery.
Revision surgery	A second or succeeding surgery performed for an unstable, loose, or painful joint replacement.
Total hip replacement (THR) or total hip arthroplasty (THA)	Replacement of the femoral head and the acetabular articular surface.
Hemiarthroplasty	Replacement of the femoral head only.
Bipolar hemiarthroplasty	A specific form of hemiarthroplasty using a femoral prosthesis with an articulating acetabular component. The acetabular cartilage is not replaced. This procedure aims to decrease the frictional wear between the femoral head prosthesis and the cartilage of the acetabulum.

POLICE	An acronym for treating acute injuries that replaced the former acronym PRICE (protection, rest, ice, compression, elevation) with protection, optimal loading, ice, compression, and elevation.

Gentle manual techniques (grade I or II joint mobilizations) may also help with the pain. As the patient progresses, gentle passive muscle stretching may be introduced. Self-stretching and self-mobilization techniques are taught to the patient at the earliest and appropriate opportunity.

The goals of the acute phase should include the following:

- Maximizing patient comfort by decreasing pain and inflammation.
- Protection of the injury site.
- Restoration of pain-free ROM throughout the entire kinetic chain.
- Retardation of muscle atrophy.
- Minimizing the detrimental effects of immobilization and activity restriction.
- Attainment of early neuromuscular control.
- Improving soft tissue extensibility.
- Increasing functional tolerance.
- Maintaining general fitness.
- Appropriate management of scar tissue.
- Encouraging the patient toward independence with the home exercise program.
- Progression of the patient to the functional stage.

PROMOTE AND PROGRESS HEALING

The promotion and progression of tissue repair involve a delicate balance between protection and the control of functional stresses to the damaged structure. These stresses can be in the form of manual techniques and/or therapeutic exercises. Although physical therapy cannot accelerate the healing process, it can ensure that the healing process is not delayed or disrupted and occurs in an optimal environment. In addition to excess stress, detrimental environments include prolonged immobilization, which must be avoided. The rehabilitation procedures chosen to progress the patient will depend on the type of tissue involved, the extent of the damage, and the healing stage. The intervention must be related to the signs and symptoms present rather than the actual diagnosis.

The functional phase addresses any tissue overload problems and functional biomechanical deficits. The goals of the functional phase should address the following:

- Attainment of the full range of pain-free motion.
- Restoration of normal joint kinematics.
- Improvement of muscle strength to within normal limits.
- Improvement of neuromuscular control.
- Restoration of normal muscle force couples.
- Correction of any deficits in the whole kinetic chain that are involved in an activity to which the patient is planning to return.
- Performance of activity-specific progressions before full return to function.

The selection of intervention procedures, and the intervention progression, must be guided by continuous reexamination of the patient's response to a given procedure, making the reexamination of patient dysfunction before, during, and after each intervention essential. There are three possible scenarios following a reexamination:

1. The patient's function has improved. In this scenario, the intensity of the intervention may be incrementally increased.

2. The patient's function has diminished. In this scenario, the intensity and the focus of the intervention must be changed by discussing with the physical therapist. Further review of the home exercise program may be needed. The patient may require further education on activity modification and the use of heat and ice at home. The working hypothesis must be reviewed. Further investigation is needed.

3. There is no change in the patient's function. Depending on the elapse of time since the last visit, there may be a reason for the lack of change. This finding may indicate the need for a change in the intensity of the intervention. If the patient is in the acute or subacute stage of healing, a decrease in the intensity may be warranted to allow the tissues more of an opportunity to heal. In the chronic stage, an increase in intensity may be warranted.

TENDON INJURY

For the treatment of a tendon injury, the following five-step plan is recommended:

1. The principles of POLICE to aid healing.
2. A gradual progression of therapeutic exercise, focusing on progression toward eccentric exercises and removing intrinsic deficits: increasing flexibility and correcting muscle imbalances.
3. Removal of extrinsic factors (damaging stimuli). This often involves absence from abuse rather than absolute rest.
4. Identification of any faulty mechanics/technique. When treating overuse injuries, the clinician must limit both the chronic inflammation and degeneration by working on both sides of the problem—tissue strength should be maximized through proper training, and adequate healing time must be allowed before returning to full participation.
5. Application of cross-section massage to the tendon as tolerated.

LIGAMENT INJURY

Intervention in the acute stage centers around aggressive attempts to do the following:

- Minimize effusion to speed healing (cryotherapy, compression, and elevation).
- Promote early protected motion and early supported/protected weight-bearing as tolerated/appropriate using low load cyclic loading. For example, with an ankle sprain, protected weight-bearing with an orthosis is permitted, with weight-bearing to tolerance as soon as possible.
- Protected return to activity. As the healing progresses and the patient can bear more weight through the joint, there is a corresponding increase in weight-bearing (closed chain) exercises.
- Prevention of reinjury.

BURSITIS

Most forms of bursitis are treated conservatively to reduce inflammation. Conservative treatment includes rest, cold and heat treatments, elevation, and NSAIDs. Patients with suspected septic bursitis are treated with antibiotics while awaiting culture results.

ORTHOPEDIC SURGICAL REPAIRS

Lumbar Diskectomy

Lumbar diskectomy involves removing a small window of bone in the spine, moving the nerve to one side, and removing either some or the entire herniated disk. Percutaneous diskectomy uses an x-ray and a video screen to guide small instruments toward the disk. Postoperative recovery is relatively fast, with relief from nerve root compression often immediate.

Laminectomy

Laminectomy is the most commonly performed surgery on the lower spine and involves removing part or all of the lamina to remove pressure on one or more nerve roots. Because the procedure requires an incision of 2 more in, a hospital stay is required.

Vertebroplasty

This procedure, usually performed on an outpatient basis, is used to repair a fractured vertebra. A small incision is made in the skin over the affected area, and a cement-like mixture is injected into the vertebra. The cement hardens to stabilize the bones of the spine.

Kyphoplasty

Kyphoplasty is similar to vertebroplasty and involves making a small incision in the back and injecting a cement-like material to repair a fractured vertebra(e). However, before injecting the cement in kyphoplasty, the surgeon inserts a balloon device to help restore the height and shape of the spine.

Foraminotomy

This procedure, used to enlarge the foramen, involves removing any bone or tissue obstructing the foramen and compressing the nerve root. This procedure is often combined with other procedures such as a laminectomy.

Total Joint Replacement

Total joint replacement (arthroplasty) represents a significant advance in treating painful and disabling joint pathologies. Total joint replacement can be performed on any joint of the body, including the hip, knee, ankle, foot, shoulder, elbow, wrist, and fingers. Cemented joint replacement or arthroplasty is when bone cement or polymethylmethacrylate (PMMA) is used to fix the prosthesis in place in the joint. Ingrowth or cementless joint replacement or arthroplasty does not involve bone cement to fix the prosthesis in place. Instead, an anatomic or press fit with bone ingrowth into the prosthetic surface leads to a stable fixation. This procedure is based on a fracture-healing model.

Of the total joint replacement procedures, hip and knee total joint replacements are the most common.

Standard precautions given to patients to prevent posterior hip dislocation include the following for 3 months postsurgery:

- Maintain appropriate weight-bearing status.
- Do not cross legs (avoid hip adduction) when sitting or lying.
- Put a pillow between legs if lying on the side.
- Do not turn leg inward (avoid internal rotation of the hip).
- Do not pivot toward the surgical side.
- Sit only on elevated chairs or toilet seats.
- Do not lean forward to get up from a chair.
- Do not bend over from the hips toward the ground to reach objects or tie shoes.

With an anterior approach, the surgery is performed without violating any of the hip's posterior structures, and thus hip precautions are not required.

Flexor Tendon Repair

One of the hand's main purposes is to grasp; therefore, the loss of flexor tendons imposes a devastating functional loss. The purpose of a flexor tendon repair is to restore maximum active flexor tendon gliding to ensure effective finger joint motion.

Most flexor tendon ruptures occur silently after prolonged inflammatory tenosynovitis, although the causes also can be traumatic. Researchers have shown that early mobilization can prevent scar tissue formation without jeopardizing tendon healing, and they have

TABLE 3-51 • Drugs for Inflammation and Fever.	
Therapeutic Class: Anti-inflammatory, antipyretic	
Pharmacology class: Nonsteroidal anti-inflammatories (NSAID)	**Indications*:** Inflammation, fever, itching *Nonsteroidal anti-inflammatories prescribed vary by diagnosis **Adverse effects:** Gastrointestinal upset, dizziness, drowsiness
Medications: Generic names (trade names)	
Aspirin (acetylsalicylic acid [ASA]) Celecoxib (Celebrex) Diclofenac (Cataflam, Solaraze, Voltaren) Diflunisal Etodolac Fenoprofen (Nalfon) Flurbiprofen (Ansaid) Ibuprofen (Advil, Motrin) Ketoprofen Meloxicam (Mobic) Nabumetone (Relafen) Naproxen (Naprosyn), naproxen sodium (Aleve, Anaprox) Oxaprozin (Daypro) Piroxicam (Feldene) Tolmetin (Tolectin)	
Pharmacology class: Corticosteroids	**Indications*:** Severe inflammation, pain *Corticosteroid prescribed varies by diagnosis **Adverse effects:** Long-term use, Cushing syndrome, high blood sugar, gastric ulcers, risk of infections, tendon rupture
Medications: Generic names (trade names)	
Betamethasone (Celestone, Diprolene) Cortisone Dexamethasone Hydrocortisone (Cortef, Hydrocortone, Solu-Cortef) Methylprednisolone (Depo-Medrol, Medrol) Prednisolone (Prelone) Prednisone Triamcinolone (Aristospan, Kenalog) Betamethasone (Celestone, Diprolene)	
Pharmacology class: Antipyretics	**Indications*:** Fever *Antipyretic prescribed varies by diagnosis **Adverse effects:** Acute acetaminophen poisoning symptoms anorexia, vomiting, dizziness, lethargy, diaphoresis, chills, abdominal pain, and diarrhea
Medications: Generic names (trade names)	
Acetaminophen (Tylenol)	

developed many different forms of early mobilization programs. In addition, several post-surgical protocols and modifications exist based on individual characteristics, the zone involved, the suture strength, and physician preferences.

SKILL KEEPER QUESTIONS

1. What are the different findings you would see with bicep tendinopathy and a bicep muscle strain?

2. Your patient can walk on an incline longer than on a flat surface. Does this suggest vascular or neurogenic claudication?

_____

_____

_____

_____

3. Compare and contrast the neurovascular differences with entrapment of the median nerve versus spinal cord compression at the C5-C6 level.

_____

_____

_____

_____

SKILL KEEPER ANSWERS

1. Both are contractile tissues so would likely have pain with contraction (MMT), pain with lengthening the tissues (in the case of a bicep tendon or muscle involvement, lengthening with elbow extension, pronation, and shoulder extension), and pain with palpation over the involved area. The best way to differentiate which is the culprit is to palpate the location; the tendon will be painful with tendinitis, and the bicep muscle belly will be tender with a muscle strain.

2. Neurogenic claudication, because the incline would cause a positional change in the spine to a more flexed posture, decreasing venous congestion due to the stenosis. A person's vascular claudication symptoms would worsen, as the incline requires more intensity, which increases the oxygen demand to the muscles, and therefore, the paresthesia would worsen.

3. This is comparing an LMN and a UMN presentation. (See Table 3-49 for details on LMN versus UMN signs, symptoms, and findings.)

■ RELEVANT PHARMACOLOGY

In addition to the expanded pharmacology section in Appendix D, Table 3-51 outlines the more common drugs prescribed for patients with musculoskeletal conditions

CHECKLIST

When you complete this chapter, you should be able to:

❏ Describe the various structures of the musculoskeletal system.

❏ Describe the axes and planes of motion about which body movements occur.

❏ Differentiate between osteokinematic and arthrokinematic motion.

❏ Explain the importance of the concave-convex rule as it pertains to joint mobilizations.

❏ Describe how the various musculoskeletal tissues respond to injury.

❏ Describe the various clinical signs and symptoms seen during the healing process of each of the musculoskeletal tissues.

❏ Describe how each of the various energy systems produces energy.

❏ Describe how each of the various energy systems work together during various levels of exercise intensity.

❏ Describe the functional anatomy and biomechanics of all of the major joints in the body.

❏ List the various components of a musculoskeletal physical therapy examination.

❏ Be able to recognize the various special tests designed for each of the major regions.

❏ Have a working knowledge of the more common orthopedic conditions in terms of their clinical significance and each intervention.

❏ Describe the various intervention principles used to treat orthopedic conditions.

❏ Outline the different kinds of orthopedic surgical repairs.

REFERENCES

1. American Physical Therapy Association. Guide to Physical Therapist Practice 3.0. Alexandria, VA: American Physical Therapy Association; 2014.

2. Castillo C, Mendez M. Slipped capital femoral epiphysis: a review for pediatricians. *Pediatr Ann.* 2018;47:e377-e380.

3. Uvodich M, Schwend R, Stevanovic O, Wurster W, Leamon J, Hermanson A. Patterns of pain in adolescents with slipped capital femoral epiphysis. *J Pediatr.* 2019;206:184-189.

4. Peck DM, Voss LM, Voss TT. Slipped capital femoral epiphysis: diagnosis and management. *Am Fam Physician.* 2017;95:779-784.

5. Leroux J, Abu Amara S, Lechevallier J. Legg-Calve-Perthes disease. *Orthop Traumatol Surg Res.* 2018;104:S107-S112.

6. Mills S, Burroughs KE. *Legg Calve Perthes Disease (Calves Disease).* Treasure Island, FL: StatPearls; 2018.

7. Burnett RS, Della Rocca GJ, Prather H, Curry M, Maloney WJ, Clohisy JC. Clinical presentation of patients with tears of the acetabular labrum. *J Bone Joint Surg Am.* 2006;88:1448-1457.

8. Standring S, Gray H. *Gray's Anatomy: The Anatomical Basis of Clinical Practice.* 41st ed. London: Elsevier; 2015.

9. Whitmore A. Osgood-Schlatter disease. *JAAPA.* 2013;26:51-52.

10. Tippett SR. Considerations for the pediatric patient. In: Voight ML, Hoogenboom BJ, Prentice WE, eds. *Musculoskeletal Interventions: Techniques for Therapeutic Exercise.* New York, NY: McGraw-Hill; 2007:803-820.

11. Jull G, Falla D, O'Leary S, McCarthy C. Cervical spine: idiopathic neck pain. In: Jull G, Moore A, Falla D, Lewis J, McCarthy C, Sterling M, eds. *Grieve's Modern Musculoskeletal Physiotherapy.* 4th ed. London: Elsevier; 2015:410-422.

12. McKenzie RA, May S. *The Cervical and Thoracic Spine: Mechanical Diagnosis and Therapy.* Waikanae, NZ: Spinal Publications; 2006.

13. Nassif NJ, Al-Salleeh F, Al-Admawi M. The prevalence and treatment needs of symptoms and signs of temporomandibular disorders among young adult males. *Journal of oral rehabilitation.* 2003;30:944-950.

14. Tasaki MM, Westesson PL. Temporomandibular joint: diagnostic accuracy with sagittal and coronal MR imaging. *Radiology.* 1993;186:723-729.

15. Hundozi-Hysenaj H, Dallku IB, Murtezani A, Rrecaj S. Treatment of the idiopathic scoliosis with brace and physiotherapy. *Niger J Med.* 2009;18:256-259.

16. Newman PH. The etiology of spondylolisthesis. *J Bone Joint Surg.* 1963;45B:39-59.

17. Wang YC, Hart DL, Mioduski JE. Characteristics of patients seeking outpatient rehabilitation for pelvic-floor dysfunction. *Phys Ther.* 2012;92:1160-1174.

18. Markwell SJ. Physical therapy management of pelvi/perineal and perianal pain syndromes. *World J Urol.* 2001;19:194-199.

19. Urinary incontinence. Know your drug options. *Mayo Clin Health Lett.* 2005;23:6.

20. Blackwell RE. Estrogen, progestin, and urinary incontinence. *JAMA.* 2005;294:2696-2697; author reply 7-8.

21. Bren L. Controlling urinary incontinence. *FDA Consum.* 2005;39:10-15.

22. Castro-Diaz D, Amoros MA. Pharmacotherapy for stress urinary incontinence. *Curr Opin Urol.* 2005;15:227-230.

23. Kelleher C, Cardozo L, Kobashi K, Lucente V. Solifenacin: as effective in mixed urinary incontinence as in urge urinary incontinence. *Int Urogynecol J Pelvic Floor Dysfunct.* 2006;17:382-388.

24. Hsu LF, Liao YM, Lai FC, Tsai PS. Beneficial effects of biofeedback-assisted pelvic floor muscle training in patients with urinary incontinence after radical prostatectomy: a systematic review and metaanalysis. *Int J Nurs Stud.* 2016;60:99-111.

25. Ohtake PJ, Borello-France D. Rehabilitation for women and men with pelvic-floor dysfunction. *Phys Ther.* 2017;97:390-392.

4

Cardiac, Vascular, and Pulmonary Systems

MELISSA SCHNEIDER

CHAPTER TABLE OF CONTENTS

OVERVIEW

The human body and its ability to function proficiently depends highly on the principles of moving blood, nutrients, ions, oxygen (O_2), carbon dioxide (CO_2), metabolic by-products and waste, producing electrical gradients, and generating pressure differences. These principles are fundamental in the functioning of the cardiac, vascular, and pulmonary systems. However, in terms of physiology, the action at the cellular level of these organ systems allows for the transport, movement, and functioning of the systems in everyday life, activity, and exercise. In addition, the use of pharmacologic agents influences the movement of these systems when needed in instances of pathology and/or disease.

▲ HIGH-YIELD TERMS

Action potential	The basis for nerve impulses when cell membrane reaches threshold potential.
Angina pectoris	Chest pain related to ischemia of the myocardium.
Apnea	Cessation of breathing after an expiration, interrupted by eventual inspiration, or it becomes fatal.
Atherosclerosis	A disease of the arteries characterized by plaque deposits of fatty materials on the vessel's inner walls.
Automatic rhythmicity	Property of cardiac nodal tissue to self-excite, which leads to automatic action potentials and heart contraction.
Bradypnea	Slow rate, shallow or normal depth, regular rhythm (as in drug overdose).
Chronotropy	Changes or influences that increase or decrease heart rate.
Cor pulmonale	Right-side heart failure due to pulmonary hypertension, causing acute and chronic pulmonary disease.

Crackles/rales	Adventitious breath sounds heard over areas of the lung where there are accumulated fluids or collapsed alveoli.
	There is a partial reopening of the alveoli during inspiration.
Cyanosis	Bluish coloration of the skin, tissues, or membranes.
Dead space	Where air does not reach into the alveoli or airways within the lungs.
Dyspnea	Shortness of breath.
Effective refractory period	The time frame when tissue cannot generate additional incoming action potentials.
Eupnea	Normal rate, depth, and rhythm of breathing.
Frank–Starling law	The observation that increased stretching and preloading of the heart causes an increase in heart contractility.
Hemoptysis	Presence of blood produced from coughing.
Hyperpnea	Increased breathing due to increased depth, but usually not increased rate.
Ionotropy	Changes or influences that increase or decrease heart contractility.
Orthopnea	Shortness of breath caused by lying flat.
Oxygen diffusing capacity	A measure of the rate at which oxygen can diffuse from the pulmonary alveoli into the blood.
Pulmonary ventilation	The process of drawing air into and out of the lungs.
Perfusion	Amount of blood flow to a given region.
Respiration	The process of gas exchange with the atmosphere and cells of the body.
Shunt	When blood does not flow to a region.
Sinus rhythm	Any rhythm of the heart established by impulses from the SA node.
Stridor	A high-pitched sound caused by obstruction of the larynx or trachea heard during inspiration and expiration.
Tachypnea	Increased breathing rate, usually shallow with regular rhythm (as in restrictive lung pathologies).
Wheezing	A music-pitch-like continuous sound heard due to narrowing in the airway.

■ ANATOMY AND PHYSIOLOGY OF THE CARDIOVASCULAR SYSTEM

HEART TISSUE

It is important to understand the topology of the heart. Heart tissue comprises the pericardium, epicardium, myocardium, and endocardium.

- Pericardium: The outermost double-walled connective tissue sac surrounding the heart and vessels.
- Epicardium: The inner layer of the pericardium.
- Myocardium: The middle layer, contractile muscle tissue (has a considerable thickness compared to the other layers of the heart tissue).
- Endocardium: The endothelial tissue lining the inside heart chambers and valves.

Heart Chambers and Valves

Chambers. There are four chambers of the heart. The chambers on the right side of the heart are the right atrium (RA) and right ventricle (RV) and serve as pumps to the lungs (pulmonary circulation) (Figure 4-1). The left-sided chambers are the left atrium (LA) and left ventricle (LV) and serve as pumps to the rest of the body (systemic circulation).

Valves. There are four valves within the heart; two semilunar (SL) valves and two atrio-ventricular (AV) valves. The function of each valve is to prevent the backflow of blood from the previous chamber, assuring one-directional blood flow through the heart. The two AV valves are located between the atria and ventricles on each side of the heart and are rein-forced by structures called chordae tendineae and papillary muscles. The tricuspid valve is found on the right side between the RA and RV, while the bicuspid valve (also referred to as mitral valve) is located on the left side of the heart between the LA and LV. The semilunar

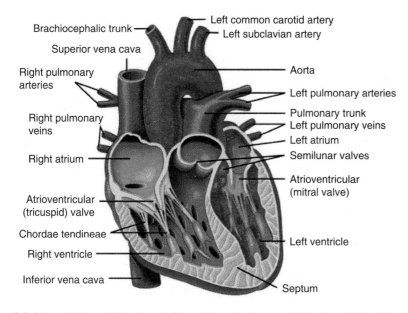

Figure 4-1. **Internal view of the heart.** (Reproduced with permission from Burke-Doe A, Dutton M, eds. *National Physical Therapy Examination and Board Review.* 2019. Copyright © McGraw Hill LLC. All rights reserved. https://accessphysiotherapy.mhmedical.com.)

valves prevent the backflow of blood into the ventricles. The right semilunar valve (also known as the pulmonary valve) is located between the RV and pulmonary artery trunk, while the left semilunar valve lies between the LA and the aorta.

CIRCULATION OF BLOOD WITHIN THE HEART

Venous blood enters the RA by way of the superior and inferior vena cava. Blood then flows through the tricuspid valve, when opened, into the RV. Once the tricuspid valve is closed, contraction of the RV occurs, pumping blood through the pulmonary valve into the pulmonary trunk. The pulmonary trunk branches into the right and left pulmonary arteries, bringing blood to the respective lungs, where it becomes oxygenated by way of the pulmonary capillaries within the alveolar sacs of the lungs. Once perfusion has occurred, the newly oxygenated blood is brought back to the LA by the right and left pulmonary veins. Blood then flows into the LV through the bicuspid valve (mitral valve). After the bicuspid valve closes, the LV contraction delivers blood to the aorta, followed by continued arterial systemic circulation to the body.

MOVEMENT OF IONS, ELECTRICAL ACTIVITY, AND CONDUCTION OF THE HEART

Cardiac tissues of the heart maintain levels of ionic gradients. Calcium (Ca), potassium (K^+), sodium (Na^+) ions, together with proper levels of magnesium, have varying roles in heart activity. Cardiac muscle tissue requires the appropriate calcium, potassium, sodium, and magnesium levels for normal conduction. The action of active and passive ion pumps regulates heart contraction and conduction. The movement of these ionic gradients in and out of the cardiac muscle tissue (myocytes) and nodal (nervous) tissue synapses produces continuous heart contractility and conductivity.

Muscle tissue needs to maintain proper electrolyte levels. Figure 4-2 illustrates the ionic gradient changes, which occur during ionic resting and action potentials. At rest, potential K^+ tends to efflux the cardiac cell while the gradients favor a Na^+ and Ca^+ influx.

Cardiac Nodal Tissue Action Potential

Automatic rhythmicity refers to the property of cardiac nodal tissue to self-excite, which leads to automatic **action potentials** and heart contraction (Figure 4-3). There are

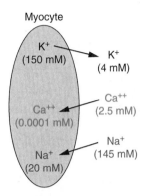

Figure 4-2. Cardiac cell ion concentration gradients. (Reproduced with permission from Burke-Doe A, Dutton M, eds. *National Physical Therapy Examination and Board Review*. 2019. Copyright © McGraw Hill LLC. All rights reserved. https://accessphysiotherapy.mhmedical.com.)

five phases (Phase 0-Phase 4) to recognize. To correlate with the normal sequence of cardiac rhythmicity, Phase 4 of nodal action potentials will be explained first, followed by Phases 0-3.

Phase 4 Resting potential: Figure 4-3 demonstrates a constant depolarization toward the threshold. Several factors contribute to this increased net positivity inside the cell. Firstly, there is a decline in the efflux of K^+ due to decreased K^+ permeability that causes a climb in intracellular positivity. Secondly, there is an increase in Na^+ permeability, which causes an influx of Na^+, which further increases the net positivity within the cell. Further, the contributions of K^+ and Na^+ cause the biased opening of voltage-gated Ca^+ channels, leading to the next phase.

Phase 0 Upstroke: Figure 4-3 shows an increased positive movement from the threshold at approximately −40 mV. The opening of voltage-gated Ca^+ channels brings on depolarization. The influx of Ca^+ causes depolarization beyond the threshold toward the top of the action potential.

Phase 1 Spike: This phase is absent in cardiac nodal tissue but is present in cardiac muscle tissue action potentials.

Phase 2 Plateau: In Figure 4-3, at the top of depolarization is a relative "flattening" of the wave pattern, a prolonged plateau phase, caused by the continuing influx of Ca^+ that is countered by the opening of K^+ channels that cause K^+ efflux.

Phase 3 Repolarization: In Figure 4-3, the decline and drop toward resting potential is from the continued efflux of K^+. At the end of repolarization, Na^+/K^+ pumps and Ca^+ pumps return the cell to resting potential.

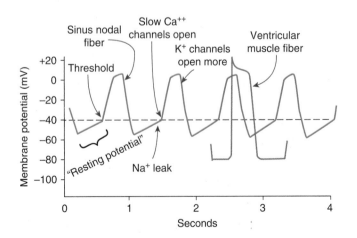

Figure 4-3. Rhythmical discharge of sinus nodal fiber. (Reproduced with permission from Hall JE. *Guyton and Hall Textbook of Medical Physiology*, 12th ed. 2011. Copyright © Saunders Elsevier. All rights reserved.)

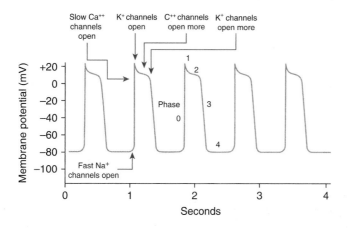

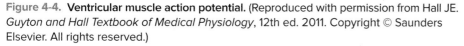

Figure 4-4. Ventricular muscle action potential. (Reproduced with permission from Hall JE. *Guyton and Hall Textbook of Medical Physiology*, 12th ed. 2011. Copyright © Saunders Elsevier. All rights reserved.)

Cardiac Muscle Tissue Action Potential

The characteristics of depolarization and repolarization in cardiac muscle tissues differ from those of nodal tissue. There are five phases, described below, in a ventricular muscle action potential.

Phase 4 Resting potential: Figure 4-4 demonstrates a lower resting potential in cardiac muscle tissue than cardiac nodal tissue. Several factors contribute to this increase in negativity inside the cell. There is an increase in K^+ permeability, which results in an efflux of K^+. This loss of positive charge causes the intracellular membrane to become more negative. Second, there is a slight increase in permeability to Na^+ and Ca^+, which causes an influx of these ions. This aids in preventing the resting potential from becoming increasingly more negative or hyperpolarized due to the loss of K^+.

Phase 0 Upstroke: Since we are now looking at cardiac muscle tissue, there is no inherent property for automatic rhythmicity. Therefore, the arrival of a stimulus or action potential from nodal tissue is required for cardiac muscle to undergo an action potential. However, unlike nodal tissue, the opening of the fast voltage-gated Na+ channels causes the upstroke in the action potential.

Phase 1 Spike: Figure 4-4 shows the characteristic spike that represents this phase. At the depolarization peak in Phase 0, there is a brief opening of K^+ channels, and then the channels mostly close. This brief window causes K^+ to efflux, and there is a drop in positive charge within the tissue.

Phase 2 Plateau: At the end of Phase 1, there is relative "flattening" of the wave pattern, a prolonged plateau phase caused by increasing permeability to Ca^+, and this influx of Ca^+ is countered by the opening of K^+ channels, which cause a K^+ efflux. The plateau phase is an important feature in cardiac muscle physiology that increases the time for the **effective refractory period**, also known as the absolute refractory period. If there were an arrival of another **action potential** during the refractory period, this would not cause another heart contraction. The absolute refractory period prevents summation and tetany of cardiac muscle, which would have consequential effects on heart function if it were to occur.

Phase 3 Repolarization: In Figure 4-3, the decline and drop toward resting potential is from the continued efflux of K^+. At the end of repolarization, Na^+/K^+ pumps and Ca^+ pumps return the cell to resting potential.

Conduction System

Contraction of the ventricles will only occur when there is appropriate electrical conduction within the heart. Appropriate conductivity creates the depolarization of the myocardium and relative repolarization, together creating normal sinus rhythm. The conduction system of the heart is illustrated in Figure 4-5.

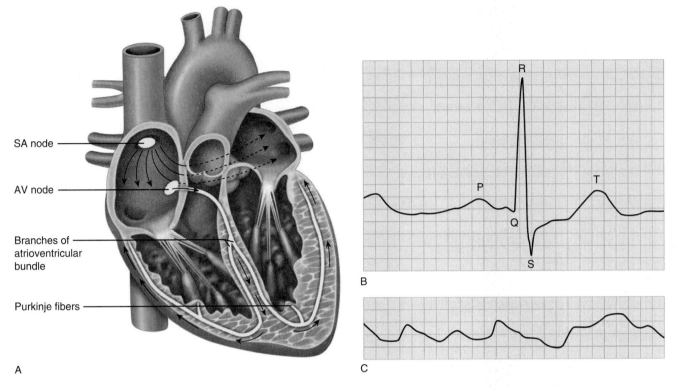

Figure 4-5. Conduction system of the heart. AV, atrioventricular; SA, sinoatrial. (Reproduced with permission from Burke-Doe A, Dutton M, eds. *National Physical Therapy Examination and Board Review.* 2019. Copyright © McGraw Hill LLC. All rights reserved. https://accessphysiotherapy.mhmedical.com.)

Sinoatrial Node. The sinoatrial (SA) node is an area of specialized tissue located on the RA near the opening of the superior vena cava. Also known as the heart's pacemaker, the SA node automatically creates **action potentials** 70 to 80 times per minute in the normal adult.

Atrioventricular Node. Conduction continues along internodal pathways from the SA node to another area of specialized tissue called the AV node. There is a 0.1-second delay that occurs that allows the atria to contract first to empty all blood into the ventricles before the ventricles contract.

Atrioventricular Bundle. The distal portion of the AV node passes into the area known as the AV bundle, also known as the bundle of His, located at the interventricular septum. Gap junctions do not connect the atria and ventricles. The only conduction between the atria and ventricles is via the AV bundle.

Right and Left Bundle Branches. The AV bundle divides into the right and left bundle branches and follows along the length of the interventricular septum and toward the apex of the heart.

Purkinje Fibers. The right and left bundle branches continue into enlarged Purkinje fibers that extend from the apex and around the ventricles and lateral heart walls. Thus, the conduction system causes heart contraction from the apex and then up in a superior direction to direct blood toward the aorta and the pulmonary trunk.

Electrocardiogram

Conduction of the heart can be viewed through an electrocardiogram (ECG or EKG).

An ECG is performed by placing electrodes on a patient's chest with wire leads connected to a recording device. The device provides an image of the heart's electrical waveform visually and/or on a paper strip. Figure 4-6 provides a schematic of a normal sinus rhythm waveform.

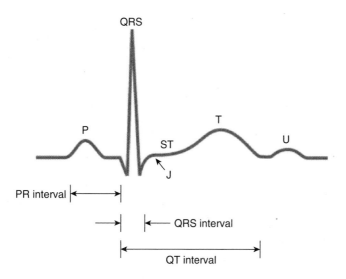

Figure 4-6. Electrocardiogram normal waveform. (Reproduced with permission from Burke-Doe A, Dutton M, eds. *National Physical Therapy Examination and Board Review*. 2019. Copyright © McGraw Hill LLC. All rights reserved. https://accessphysiotherapy.mhmedical.com.)

- P-wave depicts sinus node and represents atrial depolarization.
  - The PR interval denotes AV node conduction, represents the time current travels from the atria to the Purkinjean fibers. The QRS wave or complex represents ventricular depolarization (the QRS wave masks atrial repolarization).
- The ST segment shows the start of ventricular repolarization.
  - The T-wave represents ventricular repolarization.
- The QT interval represents the time of ventricular activity from depolarization to repolarization.

CORONARY ARTERY CIRCULATION

The coronary arteries deliver blood to the heart muscle for oxygenation of the tissues. Figure 4-7 shows the right and left coronary arteries and their branches.

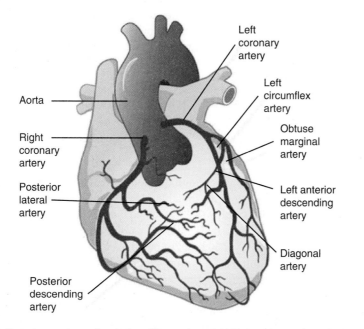

Figure 4-7. Coronary artery circulation. (Reproduced with permission from Longnecker DE, Mackey SC, Newman MF, et al., eds. *Anesthesiology*, 3rd ed. 2017. Copyright © McGraw Hill LLC. All rights reserved. https://accessanesthesiology.mhmedical.com.)

AUTONOMIC NERVOUS SYSTEM REGULATORY INFLUENCES ON THE HEART

Sympathetic Innervation. The cardiac acceleratory center (CAC) is a specialized area located in the medulla oblongata. When the body requires increased blood flow, such as in exercise or the fight-or-flight response, there are several areas that the CAC can affect. With influences over the SA and AV node, the CAC can increase heart rate (HR), known as a positive **chronotropic** effect. In addition, influences over the cardiac muscle can increase the strength of heart contraction; this is termed a positive **ionotropic** effect.

Parasympathetic Innervation. The cardiac inhibitory center (CIC) is located in the medulla oblongata and influences the heart via the vagus nerve (cranial nerve X). The primary influence of the CIC is directed only toward the SA and AV node and regulates HR. Unlike the CAC, the CIC does not have direct links to cardiac muscle to affect contractile strength. With increased parasympathetic input, the HR decreases, which produces a negative chronotropic effect.

Sensory Input. Sensory input for regulation of the cardiovascular system is received through several sensory receptors. Central and peripheral chemoreceptors and baroreceptors help monitor the changing needs of blood volume, O_2, and arterial pressure.

Peripheral chemoreceptors are located in the aorta and carotid artery. These receptors detect changes in blood pH, hydrogen (H^+), O_2, and CO_2. When CO_2 increases and/or O_2 decreases, pH levels decrease, indicating signs of respiratory acidosis (also referred to as pH acidosis). When the pH increases, there is an increase in cardiac output. Conversely, when CO_2 decreases and/or O_2 increases, pH levels increase, indicating signs of respiratory alkalosis (also referred to as pH alkalosis), which calls for a decrease in cardiac output.

Central chemoreceptors are located in the medulla and are sensitive to changes in H^+ ion concentration. Only dissolved gases can diffuse past the blood–brain barrier. In the presence of increased CO_2 levels in the peripheral blood, CO_2 can cause an increase in H^+ ion concentrations in the brain. Central chemoreceptors would detect these changes in H^+ concentrations.

Baroreceptors are located in the carotid artery and aorta. Changes in blood pressure (BP) and blood volume cause a response to counter these changes. The body's response has several mechanisms that counter these changes in several ways, including increasing or decreasing cardiac output, heart contractility, HR, vasoconstriction, and vasodilation.

THE CARDIAC CYCLE

A cardiac cycle is a group of cardiac events from the beginning of one heartbeat to the next beat. Two phases of the cycle, diastole (the relaxation period of the heart) and systole (the contraction period) are illustrated in the Wiggers diagram in Figure 4-8.

Cardiac Hemodynamics

Cardiac Output. The heart helps to continue blood circulation to the body, meeting metabolic demands. The amount of measured blood ejected from a single ventricular contraction is referred to as stroke volume (SV) and expressed in milliliters per minute. Cardiac output is a product of SV and HR. The normal cardiac output at rest is approximately 4 to 6 L/min. A person with a HR of 60 beats/min and SV of 70 mL per stroke would have a cardiac output of 4200 mL/min or 4.2 L/min. By increasing either the SV (or increasing heart contractility) or the HR, cardiac output correspondingly increases.

It is also important to note that SV is a product between end-diastolic volume (EDV) and end-systolic volume (ESV). This amount is normally 120 mL. Whereas EDV is the amount of blood that enters the ventricle at the end of diastole, ESV is the amount of blood remaining in the ventricle after a full contraction. This range is normally 70 mL. Therefore, SV is

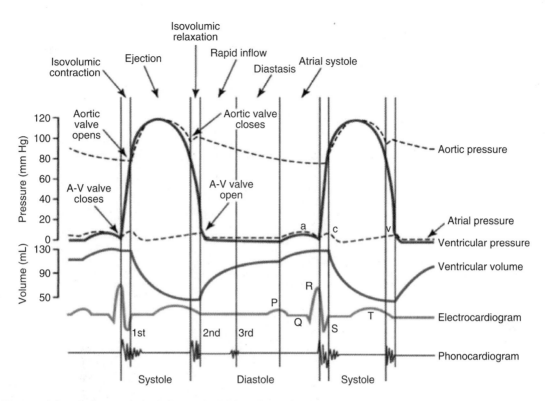

Figure 4-8. Events of the cardiac cycle for left ventricular function—also known as Wiggers diagram. (Reproduced with permission from Guyton AC, Hall JE. *Textbook of Medical Physiology*, 11th ed. 2006. Copyright © Saunders. All rights reserved.)

approximately 70 mL. Many varying factors can play a role in cardiac output dynamics that can increase or decrease EDV or ESV, affecting SV.

Preload. Preload is the amount of blood volume entering the ventricle at the end of the ventricular diastole. The degree to which the heart muscle can stretch just before a contraction influences preload. To a certain extent, within physiologic limits, an increase in preload will have a net increase in SV. This phenomenon is known as the **Frank–Starling law** of the heart, where it was observed that increased stretching and preloading of the heart causes an increase in heart contractility. The primary factor that can drive preload is the amount of venous return received by the ventricles.

Heart Contractility. Contractility is described by the contractile force exerted at a given muscle length. The ventricle at rest is shorter than the optimal length for a contraction. As previously described, stretching the ventricle by increasing preload will positively create a stronger contraction and larger SV. Other extrinsic and intrinsic factors can influence contractility. In a sympathetic response, there is increased contractility. Other influences such as certain hormones, ions, and pharmaceutical agents can also regulate contractility.

Afterload. Whereas preload is a measure of the amount or volume of blood, afterload is a distinctly different measure by looking at the amount of pressure exerted from the pulmonary and arterial system back toward the aortic and pulmonary SL valves. Therefore, afterload represents the amount of force that must be overcome to open these valves to eject blood. Normally, this pressure is 80 mm Hg in the aortic valve and 10 mm in the pulmonary trunk.

CIRCULATORY SYSTEM

Blood is moved through the body along two major circuits that deliver nutrients, oxygenated enriched blood, and return deoxygenated blood to the heart via systemic circulation. There are five major blood vessels within the circulatory system: arteries, arterioles, capillaries, venules, and veins. Figure 4-9 illustrates the cardiovascular circulatory system.

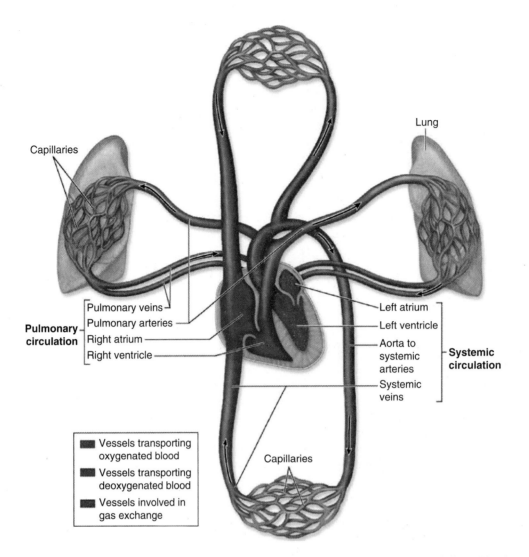

Figure 4-9. **Cardiovascular circulatory system.** (Reproduced with permission from Mescher AL. *Junqueira's Basic Histology*, 13th ed. 2013. Copyright © McGraw Hill LLC. All rights reserved.)

The venous circulation utilizes venules and veins to carry deoxygenated blood toward the heart from the peripheral tissues. Arterial circulation carries oxygenated blood away from the heart through branching arteries, arterioles, and capillaries, distributing oxygen to all areas of the body.

The concept of veins carrying deoxygenated blood and arteries carrying oxygenated blood differs with blood travel between the heart and lungs. The deoxygenated blood traveling from the RV to the lungs flows through pulmonary arteries. The oxygenated blood traveling from the lungs to the heart flows through pulmonary veins.

Arteries

Arteries consist of the aorta and the main peripheral branching arteries. These vessels carry O_2 from high-pressure areas to low-pressure areas, carrying vital O_2 to the tissues throughout the body. There are varying amounts of elasticity and extensibility in arteries. The pulmonary artery carries deoxygenated blood from the RV to the lungs for oxygenation.

Arterioles

Arterioles are the smallest of the arteries, measuring between 0.3 and 10 mm in diameter. Their most important feature is the vascular smooth muscles that can change the diameter and regulate blood flow. This ability is an important regulator of blood pressure and flow by changing the vessel diameter to direct and reroute blood flow using the properties of vasodilation and vasoconstriction where needed.

Capillaries

Capillaries are the smallest vessels that allow for the exchange of gases, fluids, ions, and nutrients to and from the blood to the tissues and cells throughout the body.

Venules

Venules receive unoxygenated blood from the capillaries and deliver this blood to the veins that transport blood back to the heart. Venules and veins have a large capacity to hold blood and serve as the primary blood reservoir; 64% of the systemic circulation is found in these vessels.

Veins

Blood pressure in veins is very low when compared to the arterial system. Therefore, an important feature of one-way valves is that they help prevent any backflow and pooling of blood en route to the heart's RA. There are both superficial and deep veins, with the deep veins corresponding with an artery in the same area and often sharing the same name (ie, femoral, axillary, tibial, etc). The blood returned through venous circulation is aided by skeletal muscle contractions, gravity, and the movement from respiratory function.

■ ANATOMY AND PHYSIOLOGY OF THE PULMONARY SYSTEM

The pulmonary system has several components, which perform unique functions. The components of the pulmonary system include the bony thorax, the muscles of ventilation, the upper and lower airways, and the pulmonary circulation. Sometimes referred to as the respiratory system, it works alongside the cardiovascular system to effectively move and exchange gases, assist with fluid exchange within bodily tissues, and helps maintain adequate blood volume levels. **Respiration** is defined as the movement of air or dissolved gases into and out of the lungs. For respiration to occur, the cardiac and the pulmonary systems move and exchange gases from the atmosphere to the tissues. Several exchanges occur in the processes of external and internal respiration.

EXTERNAL AND INTERNAL RESPIRATION

External respiration involves the drawing of air in and out of the lungs, also called **pulmonary ventilation**. Air is drawn into the lungs during inspiration and removed from the lungs during expiration. Gas exchange occurs in the lungs with the movement of O_2 into and removal of CO_2 out of the blood. The cardiac system carries oxygenated blood to the body, and CO_2 is transported from the body tissues to the lungs. The delivery of O_2 and CO_2 between body tissue cells and the blood is called internal respiration. Cellular respiration is when there is cellular processing of O_2 and CO_2.

GENERAL ANATOMY AND STRUCTURE

The right lung is larger and has three lobes (superior, middle, and inferior) separated by a horizontal and oblique fissure. The left lung is smaller due to the accommodation of the heart within the cardiac notch. The oblique fissure separates the two left lobes (superior and inferior). The diaphragm borders the inferior aspect of the lungs. This large dome-shaped muscle is the major muscle involved in inspiration. Figure 4-10 represents the surface anatomy of the lungs.

Atmospheric air is inspired and expired in the upper airways of the nose or mouth. Air is warmed and filtered by the mucosal layers in the nasal cavity. The nose and mouth come together in the pharynx. The larynx leads to the trachea, with the epiglottis serving as a flap to direct only air into the trachea and the lungs. Vocal cords in the larynx are involved in the formation of speech.

The trachea divides into primary left and right bronchi that enter each lung. Each bronchus has multiple divisions transforming to bronchioles forming the bronchial tree. At the level of respiratory bronchioles, alveolar sacs and alveoli comprise the respiratory unit where respiration occurs.

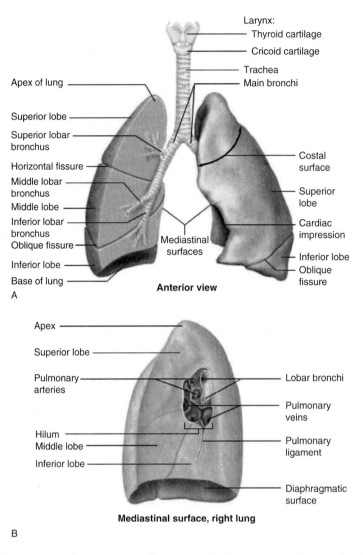

Figure 4-10. Lungs—surface anatomy. (Reproduced with permission from Burke-Doe A, Dutton M, eds. *National Physical Therapy Examination and Board Review*. 2019. Copyright © McGraw Hill LLC. All rights reserved. https://accessphysiotherapy.mhmedical.com.)

Pleura of the Lungs

The innermost layer that directly lines the lungs is called the visceral pleura. The outermost layer that interfaces with the inner surface of the rib cage, diaphragm, and mediastinum is called the parietal pleura. The potential space between these layers is the intrapleural space, and a serous pleural fluid aids in the movement of these layers across each other during respiration.

BREATHING MECHANICS

Inspiration

Ventilation is the process of moving air into and out of the lungs. The diaphragm plays the principal role in inspiration. The dome shape of the diaphragm contracts, flattens, and moves downward when the phrenic nerve innervates it. Contributing to inspiration are the external intercostals that pull the rib cage upward and outward, creating increased volume in the thoracic cavity and pressure inversely decreases. This internal negative pressure draws air into the lungs.

When more air is required due to increased workload, accessory muscles contribute to deeper breathing and increased breathing rate. Although the intercostal muscles and the diaphragm are the primary muscles for inspiration, a patient who suffers from chronic obstructive pulmonary disease (COPD) often depends on both primary and accessory muscles to ensure adequate ventilation. The scalenes and sternocleidomastoid serve as accessory inspiration muscles, as does the upper trapezius, levator scapulae, serratus anterior, and pectoralis muscles.

Expiration

In normal resting expiration, it is important to note that there is no active muscle involvement. Passive forces allow the lungs to deflate and expire air. There is a normal elastic recoil in the lung tissue due to elastic fibers stretched on inspiration. Surface tension along the alveoli also contributes to the tendency of the lungs and alveoli to deflate.

When increased demand for respiration and air needs to be quickly expelled, the internal intercostals, abdominal muscles, and quadratus lumborum can aid as accessory muscles to expiration. Purposeful contraction of the expiration accessory muscles during expiration is encouraged with various breathing exercises to improve lung volumes and capacity.

LUNG VOLUMES AND CAPACITIES

SKILL KEEPER: LUNG VOLUMES

When a patient starts to exercise, breathing rate and depth increase. What are the changes that occur to the different lung volumes with increased activity in healthy individuals?

_____

_____

_____

_____

SKILL KEEPER ANSWERS

Vital capacity, and exercise tolerance, are greater in healthy individuals. During exercise, with an increased workload for both inspiration and expiration, accessory muscles will aid in effective ventilation. The healthier individual exhibits greater efficiency in the ventilation and perfusion processes than someone who suffers from a chronic obstructive pulmonary disease.

Figure 4-11 shows the maximum lung volumes and capacities. The normal ranges for lung volumes and capacities measured in liters of oxygen of a healthy individual are presented in the chart below.

Lung Volumes	Normal Ranges
Tidal volume (TV)	0.4-1.0 L
Inspiratory reserve volume (IRV)	2.5-3.5 L
Expiratory reserve volume (ERV)	1.0-1.5 L
Residual volume (RV)	0.8-1.4 L

Lung Capacities	Normal Ranges
Inspiratory capacity (IC) • TV + IRV	2.9-4.5 L
Functional residual capacity (FRC) • ERV + RV	1.8-2.9 L
Vital capacity (VC) • TV + IRV + ERV	3.0-5.0 L
Total lung capacity (TLC) • TV + IRV + ERV + RV	4.7-6.4 L

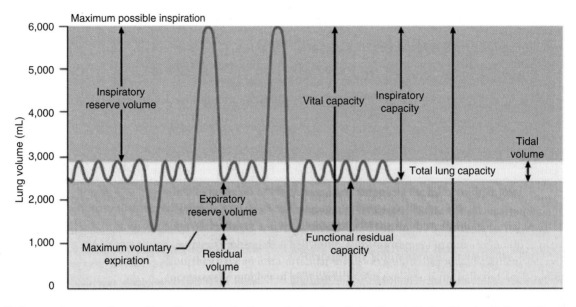

Figure 4-11. Lung volumes and capacities. (Reproduced with permission from Burke-Doe A, Dutton M, eds. *National Physical Therapy Examination and Board Review*. 2019. Copyright © McGraw Hill LLC. All rights reserved. https://accessphysiotherapy.mhmedical.com.)

GAS EXCHANGE

At sea level, the pressure surrounding us is 760 mm Hg, sometimes expressed as 1 atmospheric unit. Atmospheric air has a composition of 78% nitrogen, 21% O_2, and 0.4% CO_2, in addition to other trace amounts of gases. The represented amount of pressure of each gas is termed the partial pressure of that gas. For instance, O_2 is 21% of atmospheric pressure. Atmospheric pressure is 760 mm Hg, and O_2 represents 21% of the composition. Therefore, O_2 is 160 mm Hg of atmospheric pressure. The pH of blood indicates the presence or absence of H^+ ions in the body. The normal range for blood pH is 7.36 to 7.44. The normal range for CO_2 in the blood is 36 to 44 mm Hg. Bicarbonate (HCO_3^-) is normally 23 to 30 mEq/mL. An increase in HCO_3^- increases pH, and a decrease in HCO_3^- decreases body pH.

Ventilation and Perfusion

Optimal respiration occurs when there is adequate ventilation and perfusion. Ventilation (Ve) occurs when air enters the alveoli. **Perfusion** (Q) represents the amount of blood flow to an area.

Some air does not reach the alveoli or to the terminal ends of the bronchial tree where respiration occurs, referred to as anatomic **dead space**. However, some air does reach the alveoli, possibly with poor perfusion to this area, and is referred to as alveolar dead space or physiologic dead space.

Anatomic **shunt** refers to blood vessels that do not interact with the terminal respiratory units of the bronchial tree, where there is no gas exchange. Physiologic shunt occurs when there is good perfusion at the alveoli, but the alveoli do not have ventilation.

The relationship between ventilation and perfusion can be expressed as a ratio of V/Q. Position of the body and various disease states can affect this ratio. In the upright position, the top of the lungs, or apex, receives greater ventilation. The bottom of the lungs has decreased ventilation. Conversely, perfusion, which is gravity-dependent, is greater at the base of the lungs and less at the top (apex) of the lungs. Changing positions (ie, supine and sidelying) change these zones and ratios of V/Q.

Oxygen and Carbon Dioxide Transport

Oxygen is not as soluble in water as CO_2. Therefore, approximately less than 2% of O_2 is dissolved in the blood plasma. Hemoglobin is a specialized protein that contains iron that helps to bind and carry O_2. Ninety-eight percent of the body's O_2 is carried by hemoglobin. The combination of O_2 and hemoglobin is called oxyhemoglobin.

CO_2 is transported in the body through several different mechanisms. The following chemical equation describes CO_2 transport:

$$H_2O + CO_2 \leftrightarrow H_2CO_3 \text{ (carbonic acid)} \leftrightarrow H^+ \text{ (hydrogen ion)} + HCO_3^- \text{ (bicarbonate)}$$

Carbon dioxide has a higher solubility than O_2, and therefore it can dissolve directly into the plasma. Some of the CO_2 is converted to H^+ and HCO_3^- which are directly dissolved in the plasma. CO_2 is also able to bind to hemoglobin, and 23% of CO_2 is transported as carbaminohemoglobin. Most CO_2 is transported as HCO_3, produced from the red blood cells through carbonic enzyme anhydrase. Seventy percent of CO_2 transport occurs from this process.

CONTROL OF BREATHING

Specialized groups of neurons gather in the pons and the medulla to regulate breathing, as shown in Figure 4-12. These centers are categorized as the dorsal respiratory group (DRG) and the ventral respiratory group (VRG), both located in the medulla. The pneumotaxic center and the apneustic center are located in the pons.

SKILL KEEPER: NEUROLOGIC CONTROL OF BREATHING

A patient has sustained a traumatic brain injury from a motor vehicle accident. If the patient experiences an erratic and random breathing rate and depth, the physical therapist assistant (PTA) can suspect the patient has what type of injury?

_____

_____

_____

_____

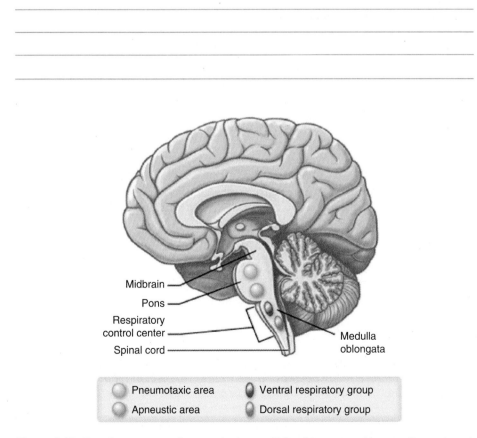

Midbrain

Pons

Respiratory control center

Spinal cord

Medulla oblongata

| Pneumotaxic area | Ventral respiratory group |
| Apneustic area | Dorsal respiratory group |

Figure 4-12. Respiratory control center in the medulla oblongata and pons. (Reproduced with permission from Porcari JP, Bryant CX, Comana F, et al., eds. *Exercise Physiology*. 2015. Copyright © FA Davis. All rights reserved. https://fadavispt.mhmedical.com.)

Vital capacity and exercise tolerance are greater in healthy individuals. During exercise, with an increased workload for both inspiration and expiration, accessory muscles will aid in effective ventilation. The healthier individual exhibits greater efficiency in the ventilation and perfusion processes than someone who suffers from a chronic obstructive pulmonary disease.

Dorsal Respiratory Group and Ventral Respiratory Group

The DRG is involved in inspiration by causing excitation of the diaphragm via the phrenic nerve and the external intercostals via the external intercostal nerve. These are the primary muscles in normal inspiration. The VRG is involved in motor control of expiration and inspiration when there is increased demand for respiration, such as in exercise. Recall that expiration in normal rested conditions is a passive process, and no muscle activity is needed in the lungs for recoil and expelling of air under normal breathing conditions.

Pneumotaxic Center and Apneustic Center

The pneumotaxic center controls the rate and depth of breathing by inhibiting the activity of the DRG. The pneumotaxic center essentially serves as an on/off switch for the DRG. In addition, the pneumotaxic center inhibits apneustic center activity. The apneustic center prolongs the activity of the DRG by increasing the depth and slowing the rate of inspiration.

Sensory Input

Various receptor types monitor the environment of the body to regulate breathing dynamics. For example, baroreceptors monitor pressure changes, and chemoreceptors are sensitive to H^+, HCO_3^-, O_2, and CO_2 levels. Input from irritant receptors and stretch receptors also regulate ventilation and respiration. Various reflexes and responses from the input of these receptors are relayed to the brain for adjustments in breathing.

CARDIOVASCULAR/PULMONARY SYSTEM PHARMACOLOGY

There are numerous medications prescribed for patients with cardiovascular conditions[1] (see Appendix D and Relevant Pharmacology section).

What are the mechanisms of diuretic medications that are used to manage HTN? When diuretics are not effective in managing chronic HTN, what other medications might be prescribed and what are their effects?

_____

_____

_____

_____

Diuretics help control HTN by decreasing the excessive effect of blood volume within the arterial tissues. In addition, diuretics assist the kidneys in the excretion of excess fluid.

Other medications which help with chronic HTN include beta-blockers and calcium channel blockers. All medications are prescribed on an individual basis according to the need of the patient.

Primary or Essential Hypertension Medications

Various drugs, classified by the mechanism of action, are employed to address hypertension (HTN). The action of the pharmaceutical intervention may affect (a) blood volume, (b) vascular smooth muscle tone, (c) angiotensin, and (d) sympathetic nervous system effects.

Diuretics. Loss of fluid from the blood has a decreased net effect on blood volume and lowers blood pressure.

- Thiazide group.
  - Hydrochlorothiazide for mild-to-moderate HTN.
- Loop diuretics.
  - Furosemide (Lasix).
  - Bumetanide (Bumex).

Sympathetic Nervous System Control. Pharmacologic drugs will regulate the amount of sympathetic flow to the cardiovascular system. This influence controls several aspects, including HR, contractile force of the cardiac muscle, cardiac output, venous tone, and total peripheral resistance.

- Central nervous system sympathetic regulation of cardiac output and vascular resistance.
  - Examples: Clonidine, methyldopa.
  - Side effects: Salt retention.
- Beta-blockers.
  - Examples: Propranolol, atenolol, metoprolol, carvedilol, and newer drug nebivolol.
  - Affect cardiac output.

Vasodilators. Vasodilation is achieved by affecting the tone in the vascular system's smooth muscles. Factors that cause vasodilation include blocking of Ca^+ channels, increase in nitric oxide (NO), opening K^+ channels (which leads to increased hyperpolarization within the cell), or activation of dopamine receptors.

- Calcium channel blockers.
  - Examples: Nifedipine, verapamil, diltiazem.
  - Compensatory salt retention of the body is decreased with the use of these drugs, and therefore they are often used for the treatment of chronic HTN.
- Infused intravenous (IV) drugs used in emergency cases.
  - Nitroprusside, diazoxide, and fenoldopam.
  - Cause membrane hyperpolarization or dopamine receptor activation.

Angiotensin and Renin Inhibitors

- Angiotensin-converting enzyme (ACE) inhibitors: Decrease amount of angiotensin II and decrease vasoconstriction and production of aldosterone (a hormone from the kidneys that promotes salt and water retention).
  - Examples: Lisinopril, captopril, benazepril (Lotensin).
  - Side effects: Chronic cough, hyperkalemia, and possible renal damage.
  - Contraindications: During pregnancy due to damage to the renal system of developing fetus.
- Angiotensin II blockers.
  - Valsartan, irbesartan, and candesartan.

Medications used for Angina Pectoris

Nitrates

- Nitrates are the most important therapeutic drug in treating insufficient O_2 delivery to the coronary arteries.
- Duration: Can range from 10 to 20 minutes to 8 to 10 hours.

- Delivery route: Sublingual or transdermal.
- Action.
  - Release of NO within the smooth muscle. Relaxation of the muscle in the vascular system causes vasodilation.
  - Most importantly, the effect is more on the venous system than on the arterial vessels. Increasing venous diameter causes more blood to stay within the venous system, which reduces the amount of blood returning to the RA, causing a decrease in preload, and the heart has to work less, resulting in an ultimate decrease in O_2 need for the heart.
  - Relaxation of the arterial vessels decreases total peripheral resistance, and there is a decrease in afterload. In response, the heart has to work less to deliver blood from the ventricles. A decrease in heart work also decreases the O_2 demands of the heart.
  - To a lesser degree, nitrates can also cause dilation of the coronary vessels and reverse the spastic restrictions to the coronary arteries delivering blood and O_2 to the heart.

Calcium Channel Blockers. These drugs were discussed earlier in the treatment of HTN due to the ability to cause vasodilation. These drugs also are effective in the treatment of **angina pectoris**.

- Examples: Nifedipine, diltiazem, verapamil.
- Specifically, these drugs block L-type Ca^+ channels. Calcium is important in the interaction of actin and myosin in muscle contraction. The decreased presence of intracellular Ca^+ causes decreased interaction of these filaments and thus promotes decreased muscle contraction in smooth muscle. The net effect is vasodilation.
- A newer drug, ranolazine, affects Ca^+ but is not a Ca^+ channel blocker like the drugs described above. Instead, this medication decreases intracellular Na^+, which also causes the cell to remove intracellular Ca^+ and therefore decreases heart contractility.

Beta-blockers

- This class of drugs was discussed in the treatment of HTN as well.
- Examples: Propranolol, atenolol.
- Block sympathetic nervous system flow and decrease HR and contraction and cardiac output. Decreased heart work also decreases the pressure exerted by the heart.
- In the same manner, beta-blockers provide antianginal benefits by decreasing the O_2 demands of the heart. Though not effective in acute angina, these medications are used in prophylactic treatment in conjunction with nitrates, which may help mitigate angina during exercise.

Heart Failure Medications

Heart Failure is when the heart function has a progressive decline due to disease, with a resultant decrease in cardiac output. The various intervention pathways include diuretic use to remove salt and water, reduce afterload with ACE inhibitors, decrease sympathetic input through beta-blockers, and decrease preload and afterload by promoting vasodilation.

Digoxin

- Digoxin is also known as digitalis and is one of the most commonly used medications for heart failure.
- Action.
  - Decreases activity of the Na^+/K^+ ATPase, which affects the Na^+ pump of the cell.
  - Decreases the removal of Na^+ and increases its intracellular presence.
  - Increases intracellular Ca^+ and is stored in the sarcoplasmic reticulum.
  - Increases strength of heart contraction.
  - Increases HR (**chronotropy**) and the rate of fire in the electrical properties of the heart. Though there is increased **inotropy**, digoxin has not demonstrated decreases in mortality rate.

- Prescribing the use of other medications such as diuretics, ACE inhibitors, and vasodilators is more effective with less risk of undesired side effects and toxicity. Some toxic side effects include heart arrhythmias, nausea, vomiting, and diarrhea. Cardiac depression may also occur, leading to cardiac arrest.

Diuretics

- Classification of drugs differs for various heart pathologies.
- Diuretics are considered first in cases of systolic and diastolic heart failure.
- Furosemide is used immediately for severe edema or pulmonary congestion.
- Thiazide is used for milder cases of heart failure.

Angiotensin Antagonists

- Used for HTN but also for heart failure.
- Examples: Losartan, captopril.
- Reduce aldosterone, vasoconstriction, and amount of heart work via lower blood volume and afterload resistance.

Beta-Blockers

- Seem counterproductive to decrease heart contraction in heart failure; however, long-term studies show these drugs slow the progression of chronic heart failure.
- Can be used in cardiomyopathy.
- Not used for the treatment of acute heart failure.

Vasodilators

- Used in acute severe failure with congestion.
- Increasing preload through increased venous return and decreasing afterload resistance result in increased efficiency of the heart.
- Especially effective when heart failure is a result of chronically increased afterload, such as hypertension and a recent myocardial infarct.
- Examples: Hydralazine, isosorbide dinitrate.
- Shown effective in treating heart failure in African Americans.

Antiarrhythmic Drugs

An abnormality in automaticity or conduction causes arrhythmias. Pharmacologic agents are classified or grouped by the ion channels influenced by the drug's mechanism of action. These include (a) Na^+ channel blockers, (b) beta-adrenoreceptor blockers, (c) K^+ channel blockers, and (d) Ca^+ channel blockers.

Sodium Channel Blockers

- Sodium channel blockers can shorten **action potentials** (APs) or lengthen APs in heart conduction.
- Examples:
  - Amiodarone slows the speed of conduction and prolongs APs. Therefore, this drug is classified as both a Na^+ channel blocker and a K^+ channel blocker.
  - Lidocaine is introduced by IV or via intramuscular injection.

Beta-Blockers

- Used to treat arrhythmias after myocardial infarction (MI).
- Decrease movement of Ca^+ and Na^+ and reduce abnormal pacemakers.
- Are effective in reducing chronic heart failure.
- Examples: Propanolol, esmolol.

Potassium Channel Blockers

- The blocking of K$^+$ channels prolongs AP, increases the time for repolarization, and increases the **effective refractory period**, preventing the heart from responding to additional APs such as ventricular tachycardia.
- Example: Amiodarone.
- Side effects: Depositing microcrystals in the cornea and skin affects the thyroid, leading to paresthesia and tremors.

Calcium Channel Blockers

- Effective at managing AV nodal tachycardia.
- Examples: Verapamil, diltiazem.
- Side effects: Decreased cardiac contractility, prolonged AV conduction, and decreased blood pressure.
- Should not be used in cases of ventricular tachycardia.

Asthma and Chronic Obstructive Pulmonary Disease Medications

Acute bronchoconstriction can be treated with various classifications of drugs. Bronchodilators such as β_2-agonists, muscarinic antagonists, and theophylline are used effectively to manage these pathologies. In cases of chronic asthma, long-term management with corticosteroids is employed.

Beta-Adrenoreceptor Agonists

- Delivery route: Inhalation via pressurized canister or nebulizer treatment.
- Side effects: Skeletal muscle tremor, tachycardia, and cardiac arrhythmias.
- Short-acting:
  - Examples: Albuterol, terbutaline, metaproterenol.
  - Duration: No more than 4 hours.
- Long-acting:
  - Examples: Salmeterol, formoterol, indacaterol, vilanterol.
  - Duration: Up to 12 hours.
  - Recommended for prophylactic intervention.

Methylxanthines

- Naturally occurring forms: Caffeine from coffee, theophylline from tea, and theobromine from cocoa.
- Theophylline prescribed medically for asthma and COPD.
- The result produced by theophylline is bronchodilation and increased contractile force of the diaphragm.
- Examples: Aminophylline, roflumilast, pentoxifylline.
- Side effects: GI irritation and tremors. More severe effects in overdosage may include insomnia, nausea, arrhythmias of the heart, and seizure activity.

Muscarinic Antagonists

- Block muscarinic receptors, inhibit bronchoconstriction; mediated by the vagus nerve (parasympathetic nervous system).
- First-response drugs in acute bronchoconstriction are beta-agonist drugs such as albuterol. However, muscarinic antagonists may be preferred in COPD and may be more effective with fewer side effects.
- Delivery route: Aerosol.
- Examples: Ipratropium, tiotropium, aclidinium.

Corticosteroids

- Commonly considered first-line pharmaceutical interventions to treat moderate-to-severe asthma.

- Decrease inflammation and allergic response by minimizing bronchoconstriction.
- Used for children who do not respond to the use of beta-agonists. Considered appropriate to mitigate deleterious chronic inflammation and damage from long-standing asthma.
- Delivery route: Aerosol.
- Examples: Beclomethasone, budesonide, dexamethasone, flunisolide, fluticasone, mometasone.
- Less harmful than prednisone and hydrocortisone:
  - Prednisone and hydrocortisone are used in severe cases and when other interventions are unsuccessful.
  - These drugs act by reducing the arachidonic acid synthesis and inhibiting COX-2 expression.
  - Side effects: Frequent use may cause adrenal suppression and changes in the natural pharynx bacteria, leading to candidiasis. These effects can be countered by alternating the dosage of the medication to higher doses every other day.

Leukotriene Antagonists

- Receptor blockers that inhibit leukotrienes that are involved in the late inflammatory response.
- Prevent bronchoconstriction during exercise and antigen reaction.
- Examples: Montelukast, zafirlukast.
- These drugs are not as effective in managing severe asthma; therefore, corticosteroids are more commonly used.

■ EFFECTS OF ACTIVITY AND EXERCISE ON THE CARDIOVASCULAR/PULMONARY SYSTEM

Exercise affects the body in many ways. To best understand the benefits, progressions, and limitations of treating patients, it is important to recognize how exercise affects the cardiovascular and pulmonary systems.

EXERCISE EFFECTS ON RESPIRATION

Oxygen use and pulmonary ventilation during exercise—The resting O_2 consumption for a young male at rest is approximately 250 mL/min, which can be increased on average to the numbers in the following chart:

	mL/min
Untrained average male	3600
An athletically trained average male	4000
Male marathon runner	5000

From Hall JE. *Guyton and Hall Textbook of Medical Physiology.* 12th ed. Philadelphia, PA: Saunders Elsevier; 2011:1036.

The chart demonstrates that O_2 consumption can be increased significantly by nearly 20-fold when comparing an average male to a well-conditioned athlete.[2]

VO$_2$ MAX AND EFFECTS OF EXERCISE TRAINING

In a study of gains in VO_2 max by Fox in 1979, the effects of progressive athletic training on VO_2 max were measured at 7 and 13 weeks. It was surprising that results demonstrated only an increase of approximately 10% of VO_2 max overall. Also, there was little variance in training frequency when comparing two to five times a week. Marathon runners can improve O_2 consumption by up to 45% more than the untrained athlete, which may be linked by genetic determination, body type, and the relative ratio of body mass to lung capacity. Individuals with distinct advantages may self-select for marathon and longer-distance sports.

However, years of training may likely account for large increases in VO_2 for marathon runners versus short-term training, as demonstrated in the study.[3]

The oxygen-diffusing capacity of athletes—The measure of the **O_2-diffusing capacity** is the amount of O_2 that crosses through the respiratory membrane and enters into the blood each minute. The following chart demonstrates diffusing capacities in various individuals:

	mL/min
Nonathlete at rest	23
Nonathlete during maximal exercise	48
Speed skaters during maximal exercise	64
Swimmers during maximal exercise	71
Oarsman during maximal exercise	80

From Hall JE. *Guyton and Hall Textbook of Medical Physiology*. 12th ed. Philadelphia, PA: Saunders Elsevier; 2011:1037.

There are several significant findings. The first is the greater than twofold increase from a nonathlete at rest to during maximal exercise. Physiologically, this occurs because many pulmonary alveoli are poorly perfused or not perfused at all at rest. During exercise, there is a large increase in blood flow. In maximal exercise, all pulmonary capillaries are perfused, increasing the surface area exposing blood to O_2. Second, there is a threefold or greater increase in O_2-diffusing capacity in well-trained athletes. Is this because persons with higher O_2-diffusing capacities choose these sports, or is it because endurance training improves this ability? The mechanisms of how this occurs are unknown; however, it is most likely linked to the effects of long-term endurance training activities that increase a person's O_2-diffusing capacity.[2]

Exercise effects on blood gases—During exercise, there is an increased demand for O_2 by muscles throughout the body. It might be thought that this increase in demand would cause a decrease in O_2 levels and an increase in CO_2 in the blood. However, this is not normally what occurs as O_2 and CO_2 levels remain near normal, demonstrating the body's increased respiratory capacity to adjust in a large range to maintain adequate aeration. Significant changes in blood gases are not necessary to prompt a change in respiration. Instead, stimulation of the respiratory centers at the brainstem can regulate these changes. Movement of the joints and muscles can cause sufficient sensory input to the respiratory centers, and in turn, the brain can match the exact needs to maintain blood gas levels at or near normal.[2]

EXERCISE EFFECTS ON THE CARDIOVASCULAR SYSTEM

Effects of training and exercise on the heart and cardiac output—The tables below compare cardiac output, HR, and SV among various individuals and circumstances. From rest to exercise, cardiac output in an untrained individual can be increased more than four times resting. An average marathoner can increase this almost six times greater, while well-seasoned athletes can increase this to nearly seven to eight times more, ranging from 35 to 40 L/min.[2]

	L/min
Cardiac output in a young man at rest	5.5
Maximal cardiac output during exercise in young untrained man	23
Maximal cardiac output during exercise in average male marathoner	30

From Hall JE. *Guyton and Hall Textbook of Medical Physiology*. 12th ed. Philadelphia, PA: Saunders Elsevier; 2011:1038.

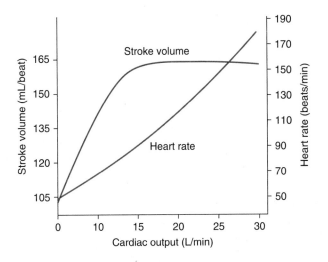

Figure 4-13. Approximate stroke volume output and heart rate at different levels of cardiac output in a marathon athlete. (Reproduced with permission from Burke-Doe A, Dutton M, eds. *National Physical Therapy Examination and Board Review*. 2019. Copyright © McGraw Hill LLC. All rights reserved. https://accessphysiotherapy.mhmedical.com.)

	Stroke Volume (mL)	Heart Rate (beats/min)
Resting		
Nonathlete	75	75
Marathoner	105	50
Maximum		
Nonathlete	110	195
Marathoner	162	185

From Hall JE. *Guyton and Hall Textbook of Medical Physiology*. 12th ed. Philadelphia, PA: Saunders Elsevier; 2011:1039.

According to the data, marathoners have about a 40% greater maximum cardiac output than untrained persons. There is hypertrophy of the skeletal muscle during exercise and a 40% increase in heart chamber size and mass. The enlarged heart affords decreased HR for marathon athletes because the SV is greater when compared to the nonathlete.[3]

SV increases from 105 to 162 mL during exercise, while HR increases from 50 to 185 beats/min. These changes represent an increase of 50% and 270%, respectively, and demonstrate that HR by and large accounts for the greater contribution in increasing cardiac output during strenuous exercise. SV reaches a ceiling effect at approximately 50% of the maximum HR. Therefore, any remaining increase in cardiac output is attributed to increased HR. Figure 4-13 shows the approximate SV and HR at different levels of cardiac output in a marathon athlete.[2]

Relationship of cardiac performance and VO₂ max—The respiratory system has a much greater capacity and reserve than the cardiovascular system. In maximal exercise, the cardiovascular system is at nearly 90% of capacity. In contrast, the respiratory system is about 65% of maximum ventilation. Because of this, the cardiovascular system is the primary limiter of VO_2 max. The 40% gains in cardiac output in marathon runners serve as the single most important physiologic benefit of the training regimen of marathon runners.[2]

■ PATIENT ASSESSMENT

The physical therapist and physical therapist assistant use the results of tests and measures to determine whether an individual has an adequate ventilatory pump and O_2 uptake/CO_2 elimination system to meet O_2 demands at rest, during movement, and during the performance of purposeful activity as well as whether the cardiovascular pump, circulation, O_2 delivery, and lymphatic drainage system are adequate to meet the body's demands at rest and with activity. Responses are monitored at rest, during activity, and after activity and may indicate the presence or severity of an impairment, activity limitation, participation restriction, or disability.

VITAL SIGN ASSESSMENT

Heart Rate or Pulse

- Locations: Heart rate is most accurately measured at the cardiac apex, where the point of maximal impulse (PMI) can be palpated. Pulses should be palpated using two to three fingers (not the thumb) at various locations: carotid, axillary, brachial, radial, femoral, popliteal, posterior tibial, and dorsalis pedis pulse, and can be graded on a four-point scale as seen in Table 4-1.
- Tachycardia is defined as greater than 100 beats/min and can be a normal response to exercise or abnormal with disease processes. Bradycardia is defined as less than 60 beats/min, but athletes may have lower resting heart rates.

Respiration

- Observe the rate, depth, and rhythm of breathing.
- Normal respiratory rate in adults is 12 to 20 beats/min. Late childhood is 15 to 25 beats/min. Early childhood is 20 to 40 beats/min. Newborns are 30 to 60 beats/min.
- Various breathing patterns: **Eupnea** (normal), **bradypnea**, **tachypnea**, **hyperpnea**, Cheyne–Stokes, air trapping, apneustic, pursed-lip, Kussmaul, Biot, and ataxic.

Pulse Oximetry (SpO$_2$)

- A specialized sensor typically placed on the finger or earlobe measures arterial O$_2$ saturation.
- Normal ranges are 96% to 100%.
- Activity should stop if SpO$_2$ drops below 90% in acutely ill patients. Patients with chronic lung disease should stop if below 85% to 88%.
- Consult with the supervising physical therapist and physician for the possible need for supplemental O$_2$ for patients with low SpO$_2$ levels during activity or mobility tasks.

Blood Pressure

- Hypotension results when blood pressure is lower than the expected normal. Blood pressure is not adequate to maintain proper perfusion/oxygenation. Low blood pressure may be caused by bed rest, drugs, shock, heart arrhythmias, or myocardial infarction.
- Orthostatic hypotension is considered a drop in systolic blood pressure (SBP) of more than 20 mm Hg or a diastolic drop of more than 10 mm Hg when a patient moves from supine to standing. Healthy and unhealthy blood pressure ranges are presented in Table 4-2.

Temperature

- The body may experience temperature changes, which may include either increased warmth or areas that are cool to touch.
- Changes in skin coloration or hair loss may also accompany temperature differences in the skin or the extremities.

TABLE 4-1 • Pulse Four-Point Scale.

Grade	Description
0	Absent
1+	Palpable, but thready and weak; easily obliterated
2+	Normal, easily identified; not easily obliterated
3+	Increased pulse; moderate pressure for obliteration
4+	Full, bounding; cannot obliterate

TABLE 4-2 • Healthy and Unhealthy Blood Pressure Ranges.

Blood Pressure Categories

American Heart Association.

BLOOD PRESSURE CATEGORY	SYSTOLIC mm Hg (upper number)		DIASTOLIC mm Hg (lower number)
NORMAL	LESS THAN 120	and	LESS THAN 80
ELEVATED	120-129	and	LESS THAN 80
HIGH BLOOD PRESSURE (HYPERTENSION) STAGE 1	130-139	or	80-89
HIGH BLOOD PRESSURE (HYPERTENSION) STAGE 2	140 OR HIGHER	or	90 OR HIGHER
HYPERTENSIVE CRISIS (consult your doctor immediately)	HIGHER THAN 180	and/or	HIGHER THAN 120

© American Heart Association. DS-16580 8/20

heart.org/bplevels

Reprinted with permission https://www.heart.org/-/media/files/health-topics/high-blood-pressure/hbp-rainbow-chart-english.pdf. ©American Heart Association, Inc.

Angina Pectoris (Chest Pain)

A patient with cardiovascular disease may experience chest pain when having an acute coronary syndrome (otherwise known as a myocardial infarction). The PTA should understand the various signs and symptoms of chest pain. The medical term for cardiac-based chest pain is *angina pectoris*. Common types of angina pectoris include stable angina, unstable angina, and Prinzmetal (variant) angina and will be presented later in this chapter.

- Differentiate between noncardiac-origin or cardiac-origin pain.
- Assess patient's complaint of angina such as:
  - Description (throbbing, aching, strong, sharp, dull).
  - Frequency.
  - Onset.
  - Triggering events.
  - Time of day.
  - What alleviates symptoms (activity, cessation of activity, medication).
  - Take special note of any referred pain symptoms that could be cardiac in nature.

Patients can rate angina using a standardized scale, as shown in Table 4-3. Patients can also rate exertion using the Borg scale or modified Borg scale to rate exertion during activity (Table 4-4).

HEART SOUNDS AND LUNG SOUNDS

Heart Sounds

Heart sounds provide detail about a patient's cardiopulmonary status. When auscultating for heart sounds, the stethoscope's diaphragm is used for high-pitched sounds (S1 and S2); the bell portion is used for lower-pitched sounds (S3 and S4).

TABLE 4-3 • Angina Rating Scale.

1. Mild, barely noticeable
2. Moderate, bothersome
3. Moderately severe, very uncomfortable
4. Most severe or most intense pain ever experienced

This scale is used in rating the subjective pain associated with myocardial insufficiency.

Data from American College of Sports Medicine 2006.

TABLE 4-4 · Versions of the Modified Borg Scale Used to Evaluate Dyspnea.	
A. Angina Rating Scale—O'Sullivan et al.[a]	
0	No complaints of angina or chest pain
1	Complaints of light pain yet barely noticeable
2	Moderate complaints of bothersome chest pain
3	Severe complaints causing the patient to be very uncomfortable (pre-infarction pain)
4	Infarction pain being the most pain every experienced
(Patient used this scale to provide subjective pain associated with myocardial infarction)	
B. Modified Borg Scale—Kendrick et al.[b]	
0	No breathlessness at all
0.5	Very, very slight (just noticeable)
1	Very slight
2	Slight breathlessness
3	Moderate
4	Somewhat severe
5	Severe breathlessness
6	
7	Very severe breathlessness
8	
9	Very, very severe (almost maximal)
10	Maximal

[a]*Data from O'Sullivan S, Schmitz T, Fulk G. Physical Rehabilitation, 7th ed. 2019. Copyright © F.A. Davis. All rights reserved.*

[b]*Reproduced with permission from Kendrick KR, Baxi SC, Smith RM, et al. Usefulness of the modified 0-10 Borg scale in assessing the degree of dyspnea in patients with COPD and asthma. J Emerg Nurs. 2000;26(3):216-222.*

A PTA should listen for intensity, quality, and timing during the cardiac cycle while also listening for additional sounds or abnormal sounds.

- Normal heart sounds:
  - S1 heart sound: The "Lub" sound corresponds to the closure of the AV valves and is the start of ventricular systole.
  - S2 heart sound: The "Dub" sound corresponds to the closure of the aortic and pulmonic SL valves; best heard at Erb point.
- Abnormal heart sounds:
  - Gallop's heart sounds: Additional sounds heard accompanying S1 and S2. Sounds like the galloping rhythm of a horse.
- S3 heart sound: "Ventricular gallop" is heard after S2 and corresponds with an early and rapid filling of the ventricles during diastole. It can be heard in normal conditions or can be abnormal or pathologic.
  - Cadence is like saying "Kentucky" ("Ken-tu-cky" = S1-S2-S3).
  - May indicate congestive heart failure (CHF).
- S4 heart sound: "Atrial gallop" is heard before S1 and corresponds with ventricular filling due to atrial systole ("atrial kick"). It is rarely considered normal and usually indicates pathology.
  - Cadence is like saying "Tennessee" ("Ten-nes-see" = S1-S2-S4).
  - May indicate HTN, coronary artery disease (CAD), post-MI, aortic stenosis, changes in compliance to the heart.

TABLE 4-5 • Grading Systolic Murmurs.	
Intensity	**Description**
Grade I/VI	Barely audible
Grade II/VI	Audible, but soft
Grade III/VI	Easily audible
Grade IV/VI	Easily audible and associated with a thrill
Grade V/VI	Easily audible, associated with a thrill, and still heard with the stethoscope only lightly on the chest
Grade VI/VI	Easily audible, associated with a thrill, and still heard with the stethoscope off of the chest

Grading Systolic Murmurs. *Learn the Heart.* https://www.healio.com/cardiology/learn-the-heart/cardiology-review/topic-reviews/grading-systolic-murmurs. Reprinted with permission from SLACK Incorporated.

- Other abnormal findings:
  - Systolic murmur: If auscultation reveals AV valve murmur, this could represent regurgitation, as the AV is not closing properly. If auscultation reveals aortic or pulmonary SL valve murmur, this could represent stenosis of the valve because the valve is not opening when needed. It could also indicate mitral valve prolapse. A grading scale for the intensity of systolic murmurs is presented in Table 4-5.
  - Diastolic murmur: If auscultation reveals AV murmur, it could represent stenosis, as the AV valve is not opening when needed. If auscultation reveals an SL valve murmur, this could represent regurgitation, as the SL valve is not closing properly. Figure 4-14 illustrates the location for auscultating each heart valve.
  - Thrill: Palpable tremor due to movement of blood and accompanies extra sound or murmur.

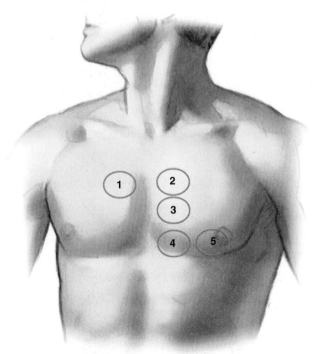

Figure 4-14. Areas of auscultation. The five classic areas of cardiac auscultation: (1) aortic (second intercostal space at the right parasternal line), (2) pulmonic (second intercostal space at the left parasternal line), (3) accessory aortic area (third intercostal space at the left parasternal line), (4) tricuspid (fifth intercostal space at the left parasternal), and (5) mitral (over the apical impulse). (Reproduced with permission from Fuster V, Harrington RA, Narula J, et al., eds. *Hurst's The Heart,* 14th ed. 2017. Copyright © McGraw Hill LLC. All rights reserved. https://accessmedicine.mhmedical.com.)

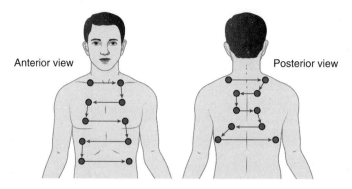

Respiratory patterns	
Normal (eupnea)	Regular and comfortable at 12-20 breaths/min.
Tachypnea	20 breaths/min.
Bradypnea	<12 breaths/min.
Hyperventilation	Repid, deep respiration >20 breaths/min.
Apneustic	Neurologic—sustained inspiratory effort.
Cheyenne-Stokes	Neurologic—alternating patterns of depth separated by brief periods of apnea.
Kussmaul	Rapid, deep, and labored—common in DKA.
Air trapping	Difficulty during expiration—emphysema.

Figure 4-15. Order of auscultating lung sounds. DKA, diabetic ketoacidosis. (Reproduced with permission from Burke-Doe A, Dutton M, eds. *National Physical Therapy Examination and Board Review.* 2019. Copyright © McGraw Hill LLC. All rights reserved. https://accessphysiotherapy.mhmedical.com.)

Lung Sounds

The following are the types of sounds heard through lung auscultation:

Normal Lung Sounds

- Normal or vesicular: Soft, low-pitched, rustling, wispy sound, which can be heard in most lung fields, especially the periphery, during inspiration and the first part of expiration.
- Bronchovesicular: Combination of vesicular and bronchial sounds heard in the large central airways over the manubrium, main stem, and segmental bronchi.
- Bronchial: Harsh, hollow, high-pitched sound, which can be heard during inspiration and expiration and is normally heard over the manubrium and trachea. Figure 4-15 shows the order of auscultating lung sounds.

Abnormal Breath Sounds

- Absent or diminished sounds: Pleural effusion, hemothorax, pneumothorax, obesity.
- Adventitious breath sounds.
- Abnormal sounds heard that are continuous or discontinuous with either inspiration or expiration.

Added or Adventitious Breath Sounds

- Crackles (formerly rales): High-pitched or medium-to-low-pitched discontinuous sound, which can indicate atelectasis, pulmonary fibrosis (PF), or secretions.
- Rhonchi: Described as having a snoring or gurgling sound, low-pitched in sound, and can be heard on inspiration or expiration.
- Wheezes: Mono- or polyphonic low-, medium-, or high-pitched sound indicating bronchospasm, asthma, COPD, or secretions in the larger airways.
- Vocal sounds: Normally, sounds are not transmitted in the lungs, and sound is muffled and inaudible.
  - Bronchophony: Can audibly hear patient saying "99."

TABLE 4-6 • Pitting Edema Scale Indentation Depth.				
Scale	Edema	English Units	Metric Units	Time to Baseline
0	None	0	0	
1+	Trace	0-0.25 in	< 6.5 mm	Rapid
2+	Mild	0.25-0.5 in	6.5-12.5 mm	6.5-12.5 mm
3+	Moderate	0.5-1 in	12.5 mm-2.5 cm	1-2 min
4+	Severe	>1 in	> 2.5 cm	2-5 min

Reproduced with permission from Urden, LD, Stacy KM, Lough ME. *Priorites in Critical Care Nursing*, 7e. 2016. Copyright © Elsevier, Inc. All rights reserved.

- Egophony: The "A" sound is heard when the patient says "E."
- Whispered pectoriloquy: When auscultating, can distinguish and audibly hear even when patient whispers.

PERIPHERAL CIRCULATION

- Assess all peripheral pulses of the arms and legs and include carotid artery. Note pulse rate, strength, and auscultation for abnormal sounds.
- Visual inspection for skin color changes (**cyanosis**, redness, pallor), trophic changes (skin is shiny, thin, pale, hairless), presence of skin lesions (ulcers, wounds), changes in the nail bed (bulbous thickening or clubbing at proximal nail bed).
- Doppler/ultrasound flowmetry: Ultrasound frequency can be used to listen to circulation difficult to palpate or auscultate.
- Edema: Can indicate heart or vascular disease.
  - Girth measurements can be measured with a tape measure or volumetric readings (measuring water displacement).
  - Scale for measuring the severity of edema is seen in Table 4-6.

Assessment of Peripheral Circulation

- Capillary refill: Pressure applied to the fingernail or toenail. Normally, the nail will blanch (whiten), then color returns within 3 seconds after pressure release. Delay can indicate arterial insufficiency.
- Intermittent claudication: The patient may complain of pain in the lower extremity (usually in the calf, foot, thigh, or buttocks) during ambulation or going up an incline or steps.
- Rubor of dependency: While the patient is in the supine position, the upper extremity (UE) or lower extremity (LE) is elevated to 45 degrees. Changes in skin color are noted. Normally, the color remains the same or may blanch slightly. If circulation is compromised, the leg will become pale or grayish. Next, the extremity is placed in a dependent position. A normal response is when there is a return to normal color or pinkish coloration. If an arterial disease is present, the extremity will become bright red (dependent rubor).
- Ankle-brachial index (ABI): The ankle-brachial index test compares blood pressures at the ankle and arm to check for peripheral artery disease.
  - Blood pressures are taken at the brachial arteries bilaterally and the posterior tibialis arteries bilaterally. A sphygmomanometer and handheld Doppler ultrasound flowmeter are used.
  - The ABI is calculated by dividing the higher of the two ankle blood pressures by the higher of the two systolic blood pressure measurements of the arm. The interpretation of an ABI and the severity of vascular compromise is listed in Table 4-7.

PERCUSSION

Regarding pulmonary conditions, the term percussion has multiple meanings. The physical therapist may use a percussion technique to assess abnormal lung findings, which will be further explained. The PTA may use a percussion technique when performing postural drainage amid a chest therapy intervention, and this will be further reviewed later in the chapter.

TABLE 4-7 · Interpretation of Ankle-Brachial Index (ABI).		
Generally normal	0.91-1.3	
Mild–moderate disease	0.41-0.90	Pain in the foot, leg, or buttock may occur during exercise due to some narrowing of the arteries
Severe disease	≤ 0.40	Symptoms may occur even while resting; danger of limb loss
Rigid arteries	> 1.3	Calcified vessels: Need an ultrasound test to check for peripheral artery disease instead of an ABI test

Data from Grenon SM, Gagnon J, Hsiang Y. Ankle-brachial index for assessment of peripheral arterial disease. *N Engl J Med* 2009; 361:e40 and http://www.educatehealth.ca.

When assessing possible abnormal lung findings, the physical therapist will percuss (tap) one finger over the other along areas of the rib cage and thorax to assess the sound produced. Well-ventilated lung tissue will produce a low-pitched resonant sound, like a muffled drum.

Dense tissue such as the liver, heart, and visceral organs will have a duller sound. Hollower organs produce a more resonant or tympanic sound, whereas a higher-pitched, dull "thud" sound could indicate increased density, such as in atelectasis, consolidation, or pleural effusion. Finally, a hyperresonant sound may indicate decreased density, such as a pneumothorax or hyperinflated lung.

RIB CAGE MOVEMENT AND EXCURSION

Due to the shape of the rib cage, with inspiration, the upper ribs move in a pump handle-like motion, increasing the anteroposterior (AP) diameter of the chest. The lower ribs (7th-10th) move in the bucket-handle movement. AP motion is more limited, resulting in ribs swinging out and up, increasing the transverse diameter of the rib. Rib cage expansion can be measured with a tape measure at the chest circumference. The patient exhales maximally, and a measurement is recorded, then the patient inhales maximally, and a measurement is recorded. The difference between the two measurements indicates total chest expansion. Measurements can be taken at the level of the xiphoid process and the axillary line. Upper, middle, and lower lobes are assessed. Movement should be equal, and the examiner's thumbs should move apart. Figure 4-16 shows the proper hand positioning to evaluate chest wall excursion.

EXERCISE TESTING

Exercise testing of the cardiopulmonary system can serve several purposes:

- As a diagnostic tool.
- To determine severity or involvement of a disease or prognosis.
- As objective assessment of disability and to measure progress.
- As a part of a treatment or training program.
- To improve fitness in healthy individuals as well as those diagnosed with pathology or disease.

With any exercise testing, there are indications for terminating exercise as listed in Table 4-8.

Walking Tests

The 6-minute walk test is one of the standardized walking exercise tests. The patient walks for 6 minutes, and the total distance is measured, and the symptoms the patient experiences are recorded.

Another test is the 10-m shuttle walk test, in which the pace is incrementally increased. The patient walks between two cones placed 10 m apart. The number of shuttles between cones is recorded, and an audiotape "beeps" indicates the time/cadence for the patient to start

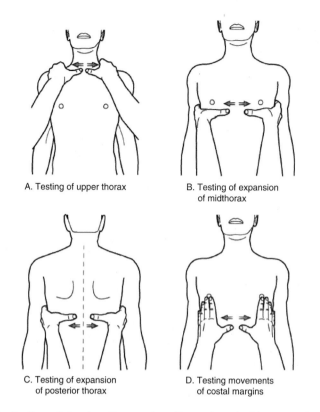

A. Testing of upper thorax

B. Testing of expansion of midthorax

C. Testing of expansion of posterior thorax

D. Testing movements of costal margins

Figure 4-16. Evaluation of chest wall excursion. (Reproduced with permission from Suneja M, Szot JF, LeBlond RF, et al., eds. *DeGowin's Diagnostic Examination*, 11th ed. 2020. Copyright © McGraw Hill LLC. All rights reserved. https://accessmedicine.mhmedical.com.)

and stop. At each level, the cadence is increased, and the number of completed shuttles increases to progress patient pace.

ELECTROCARDIOGRAM

SKILL KEEPER: ECG/EKG READINGS

When analyzing an ECG/EKG strip, the physical therapist notes a depression in the ST segment. What are the possible causes for this? What are other possible changes to the ST segment? What possible changes on an ECG/EKG reading might one expect to see for a patient taking calcium channel blockers?

TABLE 4-8 • Ankle-Brachial Index Measures	
ABI Value	**Interpretation of ABI Value**
>1.2	Falsely elevated yet considered abnormal, arterial disease, common in advanced diabetes mellitus
1.19–0.95	Normal
0.94–0.75	Mild arterial insufficiency, intermittent claudication (some patients are asymptomatic)
0.74–0.50	Moderate atrial insufficiency, pain with rest (minimal perfusion)
<0.50	Severe arterial insufficiency (wound healing is unlikely)
<0.40	Critical arterial insufficiency (possible necrosis may occur)

Data from O'Sullivan S, Schmitz T, Fulk, G. *Physical Rehabilitation*, 7th ed. 2019. Copyright © F.A. Davis. All rights reserved; Fruth S, Fawcett C. *Fundamentals of Tests and Measures for the Physical Therapist Assistant*. 2020. Copyright © Jones & Bartlett Learning. All rights reserved.

SKILL KEEPER ANSWERS

a. *Possible causes for the ST-segment depression may be caused by digitalis toxicity, or it could mean the patient suffers from stable angina. In either case, the patient should be evaluated for possible coronary artery disease. Generally speaking, the depressed ST segment is not an indication of an acute syndrome, yet it is a condition that requires evaluation by the cardiologist promptly.*

b. *There are two types of calcium: (1) intracellular calcium, which is stored within the sarcoplasmic reticulum, and (2) extracellular calcium within the plasma. The coronary arteries and peripheral vascular system depend on one type of calcium for a contraction, while the SA and AV nodes depend on the other calcium levels. Therefore, when the cardiac system experiences varied calcium levels, it may cause cardiac arrhythmias, which may be seen on the ECG/EKG reading.*

An ECG (also called EKG) is a medical device that records the heart's electrical activity. PTAs need to be aware of various heart rhythm disorders for which a patient may have symptoms, and they must also have a general knowledge of reading ECG strips (Figure 4-17). It is important to follow a systematic approach to avoid misreading or missing important key signs of various heart conditions. Figure 4-17 provides a normal ECG reading and an abnormal reading.[4]

Various approaches can be utilized to help determine heart activity through reviewing the ECG strip:

- Use the appropriate method to calculate the heart rate.
- What is the rhythm of the pattern? Classification of patterns can include regularly regular, regularly irregular, and irregularly irregular. Observation of the space between R waves indicates the regularity of patterns.
- Is there a P wave before each QRS complex? Is there a QRS complex after every P wave? These are indicators of atrial and ventricular activity.
- What is the duration of the PR interval? Increased length of the PR interval may indicate blocks in conduction through the nodal system.
- What is the size, shape, and duration of the QRS complex?
- Assess the ST-segment shape and duration. Is it elevated or depressed?

Determining Heart Rate

Various methods can be used to measure heart rate based on ECG/EKG strip readings.

- **Method 1:** Using the quick-count method, find an R wave that falls on the heavy dark line. After that, each heavy line can be marked and counted down with the following

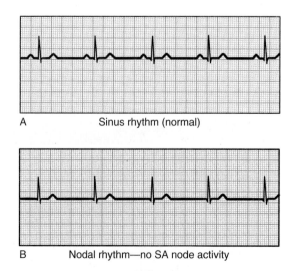

A   Sinus rhythm (normal)

B   Nodal rhythm—no SA node activity

Figure 4-17. ECGs: normal and abnormal. (Reproduced with permission from Burke-Doe A, Dutton M, eds. *National Physical Therapy Examination and Board Review.* 2019. Copyright © McGraw Hill LLC. All rights reserved. https://accessphysiotherapy.mhmedical.com.)

numbers: 300, 150, 100, 75, 60, 50, 43, and 37. The next R wave would be estimated to fall either on or between the heavy lines marked. For example, if the next wave fell directly on the fourth heavy line, the heart rate would be estimated at 75 beats/min. However, if the next R wave fell directly between the second and third heavy line, the heart rate would be between 100 and 150 beats/min and would be estimated at 125 beats/min.[3]

- **Method 2:** Count the number of small boxes between two consecutive R waves. Each small box represents 0.04 seconds. There are 60 seconds in 1 minute. Sixty seconds divided by 0.04 equals 1500. Therefore, divide 1500 by the number of small boxes counted to determine heart rate. For example, if there are 22 small boxes between R waves, 1500/22 = 68 beats/min.[3]

- **Method 3:** Some ECG/EKG strips may have a rate-ruler specific to the strip and machine calibration. Instructions on the rate ruler will help determine heart rate.[3]

- **Method 4:** If the EKG has markings that indicate it is a 6-second strip and the rhythm is normal, count the number of RR intervals, then multiply by 10. For example, if there are 7 RR intervals in the 6-second range, the heart rate would be 70 beats/min.[3]

Delineating Cardiac Rhythm Patterns

Various patterns can be identified in EKG readings (Figure 4-18). They can be categorized based on location, block, or foci that cause the dysrhythmic pattern. A description of the categories and types of patterns follows together with common EKG readings of the various patterns (Figures 4-19 and 4-20).

- Supraventricular dysrhythmias arise from above the level of the ventricles, and these are further categorized as sinus rhythm, sinus bradycardia, sinus tachycardia, atrial fibrillation, and atrial flutter.

- Ventricular dysrhythmias arise due to an ectopic pacemaker occurring below the atria; categorized as premature ventricular complex (PVC), ventricular bigeminy, ventricular trigemini, or ventricular quadrigeminy (PVC occurs every second, third, or fourth beat), multifocal PVCs, ventricular tachycardia, ventricular fibrillation, or asystole.

- Conduction blocks of a first-degree mean an impairment in the SA node's conduction to the AV node. A second-degree conduction block means there is a partial block of conduction involving the AV node. Finally, a third-degree conduction block is defined as a complete conduction block of the AV node.

- Myocardial ischemia or infarction (also known as an acute coronary syndrome [ACS]).
  - An ECG strip that shows an **elevated ST segment** (beginning with the end of the S wave and ending with the beginning of the T wave) indicates acute myocardial ischemia or injury. Examples are illustrated in Figure 4-20 (I and J).

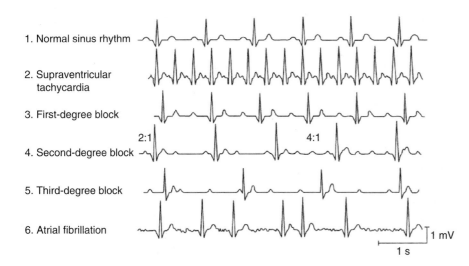

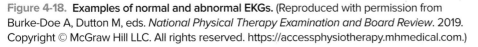

Figure 4-18. Examples of normal and abnormal EKGs. (Reproduced with permission from Burke-Doe A, Dutton M, eds. *National Physical Therapy Examination and Board Review.* 2019. Copyright © McGraw Hill LLC. All rights reserved. https://accessphysiotherapy.mhmedical.com.)

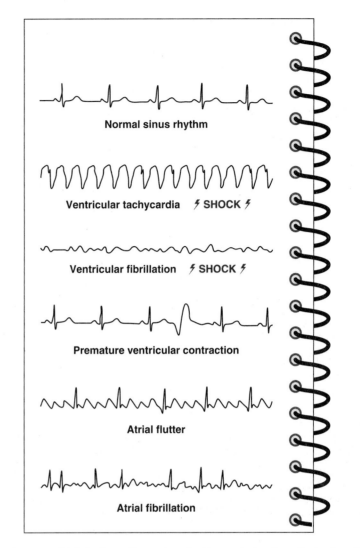

Figure 4-19. Common ECG rhythms. (Reproduced with permission from Burke-Doe A, Dutton M, eds. *National Physical Therapy Examination and Board Review*. 2019. Copyright © McGraw Hill LLC. All rights reserved. https://accessphysiotherapy.mhmedical.com.)

- ST-segment depression is illustrated in Figure 4-20 examples B and C. Although not considered acutely critical as an elevated ST segment, it is still indicative of coronary artery injury and requires a medical evaluation from a cardiac specialist, physician, physical therapist, or patient-provider.

HOLTER MONITORING

Holter monitoring allows for 24-hour noninvasive heart monitoring (Figure 4-21). Patients can also keep a log and match symptoms with daily activities. The cardiac activity is reported back to the cardiac provider to determine the patient's treatment plan.

PULMONARY FUNCTION TESTS

There are various pulmonary function tests (PFTs) that measure inspiration and expiration. Tests can be used to assess lung volumes and capacities, breathing, ventilation, pulmonary mechanics, and diffusion rates. PFTs are used for the following:

- Diagnosing lung and pulmonary pathologies.
- Screening for development of disease processes.
- Prognosis for patients diagnosed with lung pathologies.
- Measurement of progress before and after treatment intervention.

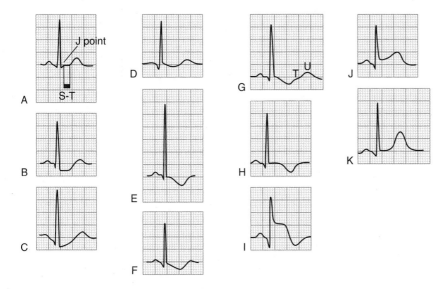

Figure 4-20. **Normal and abnormal ST segments and T waves.** (Reproduced with permission from Burke-Doe A, Dutton M, eds. *National Physical Therapy Examination and Board Review*. 2019. Copyright © McGraw Hill LLC. All rights reserved. https://accessphysiotherapy.mhmedical.com.)

Spirometry

Spirometry measures the amount of air flow and some lung volumes, and in general can indicate obstructive lung pathologies. A patient performs maximal inhalation and exhalation as quickly as possible into a spirometer. This measures the vital capacity (VC). The forced exhalation after maximal inspiration is called the forced vital capacity (FVC), and the amount of expelled air (forced expiratory volume [FEV]) in 1 second is called the FEV1. A ratio derived from the FEV1/FVC is also calculated. Together the FVC, FEV1, and the FEV1/FVC are the three important measures of spirometry. Spirometry results can be plotted on a graph linearly or in a flow-volume loop. Figure 4–22 demonstrates a spirometric flow diagram showing the flow of air during inhalation and exhalation.

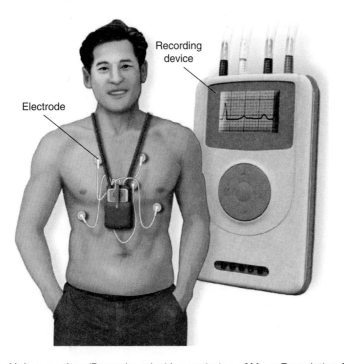

Figure 4-21. **Holter monitor.** (Reproduced with permission of Mayo Foundation for Medical Education and Research, all rights reserved.)

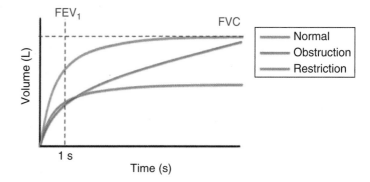

Figure 4-22. Comparison of spirograms for normal lungs, restrictive lung disease, and obstructive lung disease. FEV₁, forced expiratory volume in 1 second; FVC, forced vital capacity. (Reproduced with permission from Burke-Doe A, Dutton M, eds. *National Physical Therapy Examination and Board Review.* 2019. Copyright © McGraw Hill LLC. All rights reserved. https://accessphysiotherapy.mhmedical.com.)

Graphs also demonstrate the peak expiratory flow rate. The steepest slope represents the maximum amount of air expelled. In the presence of disease processes, changes to the peak expiratory flow, lung volumes, and the characteristic flow-volume loop can differentiate obstructive and restrictive lung pathologies. A spirogram for normal lungs, restrictive lung disease, and obstructive lung disease is presented in Figure 4-22. Figure 4-23 shows the flow-volume loop and the changes that occur with lung pathologies.

Lung Volume Tests

Lung volume tests measure various lung volumes and capacities and can effectively indicate restrictive lung diseases. Spirometry testing can measure most lung volumes and capacities; however, residual volume (RV) cannot be captured with these tests, as this is the amount of air that remains in the lungs after maximal exhalation. Therefore, RV is measured using other forms of testing such as gas dilution techniques, body plethysmography, and calculations and extrapolation of RV from chest x-rays or CT scans. RV can then calculate total lung capacity (TLC) and provide a complete picture of the patient's lung volumes and capacities.

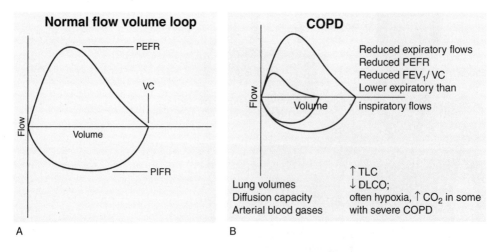

Figure 4-23. Flow-volume loop examples. **A.** Normal flow-volume loop. **B.** COPD flow-volume loop. **C.** Interstitial lung disease flow-volume loop. **D.** Restrictive lung disease flow-volume loop. **E.** Ventilatory muscle weakness flow-volume loop. COPD, chronic obstructive pulmonary disease; DLCO, diffusing capacity of the lung for carbon monoxide; FEV₁, forced expiratory volume in 1 second; PEFR, peak expiratory flow rate; PIFR, peak inspiratory flow rate; TLC, total lung capacity; VC, vital capacity. (Reproduced with permission from DeTurk WE, Cahalin LP. *Cardiovascular and Pulmonary Physical Therapy: An Evidence–Based Approach*, 3rd ed. 2017. Copyright © McGraw Hill LLC. All rights reserved. https://accessphysiotherapy. mhmedical.com.)

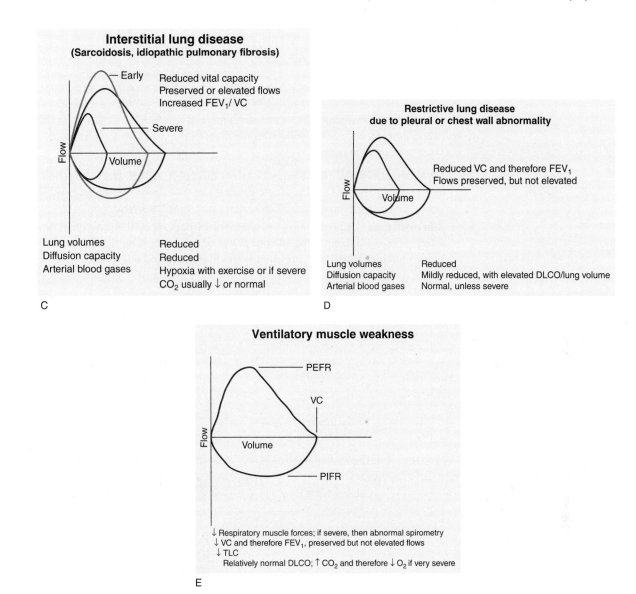

FIGURE 4-23. (Continued)

■ PATHOLOGIES/CONDITIONS OF THE CARDIOVASCULAR SYSTEM

Pathologies and conditions are described here in major categories, including ischemic conditions, CHF, cardiomyopathies, arrhythmic conditions, and heart valve disorders.

ISCHEMIC CONDITIONS OF THE HEART

SKILL KEEPER: CORONARY ARTERY DISEASE

What factors cannot be controlled that contribute to the risk of developing coronary artery disease (CAD)? What factors can be modified for which a physical therapist can make recommendations to reduce the risk of developing CAD? What can other members of the health care team contribute to making proper modifications in lifestyle for a patient?

Uncontrollable risk factors include a family history of CAD, valvular dysfunctions, congenital deformities.

Controllable risk factors are avoiding smoking, high cholesterol diets, sedentary lifestyle, acquired diabetes mellitus, high-stress lifestyle, and excessive alcohol and substance abuse.

The cardiac team members who can help contribute to lifestyle modifications include the cardiologist/physician, social worker, registered dietician, nursing staff, physical therapist and assistant, and the patient.

Coronary artery disease—Coronary artery disease (CAD) results in obstructed blood flow to the heart. CAD is the single greatest cause of death in men and women in the United States, with more than 565,000 new cases of MI each year.[4]

Atherosclerosis—Atherosclerosis is triggered by damage to the innermost layer of the artery. Figure 4-24 shows the various layers of the artery. The risk factors include cigarette smoking, high blood pressure, high cholesterol, and a sedentary lifestyle. All are modifiable factors that can reduce the risk of atherosclerosis. Nonmodifiable contributors to CAD are age, gender, race, and family history.

Atherosclerosis begins with the development of fatty streak deposits because of damage to the inner layer of the artery. Continued fatty or lipid deposits cause a buildup, and atheroma

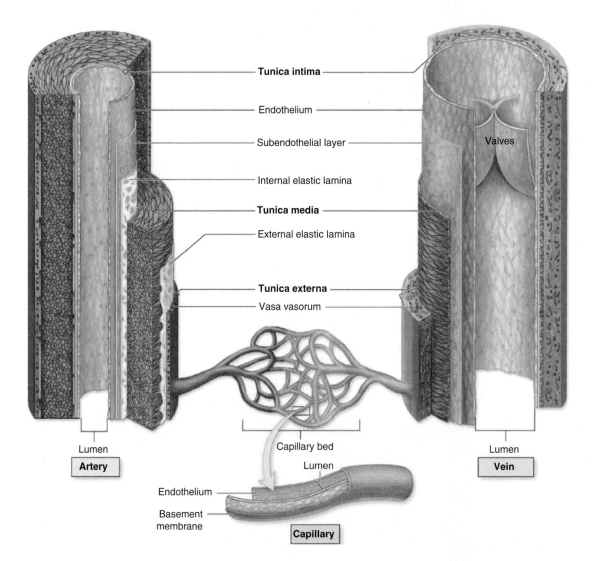

Figure 4-24. Layers of the arterial and venous vasculature. (Reproduced with permission from Burke-Doe A, Dutton M, eds. *National Physical Therapy Examination and Board Review.* 2019. Copyright © McGraw Hill LLC. All rights reserved. https://accessphysiotherapy.mhmedical.com.)

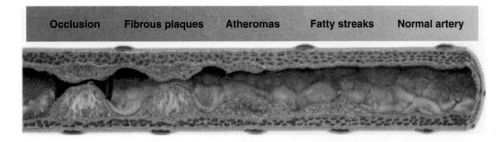

Figure 4-25. **Pathogenesis of atherosclerosis.** (Reproduced with permission from Burke-Doe A, Dutton M, eds. *National Physical Therapy Examination and Board Review*. 2019. Copyright © McGraw Hill LLC. All rights reserved. https://accessphysiotherapy.mhmedical.com.)

develops. Finally, calcification of the lesion leads to fibrous plaques and impedes blood flow to the point of occlusion. A diagrammatic look at the inside of an atherosclerotic artery is presented in Figure 4-25.

Angina pectoris—Angina pectoris is defined as chest pain related to ischemic conditions of the myocardium due to compromised coronary blood flow to the heart. Angina results when there is greater cardiac demand than available O_2 to the heart or insufficient O_2 available to the heart. Pain can be described as substernal pressure, squeezing, tightness, or heaviness. Angina can also present with referred pain patterns, with symptoms appearing at the left shoulder or arm, neck, jaw, and between the shoulder blades. Any pain above the umbilicus should be further examined for possible underlying heart conditions. The four major triggers that can lead to angina are exertion, emotional stress, extreme temperature changes (especially cold), and eating a large meal. Angina can be classified as stable, unstable, or variant (Prinzmetal angina).

Stable angina—Stable angina, also referred to as chronic angina, can be triggered by increased physical activity or stress. Symptoms may last between 5 and 15 minutes; pain is felt at the substernum and usually does not radiate. The patient's angina does not persist, and cessation from the physical activity or administration of sublingual nitrates alleviates the symptoms.

Variant (Prinzmetal) angina—Variant or Prinzmetal angina is also called atypical angina. Unlike stable angina, it occurs at night or rest. The affected coronary artery goes into vasospasm, and a high-intensity episode may lead to MI. Compared to unstable angina, variant angina may be less severe, and with low-level activity; the symptoms can be relieved (physiologic response of vasodilation by a coronary artery in response to physical activity). However, heart arrhythmias usually accompany this condition.

Unstable angina—Similar to stable angina, unstable angina can be triggered by physical activity, stress, or rest. However, symptoms are more severe, frequent, and last longer (> 15 minutes). Cessation of activity or administration of sublingual nitrates may not alleviate symptoms. Unstable angina can represent the progression of coronary heart disease (CHD), and persons are more at risk for MI. Patients may also exhibit changes in cardiac function, such as changes in blood pressure or a decline in the ability to perform previous activity levels.

Myocardial infarction—MI occurs when there is loss of blood flow to the myocardium for more than 20 minutes, resulting in necrosis of the supplied tissue. The anatomy of the coronary circulation is shown in Figure 4-26. The MI is described, and the prognosis is determined by the size and extent of the involvement.

Complications from MI include arrhythmias, cardiogenic shock, pericarditis, CHF, impaired heart function (decreased SV, contractility, output, and ejection fraction), and sudden death. Clinical manifestations include the following:

- Severe radiating or nonradiating chest pain.
- Diaphoresis.
- Dyspnea.

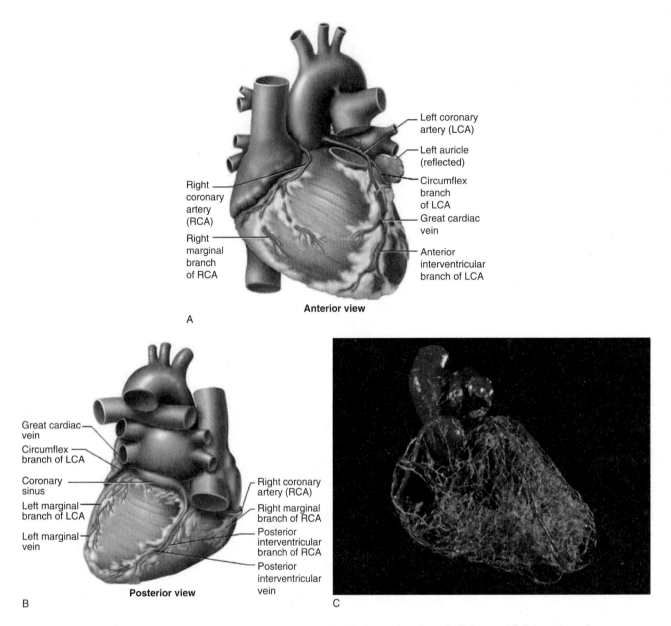

Figure 4-26. **Anatomy of the coronary circulation. A.** Anterior view. **B.** Posterior view. **C.** Enhanced 3-D imaging of coronary circulation. (Reproduced with permission from Burke-Doe A, Dutton M, eds. *National Physical Therapy Examination and Board Review*. 2019. Copyright © McGraw Hill LLC. All rights reserved. https://accessphysiotherapy.mhmedical.com).

- Nausea and vomiting.
- Light-headedness, dizziness, syncope.
- Weakness.
- ECG changes such as ST elevation or depression.
- Elevation of enzyme levels: troponin, creatine kinase, and phosphokinase.

CONGESTIVE HEART FAILURE

CHF is a group of clinical manifestations that result in pulmonary congestion from the blood that is backed up due to decreased output of the ventricle. As a result, the heart is unable to provide adequate cardiac output to meet O_2 demands. CHF can also be described by the side of the heart that is affected. Therefore, because of decreased output, blood is backed up behind the affected side. Ischemia or MI are the main causes of CHF.

Adequate cardiac output is a product of SV and heart rate and is essential in cardiovascular function. SV can be affected by three factors: the amount of blood in the ventricle after diastole (preload), the amount of pressure the ventricle must overcome to move blood into the systemic circulation (afterload), and the contractile strength of the ventricle. Therefore, any effects of these three factors may negatively impact SV and adversely decrease cardiac output.

Right ventricular failure—Right ventricular failure is usually caused by pulmonary hypertension. It can also be caused by mitral valve disease or acute and chronic lung disease such as **cor pulmonale**. When there is decreased action of the right ventricle, blood is backed up to the venous system, causing edema in the extremities. Other clinical manifestations include the following:

- Dependent edema.
- Jugular venous distension.
- Weight gain.
- Ascites.
- Cyanosis.
- Hepatomegaly.
- Anxiety.

Left ventricular failure—Left ventricular failure can be caused by atherosclerotic heart disease, cardiomyopathy, hypertension, valvular disease, arrhythmias, alcohol, and drug toxicity. Because of decreased contractility of the left ventricle, blood is backed up into the pulmonary vasculature of the lungs and causes pulmonary edema. Clinical manifestations include the following:

- Dyspnea.
- Orthopnea.
- Dry cough or spasmodic productive cough.
- Pulmonary edema.
- Pulmonary rales, wheezing ("cardiac asthma").
- Increased respiration.

CARDIOMYOPATHIES

SKILL KEEPER: CARDIOMYOPATHIES

Compare the various types of cardiomyopathies. What are the effects on ventricular filling, preload, SV, afterload, and cardiac output?

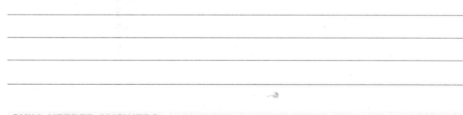

SKILL KEEPER ANSWERS

Cardiomyopathy is a term in which many cardiac dysfunctions are classified. Most commonly, cardiomyopathy refers to the myocardium tissue and relates to the ventricular function of the heart.

Ventricular filling occurs when the AV valves are open, allowing blood into the ventricles. Preload refers to the amount of blood entering the ventricle at the end of the ventricular diastole. Stroke volume is the amount of measured blood that is ejected from a single ventricular contraction. Cardiac output is the product of stroke volume and heart rate. Afterload is the amount of blood volume and pressure exerted from the pulmonary and arterial system back toward the aortic and pulmonary SL valves.

Cardiomyopathies can be classified based on a functional view and are categorized as dilated, hypertrophic, and restrictive (Figure 4-27).

Dilated cardiomyopathy—Dilated cardiomyopathy (DCM) results in dilation of the ventricle and impaired ventricular muscle function. There is little change in wall thickness; however, ventricular muscle mass does increase. An increase in the ventricular chamber also causes an increased EDV and a decreased SV. The heart cannot maintain

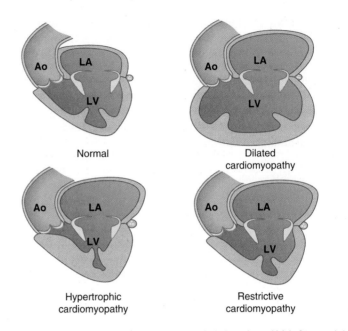

Figure 4-27. Types of cardiomyopathies. Ao, aorta; LA, left atrium; LV, left ventricle. (Reproduced with permission from Kumar V, Abbas AK, Fausto N, et al., eds. *Robbins Basic Pathology*, 8th ed. 2007. Copyright © W.B. Saunders Co. All rights reserved.)

sufficient cardiac output with exercise or increased activity, eventually leading to ventricular failure. Clinical manifestations of DCM include the following:

- Dyspnea during exertion progressing to dyspnea at rest.
- Nocturnal dry cough.
- Chest pain during exertion.
- S3 to S4 gallop.
- Resting tachycardia.
- Cardiomegaly.
- Systolic murmur from regurgitation of bicuspid or tricuspid valve.

Hypertrophic cardiomyopathy—Hypertrophic cardiomyopathy (HCM) results in increased ventricular muscle mass and no dilation of the ventricular chamber. There is decreased ventricular filling (diastolic dysfunction) and decreased compliance impairing ventricular filling. As a result, the ventricle may contract before the chamber is filled, which decreases SV. Clinical manifestations for HCM include the following:

- Dyspnea.
- Angina pectoris.
- Fatigue.
- Syncope.
- Palpitations.
- Loud S4 heart sounds.

Restrictive cardiomyopathy—Restrictive cardiomyopathy (RCM) is caused by endomyocardial or myocardial disease-causing diastolic dysfunction, stiffening of the heart walls, and decreased compliance. The rigidity of the heart walls causes decreased ventricular filling and affects the cardiac output. Bicuspid or tricuspid regurgitation, as well as pulmonary hypertension, accompany RCM. Other clinical manifestations include the following:

- Exercise intolerance.
- Weakness.
- Dyspnea.
- Edema.
- Enlarged liver.
- Symptoms of CHF.
- Cardiac arrhythmias.

ARRHYTHMIC CONDITIONS

Cardiac arrhythmic conditions affect heart rate, rhythm, or impulse condition. Classification of cardiac arrhythmias can be based on (a) origin (atria, also called supraventricular or ventricles), (b) type of pattern or rhythm (fibrillation or flutter), and (c) effect on rate or speed (tachycardia or bradycardia). Cardiac arrhythmias can vary in severity from asymptomatic and mild, requiring no intervention, severe and life-threatening, requiring resuscitation or immediate medical intervention.

Type of pattern or rhythm—Atrial fibrillation is the most common type of supraventricular tachycardia (SVT). The muscles of the atria quiver or flutter instead of producing one coordinated contraction, causing pooling of blood in the atria chamber and decreased filling of the ventricle. This reaction results in decreased O_2 levels and can cause shortness of breath, fatigue, palpitations, and in some instances, syncope. In addition, since blood remains in the atria, there is an increased risk for thrombus formation and emboli, leading to a cerebral vascular accident (also known as stroke).

Electrical disturbances cause ventricular fibrillation (VF), and there is a flutter of the ventricular muscles of the heart, causing cessation of cardiac output. VF often leads to cardiac arrest, and immediate medical attention is needed with defibrillation of the heart to end the erratic heart activity and allow for normal electrical conduction to resume.

Heart block is caused by an interruption to the normal conduction pathway in the heart. There are three types of heart block: first-degree, second-degree, and third-degree (complete). Heart block can be caused by CAD, HTN, myocarditis, or overdose of heart medications such as digitalis or beta-blockers. Patients may present with dizziness, syncope, light-headedness, and fatigue. Medication management or placement of a pacemaker are often used to manage these conditions.

Effect on rate or speed—Normal heart rate averages from 60 to 100 beats/min. The two rate arrhythmias are tachycardia (> 100 beats/min) and bradycardia (< 60 beats/min). Increased sympathetic stimulation results in tachycardia and can be caused by multiple factors, including pain, fear, emotions, exercise, or artificial stimulants (such as caffeine, nicotine, amphetamines). Abnormal conditions may include MI, fever, CHF, infection, and anemia. Bradycardia is normal in well-trained athletes. Patients taking beta-blockers also have decreased heart rates.

Signs and symptoms can range from asymptomatic to severe and may also include the following:

- No symptoms.
- Palpitations or flutter.
- Light-headedness or dizziness.
- Syncope.
- Chest discomfort.
- Weakness or fatigue.
- Dyspnea.
- Anxiety.
- Irregular or weak pulse.

HEART VALVE DISORDERS

Heart valve disorders are classified as either acquired or congenital. These disorders may lead to cardiac muscle dysfunction due to compensatory mechanisms to increase cardiac output, including ventricular hypertrophy and chamber dilation. The following characteristics or causes define them:

- Atresia: Congenital absence or closure.
- Prolapse: Cusp of the heart valve (usually bicuspid/mitral valve) falls back into the atrial chamber.

- Regurgitation: Backflow of blood due to incomplete valve closure.
- Stenosis: Fibrotic changes and stiffening of the heart valve causing decreased blood flow between chambers.

■ PATHOLOGIES/CONDITIONS OF THE PULMONARY SYSTEM

Injury to the lungs can occur via several means: (a) exposure to toxins or irritants, (b) pathogens, or (c) autoimmune disorders. In response, the lungs initiate acute inflammatory responses with cytokines and inflammatory mediators. The results will either be a resolution of the injury, tissue breakdown, tissue destruction, or scarring (fibrosis).

Diseases of the pulmonary system can be classified as (a) acute or chronic, (b) obstructive or restrictive, or (c) infectious or noninfectious. Common conditions of any pulmonary disease include cough or **dyspnea**. Other conditions or symptoms may include chest pain, sputum production, **cyanosis**, **hemoptysis**, changes in breathing patterns, abnormal lung sounds, respiratory gas changes, and clubbing of the fingers.

ACUTE DISEASES

Pneumonia

- Pneumonia is a state of inflammation of the lung parenchyma.
- Viral, bacterial, fungal.
  - Viral pneumonia: Influenza virus, adenovirus, measles, herpes, and cytomegalovirus.
  - Bacterial pneumonia: Gram-positive pneumococcal pneumonia (streptococcal) is the most common agent; gram-negative organisms such as *Klebsiella*, *Pseudomonas aeruginosa*, and *Haemophilus influenza* are found in compromised individuals such as those with severe illness or those receiving antibiotic therapy.
- Inhalation of allergens such as smoke, dust, irritants, and gas.
- Aspiration of food, fluids, or vomitus.
  - Aspiration pneumonia is present for persons with swallowing disorders caused by neurologic or muscular disease, or altered consciousness.
  - Pneumonia symptoms are generally mild and resolve in 1 to 2 weeks.
  - Manifestations may include the following:
    - Productive or nonproductive cough.
    - Pleural chest pain.
    - Rust- or green-colored sputum.
    - Dyspnea and tachypnea.
    - Headache, fevers, chills, and generalized aches and fatigue.

Pneumocystis carinii Pneumonia

- Unknown origin but possibly linked environmentally with transmission by other humans, animals, or another infected host.
- Common in immune-compromised individuals: Immune-suppressing drugs after transplant surgery or postchemotherapy. Prior increased prevalence for individuals with AIDS. Recent drug advances have limited these incidences.
- Symptoms of *Pneumocystis carinii* pneumonia (PCP) may include the following:
  - Fever.
  - Progressive dyspnea.
  - Nonproductive cough.
  - Fatigue.
  - Tachypnea.
  - Weight loss.

Tuberculosis

- Primary tuberculosis (TB): Exposure to *Mycobacterium tuberculosis*; lasts 10 to 14 days.
- Secondary TB: Occurs at any time after reactivation of the dormant bacteria encapsulated in the lungs. Symptoms do not usually occur during early exposure.

However, later-onset symptoms (as late as a year postexposure) may include the following:

- Productive cough and hemoptysis.
- Accompanying night sweats.
- Weight loss.
- Fatigue.
- Abnormal lung sounds such as **crackles**/rales and bronchial breath sounds.

TB exposure results in a positive skin test at initial exposure. Late TB is confirmed by chest x-ray and would show upper lobe involvement with air spaces and segmental lobe consolidation.

CHRONIC OBSTRUCTIVE DISEASES

Chronic Obstructive Pulmonary Disease (COPD)

There are many pulmonary conditions often classified as COPD.

COPD is characterized by chronic limitations to airflow.

Airflow can be caused by the following factors:

- Accumulation of mucus or secretions.
- Bronchospasm.
- Inflammation of the bronchioles.
- Fibrosis of bronchioles.

Over time, there is increased lung compliance resulting in air trapping and overstretched alveoli, floppy bronchiole airways, and hyperinflation of the lungs, resulting in abnormal pulmonary function tests. Patients may exhibit multiple symptoms or be diagnosed with several of the obstructive lung disease processes. In these instances, the general term of COPD is often used.

Asthma

- Reversible obstructive lung disease described by obstruction of the airway from inflammation and increased smooth muscle activity causing bronchospasm.
- There are two types of exacerbations or reactions:
  - Extrinsic (allergic).
  - Intrinsic (nonallergic).

Physical findings with asthma may include the following:

- Inspiratory and expiratory wheezing.
- Chest tightness.
- Dyspnea.
- Anxiety.
- Tachycardia.
- Tachypnea.
- Restlessness.
- Increased accessory muscle use.
- Nonproductive cough progressing to a productive cough with sputum.

Bronchiectasis

- Congenital or acquired disease resulting in an abnormal dilation of the bronchi.
- Usually caused by bacterial infections.
- Loss of elastic and muscle tissues of the bronchi and bronchioles.
- Increased sputum production; accumulation of wet secretions and mucus causes bronchospasm, which exacerbates airway obstruction.

- Common symptoms may include the following:
  - Productive cough with purulent sputum.
  - Hemoptysis.
  - Crackles and wheezing.
  - Clubbing of digits.
  - Dyspnea.
  - Hypoxemia and hypercapnia.

Chronic Bronchitis

- Irritation of the airways from smoking, air pollutants, occupational exposure, or infection.
- Chronic cough and excessive production of mucus.
- Diagnosis: Must have symptoms on most days for at least 3 months and two or more consecutive years.
- Term "blue bloaters" is often used to describe patient symptoms.
- Other clinical manifestations may include the following:
  - Smoker's cough progressing to productive cough.
  - Dyspnea on exertion.
  - Respiratory sensitivity to irritants and cold or damp weather.
  - Crackles and wheezing.
  - Prolonged expiration.

Cystic Fibrosis

- Genetic disorder with overproduction of mucus from the exocrine glands.
- Causes presence of thick mucus, decreased ciliary transport, and poor cough clearance, causing chronic lung infections and tissue damage.

Emphysema

- Pathologic destruction of the elastic fibers of the lung tissues.
- Results in accumulation of air due to destruction of the air spaces distal to the terminal bronchioles.
- History of long-term smoking.
- Nonsmoking cases of alpha antitrypsin deficiency emphysema caused by lack of an enzyme that prevents trypsin, which causes alveolar damage.
- Term "pink puffers" is often used to describe patient symptoms.
- Other common characteristics include the following:
  - Barrel chest.
  - Marked exertional dyspnea progressing to dyspnea at rest.
  - Effort-filled breathing.
  - Posturing to use accessory muscles to aid in breathing.
    - Prefers sitting in the recovery position when short of breath; seated, leaning forward with their hands on thighs or elbows on thighs.
  - Prolonged expiration.
  - Wheezing.
  - Clubbing.
  - Anxiety and distress.

CHRONIC RESTRICTIVE DISEASES

Chronic restrictive diseases encompass a range of diagnoses in which there is a decreased lung volume or decreased compliance causing stiffness in lung tissue. General categories or major classifications include the following:

- Connective tissue (rheumatoid arthritis, lupus, scleroderma, polymyositis).
- Pulmonary (asbestosis, pneumonia, acute respiratory distress syndrome, pleural effusion).

- Cardiovascular (pulmonary emboli [PE], pulmonary edema).
- Neuromuscular (spinal cord injury, head injury, amyotrophic lateral sclerosis, Guillain–Barre syndrome, muscular dystrophy, polio).
- Musculoskeletal disorders (ankylosing spondylitis, scoliosis, chest injuries, trauma, pectus carinatum/excavatum, chest or abdominal surgery, obesity).

Generalized physical findings for the range of restrictive lung disease may include the following:

- Dyspnea on exertion.
- Decreased exercise tolerance.
- Usually nonproductive and dry cough.
- Tachypnea.
- Decrease in most lung capacity measures.
- Weight loss.

Specific restrictive lung diseases are described below.

Atelectasis

- Alveolar collapse from pathologic or mechanical blockages of the bronchial airway:
  - Mucus or tumor.
  - Compression from fluid or pneumothorax.
  - Lack of surfactant.
  - Postoperation of the abdomen or thorax.
  - Neuromuscular diseases causing weakness of the respiratory muscles.
- Atelectasis physical findings are more pronounced if a large area is affected, including the following:
  - Profound dyspnea.
  - Hypoxia.
  - Tracheal or mediastinal shift toward the affected side.
  - Crackles or wheezes.

Chest Trauma

- Rib fractures, flail chest, lung contusion.
- Penetration wounds can cause pneumothorax, hemothorax, or pulmonary laceration.
- Flail chest occurs when there are multiple fractures of two or more ribs. Paradoxical movement, or opposite from normal movement, of breathing at the fracture site (inward movement of the flail segment with inspiration and outward movement with expiration) is seen and can cause significant pain, further compromising breathing.
- Other symptoms involved with chest trauma include the following:
  - Chest pain, especially with inspiration.
  - Tachypnea.
  - Hypoxia and hypercapnia.
  - Weak cough.
  - Tachycardia.

Pneumothorax

- Air or gas in the pleural space that causes collapse of the lung tissue beneath the affected area.
- Hemothorax with an entire collapse of the right or left lung.
  - Causes increase in thoracic pressure.
  - Mediastinal and tracheal shift away from the collapsed area.

- Symptoms and findings with pneumothorax may also include the following:
  - Unilateral chest pain.
  - Dyspnea.
  - Tachycardia.
  - Chest x-ray shows dense-appearing lung tissue, absence of lung tissue in the area of the pneumothorax, possible expansion of the rib cage due to lack of negative pleural pressure, flattening of the diaphragm on the side of the affected lung.

Pulmonary Effusion

- Excess fluid in the pleural space.
- Transudate: Fluid from increased pressure in the lung from CHF, renal disease, or pulmonary embolus.
- Exudate: Fluid from infection, malignancy, infarct, toxic drugs, or rheumatoid arthritis.
- Physical findings with pulmonary effusion may include the following:
  - Dyspnea.
  - Chest pain from the pleura varying from deep diffuse pain to sharp, stabbing pain.
  - Pleural rubbing.
  - Fever, chills, and night sweats.

Pulmonary Fibrosis

- Diseases of the lung parenchyma and pleura also called interstitial lung disease.
- Damaged epithelium and chronic inflammation leading to scar formation (fibrosis).
- Damage from prolonged asbestosis exposure is a PF disease.
- Physical findings relative to pulmonary fibrosis may include the following:
  - Dyspnea.
  - Hypoxemia and hypocapnia.
  - Crackles.
  - Clubbing.
  - Dry cough.
  - Cyanosis.
  - Chest x-rays show increased thickening of the lung pleura due to proliferation of fibroblasts; damage at the alveolar level causes shrinking of the lung and decreased compliance, resulting in the lung becoming stiff.

OTHER PULMONARY ABNORMALITIES

Pulmonary Edema

- Accumulation of fluid in the alveolar spaces from cardiogenic processes with increased pressure, such as in hypertension reflecting from the heart, causing a fluid backup to the pulmonary capillaries.
- Other cardiogenic abnormalities include CAD, cardiac valvular disease, and cardiomyopathy.
- Noncardiogenic pathologies include acute lung injury and inflammation, causing leakage into the lung tissues, such as in acute respiratory distress syndrome.
- Symptoms of pulmonary edema include the following:
  - Dyspnea.
  - Orthopnea, paroxysmal nocturnal dyspnea (shortness of breath causing awakening at night).
  - Pallor and cyanosis.
  - Diaphoresis.
  - Tachycardia and heart arrhythmias.
  - Anxiety or agitation.
  - Chest x-ray shows lung congestion or central infiltrates.

Pulmonary Emboli or Infarction

- Sudden blockage of the pulmonary artery usually from deep vein thrombosis (DVT); DVT usually occurs in the lower extremity then travels through the venous pathway toward the heart causing blockage of the pulmonary artery.
- Other causes: PE at the right side of the heart caused by fat, air, or bone.
- PE has a high rate of morbidity and mortality.
- Signs and symptoms of DVT or PE can include the following:
  - Acute dyspnea or tachypnea.
  - Chest pain.
  - Cough with hemoptysis.
  - Tachycardia and weak, feeble pulse.
  - Hypotension, light-headedness, dizziness.
  - Syncope.
  - Upon development of PE, the patient may have complaints of lateral neck pain.

◼ DIFFERENTIAL DIAGNOSES RELATED TO PATHOLOGIES OF THE CARDIAC, VASCULAR, AND PULMONARY[5]

CHEST PAIN/DISCOMFORT

- MI/ischemia.
- Pericarditis.
- Mitral valve prolapse.
- CAD.
- Pleurisy.
- Pulmonary embolism.
- Pneumothorax.
- Pulmonary hypertension.
- Lung cancer or other pulmonary metastatic diseases.
- Dissecting aortic aneurysm.
- Referred from the esophagus; "heartburn."
- Epigastric pain.
- Herpes zoster.

COUGH

- Pulmonary infection.
- Pulmonary inflammation.
- Tumor, foreign body, aspiration.
- Left ventricular failure.
- Thoracic aortic aneurysm.
- Postnasal drip.
- Gastroesophageal: Nonproductive cough at night or after meals; microaspiration causing irritation and cough.
- Medications such as ACE inhibitors, beta-blockers, chemotherapeutic drugs.

DYSPNEA OR SHORTNESS OF BREATH

- CAD, CHF, dilated cardiomyopathy, valvular disease.
- Left ventricular hypertrophy, restrictive cardiomyopathy, constrictive pericarditis.
- COPD.
- Restrictive lung disease.

- Pulmonary edema.
- Anemia.
- Sepsis.
- Peripheral arterial disease.
- Deconditioning.
- Psychogenic.

EDEMA AND SWELLING WITH WEIGHT GAIN GREATER THAN 3 POUNDS IN 1 DAY

- Right ventricular or left and right ventricular failure (CAD, CHF, valvular disease, cardiomyopathy, pulmonary HTN, **cor pulmonale**).
- Fluid overload or kidney failure.
- Venous disease (compromised valves in veins, obstruction, thrombophlebitis).
- Lymphatic pathology.
- Medication.
- Cirrhosis.
- Anemia.

FATIGUE OR WEAKNESS

- Left ventricular compromise (CAD, CHF, valvular disease, cardiomyopathy, myocarditis).
- Heart arrhythmic disorders.
- Cor pulmonale.
- Emotional factors: Depression, anxiety, stress.
- Sleep disorders or deprivation.
- Inadequate nutrition.
- Medications such as beta-blockers or other antihypertensive medication.
- Chemotherapy or radiation treatment.
- Chronic fatigue syndrome.
- Mitral valve prolapse.
- Deconditioning.

HEMOPTYSIS

- Pulmonary infections.
- TB.
- Bronchogenic carcinoma.
- Pulmonary infarction.
- Mitral stenosis.
- Eisenmenger syndrome.
- Aortic aneurysm.

LEG PAIN DURING ACTIVITY

- Peripheral artery disease.
- Arthritis of the hip, knee.
- Stress fractures or other musculoskeletal injuries (meniscal tear, muscle injury).
- Radiculopathy (sciatica, degenerative disk disease, disk herniation or bulge, spinal stenosis).
- Venous insufficiency.
- Anterior compartment syndrome.
- Neuropathy (neurologic disease such as peripheral vascular disease due to diabetes mellitus).

LIGHT-HEADEDNESS OR DIZZINESS

- Hypotension.
- Impaired cardiac output.
- Excess vasodilation that decreases venous return and cardiac output.
- Cerebral or vertebral artery insufficiency.
- Low blood sugar.

PALLOR OR CYANOSIS

- Decreased cardiac output.
- Decreased peripheral perfusion.
- Hypoxemia.
- Pulmonary disease.
- Congenital heart disease.
- Anemia.

PALPITATIONS

- Premature atrial contractions.
- PVCs.
- Atrial or ventricular tachycardia.
- Atrial fibrillation or flutter.

SYNCOPE

- Severe compromise of cardiac output.
- Cardiac arrhythmias.
- LV failure, obstruction, aortic stenosis, obstructive cardiomyopathy.
- Aortic dissection.
- Orthostatic hypotension, vasovagal reflex, Valsalva maneuver.
- Pulmonary embolus.
- Pulmonary hypertension.
- CVA.
- Hyperventilation.
- Low blood sugar.

■ DIAGNOSTIC TESTS AND IMAGING OF THE CARDIOVASCULAR/PULMONARY SYSTEMS

CHEST X-RAY (RADIOGRAPH)

- Reveals rib cage for possible fractures, size of heart, vessels, and respiratory airways.
- Can look at the clarity of lungs and can show evidence of fluid.
- Reveals abnormal tissues, densities, infection, or foreign materials.
- Lung volumes can be analyzed; rib cage expansion can show possible pneumothorax, collapse, hemothorax, or effusion. Overinflation from disease processes can be seen. For comparison, a normal chest x-ray is shown in Figure 4-28.

COMPUTED TOMOGRAPHY

- Computed tomography (CT) scans can be used for specific diseases or diagnostic procedures.
- Uses the same ionizing radiation as radiographs but is more rapid and more detailed. Image slices are created in an axial plane. Figure 4-29 illustrates a CT scan of the chest.

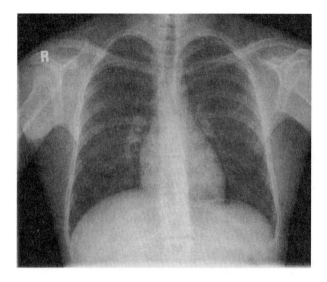

Figure 4-28. **Normal chest x-ray.** (Reproduced with permission from Burke-Doe A, Dutton M, eds. *National Physical Therapy Examination and Board Review*. 2019. Copyright © McGraw Hill LLC. All rights reserved. https://accessphysiotherapy.mhmedical.com.)

- Provides excellent images of lungs, vasculature, and heart.
- Newer software can produce three-dimensional images and detect small calcification buildup in the coronary arteries (Figure 4-30).

ECHOCARDIOGRAM

- Noninvasive procedure that uses ultrasound to produce images.
- Air affects the transmission of ultrasound waves, and therefore it is limited in use for the chest; it is primarily used for heart imaging.

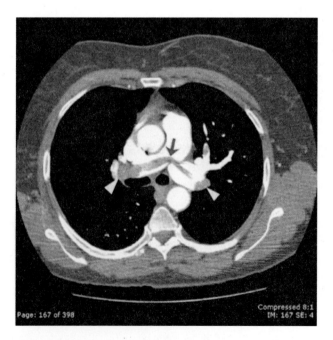

Figure 4-29. **Example of contrast CT angiogram of the chest. Contrast CT angiogram of the chest showing a "saddle" pulmonary embolism (red arrow) as well as filling defects in the left and right pulmonary artery branches (yellow arrowheads) secondary to obstruction by thromboembolic materials.** (Reproduced with permission from Lechner AJ, Matuschak GM, Brink DS, et al., eds. *Respiratory: An Integrated Approach to Disease*. 2012. Copyright © McGraw Hill LLC. https://accessmedicine.mhmedical.com.)

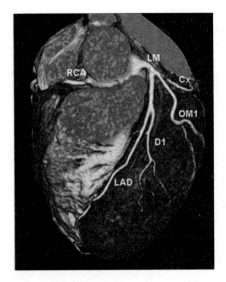

Figure 4-30. **3D image of the heart.** (Reproduced with permission from De Cecco CN, Meinel FG, Chiaramida SA, et al. Coronary Artery Computed Tomography Scanning. *Circulation*. 2014:129:1341-45.)

- Produces real-time video of internal heart structures, size of heart chambers, valve function, and normal or abnormal heart wall movement.

RADIONUCLIDE IMAGING

- Ventilation-perfusion (V/Q) scanning is used to diagnose pulmonary embolism.
- Radioactive tracers are introduced into the bloodstream, and images reveal areas of perfusion. Inert gases are inhaled to show areas of ventilation.
- Images are compared to show where there is a mismatch of V/Q.
- Positron emission tomography (PET) scans are a type of radionuclide scanning and are primarily used to detect the spread of lung cancer to the lymph nodes.

CARDIAC CATHETERIZATION

- Hollow tube (catheter) is introduced to the brachial or femoral artery and is guided toward the aorta and heart vessels and then into the coronary arteries.
- Contrast dye is injected into the catheter, and x-rays are taken.
- Heart vessels, chambers, walls, and valves can be examined and the determination of ejection fraction percentage.

SWAN–GANZ CATHETER

- A central catheter is introduced from the venous system to the right side of the heart (Figure 4-31).
- Pressures can be monitored, such as central venous pressure (CVP) and pressures at the pulmonary artery.

MAGNETIC RESONANCE IMAGING

- Usedhh primarily to evaluate soft tissues of the chest cavity. Figure 4-32 shows a gated-3D-MRA image of the chest.
- Using magnetic energy instead of ionizing radiation.
- Produces higher-quality images in various planes (axial and coronal) but takes more time (up to an hour) than less than a minute for CT scan and considered to be more financially costly than other imaging tests.

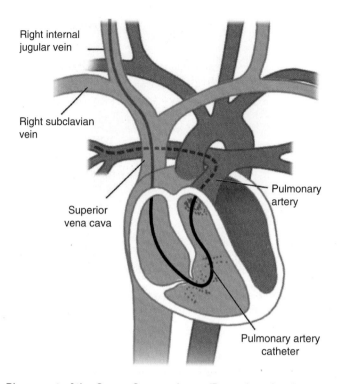

Figure 4-31. Placement of the Swan–Ganz catheter. (Reproduced with permission from Reichman EF, ed. *Reichman's Emergency Medicine Procedures*, 3rd ed. 2019. Copyright © McGraw Hill LLC. All rights reserved. https://accessemergencymedicine.mhmedical.com.)

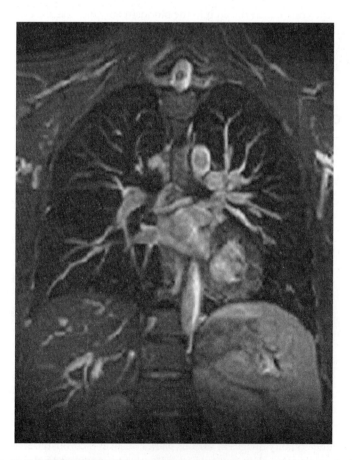

Figure 4-32. Gated-3D-FSE MRA image of the chest. (Reproduced with permission from Allen D. Elster, MRIQuestions.com.)

■ MEDICAL MANAGEMENT OF THE CARDIOVASCULAR/ PULMONARY SYSTEM

The following conditions explain the medical management for common cardiopulmonary pathologies. A patient may be diagnosed with one of the following conditions; however, it is common for aging patients with diabetes mellitus and obesity to have multiple cardiopulmonary diagnoses.

PERCUTANEOUS CORONARY INTERVENTION

- Percutaneous coronary intervention (PCI) is known as percutaneous transluminal coronary angioplasty (PTCA).
- Used for increasing blood flow and revascularization in instances of blockage of the coronary arteries.
- A balloon-tipped catheter is placed into the heart vessel and is inflated, increasing vessel diameter. Improved blood flow decreases angina, improves the effects of CAD with increased coronary blood flow.
- The walls may be reinforced with intravascular stents (wire mesh).

CORONARY ARTERY BYPASS GRAFT

- Vessels from another site (L or R internal thoracic, radial, or femoral artery) are used to bypass an area of blockage. Grafted tissue from the saphenous vein is also common; however, it has led to some concerns with graft site atherosclerosis during cardiac rehabilitation and disease prevention phases.
- Two types of CABG are performed:
  - Traditional CABG.
    - Sternotomy is required; the patient is placed on a heart-lung machine, and the heart is emptied and stopped.
    - Heart is protected via hypothermia in cardioplegic solution (K^+ with oxygenated blood) at a temperature of 4°C.
  - Mid CABG.
    - Sternotomy is not required.
    - Heart-lung machine is not used.
    - Cardioplegia is not used, and surgery is performed while the heart is still beating.

INTRA-AORTIC BALLOON PUMP

- Assists in blood flow from the left ventricle. Essentially creates suction to draw blood from the LV to increase systemic and coronary blood flow. Figure 4-33 presents a diagram of an intra-aortic balloon pump (IABP) with inflation of the balloon during diastole and deflation during systole.

LUNG SURGERIES

- Pneumonectomy: Removal of entire left or right lung.
- Lobectomy: Removal of one lobe section of a lung.
- Thoracotomy: Incision used to perform lung resections at the fourth intercostal space.

HEART AND LUNG TRANSPLANTS

Heart and lung transplants can be performed by replacing the recipient's heart and lung with donor organs. Complications from heart and lung transplant are tissue rejection, infection, and compromised immune response due to patients taking immunosuppressive drugs.

- Heart transplant: Utilized in cases of an end-stage disease process such as severe damage from MI, valvular disease, or cardiomyopathy. There are two types of heart transplantation surgery:

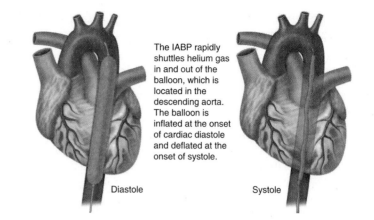

The IABP rapidly shuttles helium gas in and out of the balloon, which is located in the descending aorta. The balloon is inflated at the onset of cardiac diastole and deflated at the onset of systole.

Diastole   Systole

Figure 4-33. **The ins and outs of the intra-aortic balloon pump (IABP).** (Reproduced with permission from Burke-Doe A, Dutton M, eds. *National Physical Therapy Examination and Board Review*. 2019. Copyright © McGraw Hill LLC. All rights reserved. https://accessphysiotherapy .mhmedical.com.)

- Heterotopic transplantation:
  - Rarely performed; used in instances of cardiac dysfunction and pulmonary hypertension.
  - Recipient heart is left in place, and a donor's heart is placed in a "piggyback" procedure in the right chest.
- Orthotopic:
  - Most common.
  - Diseased heart is removed and replaced with a donor's heart.
  - Midsternotomy incision is utilized by creating an incision down the length of the sternum, and the chest cavity is opened. The sternum is wired after surgery, and sternal precautions are observed postsurgery.
- Lung transplant:
  - Single-lung or double-lung/bilateral sequential lung transplantation can replace the recipient lung with the donor organ.

■ COMMON LABORATORY TESTS AND VALUES

Clinical laboratory studies assist the practitioner in determining the clinical status of a patient. Tables 4-9 through 4-11 provide values for laboratory tests typically used in assessing patients with cardiac dysfunction.

■ INTERVENTIONS

Physical therapists and physical therapist assistants, as movement specialists, are essential in mobilization and exercise as early as possible in the rehabilitation process. Bed exercises, bed mobility, transfers, ambulation, and functional activities significantly help to decrease the negative effects of bed rest and immobility.

AEROBIC CARDIAC EXERCISE PRESCRIPTION

The cardiac patient must participate in aerobic exercise regimens specific to their diagnosis. In general, the cardiac patient (being monitored by a cardiologist, nurse practitioner, or physician assistant) rehabilitating from cardiac surgery, myocardial infarction, or other cardiopulmonary condition will participate in a rehabilitation program. The following information provides general exercise regimens specific to cardiac rehabilitation.

Adequate Warm-Up

- Mode: Light-intensity aerobic (walking), light calisthenics, and stretching.
- Duration: 5 to 10 minutes.

TABLE 4-9 • Laboratory Tests and Values	
Test	**Referenced Normal Value**
CBC (Complete Blood Count)	
RBC (red blood cell)	Male: 4.35–5.65 trillion cells/L[a] Female: 3.92–5.13 trillion cells/L
Hgb (hemoglobin)	Male: 13.2–16.6 g/dL[b] Female: 11.6–15 g/dL
Hct (hematocrit)	Male: 38.3–48.6 percent Female: 35.5–44.9 percent
WBC (white blood cell)	3.4–9.6 billion cells/L
Platelet count	Male: 135–317 billion/L (135,000–317,000/mcL[c]) Female: 157–371 billion/L (157,000–371,000/mcL)
BMP (Basic Metabolic Panel)	
Calcium	9–11 mg/dL
Chloride	95–105 mEq/L[d]
Sodium	135–145 mEq/L
Potassium	3.5–5.0 mEq/L
Creatinine	0.5–1.2 mg/dL
BUN (blood urea nitrogen)	10–20
Albumin	3.2–4.8 g/L
Glucose	70–110 mg/dL
Magnesium	1.5–2.5 mEq/L
Anticoagulant and Clotting Factors	
PT	9.0–11.7 seconds
PTT (heparin monitoring)	55.0–75.0 seconds
INR	≤ 1.1 normal (2.0–3.0 is general effective therapeutic range when taking warfarin for A-fibrillation or blood clot in the leg or lung)
ABG (Arterial Blood Gas) values	
pH (blood acid-base balance)	Normal value 7.40 Normal adult range 7.35–7.45 Patient will have **acidemia** with pH < 7.35 and **alkalemia** with pH >7.45.
$PaCO_2$ (mm Hg) (alveolar hyperventilation value)	Normal value 40 Normal adult range 35–45 (**eucapnia**) Elevated $PaCO_2$ is referred to as **hypercapnia.** Low $PaCO_2$ is referred to as **hypocapnia.**
PaO_2 (mm Hg) (alveolar hypoventilation value)	Normal value 97 Normal range >80 Low PaO2 is referred to as **hypoxemia.** **Hypoxia** means a patient has low level of O2 in tissue yet adequate perfusion of tissue.
HCO_3 (mEq/L) (bicarbonate)	Normal value 24 Normal adult range 22–28
SaO_2 (percent oxygen saturation of hemoglobin)	95–98%

[a]L = Liter.

[b]dL = deciliter.

[c]mcL = microliter.

[d]mEq/L = milliequivalents per liter.

TABLE 4-10 • Cardiac Enzymes.

	Normal Serum Level Values (IU)[a]	Onset of Rise (hours)	Time of Peak Rise (hours)	Return to Normal (days)
CPK	55-71[b]	3-4	33	3
LDH	127[c]	12-24	72	5-14
SGOT	24	12	24	4
Troponin I	< 0.1 ng/mL	4-6	12-24	4-7
Troponin T	< 0.2 ng/mL	3-4	10-24	10-14

CPK, creatine phosphokinase; LDH, lactic dehydrogenase; SGOT, serum glutamic oxaloacetic transaminase.

[a]*1 IU is the amount of enzyme that will catalyze the formation of 1 μmol of substrate per minute under the conditions of the test.*

[b]*CPK-MB, 0%-3%.*

[c]*LDH-1, 14%-26%.*

Data from Smith AM, Theirer JA, Huang SH. Serum enzymes in myocardial infarction. *Am J Nurs.* 1973;73(2):277.

- Benefits: Gradually increases breathing, BP, and HR; decreases musculoskeletal injury while increasing muscle and tissue extensibility, flexibility, and range of motion (ROM). Patients with CV pathology may have decreased exercise response and delayed or impaired heart, lung, or vascular response.

Adequate Cool-Down Period

- Mode: Light aerobic activity such as walking or slow cycling.
- Duration: 5 to 10 minutes.
- Benefits: Return of breathing, HR, and BP to normal levels; prevents venous pooling, decreases lactic acid buildup.

MODE

The type of aerobic activity should be based on what a patient would enjoy and therefore be more motivated to participate in the exercise prescription. Aerobic exercise should incorporate large muscle groups used continuously in a rhythmical pattern.

- Walking, jogging on ground or treadmill.
- Cycling (stationary, recumbent, bike path/trail).
- Swimming.
- Aerobic equipment (elliptical, stair-stepper, rowing).
- Acute patients in hospital: Walking hospital floor, stationary bike, or treadmill at slow speeds.
- Outpatient or cardiac rehabilitation program: Incorporating multiple modes and varying exercise equipment can provide improved functional gains.

TABLE 4-11 • Normal Lipid Values.

Lipids	Low Risk (0-1 RF)	Moderate Risk (2 RF)	High Risk
Total cholesterol	< 200 mg/dL	< 200	< 200
LDL	< 160 mg/dL	< 100 optimal	< 100 (optimal < 70)
HDL	≥ 40 mg/dL Male ≥ 50 mg/dL Female		
VLDL	5-40 mg/dL		
Triglycerides	< 150 mg/dL		

HDL, high-density lipoprotein; LDL, low-density lipoprotein; VLDL, very-low-density lipoprotein.

Data from NCEP Expert Panel. Detection, Evaluation and Treatment of High Cholesterol in Adults (Adult Treatment Panel III). National Institutes on Health, Pub No.01-3670, May 2001.

Intensity

Commonly use 65% to 80% of maximum HR, approximately equal to 50% to 70% VO_2 max. Maximum HR is calculated at 220 minus patient age. Intensity can be prescribed in three categories:

- HR.
- Rate of perceived exertion (important to use for patients taking beta- or Ca^+ channel blockers).
- Metabolic equivalents (METs) of energy expenditure levels: Method that can be used to prescribe exercise and activity. The formula is based on 1 MET equaling the amount of energy used by the body at rest per kilogram of weight per minute. Walking at 3 miles/h (4.83 km/h) is equivalent to 3.3 METs.

Duration

The amount of time engaged in the exercise activity while maintaining the desired intensity.

- Acute and extremely deconditioned individuals may benefit from interval training. Two or three short bouts lasting 3 to 5 minutes with 1 to 2 minutes of rest between. Patients can add 1 to 2 minutes each session. Aim to increase to 10 minutes of continuous activity.
- Sedentary lifestyle: 10 to 20 minutes, adding 1 to 2 minutes per day.
- Goal is to increase to 20 to 30 minutes if at moderate intensity and 40 to 60 minutes if at low intensity.
- Longer duration and lower intensity are effective for patients who have goals to reduce body fat, decrease claudication, or manage HTN.

Frequency

- For patients who can tolerate moderate activity, three to five sessions per week is the goal to improve conditioning.
- If exercise is less than 15 to 20 minutes, exercise two to three times per day.
- If exercise is greater than 20 minutes, exercise once a day for 3 to 7 days per week depending on the intensity.

Strength Training

- Light strength training should be incorporated into cardiac rehabilitation.
- Goal of a single set performed two times per week to increase strength.
- Light weights or use of resistive bands, incorporated with larger muscle group movement.
- UE exercises have greater demands than LE exercises. For example, arm cycling can increase HR, BP, and O_2 demands. Therefore, the patient may have decreased tolerance on the rate of perceived exertion (RPE) or onset of angina.

CARDIAC REHABILITATION PROGRAM

Cardiac rehabilitation regimens are key in helping cardiac patients heal from an acute cardiac event. Four phases of cardiac rehabilitation are presented below, and this is not to be confused with other common sources that present two phases of cardiac rehab. It is best to consider whether the patient is undergoing care in an inpatient or outpatient setting. The heart and relatable pulmonary tissue require proper healing time, and therefore regimens will differ per patient. The best practice for the physical therapist assistant will be to follow the physical therapist's prescribed protocol and provide consistent vital sign assessment while aware of a patient presenting with adverse signs to treatment interventions.

Phase I: Acute Phase (Monitoring Phase)

- Postoperation for heart surgery.[6]
- Members of the cardiac team include the following:
  - Physician (cardiac rehabilitation specialist), nurse practitioner, physician assistant, and nursing staff, to oversee patient management and risk factor modification.

- Physical therapy for early mobilization and functional mobility and activities, exercise progression.
- Occupational therapist for self-care and management, activities of daily living, bathing, dressing, grooming, home management, occupational roles.
- Dietician for dietary modifications and risk factor management.
- Duration: Hospital stay 3 to 5 days.
- Patient is monitored closely 24 hours a day.
- Early mobilization (day 1 to 2 postoperation/event).
  - Monitor patient's response through continued use of RPE and vital sign assessment.
  - Decrease risks from bed rest (blood clots, skin breakdown, respiratory illness).
  - Spirometry.
  - Bed mobility, sitting at the edge of the bed, transfers.
  - Frequency: Mobilize two to four times per day as tolerated and prescribed by the physician and physical therapist.
- Day 3+.
  - Ambulation 2 to 3 times per day.
  - Self-care, toileting, hygiene.
  - Progress to ambulation of stairs to prepare for discharge.
  - Time: Intermittent 3- to 5-minute bouts of activity, 1 to 2 minutes rest.
- Sternal precautions.
  - No pressure on the sternum.
  - Encourage use of pillow braced against sternum if coughing or if the patient struggles with transitioning from supine to seated positions.
  - No bilateral shoulder flexion and abduction greater than 90 degrees.
  - No UE-resisted activity.
  - Avoid or be cautious of activity that causes Valsalva maneuver.
  - No car driving or passenger seat riding for 4 weeks (danger from airbag deployment).
- Care for LE incision site.
  - Patient is allowed to be weight-bearing as tolerated, and no ROM restrictions if healing normally.
  - Patient should avoid crossing legs.
  - Patient should wear compression garments and elevate legs.

Phase II: Subacute Phase (Conditioning Phase)

- Goals of Phase II[6]:
  - Improve exercise ability and endurance safely.
  - Continue exercise program and monitor CV response.
  - Prepare patient to monitor self and continue at home.
  - Educate patient on disease process, rehabilitation process, and on making changes in lifestyle.
- Mode: Common aerobic activity of walking or use of a stationary bike (biking with use of UE is appropriate if sternal precautions have been discontinued and a sternotomy has healed).
- Intensity: Interval training at 40% to 60% max HR. If the patient shows appropriate CV response, increase target HR by 10 beats/min each week.
- Frequency: Five to seven sessions of exercise done over 3 weeks.
- Duration: Initial: 10 to 15 minutes of low-level exercise in 2- to 5-minute bouts, working toward 20 to 30 minutes of continuous LE work.
- Discharge criteria:
  - Medically stable with no EKG monitor required.
  - Patient can self-monitor signs and symptoms.
  - Independent and compliant with a home exercise program (HEP).
  - Goal of 9 MET capacity (5 MET needed for self-care at home); MET levels are prescribed specifically to each patient.
  - Patient passes a maximum symptom-limited exercise test.

Phase III: Training and Maintenance Phase (Intensive Rehabilitation) and Phase IV: Disease Prevention Phase (Prevention Programs)

- Patient continues to attend outpatient centers or community centers with a cardiac rehabilitation program.[6]
- Patient is screened with an exercise stress test or can also use a 6-minute walk test.
- Frequency: 4 to 6 days/week is recommended along with the patient's HEP. If MET is less than 4, then multiple brief day sessions are recommended.
- Intensity:
  - Warm-up 5 to 10 minutes.
  - Target 40% to 60% VO_2 max to progress to 75% if able.
- Mode: Large muscle groups (walking on treadmill or track, cycling).
- Time: Accumulate 30 to 60 minutes of aerobic exercise. Low-functioning patients can use a 1:1 ratio of exercise to rest for 3 to 10 minutes.
- Goals:
  - Higher level of physical and mental functioning.
  - Continue lifelong habits of exercise and risk factor reduction.
  - Measure and assess progress and disease stability.
  - Enhance quality of life.

SPECIAL CONSIDERATIONS (PRECAUTIONS AND CONTRAINDICATIONS)

Heart Failure

- Patients may not tolerate supine or prone positions due to orthopnea and dyspnea in these positions.[6]
- Exercise can improve impaired blood flow due to vasoconstriction and impaired muscle function.
- Exercise intervals and increasing duration and number of bouts can be effective in improving exercise tolerance.

Pacemakers and Implanted Defibrillators

- Upper extremity exercises are restricted until after 6 weeks of placement or implantation.
- HR should be maintained 10 to 15 beats/min below the threshold for the device to prevent administration of shock due to tachycardia.

Arrhythmias

- Atrial fibrillation (AF) is the most common form of arrhythmia.
- New onset of AF is a contraindication to exercise.
- Ectopic ventricular beats that worsen during exercise are cause for ceasing activity and monitoring the patient.

Diabetes

- Screen the patient for vascular complications and symptoms such as retinopathy or peripheral neuropathy.
- It is important to monitor the patient's feet frequently and for the patient to wear properly fitted footwear.
- Encourage 30 g carbohydrate intake before exercise if blood glucose is less than 4 mmol/L (< 72 mg/dL).
- Intensity of 50% to 60% VO_2 max, three to four times per week for 30 to 60 minutes, has shown improved insulin sensitivity and metabolism of carbohydrates.

PULMONARY REHABILITATION AND INTERVENTIONS

Diaphragmatic Breathing

It is important to teach proper breathing techniques if improper breathing patterns are being used or an acute panic episode occurs. Diaphragmatic breathing is also called pursed-lip breathing. This technique involves first instructing the patient to place their hand on the abdomen just proximal to the umbilical area. The patient should then take a deep, slow breath to expand the abdomen, followed by an active oral exhalation through narrow pursed lips (or narrowed mouth opening). This technique can be performed in many positions, but when newly instructing a patient, it is best to start in a supine or the semi-Fowler position and progress to sitting, standing, and ambulating. For the chronic COPD patient, this technique becomes a common way to control breathing and helps to prevent or delay airway collapse allowing for better gas exchange in the lung tissue.

Postural Drainage

Postural drainage is a technique used to assist in clearing secretions from the bronchus and lung segments. The patient is placed in various positions to optimize gravity-dependent positions, and percussion, vibration, and shaking techniques can be used in conjunction to assist in clearing secretions and providing airway clearance. Positions used for postural drainage are provided in Figure 4-34.

SKILL KEEPER: POSTURAL DRAINAGE

What are precautions and contraindications for postural drainage positions where the patient has the head lowered below horizontal? What are the precautions and contraindications for percussive techniques?

_____

_____

_____

_____

SKILL KEEPER ANSWERS

Postural drainage precautions and contraindications are presented in the table titled "Precautions for Postural Drainage."

Percussion

- Used in conjunction with postural drainage.
- Hands are in a cupped position, and light percussion is performed over the treated lung segment.

Vibration and Shaking

- Also used in conjunction with postural drainage.
- Different from percussion because vibration and shaking techniques are performed while the patient exhales.
- Vibration.
  - Differs from shaking and involves a higher-frequency force.
  - Therapist can place both hands on the front and back of the chest wall or place hands on top of one another.
  - Therapist cocontracts all muscles and applies a vibration pressure through the hands and to the chest wall.
- Shaking.
  - Force is more rigorous and bouncing action against the chest wall.
  - Produces compression force on the chest wall.

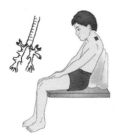

UPPER LOBES Apical segments

Bed or drainage table flat.

Patient leans back on pillow at 30° angle against therapist.

Therapist claps with markedly cupped hand over area between clavicle and top of scapula on each side.

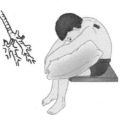

UPPER LOBES Posterior segments

Bed or drainage table flat.

Patient leans over folded pillow at 30° angle.

Therapist stands behind and claps over upper back on both sides.

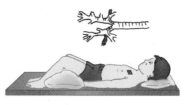

UPPER LOBES Anterior segments

Bed or drainage table flat.

Patient lies on back with pillow under knees.

Therapist claps between clavicle and nipple on each side.

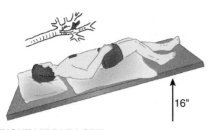
16"

RIGHT MIDDLE LOBE

Foot of table or bed elevated 16 inches.

Patient lies head down on left side and rotates 1/4 turn backward. Pillow may be placed behind from shoulder to hip. Knees should be flexed.

Therapist claps over right nipple area. In females with breast development or tenderness use cupped hand with heel of hand under armpit and fingers extending forward beneath the breast.

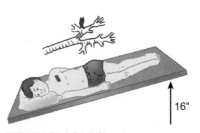
16"

LEFT UPPER LOBE Singular segments

Foot of table or bed elevated 16 inches.

Patient lies head down on right side and rotates 1/4 turn backward. Pillow may be placed behind from shoulder to hip. Knees should be flexed.

Therapist claps with moderately cupped hand over left nipple area. In females with breast development or tenderness use cupped hand with heel of hand under armpit and fingers extending forward beneath the breast.

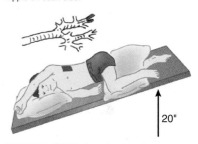
20"

LOWER LOBES Anterior basal segments

Foot of table or bed elevated 20 inches.

Patient lies on side, head down, pillow under knees.

Therapist claps with slightly cupped hand over lower ribs. (Position shown is for drainage of left anterior basal segment. To drain the right anterior basal segment, patient should be on the left side in same posture.)

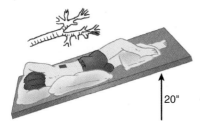
20"

LOWER LOBES Lateral basal segments

Foot of table or bed elevated 20 inches.

Patient lies on abdomen, head down, then rotates 1/4 turn upward. Upper leg is flexed over pillow for support.

Therapist claps over uppermost portion of lower ribs. (Position shown is for drainage of right lateral basal segment. To drain the left lateral basal segment, patient should lie on the right side in the same posture.)

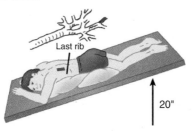
Last rib
20"

LOWER LOBES Posterior basal segments

Foot of table or bed elevated 20 inches.

Patient lies on abdomen, head down, with pillow under hips.

Therapist claps over lower ribs close to spine on each side.

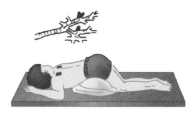

LOWER LOBES Superior segments

Bed of table flat.

Patient lies on abdomen with two pillows under hips.

Therapist claps over middle of back at tip of scapula on either side of spine.

Figure 4-34. **Positions for postural drainage and bronchial hygiene.** (Reproduced with permission from Burke-Doe A, Dutton M, eds. *National Physical Therapy Examination and Board Review*. 2019. Copyright © McGraw Hill LLC. All rights reserved. https://accessphysiotherapy.mhmedical.com.)

PRECAUTIONS FOR POSTURAL DRAINAGE

Avoid Trendelenburg position:

- When a patient has pulmonary hypertension due to CHF.
- Suffers from pulmonary edema or shortness of breath.
- Has abdominal distention, hiatal hernia, nausea, abdominal obesity, or has recently consumed food.

Possibly avoid side-lying position:

- History of axillofemoral bypass graft.
- Musculoskeletal arthritis, rib fractures, shoulder bursitis, or tendinopathy.

Avoid any position making a patient uncomfortable.

Airway Clearance and Secretion Management

SKILL KEEPER: AIRWAY CLEARANCE AND SECRETION MANAGEMENT

What is the difference between huff and cough? What are the reasons a physical therapist assistant might use one technique over the other?

_____

_____

_____

_____

SKILL KEEPER ANSWERS

A cough is a self-defense mechanism to protect the lungs and keep them free of excessive sputum and foreign particles. A huff is similar to a cough, but the glottis does not close entirely, and the exhaling pressure is a rapid and forced exhalation. Both huff and cough are presented in the corresponding section of this chapter.

- Huff.
  - Similar to coughing, but the glottis remains open.
  - Patient exhales as if trying to produce mist/condensation on a mirror.
  - It is a rapid and forced exhalation without maximal effort.
- Cough.
  - Coughing is an important self-defense mechanism to protect the lungs and the most important component of helping to keep a clean airway.
  - Consists of a voluntary closing of the glottis and the buildup of intrathoracic and intra-abdominal pressure behind the glottis. A sudden release of the pressure with the glottis opening produces the cough, which causes forceful air pressure to remove secretions or foreign particles.
  - Manually assisted cough.
    - Costophrenic assist.
    - Heimlich-type assist.
    - Anterior chest compression assist.
- Self-assisted cough.
  - Prone on elbows.
  - Long-sitting.
  - Short-sitting.
  - Rocking (hands-knees) position.

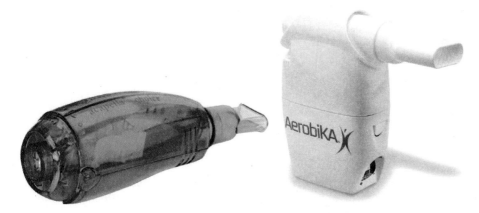

Figure 4-35. Mechanical devices for bronchial hygiene therapy. (Aerobika® Oscillating Positive Expiratory Pressure Therapy System (OPEP). Image used with permission from Monaghan Medical Corporation. © 2021 Monaghan Medical Corporation. All rights reserved; acapella® Choice Vibratory PEP Therapy System. Image used with permission from Smiths Medical. © 2021 Smiths Medical. All rights reserved.)

Mechanical Devices and Adjuncts

- Positive expiratory pressure (PEP) devices.
  - Provides constant pressure at 10 to 20 cm of H_2O.
  - Splints airways open and improves collateral ventilation.
- Oscillating PEP devices (Flutter, TheraPep, Acapella).
  - Similar to PEP device and provides positive pressure (10-35 cm of H_2O) that oscillates due to a steel ball contained in the device. Figure 4-35 illustrates various oscillating PEP (OPEP) devices for use in airway clearance.

High-Frequency Chest Compression Devices

- Mechanically powered devices are available to assist in vibration and shaking force application. For example, an inflatable vest with air channels within the material worn over the patient's thorax. The vest is connected to an air compressor, which delivers the vibration and shaking forces.
  - Pressure oscillates at varying duration rates.
  - Cough-like shear force increases mucus stabilization.

Active Cycle of Breathing Technique

The active cycle of breathing technique (ACBT) is a breathing and air clearance technique that a patient can perform independently when properly instructed. The three major components include (a) breathing control (BC), (b) thoracic expansion exercises (TEE), and (c) forced expiratory technique (FET).

- BC.
  - Patient focuses on tidal volume breaths and uses diaphragmatic breathing to focus on lower rib cage expansion.
- TEE.
  - Patient takes in a maximal inspiration.
  - Patient can hold breath for 3 seconds and add an extra inhalation through the nose (encourages collateral ventilation to help reinflate collapsed alveoli).
  - Therapist can also add vibration or shaking during expiration.
- FET.
  - Patient performs huff to assist in movement and removal of secretions followed by breathing control.

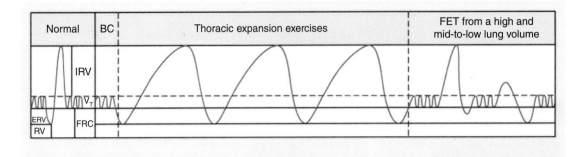

Figure 4-36. Active cycle of breathing technique (ACBT). BC, breathing control; ERV, expiratory reserve volume; FET, forced expiration technique; FRC, functional residual capacity; IRV, inspiratory reserve volume; RV, residual volume. (Reproduced with permission from, Savci S, Ince DI, Arikan H. A Comparison of Autogenic Drainage and the Active Cycle of Breathing Techniques in Patients with Chronic Obstructive Pulmonary Diseases. *Cardiopulm Rehabil.* 2000;20(1):37-43.)

- Patient performs a couple of low- to mid-volume huffs to move secretions in the periphery and from the smaller airways.
- Patient can then finish with a high-volume huff to clear the secretions in the larger airways and the upper airways.
- Cycle completes with a high-volume huff or cough.
- ACBT cycles stop when there is a nonproductive cough or patient fatigues.

Depending on which segments are involved, various forms of BC, TEE, and FET are used in combination to clear lower, mid, and upper segments as well as peripheral and central airways. In addition, external devices can be used to aid in secretion clearance. Figure 4-36 presents a diagram illustrating the components of ACBT.

EXERCISE PRESCRIPTION FOR PULMONARY REHABILITATION

Diaphragm Strengthening

- Deep breathing exercises for 10 to 15 minutes several times a day.
- Use of weights on the abdomen can give resistance to inspiration and assists in expelling air.

Thoracic Stretching

- Trunk twisting, proprioceptive neuromuscular facilitation (PNF), towel stretches, rib blocking. Figure 4-37 demonstrates a PNF exercise for stretching the thoracic cage.

Exercise for Breathing

- Resistance breathing exercises such as Active Cycle of Breathing Techniques (ACBT). (Active cycle of breathing is represented in Figure 4-38).

Aerobic Training

- Frequency: Recommended patients participate at least three times per week, two of which are supervised to monitor and increase the intensity, facilitate compliance, and encourage patient progress.
- Intensity:
  - Sixty percent maximum workforce for 30 minutes is recommended; however, patients may not tolerate this recommended intensity.

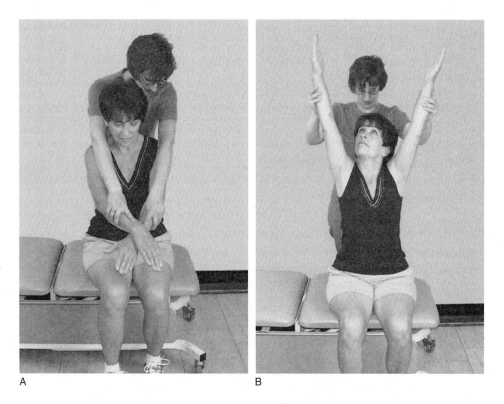

A   B

Figure 4-37. Proprioceptive neuromuscular facilitation techniques for thoracic stretching. (Reproduced with permission from O'Sullivan SB, Schmitz TJ, eds. *Improving Functional Outcomes in Physical Rehabilitation*, 2nd ed. 2016. Copyright © FA Davis. All rights reserved. https://fadavispt.mhmedical.com.)

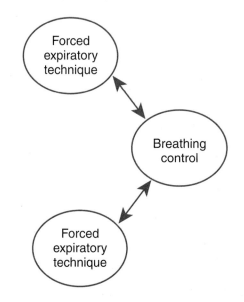

Figure 4-38. This illustration represents the active cycle of breathing. The exercise includes three phases; a breathing control phase, followed by thoracic expansion, and ends with forced expiration. (Reproduced with permission from O'Sullivan S, Schmitz T, Fulk, G. *Physical Rehabilitation*, 7th ed. 2019. Copyright © F.A. Davis. All rights reserved.)

- Interval training protocols have been developed incorporating high-intensity bouts and recovery periods.
- Eighty percent average speed achieved on 6-minute walk test or 75% peak speed on shuttle walk test.
- Sixty percent peak workforce on a cycle ergometer.
- Patients should work within a 3 to 5 on the modified (moderate to severe) Borg dyspnea scale.
- Type: Walking exercise on ground surface or treadmill and/or cycling.
- Time: Recommended 20 to 30 minutes.
- Duration: There are greater benefits for a longer-term exercise program of 6 months versus a shorter duration of 12 weeks.

Resistance Training

- Frequency: Recommend two to three times per week with a day off to allow for recovery and decrease postexercise muscle soreness.
- 50% to 60% of one-repetition maximum (RM).
- Type: Large muscle groups of the upper/lower extremity and trunk, starting with the use of light resistance (weights, resistance bands, or machines).
- Progression: Increases of 70% to 85% 1-RM performing one to two sets with 8 to 12 repetitions.

Functional Training, Work Modification, and Energy Conservation

- Teach positions that relieve dyspnea:
  - Sitting leaning forward with hands or elbows supported on thighs, or leaning forward over the table.
  - Standing and leaning forward over the table, or leaning with back against a wall with hands supported on the thighs.
  - Walking and leaning forward with forearms on a shopping cart or tall walker.
- Use of a four-wheel walker or Rollator walker allows the patient to lean on a walker for support and also provides a chair to sit on when fatigued or short of breath (SOB).
- Overhead activities or overuse of arms can cause increased SOB.
- Adapt work for improved ventilation for air movement as well as proper posture for good breathing mechanics.
- Relaxation techniques:
  - Jacobsen progressive relaxation exercises.
  - Biofeedback to control HR, breathing, BP.
  - Yoga or meditation.
  - Guided imagery or visualization.
  - Smartphone and smartwatch applications for reminders on frequent short-duration relaxation activities.

■ RELEVANT PHARMACOLOGY

In addition to the expanded pharmacology section in Appendix D, Tables 4-12 through 4-16 outline the more common drugs prescribed for patients with cardiopulmonary conditions.

TABLE 4-12 • Pulmonary Medications.

Therapeutic class: Antihistamines

Pharmacology class: H₁ receptor blockers	**Indications***: Allergic rhinitis, motion sickness, urticaria, angioedema *H₁ receptor blockers prescribed varies by diagnosis **Adverse effects:** Drowsiness, dry eyes, dry mouth, vision impairment, low blood pressure, dizziness, and headache

Medications: Generic names (trade names)

Brompheniramine (Dimetapp, others)
Chlorpheniramine (Chlor-Trimeton, others)
Clemastine (Tavist)
Dexchlorpheniramine (Dexchlor, Poladex, others)
Dimenhydrinate (Dramamine)
Diphenhydramine (Benadryl, others)
Promethazine (Phenergan)
Acrivastine with pseudoephedrine (Semprex-D)
Azelastine (Astelin, Astepro)
Cetirizine (Zyrtec)
Desloratadine (Clarinex)
Fexofenadine (Allegra)
Levocetirizine (Xyzal)
Loratadine (Claritin)
Olopatadine (Patanase)

Pharmacology class: Intranasal corticosteroids	**Indications***: Allergic rhinitis *Intranasal corticosteroids prescribed varies by diagnosis **Adverse effects:** Burning sensation after application, drying of the nasal mucosa

Medications: Generic names (trade names)

Beclomethasone (Beconase AQ, Qnasl, QVAR)
Budesonide (Rhinocort)
Ciclesonide (Omnaris, Zetonna)
Flunisolide
Fluticasone (Flonase, Veramyst)
Mometasone (Nasonex)
Triamcinolone (Nasacort AQ)

Pharmacology class: Decongestants	**Indications***: Nasal congestion *Decongestants prescribed varies by diagnosis **Adverse effects:** Rebound congestion

Medications: Generic names (trade names)

Naphazoline (Privine)	
Oxymetazoline (Afrin, Neo-Synephrine)	
Phenylephrine (Afrin, Neo-Synephrine)	
Pseudoephedrine (Sudafed, others)	
Tetrahydrozoline (Tyzine)	
xylometazoline (Otrivin)	
Pharmacology class: Beta-adrenergic agonist	**Indications***: Acute bronchospasm, asthma *Beta-adrenergic agonist prescribed varies by diagnosis **Adverse effects:** Palpitations, headaches, throat irritation, tremor nervousness, restlessness, tachycardia

(Continued)

TABLE 4-12 • Pulmonary Medications. (*Continued*)	
Medications: Generic names (trade names)	
Albuterol (Proventil HFA, Ventolin, VoSpire ER) Arformoterol (Brovana) Formoterol (Foradil, Perforomist) Indacaterol (Arcapta Neohaler) Levalbuterol (Xopenex) Olodaterol (Stiverdi Respimat) Salmeterol (Serevent) Terbutaline (Brethine)	
Pharmacology class: Anticholinergics	**Indications***: Chronic obstructive pulmonary disease (COPD) *Anticholinergics prescribed varies by diagnosis **Adverse effects:** Dry mouth, blurry vision, constipation, drowsiness, sedation
Medications: Generic names (trade names)	
Aclidinium (Tudorza Pressair) Ipratropium (Atrovent) Tiotropium (Spiriva) Umeclidinium (Incruse Ellipta)	
Pharmacology class: Xanthine	**Indications***: Acute bronchospasm, asthma *Xanthine prescribed varies by diagnosis **Adverse Effects:** Anxiety, nervousness, tremor, headache, dizziness
Medications: Generic names (trade names)	
Aclidinium (Tudorza Pressair)	
Ipratropium (Atrovent)	
Pharmacology class: Inhaled corticosteroids	**Indications***: Inflammation in asthma *Inhaled corticosteroids prescribed varies by diagnosis **Adverse Effects:** Cough, sore throat
Medications: Generic names (trade names)	
Beclomethasone (Qvar) Budesonide (Pulmicort Flexhaler) Ciclesonide (Alvesco) Fluticasone (Arnuity Ellipta, Flovent Diskus) Mometasone (Asmanex)	
Pharmacology class: Mast cell stabilizers	**Indications***: Inflammation in asthma *Mast cell stabilizers prescribed varies by diagnosis **Adverse effects:** Headaches, nasal irritation, cough, wheezing, dizziness, nausea, drowsiness
Medications: Generic names (trade names)	
Cromolyn	
Pharmacology class: Leukotriene modifiers	**Indications***: Inflammation in asthma *Leukotriene modifiers prescribed varies by diagnosis **Adverse effects:** Upper respiratory infection, fever, headache, sore throat, cough, stomach pain, diarrhea, runny nose, flu, and sinus infection
Medications: Generic names (trade names)	
Montelukast (Singulair) Roflumilast (Daliresp) Zafirlukast (Accolate) Zileuton (Zyflo)	

TABLE 4-13 · Medications for Dyslipidemia.

Therapeutic class: Antihyperlipidemic

Pharmacology class: HMG-CoA reductase inhibitors (statins)	**Indications***: Hyperlipidemia *HMG-CoA reductase inhibitors prescribed varies by diagnosis **Adverse effects:** Gastrointestinal disturbances (cramping, diarrhea, constipation), muscle injury (rhabdomyolysis)

Medications: Generic names (trade names)

Atorvastatin (Lipitor)
Fluvastatin (Lescol)
Lovastatin (Altoprev, Mevacor)
Pitavastatin (Livalo)
Pravastatin (Pravachol)
Rosuvastatin (Crestor)
Simvastatin (Zocor)

Pharmacology class: Bile acid binding drugs	**Indications***: Hyperlipidemia *Bile acid binding drugs prescribed varies by diagnosis **Adverse effects:** Gastrointestinal disturbances (constipation, bloating, gas, nausea

Medications: Generic names (trade names)

Cholestyramine (Questran)
Colesevelam (Welchol)
Colestipol (Colestid)

Pharmacology class:

Pharmacology class: Fibric acid drugs	**Indications***: Hyperlipidemia *Fibric acid drugs prescribed varies by diagnosis **Adverse effects:** Gastrointestinal disturbances (cramping, diarrhea, constipation)

Medications: Generic names (trade names)

Fenofibrate (Lofibra, Tricor)
Fenofibric acid (Fibricor, Trilipix)
Gemfibrozil (Lopid)

Pharmacology class: Other drugs for dyslipidemia

Medications: Generic names (trade names)

Alirocumab (Praluent)
Evolocumab (Repatha)
Ezetimibe (Zetia)
Icosapent ethyl (Vascepa)
Lomitapide (Juxtapid)
Mipomersen (Kynamro)
Niacin (Niaspan)
Omega-3-acid ethyl esters (Epanova, Lovaza)

TABLE 4-14 • Medications for Hypertension.

Therapeutic class: Diuretics

Pharmacology class: Diuretic	**Indications***: Mild hypertension *Diuretics prescribed varies by diagnosis **Adverse effects:** Hypotension, electrolyte imbalance (potassium, sodium, magnesium), hypokalemia

Medications: Generic names (trade names)

Amiloride (Midamor)
Bumetanide (Bumex)
Chlorothiazide (Diuril)
Chlorthalidone (Thalitone)
Eplerenone (Inspra)
Furosemide (Lasix)
Hydrochlorothiazide (Microzide)
Indapamide (Lozol)
Spironolactone (Aldactone)
Torsemide (Demadex)
Triamterene (Dyrenium)

Pharmacology Class: Angiotensin-converting enzyme Inhibitor (ACEI)	**Indications***: Hypertension and heart failure *ACEIs prescribed varies by diagnosis **Adverse effects:** Hypotension, persistent dry cough, headache, dizziness

Medications: Generic names (trade names)

Benazepril (Lotensin)
Captopril (Capoten)
Enalapril (Vasotec)
Fosinopril (Monopril)
Lisinopril (Prinivil, Zestril)
Moexipril (Univasc)
Perindopril (Aceon)
Quinapril (Accupril)
Ramipril (Altace)
Trandolapril (Mavik)

Pharmacology class: Angiotensin receptor blockers (ARBs)	**Indications***: Hypertension and heart failure *ARBs prescribed varies by diagnosis **Adverse effects:** Headache, dizziness, facial flushing

Medications: Generic names (trade names)

Azilsartan (Edarbi)
Candesartan (Atacand)
Eprosartan (Teveten)
Irbesartan (Avapro)
Losartan (Cozaar)
Olmesartan (Benicar)
Telmisartan (Micardis)
Valsartan (Diovan)

Pharmacology class: Calcium channel blocker	**Indications***: Hypertension and angina *Calcium channel blockers prescribed varies by diagnosis **Adverse effects:** Headache, dizziness, facial flushing, rebound hypotension

Medications: Generic names (trade names)

Amlodipine (Norvasc)
Diltiazem (Cardizem, Cartia XT, Dilacor XR)
Felodipine (Plendil)
Isradipine (DynaCirc)
Nicardipine (Cardene SR)
Nifedipine (Adalat CC, Procardia)
Nisoldipine (Sular)
Verapamil (Calan, Isoptin SR)

(Continued)

TABLE 4-14 • Medications for Hypertension. *(Continued)*

Pharmacology class: Adrenergic blockers and centrally acting drugs	**Indications***: Hypertension *Adrenergic blockers prescribed varies by diagnosis **Adverse effects:** Headache, dizziness, facial flushing, rebound hypotension

Medications: Generic names (trade names)

Acebutolol (Sectral)
Atenolol (Tenormin)
Betaxolol (Kerlone)
Bisoprolol (Zebeta)
Carvedilol (Coreg)
Clonidine (Catapres)
Doxazosin (Cardura)
Methyldopa (Aldomet)
Metoprolol (Lopressor, Toprol)
Nadolol (Corgard)
Pindolol (Visken)
Prazosin (Minipress)
Propranolol (Inderal, InnoPran XL)
Terazosin (Hytrin)
Timolol (Betimol, Timoptic)

Pharmacology class: Direct vasodilators	**Indications***: Hypertension *Direct vasodilators prescribed varies by diagnosis **Adverse effects:** Reflex tachycardia, sodium and water retention

Medications: Generic names (trade names)

Hydralazine (Apresoline)
Minoxidil (Loniten)
Nitroprusside (Nitropress)

TABLE 4-15 • Medications for Heart Failure.

Therapeutic class: Drugs for heart failure and hypertension

Pharmacology class: Angiotensin-converting enzyme inhibitors (ACEIs)	**Indications***: *ACEIs prescribed varies by diagnosis **Adverse effects:** Hypotension, persistent dry cough, headache, dizziness

Medications: Generic names (trade names)

Candesartan (Atacand)
Captopril (Capoten)
Enalapril (Vasotec)
Fosinopril (Monopril)
Lisinopril (Prinivil, Zestril)
Quinapril (Accupril)
Ramipril (Altace)
Valsartan (Diovan)

Pharmacology class: Diuretic	**Indications***: Mild hypertension, heart failure *Diuretics prescribed varies by diagnosis **Adverse effects:** Hypotension, electrolyte imbalance (potassium, sodium, magnesium), hypokalemia

Medications: Generic names (trade names)

Bumetanide (Burinex, Bumex)
Eplerenone (Inspra)
Furosemide (Lasix)
Hydrochlorothiazide (Microzide)
Spironolactone (Aldactone)
Torsemide (Demadex)

(Continued)

TABLE 4-15 · Medications for Heart Failure. (*Continued*)

Pharmacology class: Cardiac glycosides	**Indications***: Second-line drug for heart failure *Cardiac glycosides prescribed varies by diagnosis **Adverse effects:** Dysrhythmias, nausea, vomiting, anorexia, nervous system abnormalities (blurred vision)

Medications: Generic names (trade names)

Digoxin (Lanoxin, Lanoxicaps)

Pharmacology class: Beta-adrenergic blockers	**Indications***: Heart failure *Beta-adrenergic blockers prescribed varies by diagnosis **Adverse effects:** Back pain, bradycardia, dizziness, shortness of breath, fatigue, orthostatic hypotension, and weight gain

Medications: Generic names (trade names)

Carvedilol (Coreg)
Metoprolol (Lopressor, Toprol)

Pharmacology class: Direct-acting vasodilators	**Indications***: Heart failure *Direct-acting vasodilators prescribed varies by diagnosis **Adverse effects:** Reflex tachycardia, sodium and water retention

Medications: Generic names (trade names)

Hydralazine with isosorbide dinitrate (BiDi)
Nesiritide (Natrecor)

Pharmacology class: Phosphodiesterase inhibitors	**Indications***: Severe heart failure *Phosphodiesterase inhibitors prescribed varies by diagnosis **Adverse effects:** Ventricular dysrhythmia, headache, nausea, vomiting

Medications: Generic names (trade names)

Inamrinone (Inocor)
Milrinone (Primacor)

TABLE 4-16 · Medications for Coagulation and Hematologic Disorders.

Therapeutic class: Anticoagulants

Pharmacology class: Indirect thrombin inhibitor	**Indications***: Deep vein thrombosis, prevention of thrombi *Anticoagulants prescribed varies by diagnosis **Adverse effects:** Bleeding (gums, urine, stool), bruising

Medications: Generic names (trade names)

Antithrombin, recombinant (ATryn)
Apixaban (Eliquis)
Argatroban (Acova, Novastan)
Bivalirudin (Angiomax)
Dabigatran (Pradaxa)
Desirudin (Iprivask)
Edoxaban (Savaysa)
Fondaparinux (Arixtra)
Heparin
Pentoxifylline (Trental)
Rivaroxaban (Xarelto)
Warfarin (Coumadin)

Pharmacology class: Low-molecular-weight heparins	**Indications***: Prevention of deep vein thrombosis *Low-molecular-weight heparins prescribed varies by diagnosis **Adverse effects:** Bleeding (gums, urine, stool), bruising

(Continued)

TABLE 4-16 • Medications for Coagulation and Hematologic Disorders. (*Continued*)

Medications: Generic names (trade names)	
Dalteparin (Fragmin) Enoxaparin (Lovenox) Tinzaparin (Innohep)	
Pharmacology class: Antiplatelets	**Indications***: Essential thrombocythemia, inflammation pain, intermittent claudication, prevent thromboembolism *Antiplatelets prescribed varies by diagnosis **Adverse effects:** Bleeding

Medications: Generic names (trade names)	
Anagrelide (Agrylin) Aspirin (acetylsalicylic acid, ASA) Cilostazol (Pletal) Dipyridamole (Persantine) Vorapaxar (Zontivity)	
Pharmacology Class: Adenosine diphosphate (ADP) receptor blockers	**Indications***: Reduce the risk of stroke, myocardial infarction, and unstable angina *ADP receptor blockers prescribed varies by diagnosis **Adverse effects:** Flu-like syndrome, headache, diarrhea, dizziness, bruising, upper respiratory tract infection, and rash or pruritis

Medications: Generic names (trade names)	
Clopidogrel (Plavix)	
Prasugrel (Effient)	
Ticagrelor (Brilinta)	
Ticlopidine (Ticlid)	
Pharmacology Class: Glycoprotein IIB/IIIA blockers	**Indications***: Reduce the risk of cardiac events during percutaneous coronary intervention *Glycoprotein blockers prescribed varies by diagnosis **Adverse effects:** Gastric discomfort and bleeding

Medications: Generic names (trade names)	
Abciximab (ReoPro) Eptifibatide (Integrilin) Tirofiban (Aggrastat)	
Pharmacology class: Thrombolytics	**Indications***: Dissolving clots *Thrombolytics prescribed varies by diagnosis **Adverse effects:** Bruising, hematomas, nosebleeds

Medications: Generic names (trade names)	
Alteplase (Activase)	
Pharmacology class : Hemostatics	**Indications***: Control of bleeding where fibrinolysis contributes such as surgical complications prevent blood low, hemophilia *Hemostatics prescribed varies by diagnosis **Adverse effects:** Hypercoagulation

Medications: Generic names (trade names)	
Aminocaproic acid (Amicar) Thrombin (Evithrom, Recothrom, Thrombinar) Tranexamic acid (Cyklokapron, Lysteda)	

■ QUESTIONS

1. A 72-year-old patient has been diagnosed with atrial flutter and pneumonia and is resting in his room in the inpatient hospital. The physical therapist is going to evaluate the patient and is doing a chart review. In examining the patient's ECG/EKG cardiac strips, which of the following would indicate the patient's cardiac diagnosis?
   A. Sawtooth pattern
   B. Prolonged PR interval
   C. Absence of P wave
   D. Elevated ST segment

2. A 65-year-old patient is being seen at a Phase I cardiac rehabilitation program. She is being monitored for exercise response and tolerance. Which of the following symptoms would necessitate the ceasing of exercise activity?
   A. RPE of 9 (6-20 scale)
   B. Diastolic BP that remains the same level at rest and with exercise
   C. Persistent dyspnea and diaphoresis
   D. HR increases to 15 beats/min over resting rate

3. A physical therapist assistant is helping to conduct a community health education class for patients at risk for developing heart disease. One of the participants raises the question of cholesterol levels on her blood panel laboratory results and wants to understand better how the "bad" cholesterol links to atherosclerosis and CAD. Which would be the correct response?
   A. Elevated levels of high-density lipoprotein increase the risk of developing CAD.
   B. Elevated levels of low-density lipoprotein increase the risk of developing CAD.
   C. All cholesterol is bad, and totals should be below 200 mg/dL.
   D. Cholesterol is not an important factor in the risk for developing CAD, and the triglycerides should be kept low.

4. A patient is in the 4th week of Phase II of her cardiac rehabilitation program. The patient wants to engage in using the arm cycle ergometer for today's session. Which of the following responses would be expected to this exercise intervention?
   A. HR will be higher, but SBP would decrease.
   B. Exercise capacity is reduced due to higher SV.
   C. The primary effect would be increased SBP and diastolic blood pressure (DBP).
   D. Both the HR and SBP/DBP will be higher.

5. A home health physical therapist assistant works with an 85-year-old patient who returned home after a transient ischemic attack 3 days ago. The patient also has a diagnosis of HTN, dysrhythmias, COPD, osteoporosis, and mild dementia. Her husband is helping her at home, but they are confused about her discharge medications. She cannot remember if she took her BP medication earlier in the morning. Which of the following medications helps to regulate BP?
   A. Albuterol
   B. Prednisone
   C. Diltiazem
   D. Amiodarone

6. A physical therapist assistant is examining a patient who had an MI. The therapist is auscultating for the aortic valve. Which is the best placement for the stethoscope to auscultate the aortic valve?
   A. Second right intercostal space at the right sternal border
   B. Fourth intercostal space at the right sternal border
   C. Fourth intercostal space along the lower left sternal border
   D. Fifth intercostal space at the midclavicular line

7. A physical therapist assistant is working with a 20-year-old patient with cystic fibrosis. The therapist wants to use postural drainage techniques for the superior segments of the lower lobe. What is the correct position for this technique?

A. Sitting, leaning over a folded pillow at a 30-degree angle
B. Prone with two pillows under the hips
C. Supine with two pillows under knees
D. Head down on the left side, with one-quarter turn from supine

8. **A 64-year-old patient developed pulmonary embolism after right total knee replacement surgery. He presented with decreased O$_2$ saturation and hypoxemia and was admitted to the emergency department for immediate intervention. Which of the following signs is most likely to cause the hypoxemia experienced by the patient?**
   A. Retained secretions in the lungs
   B. An ineffective cough
   C. Poor ventilation in the lungs
   D. Poor perfusion in the lungs

9. **A 58-year-old man is referred to physical therapy with an excessive cough, sputum production, and SOB. The patient reports that these symptoms have persisted for the past 10 years. Therefore, the patient's symptoms are most likely indicative of which of the following?**
   A. Chronic hypoxia
   B. Chronic bronchitis
   C. Idiopathic hypoventilation
   D. Tuberculosis

10. **A physical therapist assistant attempts to prevent alveolar collapse with a patient following thoracic surgery. Which of the following breathing techniques would be most beneficial to achieve this goal?**
    A. Diaphragmatic breathing and breath control
    B. Pursed-lip breathing
    C. Forced expiratory technique (huff)
    D. Deep breathing exercises with a hold of 3 seconds, then sniff through nose

ANSWERS WITH RATIONALES

1. **The answer is A.**
   - Sawtooth patterns are a hallmark sign of atrial flutter.
   - Prolonged PR interval is indicative of block at the SA or AV node.
   - Absence of a P wave indicates lack of SA activity.
   - Elevated ST segment indicates MI or ventricular involvement.

2. **The answer is C.**
   - A patient exhibiting persistent dyspnea (difficulty breathing) and diaphoresis demonstrates inadequate compensation for exercise demands.
   - RPE of 9 represents a "fairly light" exertion perception from the patient.
   - Diastolic BP may remain the same level or may slightly elevate during exercise due to vasodilation response due to increased cardiac output, which may maintain diastolic BP, slightly decrease, or slightly increase with increased work.
   - Increase of 15 beats/min can be within an expected range of increased HR with exercise.

3. **The answer is B.** LDL levels are linked to an increased risk of developing atherosclerosis and CAD. HDL levels can reduce the risk of developing atherosclerosis and CAD.

4. **The answer is D.** Use of the arms puts increased strain on the heart, and continuous work of the arms and muscles contracting on the vascular system would increase both SBP and DBP. Patients would have decreased exercise capacity when compared to using a bike for the lower extremities.

5. **The answer is C.**
   - Diltiazem is a Ca$^+$ channel blocker that promotes vasodilation.
   - Albuterol is primarily used as a bronchodilator.
   - Amiodarone is used to manage heart arrhythmias.
   - Prednisone is a steroid used to alleviate inflammation and allergic response in the lungs.

6. **The answer is A**. The aortic valve at the second intercostal space is the only structure auscultated on the right side of the sternum. The pulmonic valve, tricuspid, and mitral valve are auscultated on the left side of the sternum.

7. **The answer is B**. The correct position for the superior segments of the lower lobe is prone with two pillows under the knees. The other positions describe positioning for other segments and lobes of the lungs.

8. **The answer is D**. Pulmonary embolism involves blockage of blood flow, which would lead to poor perfusion in the lungs. Ventilation would likely be unaffected, as airways are not blocked. Secretions can result from PE; however, the blockage of blood flow has the greatest impact on oxygenation. An ineffective cough affects the ability to clear secretions in the lungs.

9. **The answer is B**. Chronic bronchitis presents with the symptoms experienced. A patient is diagnosed with chronic bronchitis if the symptoms persist over 2 years. Chronic hypoxia may not lead to the development of a productive cough but would be compensated by other mechanisms. Idiopathic hypoventilation would also be linked to hypoxia without symptoms of sputum production. TB may have periods of no symptoms after initial exposure.

10. **The answer is D**. Deep breathing and the hold-then-sniff technique increases collateral ventilation of the alveoli. Pursed-lip breathing is used for patients who may have COPD and need extra expiration time due to decreased compliance in the lungs. Diaphragmatic breathing can inflate alveoli, but the hold-and-sniff technique inflates atelectatic alveoli. Forced huff would promote collapsing of alveoli and airways due to high pressure in the airways.

REFERENCES

1. Trevor AJ, Katzung BG, Kruidering-Hall M. *Katzung and Trevor's Pharmacology: Examination and Board Review*. 11th ed. New York, NY: McGraw-Hill Education; 2015.

2. Frownfelter D, Dean E. *Cardiovascular and Pulmonary Physical Therapy*. 4th ed. St. Louis, MO: Mosby Elsevier; 2006.

3. Hall JE, Guyton AC. *Guyton and Hall Textbook of Medical Physiology*. 12th ed. Philadelphia, PA: Saunders Elsevier; 2011.

4. Goodman CC, Boissonnault WG, Fuller KS. *Pathology: Implications for the Physical Therapist*. 2nd ed. Philadelphia, PA: Saunders; 2003.

5. Watchie J. *Cardiovascular and Pulmonary Physical Therapy: A Clinical Manual*. 2nd ed. St. Louis, MO: Saunders Elsevier; 2010.

6. Reid D, Chung F, Hill K. *Cardiopulmonary Physical Therapy: Management and Case Studies*. 2nd ed. Thorofare, NJ: Slack Incorporated; 2014.

5

Gait, Prosthetics, and Orthotics

MARK DUTTON

▲ HIGH-YIELD TERMS

Base of support (BOS)	The distance between an individual's feet while standing and during ambulation, including the part of the body in contact with the supporting surface and the intervening area. The normal BOS is considered to be between 5 and 10 cm.
Center of gravity (COG)	The point at which the three planes of the body intersect each other. That point is approximately 2 in (5 cm) anterior to the second sacral vertebra in the human.
Step length	The linear distance between the right and left foot during gait. Step length is measured as the distance between the same point of one foot on successive footprints (ipsilateral to the contralateral footfall).
Stride length	The distance between successive points of foot-to-floor contact of the same foot. One stride is a full lower extremity cycle. Two step lengths are added together to make the stride length.
Cadence	The number of separate steps taken in a certain time. Normal cadence is between 90 and 120 steps per minute.
Velocity	The distance a body moves in a given time, calculated by dividing the distance traveled by the time taken.

OVERVIEW

Normal human gait is a method of bipedal locomotion involving the complex synchronization of the neuromuscular and cardiovascular systems.[1]

▣ GAIT PARAMETERS

Walking involves the alternating action of the two lower extremities. The walking pattern is studied as a gait cycle (Figure 5-1). The gait cycle, which can be defined as the interval of time between any repetitive walking events, consists of two phases (Figure 5-1) and seven intervals (Figure 5-2). The major requirements for successful walking include the following[2]:

- Support of body mass by the lower extremities.

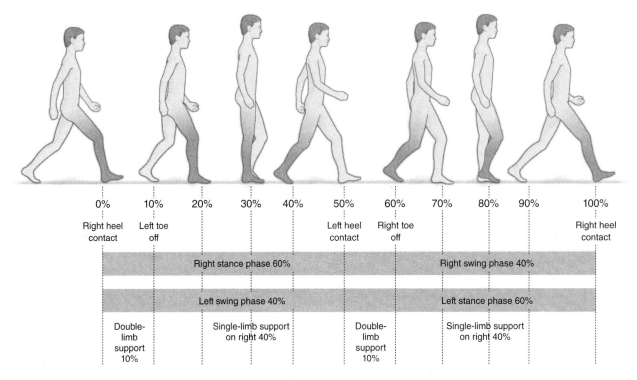

Figure 5-1. The two phases of gait. (Reproduced with permission from Dutton M. *Dutton's Orthopaedic Examination, Evaluation, and Intervention*. 5th ed. 2020. Copyright © McGraw Hill LLC. All rights reserved. https://accessphysiotherapy.mhmedical.com.)

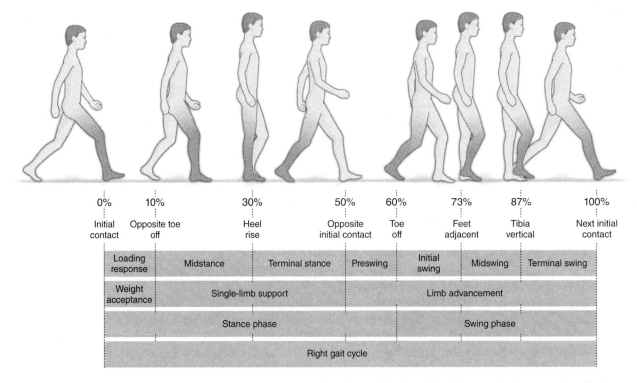

Figure 5-2. The intervals of gait. (Reproduced with permission from Dutton M. *Dutton's Orthopaedic Examination, Evaluation, and Intervention*. 5th ed. 2020. Copyright © McGraw Hill LLC. All rights reserved. https://accessphysiotherapy.mhmedical.com.)

- Production of a locomotor rhythm—the stretch reflex and the extensor thrust.[3] The stretch reflex is involved in the extremes of joint motion, while the extensor thrust may facilitate the extensor muscles of the lower extremity during weight-bearing.[4]
- Dynamic balance control of the moving body.
- Propulsion of the body in the intended direction.
- Adaptability of locomotor responses to changing tasks and environmental demands.

During the gait cycle:

- The swing of the arms is out of phase with the legs. Unless they are restrained, the arms tend to swing in opposition to the legs, the left arm swinging forward as the right leg swings forward and vice versa.[4]
- As the upper body moves forward, the trunk twists about a vertical axis. The shoulders and trunk rotate out of phase with each other during the gait cycle.[5] Although the majority of the arm swing results from momentum, the pendular actions of the arms are also produced by gravity and muscle action.[4,6]
- The thoracic spine and the pelvis rotate in opposite directions to enhance stability and balance. In contrast, the lumbar spine tends to rotate with the pelvis.
- Maximum flexion of both the elbow and shoulder joints occurs when the opposite foot initially makes contact with the ground, while maximum extension occurs when the foot on the same side initially makes contact with the ground.[7]

As gait speed increases, it develops into jogging and then running, with changes occurring with each interval. For example, as speed increases, the stance period decreases, and the terminal double stance phase disappears altogether, producing a double unsupported phase.[9]

CHARACTERISTICS OF NORMAL GAIT

Perry lists five *priorities* of normal gait[10,11]:

- Stability of the weight-bearing foot throughout the stance period.
- Clearance of the non–weight-bearing foot during the swing period.
- Appropriate prepositioning (during the terminal swing) of the foot for the next gait cycle.
- Adequate step length.
- Energy conservation.

For gait to be efficient and to conserve energy, the center of gravity (COG) must undergo minimal displacement. Therefore, during the gait cycle, the COG is displaced both vertically and laterally.

- Vertical displacement of the whole trunk occurs twice during each cycle, with the lowest in double support and the highest around midstance and midswing.[12] This vertical displacement of the COG is minimized through pelvic rotation, flexion and extension movements at the hip and knee, and rotation of the tibia and subtalar joint.[5]
- Lateral displacement. The lateral displacement of the COG occurs during the left and right stance periods.[12] Under normal conditions, the lateral displacement of the COG occurs in a sinusoidal manner. The lateral tilting of the pelvis may be accentuated in the presence of a leg length discrepancy or hip abductor weakness, the latter of which results in a Trendelenburg sign. The Trendelenburg sign is positive if standing on one leg; the pelvis drops on the side opposite the stance leg. The weakness is present on the side of the stance leg—the gluteus medius cannot maintain the COG on the stance leg's side.

When considering the energy costs of walking, the following two factors are important:

1. Any displacement that elevates, depresses, or moves the COG beyond normal maximum excursion limits, wastes energy.
2. Any abrupt or irregular movement will waste energy even when that movement does not exceed the normal maximum displacement limits of the COG.

STUDY PEARL
Individuals with muscle imbalances of the lower limbs and trunk and those with overall static-dynamic imbalances have a larger than normal base of support (BOS).[8]

The three-dimensional excursion of the COG is minimized through the intricate interactions of the lower extremity segments, especially at the knee and pelvis.[11] It has been proposed that six kinematic features, the so-called Six Determinants, are employed to reduce the energetic cost of human walking:[13,14]

1. Pelvic rotation: The pelvis rotation normally occurs about a vertical axis in the transverse plane toward the weight-bearing limb. The total pelvic rotation is approximately 4 degrees to each side.[11] Forward rotation of the pelvis on the swing side prevents an excessive drop in the body's center of mass (COM). The pelvic rotation also results in a relative lengthening of the femur, and thus step length, during the termination of the swing period.[15] If the pelvis does not rotate, the COG's position is somewhat lower during periods of double-limb support and the COG's total vertical displacement.

2. Pelvic tilt: Lateral pelvic tilting (dropping on the unsupported side) during midstance prevents an excessive rise in the body's COG. If the pelvis does not drop, the COG's position is somewhat higher during midstance, and the COG's total vertical displacement is greater.

3. Pelvic displacement: To avoid significant muscular and balancing demands, the pelvis shifts over the stance limb's support point. If the lower extremities dropped directly vertical from the hip joint, the COG would have to shift 3 to 4 in to each side to be positioned effectively over the supporting foot. The combination of femoral varus and anatomical valgum at the knee permits a vertical tibial posture with both tibias close to each other, narrowing the walking base to 5 to 10 cm (2-4 in) from heel center to heel center, thereby reducing the lateral shift required of the COG to 2.5 cm (1 in) toward either side.

4. Knee flexion during stance: In normal walking, about 60 degrees of knee motion is required to adequately clear the foot in the swing period. A loss of knee extension, which can occur with a flexion deformity, results in the hip being unable to extend fully, altering the gait mechanics. Knee motion is intrinsically associated with foot and ankle motion. At initial contact, before the elevated ankle moves into its plantarflexed position, the knee is in relative extension but flexes during loading response as the ankle plantarflexes. Midstance knee flexion prevents an excessive rise in the body's COG during that period of the gait cycle. If not for this midstance knee flexion, the COG's rise during midstance would be larger, as would its total vertical displacement. Passing through midstance as the ankle remains stationary with the foot flat on the floor, the knee extends again. As the heel comes off the floor in terminal stance, the heel begins to rise as the ankle plantarflexes and the knee flexes. In preswing, as the forefoot rolls over the metatarsal heads, the heel elevates even more as further plantarflexion occurs and flexion of the knee increases.

5. Ankle mechanism: For normal foot function and human ambulation, the amount of ankle joint motion required is approximately 10 degrees of dorsiflexion (to complete midstance and begin terminal stance) and 20 degrees of plantarflexion (for full push-off in preswing). At initial contact, the foot is in relative dorsiflexion due to the muscle action of the pretibial muscles and the triceps surae. This muscle action produces a relative lengthening of the leg, resulting in smoothing the COG pathway during the stance phase. In addition, an adaptively shortened gastrocnemius muscle may restrict normal ankle dorsiflexion during the midstance to heel raise portion of the gait cycle. This motion is typically compensated for by increased pronation of the subtalar joint, increased internal rotation of the tibia, and stress to the knee joint complex.

6. Foot mechanism: The controlled lever arm of the forefoot at preswing is particularly helpful as it rounds out the sharp downward reversal of the COG. Thus it does not reduce a peak displacement period of the COG as the earlier determinants did but rather smoothes the pathway.

JOINT MOTIONS AND MUSCLE ACTIONS DURING GAIT

The joint motions and muscle actions that occur during gait are depicted in Table 5-1.

Phase	Hip	Knee	Tibia	Ankle	Foot
TABLE 5-1 • Joint Motions and Muscle Activity During Gait.					
Initial contact/ heel strike	– Gluteus maximus and hamstrings work isometrically to resist flexion moment at the hip – Erector spinae works eccentrically to control trunk flexion Reaction force anterior to the hip joint creating a flexion moment – Hip positioned in slight adduction and external rotation	– Positioned in full extension before heel contact, but flexing as heel makes contact – Reaction force behind knee causing flexion moment – Quadriceps contracting eccentrically to control knee flexion	– Slight external rotation	– Moving into plantarflexion	– Supination
Loading response/ foot flat	– Gluteus maximus and hamstrings shift from isometric to slight concentric activation, guiding the hip toward extension – The hip begins to extend from a position of 20-40° of flexion – Hip moving into extension, adduction, and internal rotation	– In 20° of knee flexion, moving toward extension – Flexion moment – The quadriceps begin working eccentrically but, once the foot is flat, work concentrically to bring the femur over the tibia	– Internal rotation	– Plantarflexion to dorsiflexion over a fixed foot	– Pronation, adapting to support surface
Midstance	The hip approaches 0° extension, at which point the hip extensors are only slightly active (to help stabilize the hip as the body is propelled forward). This activation is minimal during slow walking on level surfaces but increases significantly with increasing speed or with an increasing slope of the walking surface. During midstance, the stance leg is in single limb support as the other leg is freely swinging toward the next step. The hip abductor muscles (eg, gluteus medius) of the stance leg are active to stabilize the hip in the frontal plane, preventing the opposite side of the pelvis from dropping excessively Pelvis rotates posteriorly – Iliopsoas contracting eccentrically to resist hip extension – Gluteus medius creating reverse action to stabilize the opposite pelvis	– Quadriceps femoris activity decreasing as the knee reaches near full extension. Because the line of gravity falls just anterior to the medial-lateral axis of rotation of the knee, the knee is mechanically locked into extension, requiring little activation from the quadriceps at this time.	– Neutral rotation	– 3° of dorsiflexion	– Neutral
Terminal stance/heel off	– Hip positioned in 10-15° of hip extension, abduction, and external rotation – Iliopsoas activity continuing – Extension moment decreases after double-limb support begins	– In 4° of flexion, moving toward extension – Maximum flexion moment – Quadriceps femoris activity decreasing	– External rotation	– 15° dorsiflexion toward plantarflexion – Maximum dorsiflexion moment	– Supination as the foot becomes rigid for push-off
Preswing/toe off	The hip continues to extend to about 10° of extension with eccentric activation of the hip flexors, particularly the iliopsoas, helping to control the rate and amount of extension – Adductor magnus working eccentrically to control the pelvis	– Moving from near full extension to 40° of flexion – Reaction forces moving posterior to the knee as the knee flexes – Flexion moment – Quadriceps femoris contracting eccentrically	– External rotation	– 20° of plantarflexion – Dorsiflexion moment	– Supination

▨ ABNORMAL GAIT SYNDROMES

In general, abnormal gait syndromes and deviations (Table 5-2) fall under four headings: those caused by weakness, abnormal joint position or range of motion (ROM), muscle contracture, and pain.[11]

- Weakness implies an inadequate internal joint moment or loss of the natural force couple relationship. In addition, neuromuscular conditions may be associated with muscle tone abnormalities, mistiming of muscle contractions, and proprioceptive and sensory disturbances, the latter of which can profoundly affect reflex postural balance.
- Abnormal joint position can be caused by an imbalance of flexibility and strength around a joint or by contracture.
- Contractures, changes in the connective tissue of muscles, ligaments, and joint capsule may produce gait changes. If the contracture is elastic, the gait changes are apparent in the swing period only. If the contractures are rigid, the gait changes are apparent during the swing and the stance periods.
- Pain can alter gait as the patient attempts to use the position of minimal articular pressure. Pain may also produce muscle inhibition and eventual atrophy. The antalgic gait is characterized by a decrease in the stance period on the involved side to minimize the force through the involved leg and use of the uninjured body part as much as possible.

Each normal gait attribute is subject to compromise by disease states, particularly neuromuscular conditions (Table 5-3).[16]

In addition to those abnormal gait syndromes listed in Table 5-3, the following two types of spastic gait are worth noting:

Hemiplegic (hemiparetic). This type of gait, frequently seen following a completed stroke, results from a unilateral upper motor neuron lesion with varying amounts of spasticity in all muscles on the involved side. During gait, the leg tends to circumduct in a semicircle, rotating outward or is pushed ahead, and the foot drags and scrapes the floor. The upper limb, held adducted at the shoulder and flexed at the elbow and wrist with the fist closed, is typically carried across the trunk for balance.

Paraparetic. This type of gait, which can result from bilateral upper motor neuron lesions (eg, cervical myelopathy in adults and cerebral palsy in children), is characterized by slow, stiff, and jerky movements—spastic extension at the knees and adduction at the hips (scissors gait).

▨ GAIT ANALYSIS

A gait examination, initially performed by the physical therapist using several methods ranging from observation to computerized analysis, involves a systematic examination of the various body parts at each point in the gait cycle. The physical therapist may also examine the patient's footwear for wear patterns. Once an overall assessment has been made of the patient's gait, the focus switches to the various segments of the lower kinetic chain (Table 5-1). Attempts are made to determine the primary cause of any gait deviations or compensations (Table 5-2). Also, a quantitative gait analysis (Table 5-4) can be used to obtain information on spatial and temporal gait variables, as well as motion patterns, although imaging-based systems are the most sophisticated (and expensive) methods of obtaining quantitative data.[17] Although a physical therapist assistant (PTA) is not responsible for the initial gait examination, understanding the differences between normal and abnormal gait and the potential causes for dysfunction is important during the intervention phase.

▨ SPECIFIC INTERVENTIONS FOR GAIT

The specific intervention for an abnormal gait varies according to severity. A graduated progression is outlined in Table 5-5.

TABLE 5-2 • Some Gait Deviations and Their Causes.	
Gait Deviations	**Reasons**
Slower cadence than expected for a person's age	Generalized weakness Pain Joint motion restrictions Poor voluntary motor control
Shorter stance phase on the involved side and a decreased swing phase on the uninvolved side	Shorter stride length on the uninvolved side Decrease lateral sway over the involved stance limb Increase in cadence Increase in velocity Use of an assistive device Antalgic gait, resulting from a painful injury to the lower limb and pelvic region
Stance phase longer on one side	Pain Lack of trunk and pelvic rotation Weakness of lower limb muscles Restrictions in lower limb joints Poor muscle control Increased muscle tone
Lateral trunk lean (to bring the center of gravity of the trunk nearer to the hip joint)	Ipsilateral lean—hip abductor weakness (gluteus medius/Trendelenburg gait) Contralateral lean—decreased hip flexion in swing limb Painful hip Abnormal hip joint (congenital dysplasia, coxa vara, etc) Wide walking base Unequal leg length
Anterior trunk leaning Occurs at initial contact to move the line of gravity in front of the axis of the knee	Weak or paralyzed knee extensors, or gluteus maximus Decreased ankle dorsiflexion Hip flexion contracture
Posterior trunk leaning Occurs at initial contact to bring the line of the external force behind the axis of the hip	Weak or paralyzed hip extensors, especially the gluteus maximus (gluteus maximus gait) Hip pain Hip flexion contracture Inadequate hip flexion in swing Decreased knee range of motion
Increased lumbar lordosis Occurs at the end of the stance period	Inability to extend the hip, usually due to a flexion contracture or ankylosis
Pelvic drop during stance	Contralateral gluteus medius weakness Adaptive shortening of quadratus lumborum on the swing side Contralateral hip adductor spasticity
Excessive pelvic rotation	Adaptively shortened/spasticity of hip flexors on the same side Limited hip joint flexion
Circumducted hip Ground contact by the swinging leg can be avoided if it is swung outward (for natural walking to occur, the leg which is in its stance phase needs to be longer than the leg which is in its swing phase to allow toe clearance of the swing foot)	Functional leg length discrepancy Painful, stiff hip or knee
Hip hiking The pelvis is lifted on the side of the swinging leg by contraction of the spinal muscles and the lateral abdominal wall	Functional leg length discrepancy Inadequate hip flexion, knee flexion, or ankle dorsiflexion Hamstring weakness Quadratus lumborum shortening
Vaulting The ground clearance of the swinging leg will be increased if the subject goes up on the toes of the stance period leg	Functional leg length discrepancy Vaulting occurs on the shorter limb side

(Continued)

TABLE 5-2 • Some Gait Deviations and Their Causes. (Continued)

Gait Deviations	Reasons
Abnormal internal hip rotation Produces a "toe-in" gait	Adaptive shortening of the iliotibial band Weakness of the hip external rotators Femoral anteversion Adaptive shortening of the hip internal rotators
Abnormal external hip rotation Produces a "toe-out" gait	Adaptive shortening of the hip external rotators Femoral retroversion Weakness of the hip internal rotators
Increased hip adduction (scissor gait) Results in excessive hip adduction during swing (scissoring), decreased base of support, and decreased progression of the opposite foot	Spasticity or contracture of ipsilateral hip adductors Ipsilateral hip adductor weakness Coxa vara
Inadequate hip extension/excessive hip flexion Results in loss of hip extension in midstance (forward-leaning of the trunk, increased lordosis, and increased knee flexion and ankle dorsiflexion) and late stance (anterior pelvic tilt), and increased hip flexion in swing	Hip flexion contracture Iliotibial band contracture Hip flexor spasticity Pain Arthrodesis (surgical or spontaneous ankylosis) Loss of ankle dorsiflexion
Inadequate hip flexion Results in decreased limb advancement in swing, posterior pelvic tilt, circumduction, and excessive knee flexion to clear foot	Hip flexor weakness Hip joint arthrodesis
Decreased hip swing through (psoriatic limp) Manifested by exaggerated movements at the pelvis and trunk to assist the hip in moving into flexion	Legg-Calve-Perthes disease Weakness or reflex inhibition of the psoas major muscle
Excessive knee extension/inadequate knee flexion Results in decreased knee flexion at initial contact and loading response, increased knee extension during stance, and decreased knee flexion during swing	Pain Anterior trunk deviation/bending Weakness of the quadriceps. The hyperextension is compensatory and places the bodyweight vector anterior to the knee Spasticity of the quadriceps. This is noted more during the loading response and the initial swing intervals Joint deformity
Excessive knee flexion/inadequate knee extension At initial contact or around midstance. Results in increased knee flexion in early stance, decreased knee extension in midstance and terminal stance, and decreased knee extension during swing	Knee flexion contracture resulting in decreased step length and decreased knee extension in the stance phase Increased tone/spasticity of hamstrings or hip flexors Decreased range of motion of ankle dorsiflexion in swing period Weakness of plantar flexors resulting in increased dorsiflexion in the stance phase Lengthened limb
Inadequate dorsiflexion control ("foot slap") during initial contact to midstance	Weak or paralyzed dorsiflexors Lack of lower limb proprioception
Steppage gait during the acceleration through deceleration of the swing phase Exaggerated knee and hip flexion are used to lift the foot higher than usual for increased ground clearance resulting from a foot drop	Weak or paralyzed dorsiflexor muscles Functional leg length discrepancy
Increased walking base (> 20 cm)	Deformity such as hip abductor muscle contracture Genu valgus Fear of losing balance Leg length discrepancy

(Continued)

TABLE 5-2 • Some Gait Deviations and Their Causes. (*Continued*)

Gait Deviations	Reasons
Decreased walking base (< 10 cm)	Hip adductor muscle contracture Genu varum
Excessive eversion of calcaneus during initial contact through midstance	Excessive tibia vara (refers to the frontal plane position of the distal 1/3 of the leg as it relates to the supporting surface) Forefoot varus Weakness of tibialis posterior Excessive lower extremity internal rotation (due to muscle imbalances, femoral anteversion)
Excessive pronation during midstance through terminal stance	Insufficient ankle dorsiflexion (< 10°) Increased tibial varum Compensated forefoot or rearfoot varus deformity Uncompensated forefoot valgus deformity Pes planus Long limb Uncompensated medial rotation of tibia or femur Weak tibialis anterior
Excessive supination during initial contact through midstance	Limited calcaneal eversion Rigid forefoot valgus Pes cavus Uncompensated lateral rotation of the tibia or femur Short limb Plantarflexed 1st ray Upper motor neuron muscle imbalance
Excessive dorsiflexion	Compensation for knee flexion contracture Inadequate plantar flexor strength Adaptive shortening of dorsiflexors Increased muscle tone of dorsiflexors Pes calcaneus deformity
Excessive plantarflexion	Increased plantar flexor activity Plantar flexor contracture
Excessive varus	Contracture Overactivity of the muscles on the medial aspect of the foot
Excessive valgus	Weak invertors Foot hypermobility
Decreased or absence of propulsion (plantar flexor gait)	An inability of the plantar flexors to fully function results in a shorter step length on the involved side

■ GAIT TRAINING WITH ASSISTIVE DEVICES

The clinician must always provide adequate physical support and instruction while working with a patient using an assistive device. A detailed description of the various assistive devices is provided in Chapter 8. Table 5-6 provides information on assistive devices for gait, including the device's appropriate measurement and the gait pattern most frequently used with it. Whichever gait pattern is chosen, it is important that the patient receives verbal and illustrated instructions for using the assistive device on stairs, curbs, ramps and doors, and transfers. These instructions should include any weight-bearing precautions the patient may have, the appropriate gait sequence, and a contact number to reach the clinician if any questions arise.

STUDY PEARL

If a patient leans over to observe the therapist while an assistive device is being measured, the device will probably be too short when fitted.

Axillary crutches that are too tall for a client can result in brachial plexus damage.

TABLE 5-3 • Gait Deviations Related to Disease.	
Deviation	**Characteristics**
Sensory taxic	Characterized by staggering and unsteadiness. As the patient is unaware of limb position, the gait is broad-based, and the patient tends to lift the feet too high and slap them on the floor in an uncoordinated and abrupt manner. The patient tends to watch the floor and the feet to maximize visual correction attempts and may have difficulty walking in the dark
Cerebellar ataxic	The site of the lesion determines the nature of the gait abnormality with a cerebellar lesion *Vermal* lesions: The gait is broad-based, unsteady, and staggering with an irregular sway. The patient is unable to walk in tandem or a straight line. The ataxia of gait worsens when the patient attempts to stop suddenly or turn sharply, with a tendency to fall *Hemispheral* lesions: The ataxia tends to be less severe, but there is persistent lurching or deviation toward the involved side
Double step	Characterized by alternate steps which are of a different length or at a different rate
Equinus (toe-walking)	One of the more common abnormal gait patterns of patients with spastic diplegia, and spastic diplegia is the most common motor impairment pattern in patients with cerebral palsy (CP).[1] In these patients, motor impairment is due to several deficits, including poor muscle control, weakness, impaired balance, hypertonicity, and spasticity[2] Equinus gait is characterized by forefoot strike to initiate the cycle and premature plantarflexion in early stance to midstance.[3] The following associated gait deviations are frequently seen at the knees, hips, and pelvis in children with CP who are walking on their toes[4]: • Increased knee flexion at initial contact and again in midstance • Diminished hip extension at terminal stance • An increased anterior pelvic tilt
Gluteus maximus	Results from a weakness of the gluteus maximus and characterized by a posterior thrusting of the trunk at initial contact in an attempt to maintain the hip extension of the stance leg and anterior tilting of the pelvis manifested in hyperlordosis of the lumbar spine
Trendelenburg	This type of gait is due to a weakness of the hip abductors (gluteus medius and minimus). The normal stabilizing impact of these muscles is absent, and the patient demonstrates an excessive lateral list in which the trunk is thrust laterally in an attempt to keep the center of gravity over the stance leg. A positive Trendelenburg sign is also present.
Quadriceps	A gait pattern caused by quadriceps weakness. Quadriceps weakness can result from a peripheral nerve lesion (femoral), a spinal nerve root lesion, trauma, or disease (muscular dystrophy). Due to the quadriceps weakness, the patient propagates forward motion by circumducting each leg and leaning the body toward the other side to balance the center of gravity, and this is repeated with each step.
Parkinsonian	The parkinsonian gait is characterized by a flexed and stooped posture with flexion of the neck, elbows, metacarpophalangeal joints, trunk, hips, and knees. The patient has difficulty initiating movements and walks with short steps with the feet barely clearing the ground, resulting in a shuffling type of gait with rapid steps. Once the patient gets moving, they may lean forward and walk progressively faster, as if chasing their center of gravity (propulsive or festinating gait). Less commonly, deviation of the center of gravity backward may cause retropulsion. There is also a lack of associated arm movement during the gait as the arms are held stiffly
Hysterical	This gait pattern is nonspecific and bizarre and does not conform to any specific organic pattern. The abnormality varies from moment to moment and from one examination to another. There may be ataxia, spasticity, an inability to move, or other types of abnormality. The abnormality is often minimal or absent when the patient is unaware of being watched or when distracted. However, while all hysterical gaits are bizarre, all bizarre gaits are not hysterical
Hemiplegic	This gait pattern is characterized by abduction and circumduction of the paralyzed limb to propel the foot forward
Scissor	This gait pattern is characterized by a crossing of the legs in midline upon advancement
Spastic	Stiff movements characterize this gait pattern, with the toes seeming to catch and drag, the hip and knee joints slightly flexed, and the legs held together
Steppage	A gait type in which elevation of the feet and toes appears exaggerated as the patient lifts the leg high enough to clear the flail foot (foot drop) off the floor by flexing excessively at the hip and knee and then slapping the sole of the foot on the floor. A foot drop results from weakness or paralysis of the dorsiflexor muscles due to an injury to the muscles, their peripheral nerve supply, or the nerve roots supplying the muscles.[5]

(Continued)

TABLE 5-3 • Gait Deviations Related to Disease. (*Continued*)

Deviation	Characteristics
Tabetic	This ataxic gait pattern, similar to the steppage gait, is characterized by a slapping of the foot on the ground
Waddling	Characterized by feet that are wide apart Associated with coax vara

Data from Blair E, Stanley F. Issues in the classification and epidemiology of cerebral palsy. *Mental Retard Devel Disab Res Rev.* 1997;3:184–93; Baddar A, Granata K, Damiano DL, et al. Ankle and knee coupling in patients with spastic diplegia: effects of gastrocnemius-soleus lengthening. *J Bone and Joint Surg.* 2002;84A:736-44; Abel MH, Damiano DL, Pannunzio M, et al. Muscle-tendon surgery in diplegic cerebral palsy: functional and mechanical changes. *J Ped Ortho.* 1999;19:366–75; Davids JR, Foti T, Dabelstein J, et al. Voluntary (normal) versus obligatory (cerebral palsy) toe-walking in children: a kinematic, kinetic, and electromyographic analysis. *J Ped Ortho.* 1999;19:461–9; Morag E, Hurwitz DE, Andriacchi TP, et al. Abnormalities in muscle function during gait in relation to the level of lumbar disc herniation. *Spine.* 2000;25:829-33.

A gait belt should be fitted around the patient's waist to enable the clinician to assist the patient. When ambulating with a patient, the clinician should be just behind the patient, standing toward the involved side, grasping the gait belt with one hand, and placing the other hand on the patient's shoulder (not their arm as this will interfere).

During ambulation, the clinician's front foot should move when the patient moves, while the back leg and the assistive device should advance together.

The appropriate gait pattern for the patient is dependent on the patient's balance, strength, cardiovascular status, coordination, functional needs, and weight-bearing status. Several gait patterns are recognized. Tables 5-7 and 5-8 provide a quick review of stair protocols and frequently used gait patterns. A more detailed description follows.

TWO-POINT PATTERN

The two-point gait pattern, which closely approximates the normal gait pattern, requires an assistive device (canes or crutches) on each side of the body. This pattern requires the patient to move the assistive device and the contralateral lower extremity simultaneously.

THREE-POINT GAIT PATTERN

The three-point gait pattern involves the use of two crutches or a walker. This pattern is used when the patient is permitted to bear weight through only one lower extremity.

The pattern is initiated with the forward movement of one of the assistive devices. Next, the involved lower extremity is advanced. Then the patient presses down on the assistive device and advances the uninvolved lower extremity.

> **STUDY PEARL**
> The three-point gait pattern requires good upper body strength, good balance, and good cardiovascular endurance.

TABLE 5-4 • Gait Variables for Quantitative Gait Analysis.

Variable	Description
Speed	A scalar quantity that has magnitude but not direction
Acceleration	The rate of change of velocity to time
Stride time	The amount of time that elapses during one stride
Step time	The amount of time that elapses between consecutive right and left foot contacts (heel strikes)
Swing time	The amount of time during the gait cycle that one foot is off the ground
Step width	The linear distance between one foot and the opposite foot
Foot angle	The angle of foot placement in relation to the line of progression (degree of toe-out or toe-in)

TABLE 5-5 • The Major Elements of Physical Therapy Intervention that Comprise Locomotor Training.	
Major Element	**Intervention—Instruction and Training in**
Preparation for locomotor training	Bridging exercises Quadruped exercises Sitting balance and perturbations Sit-to-stand activities Kneeling and half-kneeling activities Modified plantigrade exercises Standing balance and perturbations
Parallel bar progression	Moving from sitting to standing and reverse Standing balance and stability training Stepping, sidestepping, cross-stepping Use of appropriate gait pattern, forward progression, and turning Moving from sitting to stand with an assistive device, then stand to sit Standing balance and weight-shifting activities with an assistive device Use of assistive device (with appropriate gait pattern) for forward progression and turning
Indoor overground progression	Walking forward and backward with resistance Sidestepping and cross-stepping Braiding Stair climbing Falling techniques (as appropriate)
Outdoor overground progression	Opening doors and passing through thresholds Curb climbing; negotiating ramps, stairs, and sloped surfaces Walking on even and uneven surfaces Walking with imposed timing requirements Use of open community environments; outside doors, and thresholds Entering/exiting vehicles Use of elevators, revolving doors
Locomotor training using body-weight support and a motorized treadmill	Walking on treadmill using body weight support progressing to no body weight support Production of locomotor rhythm: initiating with slow speed and then progressing to faster speeds Dynamic balance control of the moving body Reciprocal stepping patterns: assisted movements to unassisted Strategies to improve speed, symmetry, and endurance
Indoor over ground progression using body weight support	Indoor walking on level surfaces with body weight support progressing to no body weight support Use of assistive devices (as indicated) for ambulation on level surfaces

- If the uninvolved lower extremity is advanced to where it is parallel to the involved lower extremity, this would be a "swing to" pattern.
- If the uninvolved lower extremity is advanced ahead of the uninvolved lower extremity, this would be a "swing through" pattern.

Modifications of the three-point gait pattern include touchdown weight-bearing (TDWB) and partial weight-bearing (PWB). This modified pattern is initiated with the forward movement of one of the assistive devices, and then the involved lower extremity is advanced. Next, the patient presses down on the assistive device and advances the uninvolved lower extremity using either a "swing to" or a "swing through" pattern.

FOUR-POINT PATTERN

The four-point gait pattern, which requires an assistive device (canes or crutches) on each side of the body, is used when the patient requires maximum assistance with either balance or stability or both. The pattern is initiated with the forward movement of one of the assistive devices, and then the contralateral lower extremity, the other assistive device, and, finally, the opposite lower extremity (eg, right crutch, then left foot; left crutch, then right foot).

TABLE 5-6 • Gait Devices.

Device	Unilateral/ Bilateral	Gait Patterns	Measurement	Typical Patient
Axillary crutches	Bilateral	Four-point Two-point Three-point Modified three-point	2 in below axilla when correctly on the floor (2-4 in lateral and 4-6 in anterior to toes) and wrist crease at the handle	Recent fracture Recent surgery Usually younger (< 65 years) Using three-point or three-point modified when WB restrictions
	Unilateral	Modified four-point Modified two-point	As above	As above, progressing to a unilateral device with no WB restrictions
Forearm or Loftstrand crutches	Bilateral	Four-point Two-point Not recommended for three-point or modified three-point	Cuff distal to olecranon wrist crease at the handle	Longer-term users such as chronic neurological patients but generally younger than 65 years
	Unilateral	Modified four-point Modified two-point	As above	As above requiring less support
Walkers Standard, front-wheeled, four-wheeled	Bilateral	Three-point or modified three-point gait just requiring the support of bilateral device with no WB restrictions; is unnamed when using a walker	Wrist crease at the handle	Generally, older than 65 years may have WB restrictions or just instability
Single-point cane	Unilateral	Modified two-point Modified four-point	Wrist crease at the handle	Adds some balance stability; least stable of all AD, used in the opposite hand to affected leg if there is one leg affected Also used as a progression from a bilateral device when no WB restrictions apply
Wide- and short-based quad canes	Unilateral	Modified two-point Modified four-point	Wrist crease at the handle	As above, but the wider base adds greater stability when there are balance deficits Often used with higher-functioning patients post CVA
Hemi-walker	Unilateral	Modified four-point Modified two-point	Wrist crease at the handle	Often used with patient post CVA for initial gait training Also used with patients post arm or shoulder injury or surgery who need increased stability using only one UE

AD, assistive device; CVA, cerebrovascular accident; UE, upper extremity; WB, weight-bearing.

SIT-TO-STAND TRANSFERS USING ASSISTIVE DEVICES

Before the patient can begin ambulation, they must first learn to transfer from a sitting position to a standing position safely. First, the bed or wheelchair wheels are locked, and the patient is reminded of any weight-bearing restrictions. Next, the patient is asked to slide to

TABLE 5-7 • Stair Protocol.

Stairs	First	Second	Third	Acronym
Ascending	Unaffected leg	Affected leg	Crutches or AD	GAS
Descending	Crutches or AD	Affected leg	Unaffected leg	SAG

AD, assistive device GAS, good affected sticks; SAG, sticks affected good.

TABLE 5-8 • Gait Patterns.

Name of Gait Pattern	Bilateral or Unilateral Device	Description of Pattern	Comments
Four-point	Bilateral	1. crutch 2. opposite foot 3. other crutch 4. other foot	Can be done with any bilateral device, but with walkers, it is not called a four-point gait unless using a reciprocal walker
Four-point modified	Unilateral	1. crutch 2. opposite foot 3. other foot	Any unilateral device can be used and is in the opposite hand to the affected LE
Two-point	Bilateral	1. crutch and opposite foot together 2. other crutch and other foot together	Can be done with any bilateral device but not called two-point if using a walker except for reciprocal walkers
Two-point modified	Unilateral	1. crutch and opposite foot together 2. other foot	Any unilateral device can be used and is in the opposite hand to the affected LE
Three-point	Bilateral	1. crutch or walker 2. affected NWB leg swings through 3. hop forward on the other leg	Only used when there is NWB on one side and must have a bilateral device—crutches or walker
Three-point modified	Bilateral	1. crutch or walker 2. foot with weight restriction 3. other foot	Used with all other weight-bearing restrictions (other than NWB) and must have a bilateral device—crutches or walker

LE, lower extremity; NWB, non–weight bearing.

Reproduced with permission from Burke-Doe A, Dutton M, eds. *National Physical Therapy Examination and Board Review.* 2019. Copyright © McGraw Hill LLC. All rights reserved. https://accessphysiotherapy.mhmedical.com.

the front edge of the chair or bed, and their weight-bearing foot is placed underneath the body so that their COG is closer to their BOS, which will make it easier for the patient to stand.

- The patient is then instructed to lean forward and push up with the hands from the bed or armrests.
- If the patient is being instructed on the use of a walker, he or she should grasp the handgrips of the walker, only after they have become upright, and should not be permitted to try to pull themselves up using the walker, as this can cause the walker to tip over, and increase the potential for falls.
- If the patient uses crutches, he or she is instructed to hold both crutches with the hand on the same side as the involved lower extremity. The patient then presses down on the handgrips of both crutches with one hand, presses down on the chair's armrest or the bed with the other hand, and comes to a standing position by pushing down the uninvolved lower extremity. Once standing, the patient then moves one of the crutches into position and begins to ambulate.
- If the patient uses one or two canes, he or she can push up with the hands from the bed or armrests. Once standing, the patient should grasp the handgrip(s) of the cane (s) with the appropriate hand and begin to ambulate.

STAND-TO-SIT TRANSFERS USING ASSISTIVE DEVICES

The stand-to-sit transfer is essentially the reverse of the sit-to-stand transfer. To sit down using an assistive device, the patient must first back up against the bed or chair's front edge. If the patient has difficulty bending the involved lower extremity, he or she is instructed to slowly advance this extremity during the sitting maneuver.

- Once in position, the patient (using a walker) reaches for the bed or armrest with both hands and slowly sits down.
- Once in position, the patient (using crutches) moves both crutches to the hand on the side of the involved lower extremity. With that hand holding onto both handgrips of the crutches, the patient reaches back for the bed or armrest with the other hand before slowly sitting down.

- Once in position, the patient (using a cane(s)) places the cane's handgrip against the edge of the chair or bed. Next, the patient reaches back for the bed or armrest and slowly sits down.

STAIR AND CURB NEGOTIATION

Ascending Stairs

To ascend steps, the patient must first move to the front edge of the step. Then, the clinician should remain behind the patient, usually toward the weaker side, and place the lead foot on the same step as the patient and the other foot one step lower.

Ascending more than two to three stairs with a standard walker is not recommended.

- To ascend steps or stairs using a walker, the patient is instructed to grasp the stair handrail with one hand and turn the walker sideways so that the walker's two front legs are placed on the first step. When ready, the patient pushes down on the walker's handgrip and the handrail and advances the uninvolved lower extremity onto the first step. The patient then advances the uninvolved lower extremity to the first step and then moves the walker's legs to the next step. This process is repeated as the patient moves up the steps.
- To ascend steps or stairs with crutches, the patient should grasp the stair handrail with one hand and grasp both crutches by the handgrips with the other hand. If the patient cannot grasp both crutches with one hand, or if the handrail is not stable, then he or she should ascend the stairs using both crutches, although this is not recommended if there are more than two to three steps. When in the correct position at the front edge of the step, the patient pushes down on the crutches and handrail, if applicable, and advances the uninvolved lower extremity to the first step. The patient then advances the involved lower extremity and finally the crutches. This process is repeated for the remaining steps.
- To ascend steps or stairs with one or two canes, the patient should use the handrail and the cane. If the handrail is not stable, then the patient should use the cane(s) only. The patient pushes down on the cane or handrail, if applicable, and advances the uninvolved lower extremity to the first step. The patient then advances the involved lower extremity. This process is repeated for the remaining steps.

Descending Stairs

A gait belt is recommended. To descend steps, the patient must first move to the front edge of the top step. The clinician should remain in front of the patient, usually toward the weaker side, and should place the lead foot on the step the patient will step on and the other foot one step lower. Descending more than two to three stairs with a standard walker is not recommended.

- Using a walker to descend, the walker is turned sideways to place the walker's two front legs on the lower step. One hand is placed on the rear handgrip, and the other hand grasps the stair handrail. When ready, the patient lowers the involved lower extremity down to the first step. Then the patient pushes down on the walker and handrail and advances the uninvolved lower extremity down the first step. This process is repeated as the patient moves down the steps.
- To descend steps or stairs with crutches, the patient should use one hand to grasp the stair handrail and the other to grasp both crutches and handrail. If the patient cannot grasp both crutches with one hand, or if the handrail is not stable, then the patient should use both crutches only, although this is not recommended if there are more than two to three steps. When ready, the patient lowers the involved lower extremity down to the first step. Next, the patient pushes down on the crutches and handrail, if applicable, and advances the uninvolved lower extremity down to the first step. This process is repeated for the remaining steps.
- To descend steps or stairs with one or two canes, the patient should use the cane and handrail. If the handrail is not stable, then the patient should use the cane(s) only.

When ready, the patient lowers the involved lower extremity down to the first step. Next, the patient pushes down on the cane(s) and handrail, if applicable, and advances the uninvolved lower extremity down to the first step. This process is repeated for the remaining steps.

■ PROSTHETICS

Similar to assistive devices, prosthetics and orthotics are implements used to support or protect weak or ineffective joints or muscles and enhance performance.[18]

AMPUTATION

The major reasons for amputation include disease (diabetes, peripheral vascular disease), infection (post joint replacement, osteomyelitis), tumor, trauma, and fracture (nonunion). Fortunately, major improvements in noninvasive diagnosis, revascularization, and wound healing techniques have lowered the overall incidence of amputations for vascular disease.[19]

Traumatic amputations may be performed at any level (Table 5-9); the surgeon tries to maintain the greatest bone length and save all possible joints.[19]

POSTOPERATIVE DRESSINGS

Soft Dressings

Elastic Wrap.   This elastic compression bandage with a sterile dressing is more commonly used during the immediate postoperative stage when a local infection is present to provide edema control, soft tissue support, and protection of the operative site.

Except for reapplication, the elastic compression bandage is normally kept in place at all times except during bathing. Then, the patient is taught how to apply compression wrapping with elastic bandages or the use of an elastic shrinker (see later).

Rewrapping should occur several times a day to maintain adequate pressure. In addition, the clinician should note the following guidelines:

- For transtibial amputations, a 3- to 4-in wrap is used, and care is taken to ensure that the anchor wrap is applied above the knee.
- For transfemoral amputations, a 6-in wrap is used, and care is taken to ensure the anchor wrap is applied around the pelvis.
- Full hip extension must be promoted following transfemoral amputations.

Rigid Dressings

A rigid dressing, the *immediate postoperative prosthesis* (IPOP), is sometimes used during the immediate postoperative stage in place of an elastic compression bandage for edema control and protection of the operative site.

- The advantages are that it allows early ambulation with a pylon, and earlier fitting of the permanent prosthesis, promotes circulation and healing, and stimulates proprioception.
- The disadvantages are that it does not permit wound inspections or daily dressing changes because this dressing is not removable.

Typically, the attending surgeon does not change the rigid cast dressing until the sutures or surgical clips are removed.

Semirigid Dressings

The classic compression treatment has been the Unna paste bandage impregnated with zinc oxide, glycerin, gelatin, and, perhaps, calamine, which dries to form a semirigid cast.

STUDY PEARL
- Amputation refers to the cutting of a limb along the long bones axis.
- Disarticulation refers to cutting off a limb through the joint.

STUDY PEARL
The specific type of surgery depends on the status of the extremity at the time of amputation. Conservation of the residual limb and uncomplicated wound healing are both important.

STUDY PEARL
Individuals not fitted with a rigid dressing or a temporary prosthesis use an elastic wrap or shrinkers to reduce the residual limb's size.

STUDY PEARL
The elastic compression bandage and sterile dressing are generally removed and reapplied a minimum of three times per day following the immediate postoperative stage and the removal of all surgical clips and sutures.

STUDY PEARL
Wrapping should be performed using either a diagonal or angular pattern, but not a circular pattern. Pressure should be applied distally to enhance shaping, and there should be no signs of wrinkles in the wrapping.

STUDY PEARL
Removable rigid dressings (RRDs) are adjustable as the limb changes and may be removed as needed for wound inspection and care.

TABLE 5-9 • Levels of Amputation.	
Level of Amputation	**Description**
Partial toe	Excision of any part of one or more toes
Toe disarticulation	Disarticulation of one or more toes at the metatarsophalangeal joint
Partial foot/ray resection	Resection of the third, fourth, and fifth metatarsals and digits
Tarsometatarsal (LisFranc) disarticulation	Disarticulation of all five metatarsals and digits.
Transmetatarsal (Chopart)	Amputation through the midsection of all metatarsals leaving only the calcaneus and talus
Syme amputation	An ankle disarticulation that can include removing both malleoli and distal tibial/fibular flares to create a smooth bony distal end with the attachment of the heel pad to the distal end of the tibia
Long transtibial (below the knee)	More than 50% tibial length
Transtibial (below the knee)	Between 20% and 50% of tibial length
Short transtibial (below the knee)	Less than 20% tibial length
Knee disarticulation	Amputation through the knee joint with shaping of the distal femur, squaring the condyles for an even weight-bearing surface. A knee disarticulation is most often used in children and young adults but is nearly always avoided in the elderly and patients with ischemic disease. Several advantages of knee disarticulation include the following: • A large distal end covered by skin and soft tissues, naturally suited for weight-bearing • A long lever arm controlled by strong muscles • Increased stability of the patient's prosthesis The main disadvantage of knee disarticulation is cosmetic—the patient's prosthetic leg has a knee that extends far beyond the other knee in the sitting position.
Long transfemoral (above the knee)	More than 60% femoral length
Transfemoral (above the knee)	Between 35% and 60% femoral length
Short transfemoral (above the knee)	Less than 35% femoral length
Hip disarticulation	An amputation through the hip joint capsule, removing the entire lower extremity, with the closure of the remaining musculature over the exposed acetabulum. A hip disarticulation is generally performed due to failed vascular procedures following multiple lower-level amputations or for massive trauma with crush injuries to the lower extremity
Hemipelvectomy (HP)	Generally, the leg, hip joint, and half of the pelvis are removed, and the remaining gluteal muscles are brought around and attached to the oblique abdominal muscles. The most common reason for HP is a rare form of connective tissue cancer known as sarcoma. There are various types of sarcomas, such as fibrosarcoma, osteosarcoma, and chondrosarcoma.
Hemicorporectomy	Involves removal of the lower limbs, the bony pelvis below the L4-L5 level, the external genitalia, the bladder, rectum, and anus Necessary life functions are maintained in the upper torso Performed for various indications, including locally invasive pelvic cancer without metastatic spread, benign spinal tumors, intractable decubitus ulcers with malignant change, paraplegia in association with intractable pelvic osteomyelitis and decubitus ulceration, and crushing trauma to the pelvis Given the high mortality following this procedure, especially when performed for visceral malignancy, the indications for its use are very restrictive

Data from Dutton M. *McGraw-Hill's NPTE (National Physical Therapy Examination)*, 2nd ed. 2012. Copyright © McGraw Hill LLC. All rights reserved. https://accessphysiotherapy.mhmedical.com.

This cast generally is changed once or twice weekly, depending on drainage and edema. The semirigid cast is useful in the initial phases of treatment for severe edema and provides protection and soft tissue support. However, after the edema decreases, the semirigid cast is not designed to accommodate limb volume changes and cannot absorb drainage from highly exudative wounds.

Elastic Shrinker. A shrinker (prosthetic compression sock) is not generally recommended until the incision line is adequately healed and there are no areas of open drainage to avoid soft tissue trauma to the distal incision line while pulling compression socks into place.

Currently available transfemoral shrinkers incorporate a hip spica, which provides good suspension except for obese individuals. Prosthetic compression socks are normally kept in place at all times except during bathing or use of a prosthesis for approximately the first 3 months following the amputation to maximize soft tissue edema control.

POSTOPERATIVE PHYSICAL THERAPY

Postoperative physical therapy begins as soon tolerated with the goal to

- Relieve postoperative stump pain.
- Promote healing of the residual limb.
- Maintain or improve strength and ROM.
- Prevent contractures.
- Promote activities of daily living training.
- Maintain stump hygiene.
- Prepare the stump for prosthetic fitting.
- Provide appropriate follow-up care.

Following the initial examination by the physical therapist, a plan of care (POC) is documented. The four main areas in the POC include desensitization, ROM exercises, positioning, and strength training.

Desensitization. The residual stumps are frequently highly sensitive postsurgically and must become tolerant to tactile stimuli and pressure. Typically, the clinician uses a progression of contact with soft materials such as cotton or lamb's wool, progressing to burlap type materials. Rubbing, tapping, and performing resistive exercises with the stump also help prepare the limb for prosthetic fitting. The traditional toughening techniques (eg, beating the stump with a towel wrapped bottle) are not recommended.

ROM exercises. Stretching and ROM exercises are extremely important postsurgically to prevent contractures.

Positioning. Contractures can develop as a result of muscle imbalance or fascial tightness, from a protective withdrawal reflex into hip and knee flexion, from loss of plantar stimulation in extension, or as a result of faulty positioning such as prolonged sitting or placing the residual limb on a pillow.[19]

- Above-knee amputee: Prevent hip flexion, abduction, and external rotation contractures.
- Below-knee amputee: Prevent hip flexion, abduction, and external rotation, and knee flexion contractures.

The clinician should emphasize correct bed and wheelchair positioning, proper stump wrapping, early ambulation, and prone lying. Supine lying with the pelvis level and hip in extension and neutral rotation can also be used. The patient should be advised to avoid prolonged sitting to help prevent hip flexor contractures.

In those who present with hip or knee flexion contractures, facilitated stretching techniques (proprioceptive neuromuscular facilitation [PNF]) are more effective than passive stretching; hold-relax and hold-relax active contractions that utilize the antagonist muscles may increase ROM, particularly at the knee.[19]

Strength training. Selected and specific strengthening exercises must be performed to increase the strength of the residual musculature. The hip extensors and abductors and knee extensors and flexors are particularly important for prosthetic ambulation. Strengthening exercises are initiated with isometrics, progressing to concentric exercises with cuff weights. As strength improves, simple adaptations with traditional weight machines may be made.

- Above-knee amputee: Hip extension, abduction, adduction, pelvic tilt exercises.
- Below-knee amputee: Hip extension, abduction, knee extension, and knee flexion exercises.

POSTOPERATIVE GAIT TRAINING

Many individuals are not fitted with any type of prosthetic appliance until the residual limb is free from edema and much of the soft tissue has shrunk, a process that can take many months of conscientious limb wrapping and exercises.[19] Early fitting with a temporary prosthesis (as soon as the wound is healed) can greatly enhance the postsurgical rehabilitation program.[19]

An understanding of the biomechanics of gait is necessary so that most problems can be discerned using observation. The components of the normal gait cycle were described earlier. Patients who have undergone amputations incorporate different muscles and adaptive strategies to ensure a smooth and well-coordinated gait pattern. As a result, the gait becomes less efficient and occurs at a higher metabolic cost than healthy intact persons, who require less endurance for any given distance (Table 5-10).[20,21]

PATIENT EDUCATION

A major component of postoperative care is patient education, which is provided by nursing and physical therapy, and typically involves the following:

- A discussion of the disease process, the physiological effects of the symptoms, and lifestyle changes to reduce risk factors.
- Methods of edema control.
- Information on the benefits of exercise.
- Hygiene and skincare: The residual limb is kept clean and dry. Care must be taken to avoid abrasions, cuts, and other skin problems.
- Limb inspection: The patient is told to inspect the residual limb with a mirror each night to ensure there are no sores or impending problems, especially in areas not readily visible. This inspection is particularly important if the person has diminished sensation.
- Residual limb wrapping.

LOWER LIMB PROSTHETIC DESIGNS

A prosthesis is an artificial replacement for a body part. Prosthetic components have advanced tremendously over the years and now provide the amputee more comfortable and responsive prosthetic choices. A primary aim of the postsurgical period is to

TABLE 5-10 • Energy Expenditure for Amputation.			
Amputation Level	**Energy Above Baseline, %**	**Speed, m/min**	**Oxygen Cost, mL/kg/m**
Long transtibial	10	70	0.17
Average transtibial	25	60	0.20
Short transtibial	40	50	0.20
Bilateral transtibial	41	50	0.20
Transfemoral	65	40	0.28
Wheelchair	0-8	70	0.16

Data from Wu YJ, Chen SY, Lin MC, et al: Energy expenditure of wheeling and walking during prosthetic rehabilitation in a woman with bilateral transfemoral amputations. *Arch Phys Med Rehabil.* 2001;82:265-269; Traugh GH, Corcoran PJ, Reyes RL: Energy expenditure of ambulation in patients with above-knee amputations. *Arch Phys Med Rehabil.* 1975;56:67-71.

TABLE 5-11 • Implications of the Various Knee, Foot, and Ankle Designs.

Component	Characteristic	Outcome
Knee joint (above knee prosthesis)	TKA line position	The more posterior the joint to the TKA line, the more knee extension is maintained. This creates a more stable leg during stance, but it is harder to initiate knee flexion for the swing phase
	Internal rotation position	Too much internal rotation creates a lateral heel whip on heel raise
	External rotation position	Too much external rotation creates a medial heel with heel raise
	Friction	Less friction makes it easier to bend the knee at heel raise but permits more terminal swing impact at heel strike
Heel	Too soft	Forces knee into extension at heel strike (can be advantageous with an above-knee socket as it speeds knee extension up) Causes premature foot slap at heel strike
	Too hard	Forces knee into flexion at heel strike (can be advantageous with a below-knee socket with patellar-bearing prosthesis)
Toe break	Too posterior	Creates early knee flexion in midstance
	Too anterior	Creates delayed knee flexion in midstance
Ankle moment	Dorsiflexed	Encourages excessive knee flexion in early stance as amputee attempts to achieve foot flat
	Plantarflexed	Encourages excessive knee extension throughout stance Creates a "hill-climbing" sensation of premature heel rise at the end of stance
	Inverted or everted	Does not affect the knee. The prosthetic foot is matched to the uninvolved foot
Foot placement	Anterior	Creates a moment that increases knee extension
	Posterior	Creates a moment that increases knee flexion
	Lateral	Creates a valgus moment at the knee
	Medial	Creates a varus moment at the knee

TKA, total knee arthroplasty.
Data from Dutton M. *McGraw-Hill's NPTE (National Physical Therapy Examination)*, 2nd ed. 2012. Copyright © McGraw Hill LLC. All rights reserved. https://accessphysiotherapy.mhmedical.com.

determine the individual's suitability for prosthetic replacement. Not all people with amputations are candidates for a prosthesis, regardless of personal desire.[19] It is not within the scope of this text to describe the various types of prosthetic devices, but a brief overview is provided (Table 5-11).

Two of the major components of a lower limb prosthesis include the interface (where the skin contacts the liner) and the pylon/frame:

Interface. The interface, where the prosthesis contacts the residual limb, can be produced from either soft or hard material. Some common interface options include thermogel/gel liners, pelite liners, urethane liners, and silicone liners.

Pylon/frame. The two main prosthetic types are the exoskeletal or endoskeletal, of which the latter, which uses pylons constructed from aluminum, titanium, stainless steel, or any hybrid of these materials, to connect the prosthetic components, is the most commonly used type of prosthetic frame.

LOWER LIMB PROSTHETIC TRAINING

The development of specific anticipated goals and expected outcomes of the individual patient with an amputation is based on the following general goals[19]:

- Reduce (or prevent) postoperative edema and promote healing of the residual limb.
- Prevent joint contractures, general debility, and integumentary disturbances.
- Maintain or regain strength in the affected lower extremity.

- Maintain or increase strength in the remaining extremity.
- Demonstrate the ability to perform a home exercise program correctly.
- Learn proper care of the remaining extremity.

The patient must learn to walk with a prosthesis, apply and remove the prosthesis, care for the prosthesis, monitor skin and any pressure points, ambulate on difficult terrain, and use the commode at night.

Donning. Correct application of the prosthesis and frequent inspection of the amputated limb are very important, especially for beginners and those with poor circulation.[22]

Proprioceptive training. This includes balance activities and mobility training. All patients must learn to balance on the amputated side. Parallel bars provide good support to both sides of the body, whereas a plinth or sturdy table offers the dual advantages of providing good support on only one side, ordinarily the contralateral side, and unidirectional control. A typical sequence is outlined below:

- Orientation to the COG and BOS: Various proprioceptive and visual feedback methods may be employed to promote the amputee's ability to maximize the displacement of the COG over the BOS.
- The amputee must learn to displace the COG forward and backward as well as from side to side.
- Single-limb standing: Single-limb balance over the prosthetic limb, while advancing the sound limb, should be practiced in a controlled manner so that, when called on to do so in a dynamic situation such as walking, this skill can be employed with relatively little difficulty. The amputee's ability to control sound limb advancement is directly related to controlling the prosthetic limb stance.
- Stool stepping: The amputee stands in the parallel bars with the sound limb in front of a 4- to 8-in stool or block (depending on the ability level). The patient is asked to slowly step onto the stool with the sound limb while using bilateral upper extremity support on the parallel bars. So the challenge can be increased by asking the patient to remove the sound side hand from the parallel bars and eventually the other hand.
- Exercises to improve the control of the stump side's musculature to maintain balance over the prosthesis.
- Exercises to enhance the patient's proprioception to detect the available sensation within the stump/socket interface.
- Visualization—the amputee must learn to visualize the prosthetic foot and its relationship to the ground.

GAIT TRAINING

Several factors determine optimal gait: pelvic rotation, pelvic obliquity, lateral displacement of the body, knee flexion in the stance phase, and foot and ankle mechanism. In addition, the common gait deviations of transtibial and transfemoral prosthetic gait are briefly addressed. PTAs need to understand gait abnormalities and probable causes with prosthetic use; see Tables 5-12 and 5-13.

UPPER LIMB PROSTHETIC DEVICES

Classification for upper limb amputees is based on the anatomic location of the amputation or surgical site. The acceptance of upper limb prosthetic devices varies depending on the amputee's age, activity level, and comfort level. As with lower limb prosthetics, there are far too many different designs to describe here. Instead, focus will be given to the various interventions.

At the earliest opportunity, the amputee must learn how to don and doff the prosthesis independently and check the fit. Correct operation of the prosthesis can take some time and patience. Typically, gross movements are taught initially, and as control of the prosthesis

TABLE 5-12 · Gait Deviations According to Prosthetic Causes and Amputee Causes.		
Deviation	**Prosthetic Causes**	**Amputee Causes**
Lateral bending of the trunk	The prosthesis may be too short Improperly shaped lateral wall High medial wall Prosthesis aligned in abduction	Poor balance Abduction contracture Improper training Short residual limb Weak hip abductors on the prosthetic side Hypersensitive and painful residual limb
Abducted gait	The prosthesis may be too long High medial wall Improperly shaped lateral wall Prosthesis positioned in too much abduction Inadequate suspension Excessive knee friction	Abduction contracture Improper training Adductor roll Weak hip flexors and adductors Pain over the lateral residual limb
Circumducted gait (this is different from above in that the foot returns to the proper position at heel strike)	The prosthesis may be too long Too much friction in the knee The socket is too small Excessive plantarflexion of the prosthetic foot	Abduction contracture Improper training Weak hip flexors Lacks the confidence to flex the knee A painful anterior distal stump Inability to initiate prosthetic knee flexion
Excessive knee flexion during stance	Socket set forward concerning the foot Foot set in excessive dorsiflexion Stiff heel Prosthesis to long	Knee flexion contracture Hip flexion contracture Pain anteriorly in the residual limb Decrease in quadriceps strength Poor balance
Vaulting	The prosthesis may be too long Inadequate socket suspension Excessive alignment stability Foot in excess plantarflexion	Residual limb discomfort Improper training Fear of stubbing the toe Short residual limb Painful hip/residual limb
Rotation of forefoot at heel strike (usually external rotation)	Excessive toe-out built-in A loose-fitting socket Inadequate suspension Rigid SACH foot	Poor muscle control Improper training Weak medial rotators Short residual limb
Forward trunk flexion	Socket too big Poor suspension Knee instability	Hip flexion contracture Weak hip extensors Pain with ischial weight-bearing Inability to initiate prosthetic knee flexion
Medial or lateral whip	Excessive rotation of the knee Tight socket fit Valgus in the prosthetic knee Improper alignment of toe break	Improper training Weak hip rotators Knee instability
Foot drag (one of the most common problems of the swing phase)	Inadequate suspension of the prosthesis A prosthesis that is too long	Weakness in the hip abductors or ankle plantarflexors on the contralateral side
Uneven arm swing (characterized by the arm on the prosthetic side held close to the body during locomotion)	An improperly fitting socket may cause limb discomfort	Inadequate balance Fear and insecurity accompanied by uneven timing

SACH, solid ankle cushion heel.

improves, finer motor movements are introduced. Use training emphasizes employing the prosthesis as an assistive device, complementing maneuvers of the sound hand. Skills to practice include the following:

- Washing the face.
- Drinking from a cup.

TABLE 5-13 • Gait Analysis of the Below-Knee Amputee.

Problem	Cause
Delayed, abrupt, and limited knee flexion after heel strike	The heel wedge is too soft; the foot is too far anterior
Toe stays off the floor after heel strike	The heel wedge is too stiff; the foot is too anterior; there is too much dorsiflexion
Extended knee throughout the stance phase	There is too much plantarflexion
"Hillclimbing" sensation toward the end of stance phase	The foot is too far anterior; there is too much plantarflexion
The knee is too forcefully and rapidly flexed after heel strike; high pressure against anterior-distal tibia at heel strike and/or prolonged discomfort at this point	The heel wedge is too stiff; the foot is too far dorsiflexed.
Hips level, but prosthesis appears short	The foot is too far posterior; the foot is too dorsiflexed
Toe off the floor as the patient stands, or the knee is flexed too much	The foot is too dorsiflexed
Uneven heel rise	The knee joint may have insufficient friction; there may be an inadequate extension aid
Foot slap	Plantarflexion resistance is usually too soft

Data from Dutton M. *McGraw-Hill's NPTE (National Physical Therapy Examination)*, 2nd ed. 2012. Copyright © McGraw Hill LLC. All rights reserved. https://accessphysiotherapy.mhmedical.com.

- Dressing, including practice with buttoning, using a zipper, and managing other garment fasteners.
- Writing.
- Dining.
- Advanced activities as appropriate (driving, bicycling, playing a musical instrument).

■ ORTHOTICS

An orthosis is an external appliance worn to restrict or assist motion or transfer load from one area to another. Orthoses are designed to promote control, correction, stabilization, or dynamic movement (Table 5-14).[23]

The design of all orthoses is based on three relatively simple principles:

- Pressure: The greater the area of the pad or plastic shell of an orthosis, the less force applied to the skin.
- Equilibrium: The force is of a magnitude and located at a point where the desired movement is either inhibited or facilitated.
- Lever arm: The farther the point of force from the joint, the greater the moment arm and the smaller the magnitude of force required to produce a given torque at the joint.

STUDY PEARL
- A splint: An orthosis intended for temporary use.
- Orthotic: An adjective, often used as a noun.
- Orthotist: The health care professional who designs, fabricates, and fits orthoses of the limbs and trunk.
- Pedorthist: The health care professional who designs, fabricates, and fits only shoes and foot orthoses.

TABLE 5-14 • Orthoses.

Type of Orthosis	Method of Control	Purpose
Ankle-foot orthosis	Limits plantar- or dorsiflexion or assists motion	Control for foot drop; prevents toe drag
Knee-ankle-foot orthosis	Controls ankle and knee and often foot	Provides stability to the knee during gait
Hip-knee-ankle-foot orthosis	Adds a pelvic band and hip joint	Adds hip control for greater stability
Trunk orthosis Corsets	Soft, nonrigid support	Primarily for abdominal compression
Rigid trunk orthosis	Rigid horizontal and vertical components	Limits movement of the trunk, often postsurgery of the spine
Cervical orthosis, soft or rigid	Fabric, foam, or a rigid plastic	Restriction of movement

Data from O'Sullivan SB, Schmitz TJ, Fulk GD. *Physical Rehabilitation*, 6th ed. 2013. Copyright © FA Davis. All rights reserved.

Other considerations include the following:

- The forces at the interface between the orthotic materials and the skin.
- The degrees of freedom at each joint.
- The number of joint segments involved.
- The level of neuromuscular control of each segment, including strength and tone.
- The material selected for orthotic fabrication.
- The activity level of the client.

Collectively, these principles have the following clinical implications:

- There is adequate padding covering the greatest area possible for comfort.
- The total force acting on the involved segment equals zero, or there is equal pressure throughout the orthoses and irritation areas on the skin.
- The length of the orthoses is sufficient to provide an adequate force to create the desired effect and avoid increased transmission of shear forces against the anatomic tissues.

FOOT ORTHOSES

The primary goal of a foot orthosis is to get the subtalar joint to function around its neutral position and facilitate pronation during the initial part of stance and supination during the latter part of stance. Also, foot orthoses can be used to treat specific symptoms or to alleviate symptoms by altering the mechanical function of the subtalar neutral position.

Foot orthoses can be classified into three general categories:

- Soft: Flexible foam-type materials provide cushioning, improve shock absorption, decrease shear forces, and are used to redistribute plantar pressures affording comfort with limited joint control.
- Semirigid: A combination of soft and rigid materials including cork, rubber, or plastics providing some flexibility and shock absorption, however, designed to balance or control the foot.
- Rigid: Strong and durable materials such as plastics or metals assist with transferring weight, stabilizing flexible deformities, and controlling abnormal motion.

Some of the modifications are available and their purposes include the following[24]:

- Arch of the orthotic shell: The arch plays an important role in capturing the inclination angle of the calcaneus and the foot's architecture; it usually does not serve as the primary corrected component.
- Heel cup: Some patients require a deep heel cup because the heel pad spreads over the edge of the shell during weight-bearing and causes discomfort.
- First-ray cut out: Used if the patient has a rigid plantarflexed first ray to increase weight-bearing under the second metatarsal head and provide room for plantarflexion of the first metatarsal.
- Thomas heel: Commonly used on the medial side of the foot to give added leverage for support under the sustentaculum tali and stabilize motion as the foot goes from heel strike to force flat.
- Sole wedge: Most commonly inserted medial to lateral and inserted with the highest part on the anteromedial corner. Serves to stabilize motion and may also shift weight from one side of the shoe to the other.

KNEE ORTHOSES

The primary purpose of most knee orthotic devices is to provide knee control in one or more planes.

- Single-axis joint: Designed to behave like a hinge, preventing movement in the coronal plane, providing medial/lateral stability, while permitting movement in the sagittal plane.

- Offset axis joint: A single-axis joint design with the axis set further posterior from the weight line than the standard single-axis joint, promoting maximal knee extension during weight-bearing without using a mechanical lock.
- Polycentric axis joint: Designed to mimic the instantaneous center of rotation present in the anatomic knee, the two-geared mechanical joint is still confined to a uniplanar path.

■ QUESTIONS

1. **A patient is transitioning from using a front-wheeled walker to a single-point cane. Which of the following gait patterns is the therapist most likely to teach the patient?**
   A. Two-point
   B. Modified two-point
   C. Three-point
   D. Modified three-point

2. **A 24-year-old patient has just had anterior cruciate ligament (ACL) surgery and is 50% partial weight-bearing. Which of the following assistive devices and gait patterns would be most appropriate for this client?**
   A. Front-wheeled walker and three-point gait
   B. Front-wheeled walker and modified three-point gait
   C. Axillary crutches and three-point gait
   D. Axillary crutches and modified three-point gait

3. **A 75-year-old patient is non–weight-bearing following an open reduction internal fixation on the right hip. Which of the following devices and gait patterns are most appropriate for this patient?**
   A. Front-wheeled walker and four-point gait
   B. Front-wheeled walker and three-point gait
   C. Crutches and four-point gait
   D. Crutches and two-point gait

■ ANSWERS WITH RATIONALES

1. **The answer is A.** This is the only gait pattern listed using a unilateral assistive device; all other patterns require bilateral support.

2. **The answer is D.** The client is young and does not need the added support of a front-wheeled walker, and 50% weight-bearing requires a modified three-point gait pattern.

3. **The answer is B.** The client is elderly, so a more stable device would be appropriate, but more importantly, a non–weight-bearing gait pattern is always a three-point pattern.

REFERENCES

1. Mann RA, Hagy JL, White V, Liddell D. The initiation of gait. *J Bone Joint Surg Am.* 1979;61:232-239.
2. Schmitz TJ. Locomotor training. In: O'Sullivan SB, Schmitz TJ, eds. *Physical Rehabilitation.* 5th ed. Philadelphia, PA: FA Davis; 2007:523-560.
3. Burnett CN, Johnson EW. Development of gait in children; I. Method; II. Results. *Dev Med Child Neurol.* 1971;13:196-206.
4. Luttgens K, Hamilton N. Locomotion: solid surface. In: Luttgens K, Hamilton N, eds. *Kinesiology: Scientific Basis of Human Motion.* 9th ed. Dubuque, IA: McGraw-Hill; 1997:519-549.
5. Richardson JK, Iglarsh ZA. Gait. In: Richardson JK, Iglarsh ZA, eds. *Clinical Orthopaedic Physical Therapy.* Philadelphia, PA: Saunders; 1994:602-625.
6. Hogue RE. Upper extremity muscular activity at different cadences and inclines during normal gait. *Phys Ther.* 1969;49:963-972.
7. Murray MP, Sepic SB, Barnard EJ. Patterns of sagittal rotation of the upper limbs in walking. *Phys Ther.* 1967;47:272-284.
8. Epler M. Gait. In: Richardson JK, Iglarsh ZA, eds. *Clinical Orthopaedic Physical Therapy.* Philadelphia, PA: WB Saunders; 1994:602-625.
9. Mann RA, Moran GT, Dougherty SE. Comparative electromyography of the lower extremity in jogging, running and sprinting. *Am J Sports Med.* 1986;14:501-510.

10. Perry J. *Gait Analysis: Normal and Pathological Function.* Thorofare, NJ: Slack Inc; 1992.

11. Gage JR, Deluca PA, Renshaw TS. Gait analysis: principles and applications with emphasis on its use with cerebral palsy. *Inst Course Lect.* 1996;45:491-507.

12. Levine D, Whittle M. Gait analysis: the lower extremities. La Crosse, WI: Orthopaedic Section, APTA, Inc.; 1992.

13. Saunders JBD, Inman VT, Eberhart HD. The major determinants in normal and pathological gait. *J Bone Joint Surg Am.* 1953;35:543-558.

14. Whitehouse PA, Knight LA, Di Nicolantonio F, Mercer SJ, Sharma S, Cree IA. Heterogeneity of chemosensitivity of colorectal adenocarcinoma determined by a modified ex vivo ATP-tumor chemosensitivity assay (ATP-TCA). *Anticancer Drugs.* 2003;14:369-375.

15. Perry J. Gait cycle. In: Perry J, ed. *Gait Analysis: Normal and Pathological Function.* Thorofare, NJ: Slack Inc; 1992:3-7.

16. Dee R. Normal and abnormal gait in the pediatric patient. In: Dee R, Hurst LC, Gruber MA, et al., eds. *Principles of Orthopaedic Practice.* 2nd ed. New York, NY: McGraw-Hill; 1997:685-692.

17. Norkin CC. Examination of gait. In: O'Sullivan SB, Schmitz TJ, eds. *Physical Rehabilitation.* 5th ed. Philadelphia, PA: FA Davis; 2007:317-363.

18. Guide to Physical Therapist Practice. 3.0. American Physical Therapy Association. Alexandria, VA 2014.

19. May BJ. Amputation. In: O'Sullivan SB, Schmitz TJ, eds. *Physical Rehabilitation.* 5th ed. Philadelphia, PA: FA Davis; 2007:1031-1055.

20. Wu YJ, Chen SY, Lin MC, Lan C, Lai JS, Lien IN. Energy expenditure of wheeling and walking during prosthetic rehabilitation in a woman with bilateral transfemoral amputations. *Arch Phys Med Rehabil.* 2001;82:265-269.

21. Traugh GH, Corcoran PJ, Reyes RL. Energy expenditure of ambulation in patients with above-knee amputations. *Arch Phys Med Rehabil.* 1975;56:67-71.

22. Edelstein JE. Prosthetics. In: O'Sullivan SB, Schmitz TJ, eds. *Physical Rehabilitation.* 5th ed. Philadelphia, PA: FA Davis; 2007:1251-1286.

23. Gailey RS. Orthotics in rehabilitation. In: Prentice WE, Voight ML, eds. *Techniques in Musculoskeletal Rehabilitation.* New York, NY: McGraw-Hill; 2001:325-346.

24. Tiberio D, Hinkebein JR. Foot orthoses and shoe design. In: Placzek JD, Boyce DA, eds. *Orthopaedic Physical Therapy Secrets.* Philadelphia, PA: Hanley & Belfus, Inc.; 2001:455-462.

6

Integumentary System

CASSADY BARTLETT

OVERVIEW

The integumentary system is the largest organ in the body and is important to our survival in many ways. The skin is an organ which acts as a barrier between the internal system and the external environment as well as plays a role in temperature regulation.

▲ HIGH-YIELD TERMS

Capillary refill	Press down on one of the patient's nails until it pales. Release the nail and observe for the pink color to return. The normal color should return in less than 3 seconds.
	Note: Capillary refill can be affected by room and body temperature, vasoconstriction from smoking, or peripheral edema.
Clubbing	Normal concave nail bases will create a small, diamond-shaped space when the nails of the index fingers of each hand are placed together. Clubbed fingers are convex at the bases and will touch without leaving a space.
	Note: Finger clubbing, a sign of chronic tissue hypoxia, occurs when the angle between the fingernail and where the nail enters the skin increases.
Cyanosis	Dark bluish or purplish discoloration of the integument and mucous membranes.
	Note: May indicate hypoxia or hematologic pathology.
Hyperthermia	Increased temperature.
	Note: May indicate localized or systemic infection, inflammation, thermal injury; hyperthyroidism or fever is generalized.
Hypothermia	Decreased temperature.
	Note: May indicate arterial insufficiency or shock.
Jaundice	Yellowish discoloration of skin and sclera.
	Note: May indicate liver disease or hemolytic pathology.
Tzanck smear	Scraping of an ulcer base to look for Tzanck cells (acantholytic cells). It is sometimes also called the chickenpox skin test or the herpes skin test.
Dermatitis	Inflammation of the skin.
Total body surface area	Used to estimate the total fluid and caloric requirements and is a predictor of mortality.
Hypertrophic scar	A raised scar that stays within the burn wound's boundaries; characteristically red, raised, firm.
Keloid scar	A raised scar extends beyond the original burn wound; red, raised, firm.
Pruritus	Itching.
Exudate	Also known as drainage, exudate is a liquid produced by the body in response to tissue damage.

Primary intention	Wound edges are approximated with sutures, staples, or adhesives. Minimal scarring and heal quickly (blisters and abrasions may fall into this quick healing).
Secondary intention	The wound closes on its own with a layer of granulation tissue filling in lost tissue space followed by wound contraction and scar tissue formation resulting in larger scars.
Tertiary intention	A delayed primary intention for cases in which a wound has been left open or the event of dehiscence (opening of the wound).

The integumentary system has two major components: the cutaneous membrane (skin), which is divided into three layers: the epidermis, the dermis, and subcutaneous tissue, and the accessory structures, which include the hair, nails, vascular supply, sweat glands, and sebaceous glands (Figure 6-1). The skin serves as a protective barrier, has immunologic functions for first-line defenses, and is involved in melanin production, vitamin D synthesis, sensation, temperature regulation, protection from trauma, and aesthetics.

Wound healing, which occurs over several phases (Table 6-1), can be affected by a wide variety of interacting elements. The patient's age, comorbidities, functional status, medications, and lifestyle may positively or negatively impact healing. The risk for delayed healing increases with elevated age, more comorbidities, history of smoking, and decreased activity level. Risk factor assessments may include *Norton Risk Assessment, Gosnell Scale-Pressure Sore Risk Assessment*, or *Braden Scale for Predicting Pressure Sore Risk* to standardize risk.[1] Additional assessment of range of motion (ROM), muscle strength, pain levels, edema, sensation, or posture may contribute to understanding risk level.

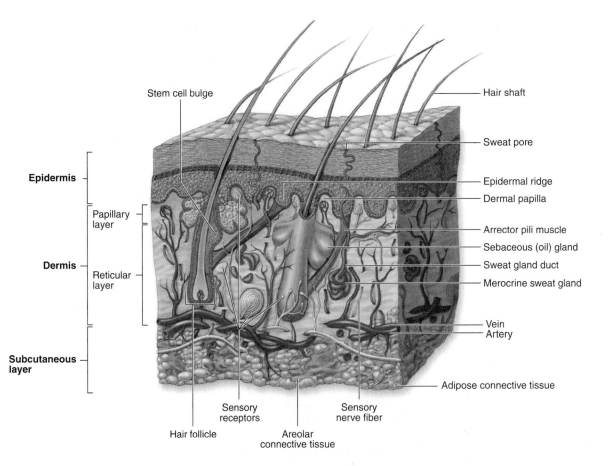

Figure 6-1. Anatomy of the skin. (Reproduced with permission from Hamm RL. *Text and Atlas of Wound Diagnosis and Treatment.* 2015. Copyright © McGraw Hill LLC. All rights reserved. https://accessphysiotherapy.mhmedical.com.)

TABLE 6-1 • Overview of Wound Healing Phases.

Inflammation phase: Immediate normal protective response to allow for initiation of the healing process. Inflammation may attack the tissue in autoimmune disorders or may become chronic, causing tissue damage.
• Days 1-6
  • Rubor (redness)
  • Edema
  • Pain
  • Heat

Proliferative phase: Occurs to cover of the wound and give strength to the tissue.
• Days 3-20
  • Epithelialization—restore epidermis
  • Collagen production—fibroblasts produce collagen fibers that create a tensile strength by crosslinking
  • Wound contraction—the wound edges are pulled together by myofibroblasts to shrink the wound opening; if uncontrolled, contractures can form
  • Neovascularization—angiogenesis occurs to provide oxygen and nutrients

Maturation phase: Goal is to restore tissue function
• Day 9 and forward
  • Longest phase—may last > 1 year
  • The scar becomes paler as collagen matures
  • Excessive collagen production may result in **keloids** extending beyond wound borders or hypertrophic scars within the wound borders that are raised. Hypertrophic scars may be treated with prolonged pressure (eg, pressure garments for burn injuries)
  • Collagen orientation may be affected by appropriately applied tension

Data from Cameron M. *Physical Agents in Rehabilitation: An Evidence-Based Approach to Practice*, 5th ed. 2018. Copyright © Elsevier. All rights reserved; O'Sullivan SB, Schmitz TJ, Fulk GD. *Physical Rehabilitation*, 7th ed. 2019. Copyright © FA Davis. All rights reserved.

■ EXAMINATION

The physical therapy examination includes taking the individual's history, conducting a standardized system review, and performing selected tests and measures to identify potential and existing movement-related disorders. The evaluating physical therapist (PT) determines if certain signs and symptoms warrant referral for additional medical evaluation. Key points for the integumentary history may include a history of the present illness, symptoms, date of onset, severity, medications, history of a previous problem, changes in size or appearance of a lesion, bleeding from the lesion, and sunscreen use. The physical therapist assistant (PTA) will document any subjective reports pertaining to the healing status or change in symptoms. Various specific tests and measures may be used in whole or portion during the examination, based on the purpose of the visit, the complexity of the condition, and the direction taken in the clinical decision-making process.

Signs and symptoms of integumentary disorders may include but are not limited to:

- Lesions of the skin (primary [Table 6-2] and secondary [Table 6-3]).
- Pigment changes (changes in color, eg, cyanosis, redness, paleness, yellowing).
- Rash/pruritus (itching, length of time present).
- Blisters.
- Bruising/bleeding.
- Nevi/moles/nodules/cysts (changes in area, border, color, diameter).
- Dryness/sweating (xerosis).
- Presence of edema.
- Changes in nail appearance.
- Changes in skin turgor, texture.

TABLE 6-2 · Primary Lesions and Their Morphology.

Terminology	Morphology	Examples
Macule	A flat, level with the surface of skin (≤ 1 cm) lesion with color change	Rubeola, rubella, scarlet fever, roseola infantum
Papule	A solid, elevated lesion, sharply circumscribed, small (1 cm) colored lesion (pink, tan, red, or any variation)	Dermatitis, ringworm, psoriasis
Wheal	An elevated white to a pink edematous lesion that is unstable and associated with pruritus that lasts < 24 hours	Mosquito bites and hives (urticaria)
Nodule	Dermal or subcutaneous solid, elevated lesion	Amelanotic melanoma
Vesicle	A bulging, small (< 1 cm) blister containing clear fluid	Herpes simplex, varicella, poison ivy, herpes zoster
Pustule	An elevated, sharply circumscribed (< 1 cm) cavity filled with pus	Impetigo, acne, *Staphylococcus* infections
Cyst	Cavity filled with pus or keratin	Epidermal cyst
Petechiae	Tiny, reddish-purple, sharply circumscribed spots of hemorrhage in the superficial layers of the skin or epidermis	Meningococcemia, bacterial endocarditis, nonthrombocytopenic purpura

Tests, measures, and screening that may be relevant to the integumentary system may include but are not limited to:

- Inspection of skin and changes (eg, color, temperature, turgor, moisture, odor, scars, masses, moles, nails, skin mobility).
- Capillary refill.
- Palpation (eg, lesion tenderness, firmness, depth).
- Measurement (length, width, depth, subcutaneous extension) using perpendicular, clock, tracing, and photographic methods.
- Location/color/shape/size (Table 6-4).
- Presence and type of exudate (Table 6-5).
- Temperature (hypothermia, hyperthermia).
- Sensation.
- Nail inspection (clubbing, discoloration, brittleness, ridging, cleanliness).
- Functional status.

■ WOUND CARE

PTs and PTAs play a vital role as members of the wound care team; however, individual state practice acts should be consulted to determine the scope of practice. Primary wound care principles include wound cleansing, management of edema and exudate, reduction of necrotic tissue, and control of microorganisms. Table 6-6 describes wound debridement techniques. The PTA is most commonly involved with nonselective debridement and application of topical agents and dressings. A review of the specific wound evaluation (example

TABLE 6-3 · Secondary Lesions and Their Morphology.

Terminology	Morphology	Examples
Crust	Dried blood, serum, scales, and pus from corrosive lesions	Infectious dermatitis
Excoriation	Mechanical removal of the epidermis leaving dermis exposed	Scratch, scrape of the original lesion
Scales	Dried fragments of sloughed dead epidermis	Seborrhea and tinea capitis
Ulcer	Destruction and loss of epidermis, dermis, and possibly subcutaneous layers	Decubitus ulceration
Fissure	A vertical, linear crack through the epidermis and dermis	
Scar	Formation of dense connective tissue resulting from destruction of skin	

TABLE 6-4 • Documentation Characteristics (Location/Color/Shape/Size).

Description	Examples
Characteristics	• Size • Shape • Color • Texture • Elevation or depression
Type	• Abrasion: A wearing away of the upper layer of the skin due to applied friction force. • Contusion (bruise): Caused when blood vessels are damaged or broken due to a direct blow to the skin. • Ecchymosis: The skin discoloration caused by the escape of blood into the tissues from ruptured blood vessels. • Hematoma: A localized collection of blood, usually clotted, in a tissue or organ. • Excoriation: Lesion of a traumatic nature with epidermal loss in a generally linear shape. • Laceration: An injury involving penetration of the skin, in which the wound is deeper than the superficial skin level. • Penetrating wound: A wound accompanied by disruption of the body surface extending into the underlying tissue or a body cavity. • Petechiae: Tiny red spots in the skin that do not blanch when pressed upon. Petechiae results from red blood leaking from capillaries into the skin (intradermal hemorrhages). Petechiae are < 3 mm in diameter. • Puncture: A wound made by a pointed object (like a nail). • Ulcer: A lesion on the skin's surface or the surface of the mucous membrane, produced by the sloughing of inflammatory, necrotic tissue.
Exudates	• Color • Odor • Amount • Consistency
Pattern of arrangement	• Annular • Grouped • Linear • Diffuse
Location and distribution	• Generalized or localized • Region of the body • Discrete or confluent

Data from Dutton M. *McGraw-Hill's NPTE (National Physical Therapy Examination)*, 2nd ed. 2012. Copyright © McGraw Hill LLC. All rights reserved. https://accessphysiotherapy.mhmedical.com.

in Table 6-7) is necessary for the PTA to become familiar to read the POC and understand the present status of wound healing. Specific wound and patient characteristics must be documented with direct references to wound location, size, tissue type, exudate, peri-wound condition, bacterial burden, pain, support needs, and quality of life (Tables 6-8 and 6-9). Dressing selection is based on optimal healing in the changing wound environment;

TABLE 6-5 • Exudate Classification.

Type of Exudate	Description
Serous	Presents as clear, light color with a thin, watery consistency. Serous exudate is considered to be normal in a healthy healing wound.
Sanguinous	Presents as red with a thin, watery consistency. Sanguinous exudate appears to be red due to the presence of blood, or it may be brown if allowed to dehydrate. This type of exudate may be indicative of new blood vessel growth or the disruption of blood vessels.
Serosanguinous	Presents as light red or pink, with a thin, watery consistency. Serosanguinous exudate can be normal in a healthy healing wound.
Seropurulent	Presents as an opaque, yellow, or tan color, with a thin, watery consistency. Seropurulent exudate may be an early warning sign of an impending infection.
Purulent	Presents as a yellow or green color with a thick, viscous consistency. This type of exudate is generally an indicator of wound infection.

Reproduced with permission from Dutton M. *McGraw-Hill's NPTE (National Physical Therapy Examination)*, 2nd ed. 2012. Copyright © McGraw Hill LLC. All rights reserved. https://accessphysiotherapy.mhmedical.com.

TABLE 6-6 · Methods of Wound Debridement.

Wound debridement can be accomplished in several ways:
- Mechanically: Whirlpool, pulsatile lavage, other forms of spray irrigation, and the traditional wet-to-dry dressing.
- Surgically: Performed by a physician with the patient anesthetized.
- Sharp debridement removes necrotic tissue using a scalpel or other sharp instrument with the patient alert.
- Chemically: The use of enzymes or other topical agents, such as Dakin's solution (weak bleach).
- Autolytically: The body does its own cleaning. This type of debridement is the least traumatic to healthy tissue but may take longer than enzymes or more invasive forms of debridement.

Data from Dutton M. *McGraw-Hill's NPTE (National Physical Therapy Examination)*, 2nd ed. 2012. Copyright © McGraw Hill LLC. All rights reserved. https://accessphysiotherapy.mhmedical.com.

a single treatment plan for any given wound will rarely remain the same throughout the healing process. Optimal dressing selection to facilitate wound healing (Table 6-10) is completed by the evaluating PT and depends on a thorough assessment of the wound. Dressing choice can vary (Table 6-11), but ideally, the dressing should create a moist environment without maceration or desiccation. Two key terms used to describe dressings are *occlusion* and *moisture*. Occlusion refers to the ability of a dressing to transmit moisture, vapor, or gases from the wound bed to the atmosphere. Occlusive dressings are completely impermeable, while nonocclusive dressings are completely permeable. The following dressings are arranged from most occlusive to nonocclusive: hydrocolloids, hydrogels, semipermeable foam, semipermeable film, impregnated gauze, alginates, and traditional gauze. Moisture dressings can be classified according to the ability to retain moisture. The following dressings are arranged from most moisture retentive to least moisture-retentive: alginates, semipermeable foam, hydrocolloids, hydrogels, and semipermeable films. Activity levels and patient goals are important for selecting the secondary dressings and interventions such as negative pressure wound therapy that may affect daily living and work demands.

◼ INTEGUMENTARY CONDITIONS

Frequently encountered integumentary conditions are described here, as are the specific intervention strategies.

HERPES ZOSTER (SHINGLES)

Herpes zoster (shingles) represents the reactivation of latent varicella (chickenpox) infection. The varicella-zoster virus may be preserved as a latent form in the dorsal root ganglia following a varicella infection. Reactivation of the virus by trauma, stress, fever, radiation therapy, or immunosuppression can result in a cutaneous eruption in the affected sensory nerve(s) distribution. In addition, direct contact with vesicular fluid can result in varicella in a susceptible person, and immunocompromised and pregnant patients are at a higher risk of severe complications if they contract varicella.

Clinical Significance

Disturbances include the following:

1. Painful skin rash with blisters in a dermatome that typically scabs in 7 to 10 days and clears within 2 to 4 weeks.
2. Persistent postherpetic neuralgia can negatively impact a patient's health and quality of life, especially in the elderly, associated with insomnia, anorexia, and depression.
3. Fever, headache, or chills.
4. Upset stomach.

Diagnostic Tests and Measures

The key diagnostic clinical features of herpes zoster are grouped painful vesicles within a dermatome.

TABLE 6-7 • Bates-Jensen Wound Assessment Tool.

Instructions for Use

General Guidelines

Fill out the attached rating sheet to assess a wound's status after reading the definitions and methods of assessment described below. Evaluate once a week and whenever a change occurs in the wound. Rate according to each item by picking the response that best describes the wound and entering that score in the item score column for the appropriate date. When you have rated the wound on all items, determine the total score by adding together the 13-item scores. The *higher* the total score, the more severe the wound status. Plot total score on the Wound Status Continuum to determine progress. If the wound has healed/resolved, score items 1, 2, 3, and 4 as = 0.

Specific Instructions

1. **Size:** Use a ruler to measure the longest and widest aspect of the wound surface in centimeters; multiply the length by width. Score as = 0 if wound healed/resolved.

2. **Depth:** Pick the depth and thickness most appropriate to the wound using these additional descriptions, score as = 0 if wound healed/resolved:
   1 = Tissues damaged but no break in skin surface
   2 = Superficial abrasion, blister, or shallow crater; even with and/or elevated above skin surface (eg, hyperplasia)
   3 = Deep crater with or without undermining of adjacent tissue
   4 = Visualization of tissue layers not possible due to necrosis
   5 = Supporting structures include tendon, joint capsule

3. **Edges:** Score as = 0 if wound healed/resolved. Use this guide:
   Indistinct, diffuse = Unable to clearly distinguish wound outline
   Attached = Even or flush with wound base, no sides or walls present; flat
   Not attached = Sides or walls are present; floor or base of wound is deeper than edge
   Rolled under, thickened = Soft to firm, and flexible to touch
   Hyperkeratosis = Callous-like tissue formation around wound and at edges
   Fibrotic, scarred = Hard, rigid to touch

4. **Undermining:** Score as = 0 if wound healed/resolved. Assess by inserting a cotton-tipped applicator under the wound edge; advance it as far as it will go without using undue force; raise the tip of the applicator so it may be seen or felt on the surface of the skin; mark the surface with a pen; measure the distance from the mark on the skin to the edge of the wound. Continue process around the wound. Then use a transparent metric measuring guide with concentric circles divided into four (25%) pie-shaped quadrants to help determine percent of wound involved.

5. **Necrotic tissue type:** Pick the type of necrotic tissue that is predominant in the wound according to color, consistency, and adherence using this guide:
   White/gray nonviable tissue = May appear prior to wound opening; skin surface is white or gray
   Nonadherent, yellow slough = Thin, mucinous substance; scattered throughout wound bed; easily separated from wound tissue
   Loosely adherent, yellow slough = Thick, stringy, clumps of debris; attached to wound tissue
   Adherent, soft, black eschar = Soggy tissue; strongly attached to tissue in center or base of wound
   Firmly adherent, hard/black eschar = Firm, crusty tissue; strongly attached to wound base and edges (like a hard scab)

6. **Necrotic tissue amount:** Use a transparent metric measuring guide with concentric circles divided into four (25%) pie-shaped quadrants to help determine percent of wound involved.

7. **Exudate type:** Some dressings interact with wound drainage to produce a gel or trap liquid. Before assessing exudate type, gently cleanse wound with normal saline or water. Pick the exudate type that is predominant in the wound according to color and consistency, using this guide:
   Bloody = Thin, bright red
   Serosanguineous = Thin, watery pale red to pink
   Serous = Thin, watery, clear
   Purulent = Thin or thick, opaque tan to yellow or green may have offensive odor

(Continued)

TABLE 6-7 • Bates-Jensen Wound Assessment Tool. (*Continued*)

Instructions for Use

8. **Exudate amount:** Use a transparent metric measuring guide with concentric circles divided into four (25%) pie-shaped quadrants to determine percent of dressing involved with exudate. Use this guide:

   None = Wound tissues dry

   Scant = Wound tissues moist; no measurable exudate

   Small = Wound tissues wet; moisture evenly distributed in wound; drainage involves < 25% dressing

   Moderate = Wound tissues saturated; drainage may or may not be evenly distributed in wound; drainage involves > 25% to < 75% dressing

   Large = Wound tissues bathed in fluid; drainage freely expressed; may or may not be evenly distributed in wound; drainage involves > 75% of dressing

9. **Skin color surrounding wound:** Assess tissues within 4 cm of wound edge. Dark-skinned persons show the colors "bright red" and "dark red" as a deepening of normal ethnic skin color or a purple hue. As healing occurs in dark-skinned persons, the new skin is pink and may never darken.

10. **Peripheral tissue edema and induration:** Assess tissues within 4 cm of wound edge. Nonpitting edema appears as skin that is shiny and taut. Identify pitting edema by firmly pressing a finger down into the tissues and waiting for 5 seconds; on release of pressure, tissues fail to resume previous position and an indentation appears. Induration is abnormal firmness of tissues with margins. Assess by gently pinching the tissues. Induration results in an inability to pinch the tissues. Use a transparent metric measuring guide to determine how far edema or induration extends beyond wound.

11. **Granulation tissue:** Granulation tissue is the growth of small blood vessels and connective tissue to fill in full-thickness wounds. Tissue is healthy when bright, beefy red, shiny, and granular with a velvety appearance. Poor vascular supply appears as pale pink or blanched to dull, dusky red color.

12. **Epithelialization:** Epithelialization is the process of epidermal resurfacing and appears as pink or red skin. In partial-thickness wounds, it can occur throughout the wound bed as well as from the wound edges. In full-thickness wounds, it occurs from the edges only. Use a transparent metric measuring guide with concentric circles divided into four (25%) pie-shaped quadrants to help determine percent of wound involved and to measure the distance the epithelial tissue extends into the wound.

Bates-Jensen Wound Assessment Tool   **Name** _____

Complete the rating sheet to assess wound status. Evaluate each item by picking the response that best describes the wound and entering the score in the item score column for the appropriate date. If the wound has healed/resolved, score items 1, 2, 3, and 4 as = 0.

Location: Anatomic site. Circle, identify right (**R**) or left (**L**), and use "**X**" to mark site on body diagrams:

___ Sacrum and coccyx	___ Lateral ankle
___ Trochanter	___ Medial ankle
___ Ischial tuberosity	___ Heel ___ Other site: ___
___ Buttock	

Shape: Overall wound pattern; assess by observing perimeter and depth. Circle and date appropriate description:

___ Irregular	___ Linear or elongated
___ Round/oval	___ Bowl/boat
___ Square/rectangle	___ Butterfly ___ Other shape: ___

Item	Assessment	Date Score	Date Score	Date Score
1. Size*	*0 = Healed, resolved wound 1 = Length × width < 4 sq cm 2 = Length × width 4-<16 sq cm 3 = Length × width 16.1-< 36 sq cm 4 = Length × width 36.1-< 80 sq cm 5 = Length × width > 80 sq cm			
2. Depth*	*0 = Healed, resolved wound 1 = Nonblanchable erythema on intact skin 2 = Partial-thickness skin loss involving epidermis and/or dermis 3 = Full-thickness skin loss involving damage or necrosis of subcutaneous tissue; may extend down to but not through underlying fascia; and/or mixed partial- and full-thickness and/or tissue layers obscured by granulation tissue 4 = Obscured by necrosis 5 = Full-thickness skin loss with extensive destruction, tissue necrosis, or damage to muscle, bone, or supporting structures			
3. Edges*	*0 = Healed, resolved wound 1 = Indistinct, diffuse, none clearly visible 2 = Distinct, outline clearly visible, attached, even with wound base 3 = Well defined not attached to wound base 4 = Well defined not attached to base, rolled under, thickened 5 = Well defined fibrotic, scarred, or hyperkeratotic			

(Continued)

TABLE 6-7 • Bates-Jensen Wound Assessment Tool. (Continued)

	Instructions for Use		
4. Undermining*	*0 = Healed, resolved wound 1 = None present 2 = Undermining < 2 cm in any area 3 = Undermining 2-4 cm involving < 50% wound margins 4 = Undermining 2-4 cm involving > 50% wound margins 5 = Undermining > 4 cm or tunneling in any area		
5. Necrotic tissue type	1 = None visible 2 = White/gray nonviable tissue and/or nonadherent yellow slough 3 = Loosely adherent yellow slough 4 = Adherent, soft, black eschar 5 = Firmly adherent, hard, black eschar		
6. Necrotic tissue amount	1 = None visible 2 = < 25% of wound bed covered 3 = 25%-50% of wound covered 4 = > 50% and < 75% of wound covered 5 = 75%-100% of wound covered		
7. Exudate type	1 = None 2 = Bloody 3 = Serosanguinous: thin, watery, pale red/pink 4 = Serous: thin, watery, clear 5 = Purulent: thin or thick, opaque, tan/yellow, with or without odor		
8. Exudate amount	1 = None, dry wound 2 = Scant, wound moist but no observable exudate 3 = Small 4 = Moderate 5 = Large		
9. Skin color surrounding wound	1 = Pink or normal for ethnic group 2 = Bright red and/or blanches to touch 3 = White or gray pallor or hypopigmented 4 = Dark red or purple and/or nonblanchable 5 = Black or hyperpigmented		
10. Peripheral tissue edema	1 = No swelling or edema 2 = Nonpitting edema extends < 4 cm around wound 3 = Nonpitting edema extends > 4 cm around wound 4 = Pitting edema extends < 4 cm around wound 5 = Crepitus and/or pitting edema extends > 4 cm around wound		
11. Peripheral tissue induration	1 = None present 2 = Induration < 2 cm around wound 3 = Induration 2-4 cm extending < 50% around wound 4 = Induration 2-4 cm extending > 50% around wound 5 = Induration > 4 cm in any area around wound		

12. Granulation tissue	1 = Skin intact or partial-thickness wound 2 = Bright, beefy red; 75%-100% of wound filled and/or tissue overgrowth 3 = Bright, beefy red; < 75% and > 25% of wound filled 4 = Pink, and/or dull, dusky red and/or fills < 25% of wound 5 = No granulation tissue present	
13. Epithelialization	1 = 100% wound covered, surface intact 2 = 75%-< 100% wound covered and/or epithelial tissue extends > 0.5 cm into wound bed 3 = 50%-< 75% wound covered and/or epithelial tissue extends to < 0.5 cm into wound bed 4 = 25%-< 50% wound covered 5 = < 25% wound covered	
Total Score		
Signature		

Wound Status Continuum

```
    <—————————————————————————————————————————————————>
    1    5    9 13 15 20   25   30   35   40   45   50   55   65
    Tissue    Healed Wound                                    Wound
    health    regeneration                                    degeneration
```

Plot the total score on the Wound Status Continuum by putting an "**X**" on the line and the date beneath the line. Plot multiple scores with their dates to see regeneration or degeneration of the wound at a glance.

© 2006 Barbara Bates-Jensen. Used with permission from Dr. Barbara Bates-Jensen.

TABLE 6-8 • Wound Colors.		
Color	**Wound Description**	**Intervention Goals**
Red	Healthy, pink granular tissue with the absence of necrotic tissue	Protect wound; maintain a moist environment
Yellow	Presence of adherent fibrinous exudates and debris (moist yellow slough)	Debride necrotic tissue; absorb drainage
Black	Presence of black, thick eschar (dried necrotic tissue), firmly adhered	Debride necrotic tissue

Data from Cozzell J. The new red, yellow, black color code. *Am J Nurs.* 1988;(88)10:1342-1346.

Other Tests

- Tzanck smear.
- Viral cultures.
- Polymerase chain reaction (PCR) testing (used to reproduce [amplify] selected sections of DNA and RNA for analysis).

Clinical Findings, Secondary Effects, Complications

1. Intense pain within a dermatome.
2. Pain may precede the eruption by one or a few days.
3. Pruritus, tingling, tenderness, or hyperesthesia may also develop.
4. Eruption presents as grouped vesicles within the dermatome of the affected nerves, usually within a single unilateral dermatome (trunk and trigeminal nerve).
5. Any area of the body may be affected, but it is seen most frequently on the trunk.

Interventions/Treatment

Medical. Oral antiviral medications, if given early, may reduce the duration of the eruption and the risk and severity of acute pain and perhaps postherpetic neuralgia. The treatments should be started within 72 hours of the symptom onset. Appropriate treatment for acute pain may be needed. Vaccination with a live zoster vaccine (Zostavax) may reduce the risk of developing herpes zoster.

Pharmacologic. Acyclovir (Zovirax), famciclovir (Famvir), valacyclovir 1000 mg (Valtrex). Treatments may include topical lidocaine or capsaicin, antidepressants (such as

TABLE 6-9 • Wound and Patient Characteristics Assessed for Treatment Decisions.	
Location	The location of the wound helps determine the secondary dressing that will best secure the primary dressing.
Size	The wound size determines the size and amount of the primary dressing required to fill and cover the wound surface adequately.
Tissue type	The tissue appearance and predominant tissue type and any exposed structures are key determinants of primary dressing selection.
Exudate	The amount and type of exudate are a fundamental consideration in both primary and secondary dressing selection.
Periwound condition	A key goal of the total dressing is to maintain the periwound skin integrity, which reduces pain and the risk of infection.
Bacterial burden	Topical agents and dressings to reduce local bioburden can reduce the number of bacteria before they replicate to a critical level.
Support needs	Compression for venous wounds, off-loading for diabetic foot ulcers, and visualization for infected wounds are examples of needs that may require special dressings.

TABLE 6-10 • Characteristics of the Ideal Wound Dressing.	
Provides a moist wound environment	By either donating or removing moisture from the wound bed, the dressing maintains the optimal moisture level, thereby preventing desiccation of the cells.
Manages exudate appropriately	The dressing adequately absorbs or manages the wound exudate so that it is sequestered in the dressing and does not exude onto the intact periwound skin, thus causing maceration or denudation.
Facilitates autolytic debridement	In the presence of necrotic tissue, the dressing creates an environment so that ambient wound fluid containing phagocytic cells and endogenous enzymes is in contact with the tissue, thus facilitating autolysis.
Provides antimicrobial properties if needed	If a wound is highly colonized or infected, the antimicrobial dressing will aid in sequestering wound fluid or providing active antimicrobial activity to reduce or eliminate bacteria.
Minimizes pain	The selected dressing material does not adhere to the wound bed and disrupts the surface, thus harming healthy cells. In addition, by not adhering, the dressing lifts from the wound and periwound easily, and as a result, does not cause the patient undue discomfort.
Prevents contamination by being impermeable to environmental bacteria	On all wounds (especially those in the sacral, coccyx, and ischial area where contamination is likely), the dressing surface is impermeable to bacteria and contamination from the environment, which is especially important for the incontinent patient.
Is compatible with support needs	The dressing can be used under support treatments such as contact casts and compression wraps that are often left in place for a full week.
Insulates and maintains an optimal temperature	The dressing allows maintenance of constant temperature without frequent cooling of the tissue that can impact healing. Frequent dressing changes can negatively impact wound healing more than the dressing selection itself.
Prevents particulate contamination or allergens from coming in contact with the wound surface	The dressing does not leave threads or pieces of adherent dressing in the wound bed, which could act as a foreign body in the tissue. Also, the dressing does not contain common allergens such as latex.
Easily applied and removed (user-friendly)	The dressing can be used by the care providers in the patient's setting, including family members at home.
Is available and cost-effective	The dressing must be available in the health care setting in which the patient resides. Choices available in a hospital or clinic may not be reimbursable for the patient at home, or they may not be on the formulary of a particular home care agency or skilled nursing facility. Therefore, flexibility in dressing selection by the prescriber is required as long as the selection meets the needs of the wound.

Reproduced with permission from Hamm RL. *Text and Atlas of Wound Diagnosis and Treatment*. 2015. Copyright © McGraw Hill LLC. All rights reserved. https://accessphysiotherapy.mhmedical.com.

amitriptyline, desipramine, and nortriptyline), and anticonvulsants (such as carbamazepine and gabapentin). Acupuncture and biofeedback may also be helpful.

Physical Therapy. As mentioned previously, the patient may complain of intense pain in a dermatomal pattern. The PTA must be aware of the signs and symptoms to identify that this pain is nonmusculoskeletal in origin. While treating a patient with herpes zoster (shingles), appropriate standard precautions should be used, especially during the blister phase of the condition.

NEUROPATHIC FOOT ULCER/PRESSURE ULCERS

Neuropathic foot ulcers are sequelae of peripheral neuropathy, often in persons with diabetes. In areas of the foot under sustained increased pressure, the absence of sensation in the area inhibits the body from relieving pressure, resulting in microtrauma, leading to tissue damage and ulceration over time. Groups of patients most susceptible include those with diabetes, but ulceration can occur in the elderly, neurologically involved, and acutely hospitalized. Motor neuron damage is common as well.

Pressure areas in the foot include the plantar surface of the foot, the big toe, and the metatarsophalangeal joints. In addition, foot cuts and bruises may lead to ulceration due to

STUDY PEARL
When assisting a patient with a shingles rash, take care to avoid placing a gait belt, manual contact, or place the patient in a position of weight-bearing over the painful area.

TABLE 6-11 • Dressing Choices.	
Wound Dressings	**Description**
Gauze	Woven or nonwoven fibers offered in pads, rolls, or sponges with characteristics of mild absorbency and nonocclusive permeability. *Pros* • Fiber gauze is effective to fill cavity space • May function as a secondary dressing • Inexpensive *Cons* • Care should be taken during removal as may have a nonselective debridement effect when adhered to wound bed that may remove healthy, viable tissue. • Avoid packing tightly into cavity space to allow proper tissue healing • May leave fibers in wound bed
Impregnated gauze	Mesh or woven synthetic fibers containing a petroleum product with characteristics of mild absorbency and nonocclusive permeability. *Pros* • Decreases adherence to tissue
Film	Transparent film with characteristics of mild absorbency and occlusive permeability. *Pros* • Provides a barrier to bacteria and external moisture • Conforms and protects the wound • Maintains a moist wound environment • Allows visibility of wound *Cons* • May adhere to wound tissue
Foam	Foam is offered in a variety of forms: pads, ropes, or sheets with or without adhesive with characteristics of high absorbency and nonocclusive permeability. *Pros* • Comfortable • Less adherent to wound tissue *Cons* • Avoid use on a dry wound due to the highly absorptive nature. May need a gel product on the wound bed to facilitate moist wound healing.
Hydrogel	Gel or sheet form made of a polymer consisting of 90% water at minimum with characteristics of moderate absorbency and nonocclusive permeability. *Pros* • Maintains moisture • Softens necrotic tissue to facilitate autolytic debridement

Hydrofiber	Synthetic hydrofibers with characteristics of moderate to high absorbency and nonocclusive permeability.
	Pros
	• Maintains moist wound environment
	• Some types may include growth factors, antimicrobial silver, or may be combined with other types of dressings
	  • For example, Hydrofiber™ in Aquacel® or Aquacel ®Ag
	  • https://www.convatec.com/advanced-wound-care/aquacel-dressings/
	Cons
	• May require secondary dressing

Hydrocolloid	Absorbent colloidal material fiber manufactured in a variety of dressing types with characteristics of moderate absorbency and semiocclusive to occlusive permeability. *Pros* • Less likely to adhere to the wound bed causing less pain with dressing changes • Maintains moist wound and facilitates autolytic debridement *Cons* • An odor may be noted along with gelatinous, yellow substance due to the combination of wound drainage with the colloidal polymer. • If not transparent, will occlude ability to visualize wound

(Continued)

TABLE 6-11 • Dressing Choices. *(Continued)*	
Wound Dressings	**Description**
Alginate	Calcium alginates from seaweed/kelp and algae are formed into woven sheets or ropes with characteristics of high absorbency (up to 30× their own weight) and nonocclusive permeability. *Pros* • Controls highly exudating wounds • Maintains moist wound environment and facilitate autolytic debridement • May contain silver for antimicrobial effects *Cons* • May require a secondary dressing to secure

Data from O'Sullivan, SB, Schmitz TJ, Fulk G. *Physical Rehabilitation*, 7th ed. 2019. Copyright © F.A. Davis. All rights reserved; and Swezey, L. Wound Dressing Selection: Types and Usage. *Wound Source.* August 4th, 2011. https://www.woundsource.com/blog/wound-dressing-selection-types-and-usage.

decreased circulation in the area and decreased healing secondary to diabetes. Complications from neuropathic foot ulcers include infections/sepsis and amputation. Clinical features of various types of ulcerations are presented in Table 6-12.

In general, pressure against the skin over a body prominence increases the risk of developing necrosis and ulceration in any area of the body. Contributing factors for ulceration can include infection, improper skin care, shear, friction, heat, maceration (softening associated with excessive moisture), medication, malnutrition, and muscle atrophy.

Clinical Significance
Disturbances include the following:

1. Symmetrical distal polyneuropathy in a stocking (lower leg and feet) distribution. The sensory loss is chronic and progressive.
2. Common complaints are persistent numbness and tingling that worsen at night.

TABLE 6-12 • Clinical Features of Ulcers.				
Clinical Features	**Venous Ulcer**	**Arterial Ulcer**	**Diabetic Ulcer**	**Pressure Ulcer**
Pulses	Normal	Poor or absent	Present or diminished	
Pain	None to aching (in the dependent position)	Often severe, intermittent claudication, progressing to pain at rest	Typically, not painful; sensory loss usually present	Painful if sensation is intact
Color	Normal or cyanotic. May see dark pigmentation (thick, tender, indurated, fibrous tissue)	Pale on elevation: dusky rubor on dependency		Red, brown/black, or yellow
Temperature	Normal	Cool		Warm if localized infection present (associated fever)
Edema	Often marked	Usually absent		
Skin changes	Pigmentation, stasis dermatitis, thickening of the skin as scarring develops	Trophic changes (thin, shiny, atrophic skin); loss of hair on foot and toes; nails thicken		Inflammatory response with necrotic tissue
Ulceration	May develop, especially on the medial ankle; wet, with a large amount of exudate	On toes or feet; can be deep	May develop due to trauma to insensitive skin	Typically occurs over bony prominences, ie, sacrum, heels, trochanter, lateral malleolus, ischial areas, elbows
Gangrene	Absent	Black gangrenous skin adjacent to ulcer can develop	May develop if left untreated	May develop if left untreated

Reproduced with permission from Burke-Doe A, Dutton M, eds. *National Physical Therapy Examination and Board Review.* 2019. Copyright © McGraw Hill LLC. All rights reserved. https://accessphysiotherapy.mhmedical.com.

3. Ophthalmoplegia affecting cranial nerve III (oculomotor) and, less frequently, cranial nerve VI (abducens) on one side.

4. Mononeuropathy of limbs or trunk, including painful lumbar radiculopathy.

5. Diabetic amyotrophy can be present with motor neuropathy of the lower limbs.

6. Symmetrical proximal weakness and atrophy.

7. Autonomic impairment.

8. Fall risk.

Diagnostic Tests and Measures

Skin assessment is vital for signs and symptoms of pressure ulcerations, as is evaluation for risk factors, including emaciation, obesity, increased age, immobilization, decreased activity, diabetes, circulatory disorders, incontinence, and decreased mental status. Pressure ulcers are graded using a four-stage system (Table 6-13). Additionally, two more levels have been added to the pressure staging criteria:

- **Deep tissue injury (DTI):** Consisting of a nonblanchable deep red, maroon, or purple discoloration with intact or nonintact skin.
- **Unstageable pressure injury:** Unable to determine the staging level as the slough or eschar may obscure. This necrotic tissue would need to be softened and removed to determine the actual staging.

Blood Test. Infection is a major risk factor with ulcers, including neuropathic foot ulcers. Blood tests, including white blood cell (WBC) count, erythrocyte sedimentation rate, and C-reactive protein level, may aid in differentially diagnosing an infection. In addition, nutritional assessment can be made by testing serum protein (albumin) and hemoglobin (anemia) levels.

Imaging. Radiography can help diagnose bone infections. Gas in soft tissues may also be detected by radiography; gas may indicate soft tissue infection due to anaerobic organisms. Nerve conduction studies and electromyography can also be useful.

Clinical Findings, Secondary Effects, Complications

1. Decreased sensation (touch, vibration, proprioception).
2. Unpleasant odor.

TABLE 6-13 · Pressure Ulcer Stages.		
Stage	**Characteristics**	**Preferred Practice Pattern According to the Guide[a]**
Stage I	An observable pressure-related alteration of intact skin whose indicators as compared to an adjacent or opposite area of the body may include changes in skin color, skin temperature (warm or cool), tissue consistency (firm or boggy), and/or sensation (pain, itching).	7B: Impaired integumentary integrity associated with superficial skin involvement
Stage II	A partial-thickness skin loss that involves the epidermis and/or dermis. The ulcer is superficial and presents clinically as an abrasion, blister, or shallow crater.	7C: Impaired integumentary integrity associated with partial-thickness skin involvement and scar formation
Stage III	A full-thickness skin loss involving damage or necrosis of subcutaneous tissue that may extend down to, but not through, underlying fascia. The ulcer presents clinically as a deep crater with or without undermining adjacent tissue.	7D: Impaired integumentary integrity associated with full-thickness skin involvement and scar formation
Stage IV	A full-thickness skin low with extensive destruction, tissue necrosis, or damage to muscle, bone, or supporting structures (eg, tendon, joint capsule). Undermining or sinus tracts may be present.	7E: Impaired integumentary integrity associated with skin involvement extending into fascia, muscle, or bone, and scar formation

[a]*American Physical Therapy Association. Guide to Physical Therapist Practice. 2nd ed. American Physical Therapy Association. Phys Ther.* 2001;81(1):9-746.

Data from Consortium for Spinal Cord Medicine Clinical Practice Guidelines. Pressure Ulcer Prevention and Treatment following Spinal Cord Injury: A Clinical Practice Guideline for Healthcare Professionals. *J Spinal Cord Med.* 2001;24(suppl 1):S40–S101.

3. Presence of pus or exudate.
4. A wound that is slow to heal.
5. Infection.
6. Poor arterial flow.
7. Charcot deformity.
8. Pain (rare, due to lack of sensation).
9. Ulcerations with prominent callus rim, with good granulation tissue and little drainage.
10. Wound skin appears dry or cracked.
11. Distal limb appears shiny and cool to touch.
12. Diminished pedal pulses.
13. Gangrene.
14. Amputation.
15. Weakness with muscle atrophy.
16. Decreased deep tendon reflexes.
17. Impaired vision.
18. Impaired balance.

Interventions/Treatment

Medical. The most direct treatment for neuropathic foot ulcers is debridement of dead tissue around the wound. Wound dressings should also be applied to assist in healing.

Pharmacologic. Antibiotics may be administered to control infection. Diabetic medications may include insulin (short-acting, long-acting), sulfonylureas to increase insulin production by beta cells of the pancreas (glyburide), biguanides to decrease liver glucose production and increase insulin sensitivity (metformin), alpha-glucosidase inhibitors, which prevent digestion of carbohydrates, and meglitinides, which lower glucose rise after a meal.

Physical Therapy. Physical therapy interventions may involve direct wound care, balance training, gait training, and improved muscle performance. In addition, the PTA can provide educational intervention to prevent the development of new ulcers (Table 6-14). Patients with diabetes or impaired sensation must be educated on proper foot and skincare (Table 6-15).

TABLE 6-14 • Pressure Ulcer Prevention.	
Prevention Technique	**Suggested Strategies**
Proper positioning in bed and wheelchair	Bony prominences protected and pressure distributed equally over large surface areas Use of pressure distribution equipment such as wheelchair cushions, custom mattresses, and alternating pressure mattress pads
Frequent changes in position	Every 2 hours when in bed Every 15-20 minutes when seated
Keep skin clean and dry	Good bowel and bladder care with immediate cleansing after an episode of incontinence Current cleansing and drying of skin at least once daily Inspect the skin for areas of redness in a.m. and p.m.
Nutrition	Diet with adequate calories, protein, vitamins, and minerals Sufficient water intake
Clothing	Avoid clothes that are either too tight or too loose-fitting Avoid clothes with thick seams, buttons, or zippers in areas of pressure
Activity	Regular cardiovascular exercise A gradual buildup of skin tolerance for new activities, equipment, and positions Avoid movements that rub, drag, or scratch the skin

Data from Cameron MH, Monroe LG, eds. *Physical Rehabilitation: Evidence-Based Examination, Evaluation, and Intervention.* 2007. Copyright © Saunders/Elsevier. All rights reserved.

TABLE 6-15 • Foot and Skin Care Tips for Patients with Diabetes or Impaired Sensation.
• Examine your feet daily, looking between toes and on soles of feet—use a mirror or family member's assistance if necessary to see all angles.
• Check for blisters, sores, corns, calluses, broken toenails, cracked skin, odor, drainage, swelling, or redness.
• Contact your health care provider if you note any of these abnormalities or if you injure your foot.
• Regular follow-up with your health care provider to monitor feet and control diabetic symptoms.
• Daily care:
• Wash feet in lukewarm water (85°F) and mild soap.
• Dry feet thoroughly with care to dry between toes.
• Use lanolin or petroleum-based lotions to soften dry skin, but not between toes.
- May use a powder or cornstarch between toes.
• Never treat corns, calluses, or toenails with any products that can cause skin injury.
• Avoid home remedies and consult with your health care provider.
• Cut toenails straight across and avoid cutting into corners.
• Use padding or lamb's wool to promote circulation.
• Daily replacement of materials is necessary for infection control.
• Apply clean socks after the footcare routine.
• Do not walk barefoot.
• Wear cotton socks if the feet are cold at night.
- Do not heat feet with a heating pad or hot water bottle.
• Check shoes for the correct size and fit.
• Avoid worn-out socks or shoes.
• Shop in the afternoon when feet are usually at the largest.
• Gradually break in new shoes.

The use of orthotics and splints may also assist in preventing the development of ulcers. Physical therapy documentation of wounds assists in monitoring healing progression. Functional activities such as bed mobility, transfers, gait, and stairs to improve mobility and reduce fall risk are essential in this patient population.

CELLULITIS

Cellulitis is an acute infection of the dermis and subcutaneous tissue. Most cases of cellulitis are caused by *Staphylococcus aureus* and group A *Streptococcus*. However, other organisms may be involved in certain situations, such as gram-negative organisms or *Haemophilus influenzae* in young infants. Cellulitis typically presents with rubor (erythema), dolor (pain), calor (warmth), and tumor (edema) and may begin with the acute onset of localized erythema and tenderness. The borders may be ill-defined, and surface crusts may develop. Other symptoms include fever, malaise, and chills. Less common findings include ascending lymphangitis and regional lymphadenopathy. Cellulitis usually presents in a unilateral distribution.

Clinical Significance

Disturbances include the following:

1. Involved site is red, hot, swollen, and tender, with the lower extremity being the most common site.
2. Borders of the involved area are not elevated or sharply demarcated.
3. Regional lymphadenopathy is present with malaise, chills, fever, and toxicity.
4. Skin infection without underlying drainage, penetrating trauma, eschar, or abscess is likely caused by streptococci; however, community-acquired methicillin-resistant *S. aureus* (CA-MRSA) is the most likely pathogen when these factors are present.
5. Cellulitis characterized by violaceous color and bullae suggests more serious or systemic infection with organisms such as *Vibrio vulnificus* or *Streptococcus pneumoniae*.

6. Lymphangitic spread (red lines streaking away from the area of infection), crepitus, and hemodynamic instability indicate severe infection, requiring more aggressive treatment.
7. Circumferential cellulitis or pain that is disproportional to examination findings should prompt consideration of severe soft tissue infection.

Diagnostic Tests and Measures

The key diagnostic clinical feature of cellulitis is a painful, warm, red, edematous plaque.

Laboratory Tests. If indicated, cultures from exudate or blistered areas can be taken with a swab, or cultures can be obtained by aspirating the affected skin. A skin punch biopsy of affected skin may also be cultured.

Imaging. Imaging studies may be needed if crepitant or necrotic cellulitis is suspected.

Clinical Findings, Secondary Effects, Complications

1. Cellulitis typically presents with rubor (erythema), dolor (pain), calor (warmth), and tumor (edema).
2. Malaise, chills, fever, and toxicity.
3. Lymphangitic spread (red lines streaking away from the area of infection).
4. Circumferential cellulitis.
5. Pain disproportionate to examination findings.

Indications for emergent surgical evaluation are as follows:

1. Violaceous bullae.
2. Cutaneous hemorrhage.
3. Skin sloughing.
4. Skin anesthesia.
5. Rapid progression.
6. Gas in the tissue.
7. Hypotension.

Interventions/Treatment

Medical. The most direct treatment for cellulitis is an oral antibiotic. Treatment for the most common forms of cellulitis likely caused by methicillin-sensitive *S. aureus* includes penicillinase-resistant penicillin, a first-generation cephalosporin, amoxicillin-clavulanate, a macrolide, or a fluoroquinolone antibiotic. Extensive disease may require intravenous (IV) antibiotics.

Pharmacologic. A culture of the infection may be necessary to determine the best pharmacologic treatment. Mild cases can be treated with antibiotics such as dicloxacillin, amoxicillin, and cephalexin. Resistant strains may need alternatives such as fluoroquinolones.

Physical Therapy. PTAs need to understand the signs and symptoms of cellulitis to refer to appropriate individuals if a patient's presentation is consistent with this diagnosis. Treatment measures may include elevation and immobilization of the involved limb to reduce swelling and functional activities as appropriate.

BURNS

Thermal injury to the skin results from direct energy to the tissue relative to temperature and contact time. Transfer of heat to cellular structures of the skin results in denaturation of proteins, vaporization of water, and thrombosis of cutaneous blood vessels, resulting in tissue and cell death. This process may be immediate with high temperature and/or prolonged contact time but may also be enhanced by the patient's premorbid condition, injury status, and local inflammatory factors.

The severity of a burn injury is determined by the depth of penetration and surface area of the injured skin relative to the patient's total body surface area (TBSA). Determination of TBSA relative to burn size for the adult can be generalized utilizing the rule of nines (Figure 6-2). More specific charts have been developed to estimate the body surface relative to age, which are more useful in the pediatric population.

Clinical Significance

Disturbances and injuries are classified as follows:

1. Superficial burns are limited to the epidermis without disruption of epithelial integrity. The skin's appearance includes erythema because of the inflammatory process. A common example would be a sunburn.

2. Superficial partial-thickness burns involve the epidermis and the superficial dermis. They are characterized by intense pain (sensate), blanching with pressure, and blistering because of the local inflammatory process between the dermis and epidermis.

3. Deep partial-thickness injuries extend into the reticular dermis and are insensate, have a mottled white appearance, and do not blanch with pressure as the result of impaired vascularity and capillary refill.

4. Full-thickness burns extend through the entire dermis and into the subcutaneous tissue. The appearance is leathery brown or black eschar with no capillary refill.

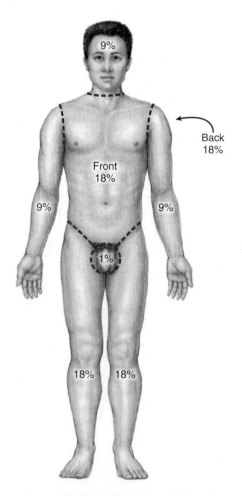

Figure 6-2. Total body surface area (TBSA) determination by the rule of nines. (Reproduced with permission from Hamm RL. *Text and Atlas of Wound Diagnosis and Treatment*. 2015. Copyright © McGraw Hill LLC. All rights reserved. https://accessphysiotherapy.mhmedical .com.)

Diagnostic Tests and Measures

Indicators of the depth of injury include biopsy, ultrasound, or perfusion. None are as reliable as physical examination at 48 to 72 hours. A quantitative biopsy diagnoses burn infection.

Blood Test. Complete blood counts should be monitored throughout treatment, including protein status.

Imaging. Ultrasound.

Clinical Findings, Secondary Effects, Complications

1. Mechanisms of burn injuries may include scalding, flame, electrical, chemical, and radiation.
2. Keloid scarring.
3. Hypertrophic scarring.
4. Pain.
5. Infection.
6. Peripheral hypoperfusion.
7. Cardiac complications (arrhythmia, hypoxia, acidosis, hyperkalemia).
8. Pulmonary complications (inhalation difficulty, distress, abnormal breath sounds).
9. Metabolic complications (hemoglobinuria, myoglobinuria).
10. Heterotrophic scarring.
11. Wound contracture.

Interventions/Treatment

Medical. Surgical removal of nonviable tissue, restoration of the immunologic barrier, and restoration of normal aesthetics as required in sensitive areas (skin grafting). Fluid resuscitation to prevent organ damage. Nutritional requirements will need to be managed for proper healing progression. Pain control for all pain types (breakthrough, background, procedural) to assist in comfortable engaging in dressing changes and participation in rehabilitation exercises.

Pharmacologic. Analgesics, anti-inflammatories, topical antimicrobial medications, silver sulfadiazine (Silvadene), mafenide acetate (Sulfamylon), silver nitrate, silver-impregnated gauze.

Physical Therapy. Treatment of the burn patient must always consider the patient's psychosocial aspects. Gentle conversation, encouragement, and an unhurried approach to therapy sessions may be beneficial. Early phases of treatment focus on minimizing edema, promoting venous return, passive ROM for all joints in all cardinal planes, and splinting to prevent wound contracture and functional limitations. The clinician may employ tubular elastic dressings, elastic wrap dressings, elevation, and retrograde massage to assist with extremity edema reduction. Proper antideformity positioning (Figure 6-3) minimizes shortening of tendons, collateral ligaments, and joint capsules; it also reduces extremity and facial edema. Positioning techniques may include removing pillows, splints, web spacers, prone position, and padded footboards. Performance of daily living activities and the impending return to play/school/work are important considerations. Scar management may be favorably influenced using pressure garments and topical silicone. Active ROM may be increased, progressing to strengthening with resistive exercises. Resisted ROM, isometric exercises, positioning/splinting, active strengthening, and gait training are important objectives.

DERMATITIS

Dermatitis pertains to the skin inflammation caused by exposure to irritants, allergies, or genetic predisposition. Examples of disorders related to dermatitis include eczema, contact dermatitis, and seborrheic dermatitis. Eczema, or atopic dermatitis, denotes the reaction of the skin to various diseases or conditions. Eczema can be accompanied by hay fever or asthma.

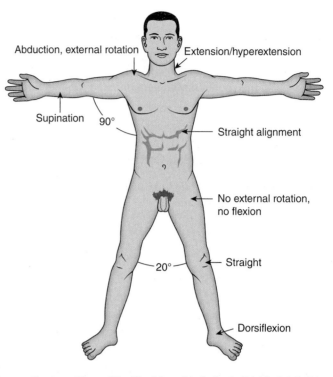
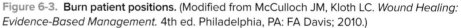

Figure 6-3. Burn patient positions. (Modified from McCulloch JM, Kloth LC. *Wound Healing: Evidence-Based Management.* 4th ed. Philadelphia, PA: FA Davis; 2010.)

It can be a long-lasting condition with flareups. Contact dermatitis results from the skin's reaction to exposure to specific substances such as metals, drugs, or poison ivy. Seborrheic dermatitis affects the oily areas of the body such as the scalp, face, sides of the nose, or ears.

Clinical Significance

1. Diagnosis is based on medical history and examination of the integument.
2. Contact dermatitis: Diagnosis is based on medical history, the appearance of the skin, and a history of exposure to irritants or allergens.
3. Seborrheic dermatitis: Diagnosis is based on history, skin appearance, physical examination, and skin biopsy.
4. Atopic dermatitis (eczema): Diagnosis is based on the history and appearance of the skin.
5. Eczema and dermatitis have three primary stages: acute, subacute, and chronic.

Diagnostic Tests and Measures

Blood Tests and Laboratory Tests. No blood test is necessary to diagnose this condition unless complications such as infections arise, in which case blood work may be necessary to diagnose the infection and identify the best course of action. In addition, skin lesion biopsies or skin cultures may be used to rule out other causes.

Imaging. No imaging is needed to diagnose this condition.

Clinical Findings, Secondary Effects, Complications

1. Redness or inflammation.
2. Dry skin.
3. Pruritus.
4. Itching that may be severe at night.
5. Elevated bumps that may ooze and crust over when scratched.
6. Localized edema.

7. Burning or tenderness.
8. Flakes on the scalp, greasy skin with yellow or white flakes (seborrheic dermatitis).

Interventions/Treatment

Medical. Dermatitis is a common skin condition that is treated based on the cause. Lifestyle changes are often recommended by applying corticosteroid creams, anti-itching products (such as calamine lotion), and oral antihistamines. In addition, applying cool compresses, taking baths, avoiding scratching, wearing cotton clothing, moisturizing the skin, and reducing stress are recommended. Exposing the skin to controlled amounts of natural and artificial light may assist in healing.

Pharmacologic. Pharmacologic management may include shampoos, creams, or gels to control inflammation.

- Antifungal medications.
- Dupilumab (Dupixent) for eczema from allergies.
- Steroid creams or ointments.
- Oral corticosteroids.
- Antihistamines.
- Anti-inflammatories.

Physical Therapy. PTAs need to be aware of the signs and symptoms of these conditions to refer these patients to appropriate medical professionals if needed. In addition, if the patient has already been diagnosed with the condition, the PTA must also be aware of any signs and symptoms of infection and refer the patient accordingly.

■ QUESTIONS

1. **A PTA inspects and palpates the skin of a patient with peripheral vascular disease. The clinician notices a dark purplish-blue discoloration of the skin. This finding may indicate which of the following?**
   A. Normal response to pressure on the skin
   B. Reflex vasoconstriction due to cold response
   C. Pathology involving the liver
   D. Tissue hypoxia or hematologic pathology

2. **On observation, a PTA notes yellowish discoloration of the skin and sclera. What medical question is most appropriate to identify a possible underlying pathology based on the observation?**
   A. Have you previously experienced difficulty in breathing or other problems affecting your lungs or respiration?
   B. Have you experienced instances where you feel that your heart is racing and your pulse is fast?
   C. Have you been diagnosed with or been told that you have a liver problem?
   D. Do you have any difficulty urinating?

3. **Which of the following statements is *true* regarding checking the nail bed for possible pathology?**
   A. Finger clubbing is a normal age-related change affecting the nails.
   B. Normal nail bases should look convex and create an oval-shaped space when nails of opposite hands are placed together.
   C. Finger clubbing refers to an increased angle between the fingernail and where the nail enters the skin.
   D. Abnormalities seen on the nail beds are not sensitive tests to indicate any systemic pathology.

4. A PTA notes a solid, elevated, sharply circumscribed, small (1 cm) colored lesion (pink, tan, red, or any variation) on the patient's lower extremities. Which of the following is the appropriate term to denote this lesion?
   A. Macule
   B. Papule
   C. Pustule
   D. Cyst

5. A clinician inspects the skin of a patient who was referred for low back pain. The clinician notes yellowish and whitish crust on the scalp, face, sides of nose, and ears. The clinician also notes that these areas appear oily. Which of the following is the appropriate diagnosis for the condition?
   A. Contact dermatitis
   B. Psoriasis
   C. Seborrheic dermatitis
   D. Eczema

6. A PTA performs ankle ROM on a patient when they note their leg feels cool to the touch, hair loss over the lower leg, and observes a small circular wound with eschar on the fifth toe. The patient also reports intense pain with prolonged walking or with the elevation of the foot. Which type of ulcer fits this description best?
   A. Arterial
   B. Venous
   C. Diabetic
   D. Pressure

7. While assisting a hospital patient with rolling in bed activities, the PTA observes a wound over the sacrum that appears as an abrasion or blister with only partial-thickness tissue loss. At what stage would this pressure wound be classified?
   A. Stage I
   B. Stage II
   C. Stage III
   D. Stage IV

8. During a wound dressing change, the PTA notes the exudate is watery pale red to pink in color and covers approximately 25% of the dressing. Which of the following would be the most accurate way to document the exudate?
   A. Scant bloody exudate is present.
   B. Small serosanguinous exudate is present.
   C. Moderate serous exudate is present.
   D. Large purulent exudate is present.

9. During wound care treatment, the wound bed is noted to be 100% covered in red granulation tissue. Which of the following would be the appropriate treatment goal?
   A. Protect wound and maintain a moist wound environment.
   B. Debride necrotic tissue and absorb any excess drainage.
   C. Protect wound bed by allowing wound bed to dry out to form a protective barrier.
   D. Debride necrotic tissue by means appropriate to the level of skill of the treating clinician.

10. The PTA reviews the treatment plan for wound care treatment on a high exudation wound. Which of the following dressing type would be most appropriately indicated?
    A. Tegaderm
    B. Duoderm
    C. Kaltostat
    D. Micropore

11. **A patient develops hypertrophic scarring after experiencing a burn across the right upper extremity. Which of the following interventions would be most appropriate for scar management?**
    A. Isometric exercise
    B. Compression garment
    C. Silvadene
    D. Antideformity positioning

■ ANSWERS WITH RATIONALES

1. **The answer is D.** A dark bluish or purplish discoloration of the integument and mucous membranes is termed cyanosis and may indicate hypoxia or hematologic pathology.

2. **The answer is C.** Jaundice, or yellowish discoloration of the skin, may indicate an underlying liver pathology.

3. **The answer is C.** Finger clubbing refers to an increased angle between the fingernail and where the nails enter the skin and may indicate chronic tissue hypoxia.

4. **The answer is B.** A papule refers to a solid, elevated lesion, sharply circumscribed, small (1 cm) colored lesion (pink, tan, red, or any variation), commonly seen in dermatitis, ringworm, or psoriasis.

5. **The answer is C.** Seborrheic dermatitis refers to yellowish and whitish flaky crust affecting the oily areas of the body such as the scalp, nose, ears, or face.

6. **The answer is A.** Arterial ulcers characteristically occur on the toes/feet, and skin shows changes with hair loss, cool skin temperature related to the lack of arterial blood flow. Venous wounds, most commonly with wet, weeping exudate often over the medial ankle, often have skin pigmentation. Pressure ulcers appear most commonly over bony prominences and may vary in appearance depending on inflammation severity, with the wound bed described as red, yellow, or black. Diabetic ulcers typically are not painful due to sensory loss.

7. **The answer is B.** The description of a partial-thickness loss involving the epidermis and/or dermis with a presentation similar to abrasion would qualify as a stage II pressure ulcer.

8. **The answer is B.** Serous exudate is clear, serosanguinous is watery pale to pink/red similar, bloody is bright red, and purulent is opaque with tan to yellow to green coloration often associated with infection. The amount of exudate is scant for a trace amount with a moist wound bed, small 0% to 25%, moderate 25% to 50%, large > 75%.

9. **The answer is C.** Kaltostat is within the calcium alginate dressing, which is indicated for highly exudating wounds due to its absorbent nature. Tegaderm (semipermeable) and Micropore (paper adhesive) are indicated for superficial or small wounds and have low absorptive qualities. Hydrocolloids such as Duoderm retain moisture but may keep the trapped exudate in contact with wound bed and periwound, causing maceration (softening of skin with prolonged moisture exposure) of the tissues.

10. **The answer is B.** Compression garments provide a pressure application to deter hypertrophic scar development. Antideformity positioning assists with edema management and prevention of contractures. Silvadene is a topical antimicrobial medication. Isometric exercises may facilitate muscle performance to facilitate functional mobility.

CHECKLIST

When you complete this chapter, you should be able to:

❑ Outline signs and symptoms of selected integumentary conditions.
❑ List general classifications of signs and symptoms associated with an integumentary disease.

❑ Identify specific clinical findings of selected pathologies affecting the integumentary system.

❑ Identify pertinent diagnostic tests and measures to confirm the presence of selected integumentary pathologies.

❑ Discuss the medical and pharmacologic management of selected integumentary conditions.

❑ Describe techniques for wound measurement.

❑ Compare dressing types for wounds with increased exudate.

❑ Compare selective and nonselective debridement.

❑ List wound staging classifications.

❑ Compare necrotic and granulation tissue.

❑ Discuss the role of physical therapy in the management of selected integumentary conditions.

REFERENCE

1. O'Sullivan SB, Schmitz TJ, Fulk G. *Physical Rehabilitation*. 7th ed. In: O'Sullivan SB, Schmitz TJ, Fulk G, eds. Philadelphia, PA: FA Davis; 2019.

Therapeutic Modalities

MARK DUTTON

OVERVIEW

In 2014, the American Physical Therapy Association (APTA) began recommending using the term "biophysical agents" to refer to physical agents and modalities. Also, the APTA Choosing Wisely campaign addressed the use of biophysical agents. Their first recommendation states: "Don't employ passive physical agents except when necessary to facilitate participation in an active treatment program."[1] They further state that "The use of passive physical agents is not harmful to patients except when they communicate to patients that the passive, instead of active, treatment is appropriate." These statements highlight the need to give careful consideration to the clinical indications for applying biophysical agents. The purpose of using biophysical agents is to alter pain, improve skeletal muscle activity, and promote tissue healing. The physical therapist assistant (PTA) has several adjunctive interventions at his or her disposal, each of which is determined by the physical therapist's (PT) intervention goals documented in the POC.

> **STUDY PEARL**
>
> The APTA policy statement on direction and supervision of the physical therapist assistant reads, "regardless of the setting in which the service is provided, the determination to utilize physical therapist assistants for selected interventions requires the education, expertise and professional judgment of a physical therapist as described by the Standards of Practice, Guide to Professional Conduct and Code of Ethics."

▲ HIGH-YIELD TERMS

Acoustic streaming	The atmospheric pressure at sea level, equal to 1 atmosphere absolute (ATA—760 mm Hg).
Accommodation	The increased threshold of excitable tissue when a slowly rising stimulus is used. The quicker the rise time, the less time the nerve has to accommodate to the impulse.
Alternating current (AC)	The uninterrupted bidirectional flow of ions or electrons that must change direction at least one time per second.
Amplitude	The magnitude of the current. Amplitude controls are often labeled intensity.
Asymmetrical waveform	A condition when the amplitude and duration characteristics between the two phases of the biphasic waveform differ in any manner.
Attenuation	A measure of the decrease in ultrasound energy by absorption, reflection, or refraction.
Beam nonuniformity ratio (BNR)	The ratio between spatial peak intensity and the average spatial intensity of an ultrasound beam.
Burst	A series of pulses or brief periods of alternating current delivered consecutively and separated from the next series.
Cavitation	Pulsation of gas bubbles in biological tissues in response to the passage of ultrasound.
Direct current	The continuous, unidirectional flow of charged particles for at least 1 second.
Duty cycle	The percentage of on-time to the total time of electrical current multiplied by 100%.
Endorphins	Endogenous opioid-like peptides that reduce the perception of pain by binding to opioid receptors. (Also referred to as opiopeptins.)

Nerve conduction	The transmission of an electrical impulse along a nerve fiber.
Piezoelectric effect	The property of generating electricity in response to a mechanical force or changing shape in response to an electrical current (as in an ultrasound transducer).
Ramp-down time	The time taken for the current to decrease from its maximum amplitude during the on-time, back down to zero.
Ramp-Up Time	The time it takes for the current amplitude to increase from zero, at the end of the off-time, to its maximum amplitude during the on-time.

The various categories of physical agents are outlined in Table 7-1.

■ THERMAL AGENTS

There are four major types of thermal modalities. These involve the transfer of thermal energy. See Table 7-2.

Cryotherapy: The use of cold to induce therapeutic and physiologic responses that result from decreased tissue temperature.

Thermotherapy: The application of therapeutic heat involving the transfer of thermal energy. Thermal effects can occur at a superficial or deep level.

The indications for cryotherapy and thermotherapy are listed in Table 7-3. The contraindications for cryotherapy and thermotherapy are listed in Table 7-4. Finally, the effects of cryotherapy and thermotherapy are listed in Table 7-5.

The main physiologic effects of cold application are vasoconstriction, reduced metabolic function, and reduced motor and sensory nerve conduction velocities. The following list describes the major physiologic effects of cold application:

STUDY PEARL
The effect of skin temperature on cutaneous blood flow involves the following:
- Normal cutaneous flow is 200 to 250 mL/min.
- At 15°C, maximal vasoconstriction is reached, with blood flow measured at 20 to 50 mL/min.
- Below 15°C, vasoconstriction is interrupted by rhythmic bursts of vasodilation occurring three to five times per hour and lasting 5 to 10 minutes. These bursts are more frequent and longer in individuals acclimated to the cold, making them less prone to frostbite injury.
- At 10°C, neurapraxia occurs, resulting in loss of cutaneous sensation.
- Below 0°C, negligible cutaneous blood flow allows the skin to freeze.
- Without circulation, skin temperature drops at a rate exceeding 0.5°C per minute.
- Smaller blood vessels (ie, microvasculature) freeze before large blood vessels.
- The venous system freezes before the arterial system because of lower flow rates.

STUDY PEARL
The use of ice by itself or in conjunction with compression has demonstrated effective minimization of edema. However, even though the immediate application of cold will help control edema if applied immediately following injury, the gravity-dependent positions should be avoided with acute and subacute injuries because of the likelihood of additional swelling.

TABLE 7-1 • Categories of Physical Agents.	

Thermal	Thermotherapy
	Superficial agents
	  Hot packs
	  Paraffin
	  Fluidotherapy
	  Warm whirlpool
	Deep heating agents
	  Ultrasound
	  Diathermy
	Cryotherapy
	  Ice pack
	  Ice massage
	  Cold whirlpool

Electromagnetic	Electrotherapy
	  TENS
	  NMES
	  IFC
	  HVPC
	  Microcurrent
	  Iontophoresis
	Diathermy (although electromagnetic, diathermy does provide deep heat)
	Ultraviolet
	Infrared

Mechanical	Traction Compression

HVPC, high-volt pulsed current; IFC, interferential current; NMES, neuromuscular electrical stimulation; TENS, transcutaneous electrical nerve stimulation.

TABLE 7-2 • Methods of Heat Transfer.		
Method	**Description**	**Examples**
Conduction	Heat is transferred by direct contact of the modality to tissue	Hot packs/heating pads Paraffin Cold packs/ice bag Ice massage Warm or cold water immersion (if there is no agitation)
Convection	Moving fluid particles contact the skin, causing heating or cooling	Fluidotherapy Warm or cool whirlpool with agitation
Evaporation	Rapid evaporation of a liquid spray causes the skin temperature to drop, resulting in decreased pain sensation	Vapocoolant sprays
Radiation	Transfer of heat from a warmer source to a cooler source through a conducting medium such as air	Infrared lamp

Reproduced with permission from Burke-Doe A, Dutton M, eds. *National Physical Therapy Examination and Board Review.* 2019. Copyright © McGraw Hill LLC. All rights reserved. https://accessphysiotherapy.mhmedical.com.

- A rapid decrease in skin temperature where the subcutaneous temperature falls less rapidly and displays a smaller temperature change. The ideal tissue temperature to achieve the optimal physiologic effects of cryotherapy is 15 to 25°C.
- A decrease in muscle and intra-articular temperature.
- Localized vasoconstriction of all smooth muscle by the central nervous system to conserve heat. Maximum vasoconstriction occurs at tissue temperatures of 15°C (59°F). Localized vasoconstriction is responsible for decreasing the tendency toward edema formation and accumulation, probably due to a decrease in local hydrostatic pressure. There is also a decrease in the number of nutrients and phagocytes delivered to the area, thus reducing phagocytic activity.

  Localized analgesia: The stages of analgesia achieved by cryotherapy are as follows:
  - Stage 1: Cold sensation, which usually occurs within 3 minutes.
  - Stage 2: Burning or aching sensation, which usually occurs between 2 and 7 minutes.
  - Stage 3: Local numbness or analgesia, which usually occurs between 5 and 12 minutes.
  - Stage 4: Deep tissue vasodilation without an increase in metabolism, which usually occurs between 12 and 15 minutes.

The timing of these stages depends on the depth of penetration and varying thickness of adipose tissue. Therefore, the patient should be advised regarding these stages, especially because the burning/aching stage occurs before the therapeutic phases. Therapeutic effects of cold application include the following:

- Decreased cell permeability and decreased cellular metabolism, which result in a decreased demand for oxygen, limiting further injury, particularly in acute tissue damage.
- Decreased muscle spasm produced through a raise in the threshold of activation of the muscle spindle.
- Decrease in the excitability of free nerve endings and peripheral nerve fibers, increasing the pain threshold.

TABLE 7-3 • Indications for Cryotherapy and Thermotherapy.	
Cryotherapy	**Thermotherapy**
• Limitation of edema formation • Pain reduction • Facilitation of skeletal muscle relaxation • Limitation of secondary hypoxic tissue injury	• Pain reduction (analgesia) • Increased joint range of motion • Decreased muscle spasm

Reproduced with permission from Burke-Doe A, Dutton M, eds. *National Physical Therapy Examination and Board Review.* 2019. Copyright © McGraw Hill LLC. All rights reserved. https://accessphysiotherapy.mhmedical.com.

STUDY PEARL

The depth of penetration depends on the amount of cold, the length of the treatment time, the intensity and duration of the cold application, and the circulatory response of the body segment exposed.

STUDY PEARL

The application of cold packs and ice bags over a superficial peripheral nerve (ie, the deep peroneal [fibular] nerve and the fibular head) can result in the nerve's temporary or permanent injury.

STUDY PEARL

The choice of thermal modality depends on the goal of the treatment and the tissue to be treated. For example, if the primary treatment goal is to increase tissue temperature and blood flow to the deeper tissues, a good choice would be a modality such as diathermy or ultrasound, both of which produce energy that can penetrate the cutaneous tissues and be directly absorbed by the deeper tissues.

STUDY PEARL

Fahrenheit = (Temperature in Celsius × 9/5) + 32 *or* (Temperature in Celsius × 1.8) + 32
Celsius = (Temperature in Fahrenheit − 32) × 5/9 *or* (Temperature in Fahrenheit − 32) × 0.55

STUDY PEARL

Before applying a cold modality, the area to be treated should be assessed for protective sensation to avoid skin damage.

STUDY PEARL

Ice chips in toweling are more effective in decreasing skin temperature than ice chips in plastic bags or cold gel packs.[2,3]

STUDY PEARL

Vapocoolant sprays, which provide superficial cooling, are often used in conjunction with passive stretching and the treatment of muscle spasms, trigger points, and myofascial referred pain.[4]

A dark red or mottled (a red area with white areas) appearance of the skin after a heat treatment indicates that too much heat has been applied and that the treatment should cease. A cold, wet towel should be applied to the area, and the supervising PT should be notified immediately.

TABLE 7-4 • Contraindications for Cryotherapy and Thermotherapy.

Cryotherapy	Thermotherapy
• Cold hypersensitivity • Cold urticaria • Cold intolerance • Cryoglobulinemia • Paroxysmal cold hemoglobinuria • Raynaud disease or phenomenon • Overregenerating peripheral nerves • Area of circulatory compromise • Peripheral vascular disease	• Potential hemorrhage • Thrombophlebitis • Vascular insufficiency • Decreased thermal sensation • Impaired mentation • Areas of infection or inflammation • Areas of malignancy • Recent application of liniments

Heat greatly influences the hemodynamic, neuromuscular, and metabolic processes of the body. Physiologic effects of local heat include the following:

- Skin temperature rises rapidly and exhibits the greatest temperature change. Subcutaneous tissue temperature rises less rapidly and exhibits a smaller change. Muscle and joint show less temperature change, if any, depending on size and structure. The increase in heat is dissipated through selective vasodilation and shunting of blood via reflexes in the microcirculation and regional blood flow.
- Increase in local nerve conduction.
- Decreased muscle spasm, thereby facilitating stretching. The muscle relaxation likely results from decreased firing rates of the efferent fibers in the muscle spindle.
- Increased capillary permeability, cell metabolism, and cellular activity can increase the delivery of oxygen and chemical nutrients to the area while decreasing venous stagnation.
- Increased analgesia through hyperstimulation of the cutaneous nerve receptors.
- An increase in tissue extensibility. To be therapeutic, the amount of thermal energy transferred to the tissue must stimulate the tissue without causing damage. In an environment of connective tissue healing, the immature collagen bonds can be degraded by heat. Thus, optimum results from stretching techniques can be obtained if the heat is applied during the stretch and the stretch is maintained until cooling occurs after the removal of the heat.

Temperature ranges for application of whirlpool treatments are listed in Table 7-6.

Hydrotherapy and fluidotherapy offer several advantages over other thermal modalities. For example, they allow the patient to mobilize the affected part during the treatment. Most of the benefits associated with these modalities are related to the physical properties of fluids.

- Buoyancy: Water provides buoyance equal to the weight of the water displaced, causing decreased weight-bearing or gravitational effect on the body part(s) submerged.
- Hydrostatic pressure: Water exerts a circumferential pressure on the submerged body part(s), decreasing edema and promoting venous return.
- Resistance: Water provides resistance to the movement of a submerged body part due to the cohesion of the water molecules and the force needed to separate them.

TABLE 7-5 • Effects of Cryotherapy and Thermotherapy.

Cryotherapy	Thermotherapy
• Vasoconstriction • Decreased local tissue metabolism • Decreased inflammation • Elevated pain threshold/analgesia • Decreased muscle spasm • Reduced muscle efficiency	• Vasodilation • Increased metabolic rate • Increased local nerve conduction • Increased collagen extensibility • Increased collagen elasticity • Decreased joint stiffness • Increased muscle flexibility

TABLE 7-6 • Clinical Applications of Whirlpool Treatment According to Temperature Ranges.		
Temperature	**Degrees**	**Use**
Very hot	104°F (40-43.4°C)	Short exposure of 7-10 minutes to increase superficial temperatures
Hot	99-104°F (37-40°C)	Increase superficial temperatures
Warm	96-99°F (35.5-37°C)	Increase superficial temperatures where prolonged exposure is wanted, such as to decrease spasticity of a muscle in conjunction with passive exercise
Neutral	92-96°F (33.5-35.5°C)	Patients who have an unstable core body temperature
Tepid	80-92°F (27-33.5°C)	It may be used in conjunction with less vigorous exercise
Cool	67-80°F (19-27°C)	It may be used in conjunction with vigorous exercise
Cold	57-67°F (13-19°C)	Used for longer exposure of 10-15 minutes to decrease superficial temperatures
Very cold	32-55°F (0-13°C)	Used for short exposures of 1-5 minutes to decrease superficial temperatures

Reproduced with permission from Burke-Doe A, Dutton M, eds. *National Physical Therapy Examination and Board Review*. 2019. Copyright © McGraw Hill LLC. All rights reserved. https://accessphysiotherapy.mhmedical.com.

A paraffin bath is a commonly used modality for stiff or painful joints and arthritis of the hands and feet due to the wax's ability to conform to irregularly contoured areas. Paraffin treatments provide six times the amount of heat available in water because the mineral oil reduces the paraffin's melting point.[5]

■ ELECTROTHERAPEUTIC MODALITIES

Electrical stimulation has a wide variety of applications in the physical therapy setting. Clinical electrical stimulation activates skeletal muscle to improve muscle performance or strengthening, decrease pain, improve blood flow, decrease edema, or facilitate tissue healing. Clinicians have a wide range of electrotherapeutic modalities at their disposal for treatment. Indications, precautions, and contraindications for electrotherapeutic modalities are listed in Table 7-7.

Two common modes of electrotherapeutic modalities are transcutaneous electrical nerve stimulation (TENS), which is used for pain control (Table 7-8), and neuromuscular electrical stimulation (NMES) (Table 7-9), commonly used to improve strength, function, and range of motion (ROM).

HIGH-VOLT PULSED CURRENT

High-volt pulsed current (HVPC), also referred to as high-voltage galvanic therapy or high-voltage pulsed galvanic stimulation (HVPGS), utilizes a twin peak, monophasic, pulsed current. There is usually one large dispersive electrode and one, two, or

TABLE 7-7 • Electrotherapeutic Modalities.		
Indications	**Precautions**	**Contraindications**
Pain control Muscle contraction to • Increase strength • Improve ROM • Improve functional activity Tissue healing Improvement of blood flow Enhancement of transdermal drug delivery Decrease edema	Cardiac disease Patients with impaired mentation or in areas with impaired sensation Malignant tumors Areas of skin irritation or open wounds	Demand cardiac pacemaker or unstable arrhythmias Placement of electrodes over the carotid sinus Areas where venous or arterial thrombosis or thrombophlebitis is present Pregnancy—over or around the abdomen or low back

Reproduced with permission from Burke-Doe A, Dutton M, eds. *National Physical Therapy Examination and Board Review*. 2019. Copyright © McGraw Hill LLC. All rights reserved. https://accessphysiotherapy.mhmedical.com.

STUDY PEARL
Although wet heat is not tolerated as well as dry heat at higher temperatures, it does produce a greater rise in local tissue temperature compared with dry heat at a similar temperature.[6]

STUDY PEARL
The risk of burn with paraffin is substantial, so the clinician should weigh the benefits between a paraffin bath and a warm whirlpool bath.

STUDY PEARL
When dipping into the paraffin, the first layer of wax should be the highest on the body segment. Each successive layer is lower than the previous one to prevent subsequent layers from getting between the first layer and the skin and burning the patient.

STUDY PEARL
The phase duration contributes to patient comfort, the chemical change in the nerves, and nerve discrimination. A 50- to 100-milliseconds duration is typically used for sensory stimulation, and 220 to 300 milliseconds is typically used for motor stimulation.

STUDY PEARL
• Very short pulse durations with low intensities can depolarize sensory nerves.
• Longer pulse durations are required to stimulate motor nerves.
• Very long pulse durations with high intensities are needed to elicit a response from a denervated muscle.

TABLE 7-8 • Transcutaneous Electrical Nerve Stimulation.

Mode of TENS	Conventional	Acupuncture-Like	Burst Train	Brief Intense
Frequency	80-110 Hz	< 10 Hz (1-4 Hz)	100 Hz delivered at 2 Hz	100-150 Hz
Pulse duration	50-100 µs	150-200 µs	150-200 µs	150-200 µs
Amplitude	Sensory Level	Motor Level	Motor Level	Noxious Level
Mechanism of analgesia	Larger-diameter peripheral nerve fibers neuromodulate pain via spinal neurochemical gating mechanism	Stimulates small diameter, high threshold peripheral afferents (A-delta) to activate extrasegmental descending pain inhibitory pathways	Simulates small diameter, high threshold cutaneous afferents (A-delta) to block transmission of nociceptive information in peripheral nerves and to activate extrasegmental analgesic mechanisms	
Advantages	Comfortable Fast-acting It can be used for acute or chronic since there is no motor response It can be worn as long as needed	The amount of carryover can be up to 4 hours Minimal adaptation	Sometimes perceived as more comfortable than acupuncture-like TENS	It can be used during short minor, painful procedures Used when other TENS modes have not been successful Fast onset of analgesia
Disadvantages	Purely chemical response, so carryover is short Adaptation to stimulus is common	Motor response required, so it may not be appropriate for acute conditions May limit functional activity Limited to 1 hour to reduce the potential of soreness from contractions The onset of analgesia delayed 20-30 minutes to allow for beta-endorphin release	Motor response required, so it may not be appropriate for acute conditions May limit functional activity Limited to 1 hour to reduce the potential of soreness from contractions The onset of analgesia delayed for 20-30 minutes to allow for beta-endorphin release	Uncomfortable Not used as the first option Pain return is quite rapid

Reproduced with permission from Burke-Doe A, Dutton M, eds. *National Physical Therapy Examination and Board Review*. 2019. Copyright © McGraw Hill LLC. All rights reserved. https://accessphysiotherapy.mhmedical.com.

TABLE 7-9 • Neuromuscular Electrical Stimulation.

	To Strengthen Weakened Muscle	To Improve ROM (1 Muscle)	To Improve ROM (2 Muscles)	Functional Electrical Stimulation (FES)
Frequency	20-100 pps	50 pps	30-50 pps	20-50 pps
Pulse duration	200-600 µs	200-600 µs	200-600 µs	200-350 µs
Amplitude	To obtain strong muscle contraction (maximum tolerated or current necessary to achieve > 50% MVC	Strong enough to move the body part through the full available range of motion	Strong enough to move the body part through the full available range of motion	To achieve −3/5 contraction
Ramp-up time	1-5 seconds	3 seconds	3 seconds	0-1 seconds
Ramp-down time	1-2 seconds	0-1 second	0-1 second	0-1 seconds
Duty cycle	1:3-1:5 with on-time up to 10 seconds and off-time up to 50 seconds	15 seconds on/ 45 seconds off	10 seconds on (each channel)/10 seconds off (each channel)	N/A stimulation is timed with the demand for functional activity
Treatment time and duration	At least 10 contractions or up to 1 h/day 3-5 times/week 4-8 weeks	30-60 minutes at least every other day	30-60 minutes at least every other day	Determined by muscle fatigue

MVC, maximum voluntary contraction; pps, pulses per second.

Reproduced with permission from Burke-Doe A, Dutton M, eds. *National Physical Therapy Examination and Board Review*. 2019. Copyright © McGraw Hill LLC. All rights reserved. https://accessphysiotherapy.mhmedical.com.

TABLE 7-10 • Interferential Current.

	Frequency	Pulse Width
Muscle contraction	20-50 pps	100-300 µs
Pain management	50-120 pps	50-150 µs

four active electrodes, with the active electrode being much smaller than the dispersive electrode.

RUSSIAN CURRENT OR MEDIUM-FREQUENCY ALTERNATING CURRENT

Russian current is a medium-frequency polyphasic waveform. The intensity is produced in a burst mode with a 50% duty cycle, with a pulse width range of 50 to 200 microseconds and an interburst interval of 10 milliseconds. Medium-frequency currents can reduce resistance to current flow, making this current more comfortable than others, especially if the current is delivered in bursts or if an interburst interval is used. In addition, Russian current is believed to augment muscle strengthening via polarizing sensory and motor nerve fibers, resulting in tetanic contractions that are painless and stronger than those made voluntarily by the patient.

INTERFERENTIAL CURRENT

Interferential current (IFC) works by combining two high-frequency alternating waveforms that are biphasic but vary in amplitude, frequency, or both. Where these two distinct currents meet in the tissue, an electrical interference pattern is created based on the summation or the subtraction of the respective amplitudes or frequencies. Parameters when using IFC can be found in Table 7-10.

IONTOPHORESIS

Transdermal iontophoresis is the delivery of ionic therapeutic agents through the skin by applying a low-level electric current. Iontophoresis has proved to be valuable in the intervention of musculoskeletal disorders. Iontophoresis causes an increased penetration of drugs and other compounds into tissues by using an applied current through the tissue. The proposed mechanisms by which iontophoresis increases drug penetration are outlined in Table 7-11.

ACOUSTIC RADIATION: ULTRASOUND

Ultrasound (US) is primarily used to deliver heat to deep musculoskeletal tissues such as tendons, muscle, and joint structures. The application of US requires a homogenous medium for effective sound wave transmission and acts as a lubricant. US produces a high-frequency alternating current. The waves are delivered through the transducer, a metal faceplate with a piezoelectric crystal cemented between two electrodes. This crystal can rapidly vibrate, converting electrical energy to acoustic (sound) energy (via the reverse piezoelectric effect) with little energy dispersion. The energy leaves the transducer in a straight line (collimated beam). As the energy travels further from the transducer, the waves begin to diverge. The sound head region that produces the sound wave is the effective radiating area (ERA) and is always smaller than the transducer.

STUDY PEARL
The effects of ultrasound are predominantly empirical and are based on reported biophysical effects within tissue, and anecdotal clinical practice experience.

STUDY PEARL
The greater the ratio difference in the beam nonuniformity ratio (BNR), the more likely the transducer will have hot spots (areas of high intensity), which will increase the likelihood of patients experiencing a burning sensation.

STUDY PEARL
The entire ultrasound head does not emit ultrasound waves, which should determine an appropriate area for treatment.

TABLE 7-11 • Mechanisms of Iontophoresis Drug Delivery.

The electrical potential gradient includes changes at the cellular level
Pore formation occurs in the stratum corneum
Hair follicles, sweat glands, and sweat ducts act as diffusion shunts for ion transport

TABLE 7-12 • Ultrasound Indications, Precautions, and Contraindications.

Indications	Precautions	Contraindications
Pain modulation Increased connective tissue extensibility Reduction of soft tissue and joint restriction Reduction of muscle spasm Remodeling of scar tissue	Acute inflammation Breast implants in the area of treatment Open epiphysis Healing fractures	Healing fractures Impaired circulation Impaired cognitive function Impaired sensation Thrombophlebitis Plastic components Area of malignancy Tuberculosis infection Hemorrhagic conditions Brain, ears, eyes, heart, cervical ganglia, carotid sinuses, reproductive organs, spinal cord, over a cardiac pacemaker, over a pregnant uterus

The depth of penetration of the US depends on the absorption and scattering of the beam. Scar tissue, tendon, and cartilage demonstrate the highest absorption. Tissues that demonstrate poor absorption include bone, blood, adipose, and muscle.

Indications, precautions, and contraindications for US can be found in Table 7-12. Depth of penetration is outlined in Table 7-13 and recommended intensities are outlined in Table 7-14.

Phonophoresis is a specific type of US application in which pharmacologic agents are driven transdermally into the subcutaneous tissues. Both the thermal and mechanical properties of US have been cited as possible mechanisms for the pharmacologic agents.

The efficacy of phonophoresis has not been conclusively established. The proposed indications include pain modulation and the decrease of inflammation in subacute and chronic musculoskeletal conditions. The method of applying phonophoresis is similar to the direct technique method of US except that a medicinal agent is used in the coupling medium to transmit the US beam. The typical treatment lasts 5 to 10 minutes and uses an intensity of 1 to 3 W/cm^2. Using lower intensity and a longer treatment time is thought to be more effective for introducing medication into the skin.

■ MECHANICAL MODALITIES

PROLOTHERAPY

Prolotherapy, also known as proliferation therapy, is a relatively controversial pain management technique used for degenerative or chronic injury to ligaments, tendons, fascia, and joint capsules. Although prolotherapy is not administered in the physical therapy clinic, patients seen in the clinic may have received a course of prolotherapy from their physician and is thus included for completeness. Prolotherapy is purported to allow rapid production of new collagen and cartilage by stimulating the immune system's healing mechanism using injections of mild chemical or natural irritants, such as dextrose sugar, manganese, and glucosamine sulfate.[9] The number of injections required per intervention is based on the type of injury.[10-12]

STUDY PEARL

The specific effects and depth of penetration when using ultrasound are influenced by the wavelength or frequency (1 or 3 MHz), the intensity (W/cm^2), contact quality of the transducer, treatment surface, and tissue type (muscle, skin, fat, etc).[7,8]

STUDY PEARL

A ground fault interrupter (GFI) is a plug-in device that constantly compares the amount of electricity streaming from the electrical outlet to the clinical unit with the amount returning to the outlet. If there is any seepage in the current flow detected, the GFI unit automatically shuts off the current flow to reduce the chances of electrical shock. A GFI should be installed at the circuit breaker at the receptacle of all whirlpools and any electrical device used near water.

TABLE 7-13 • Ultrasound Frequency.

Frequency	Depth of Penetration
1 MHz	Effective up to a depth of 5-8 cm
3 MHz	More superficial Effective to a depth of approximately 1-2 cm

The depth of penetration of the ultrasound beam is dependent on the frequency.

TABLE 7-14 • Recommended Intensity.	
Intensity W/cm²	**Purpose**
0.1-1.0	Wound healing
0.5-1.0	Pain and spasm relief
0.5-1.5	Hematoma resorption
1.0-1.5	Increased plasticity of scar and connective tissue

The amount of tissue heating is dependent on the intensity of the ultrasound.

CONTINUOUS PASSIVE MOTION

Continuous passive motion (CPM) is a postoperative treatment method designed to aid recovery after joint surgery, tendon or ligament repair, or post immobilization from a fracture, by passively moving the joint within limits set by the physician. Once the patient can participate in physical therapy, the CPM may no longer be medically necessary, although this is not conclusive.

TILT TABLE

The tilt table is used to evaluate how a patient regulates blood pressure in response to simple stresses, including gravity. The tilt table was originally designed to evaluate patients with fainting spells (syncope) but may also be useful for patients who have symptoms of severe light-headedness or dizziness. Typically, the patient is asked to lie supine on the tilt table and is secured by a series of straps or belts around the hips, knees, and trunk, if needed. First, baseline data are recorded, including pulse rate, blood pressure, and subjective reports. Next, the table's head is raised (usually in the 30-degree increments) while monitoring the vital signs. Over time or number of sessions, the tilt table is raised further while monitoring vital signs and subjective reports.

SPINAL TRACTION

Traction is a mechanical force applied to the body to separate the joint surfaces and elongate the surrounding soft tissue. Indications, contraindications, and precautions are listed in Table 7-15. Recommended dosages are listed in Table 7-16.

TABLE 7-15 • Spinal Traction.		
Indications	**Precautions**	**Contraindications**
Fluid exchange and nutrient transport within the disk Increase of intervertebral foramina dimensions Reduction of disk herniation extension Relaxation of paraspinal muscle spasm Nerve root impingement Joint hypomobility	Structural diseases or conditions affecting the spine Medial disk protrusion Claustrophobia Inability to tolerate the desired position Disorientation Chronic obstructive pulmonary disease (harnesses can be restrictive)	Acute cervical trauma Whiplash Use of steroids or other medications that tend to compromise bone integrity Osteoporosis or osteopenia Rheumatologic disorders affecting connective tissues Rheumatoid arthritis Joint hypermobility/instability Pregnancy (lumbar) Prior stabilization or decompression Spinal implants Nonmechanical pain Peripheralization of symptoms with traction Uncontrolled hypertension

TABLE 7-16 • Traction Dosage.			
	Intensity	**Duty Cycle**	**Duration**
Cervical	10-25 lb	1:1 for mobility and facet problems	10-20 minutes (generally lower duration for static)
Lumbar	Up to ½ patient body weight	3:1 or static for disk problems	

Reproduced with permission from Burke-Doe A, Dutton M, eds. *National Physical Therapy Examination and Board Review.* 2019. Copyright © McGraw Hill LLC. All rights reserved. https://accessphysiotherapy.mhmedical.com.

INTERMITTENT PNEUMATIC COMPRESSION

Intermittent pneumatic compression (IPC) is a mechanical force that increases external pressure on a body part. Indications, precautions, and contraindications can be found in Table 7-17.

There is little agreement regarding IPC pressure or treatment times. In some machines, the treatment cycles are preset, while others allow the therapist to determine the duty cycle. General guidelines accompany most machines.

■ MANUAL MODALITIES

MASSAGE

Massage is a mechanical modality that produces the following physiologic effects through different types of stroking, kneading, rubbing, slapping, and vibration:

- Reflexive effects: An autonomic nervous system phenomenon produced by stimulating the skin's sensory receptors and superficial fascia. Causes sedation, relieves tension, increases blood flow.
- Pain reduction: Most likely regulated by both the gate control theory and through the release of endogenous opiates.
- Circulatory effects: Increase lymphatic and blood flow.
- Metabolism: Indirectly affects metabolism due to the increase in lymphatic and blood flow.
- Mechanical effects: Stretching of the intramuscular connective tissue, retard muscle atrophy, increase ROM.

TABLE 7-17 • Indications, Precautions, and Contraindications for Intermittent Pneumatic Compression.		
Indications	**Precautions**	**Contraindications**
• Edema reduction • Prevention of DVT • Venous stasis ulcers • Residual limb shaping after amputation • Control of hypertrophic scarring • Lymphedema	• Impaired sensation • Impaired mentation • Uncontrolled hypertension • Cancer • Stroke or significant peripheral nerves	• Heart failure • Pulmonary edema • Recent or acute DVT, thrombophlebitis, or pulmonary embolism • Obstructed lymphatic or venous return • Severe peripheral arterial disease • Ulcers resulting from venous insufficiency • Acute local skin infection • Significant hypoproteinemia • Acute trauma or fracture • Arterial revascularization

DVN, deep vein thrombosis.

Reproduced with permission from Burke-Doe A, Dutton M, eds. *National Physical Therapy Examination and Board Review.* 2019. Copyright © McGraw Hill LLC. All rights reserved. https://accessphysiotherapy.mhmedical.com.

JOINT MOBILIZATIONS

Joint mobilization techniques improve joint mobility or decrease joint pain by restoring accessory movements to the joint, allowing unrestricted and pain-free ROM. Additional benefits attributed to joint mobilizations include decreasing muscle guarding, lengthening the tissue around a joint, beneficial neuromuscular influence on muscle tone, and increased proprioceptive awareness.[13,14] Consideration must be given to the healing stage, the direction of force, and the magnitude of force. Joint mobilizations should be performed with the joint in the loose-packed or open-packed position (Table 3-9).

Kaltenborn recommends techniques that use a combination of traction and mobilization to reduce pain and mobilize hypomobile joints. Three grades of traction are defined:

- Grade I—Piccolo (loosen): Involves a distraction force that neutralizes pressure in the joint without separating the joint surfaces. Grade I techniques are used in the inflammatory stage of healing.
- Grade II (take up the slack): Separates the articulating surfaces and eliminates the play in the joint capsule.
- Grade III (stretch): Stretches the joint capsule and the soft tissues surrounding the joint to increase mobility. These techniques are typically used during the remodeling stage of healing.

Maitland described five joint mobilization/oscillations grades, each of which falls within the available ROM at the joint—a point somewhere between the beginning point and the anatomic limit. Although the relationship between the five grades in terms of their positions within the ROM is always constant, the point of limitation shifts further to the left as the severity of the motion limitation increases.

- Grade I: A small amplitude movement at the beginning of the range of movement.
- Grade II: A large amplitude movement within the midrange of movement.
- Grade III: A large amplitude movement up to the physiologic limit in the range of movement.
- Grade IV: A small amplitude movement at the very end of the range of movement.
- Grade V: Small amplitude, quick thrust delivered at the end of the range of movement, usually accompanied by a popping sound, which is called a manipulation.

Maitland's grades I and II are used solely for pain relief and have no direct mechanical effect on the restricting barrier but have a hydrodynamic effect. Grades I and II joint mobilizations are theoretically effective in pain reduction by improving joint lubrication and circulation in the joint's tissues.[15,16] Rhythmic joint oscillations also possibly activate articular and skin mechanoreceptors that play a role in pain reduction.[17,18]

Maitland's grades III and IV (or at least III+ and IV+) stretch the barrier and have a mechanical and neurophysiologic effect. Grade III and IV joint distractions and stretching mobilizations may, in addition to the above-stated effects, activate inhibitory joint and muscle spindle receptors, which aid in reducing restriction to movement.[15-18]

■ QUESTIONS

1. **A patient has just had a cast removed 6 weeks post Colles fracture. Which of the following modalities would be the *best* modality to increase ROM in the wrist and fingers?**
   A. Fluidotherapy
   B. Heating pad
   C. Hot pack
   D. Paraffin

STUDY PEARL

The primary indications for joint mobilizations are as follows:

- Limited passive ROM.
- Limited joint accessory motion as determined with joint mobility testing.
- Tissue texture abnormality in the area of dysfunction.
- Pain.
- If the symptoms are aggravated by activity but relieved by rest.

STUDY PEARL

Kaltenborn piccolo and slack movements are generally used to treat joint problems in which the predominant feature is pain, while stretch is used to improve ROM in a joint condition whose predominant feature is stiffness.

2. **Which of the following are the optimal electrode placements for motor stimulation?**
   A. One electrode on the functional motor point and the other over a more distal site on the extremity
   B. Electrodes as far away from each other as possible
   C. Distal to the muscle fibers
   D. One electrode on the functional motor point and the other on the muscle belly

3. **A patient with severe rheumatoid arthritis has an acute exacerbation resulting in neck pain and accompanying muscle guarding and spasm. Which of the following modalities and settings would be the *best* modality for pain control?**
   A. Intermittent cervical traction at 12 lb with 1:1 duty cycle for 20 minutes
   B. Ultrasound at 1.5 W/cm^2, 1 MHz, 100% duty cycle for 7 minutes
   C. Moist hot pack to the cervical spine for 20 minutes
   D. TENS to bilateral cervical spine pulse duration 60 milliseconds, frequency 130 pulses/s with amplitude modulation set to patient comfort with sensory stimulation for 30 minutes

4. **A patient diagnosed with lateral elbow tendinopathy has completed a therapeutic exercise program. The physical therapist instructs this patient on how to apply ice massage to the affected area. Which of the following is *most* appropriate?**
   A. Continue with ice massage until a mild burning sensation is experienced
   B. Treatment time of 5 to 10 minutes
   C. Continue treatment until a response of numbness/tingling is experienced in the ring and little fingers
   D. Treatment time of 10 to 15 minutes

5. **Ultrasound applied at 1 MHz is most effective at heating which of the following tissue types?**
   A. Blood
   B. Fat
   C. Muscle
   D. Tendon

6. **Although not clinically proven, it is generally recommended that when applying intermittent pneumatic compression, inflation pressure should not exceed which of the following?**
   A. Diastolic blood pressure plus 10 mm Hg
   B. Diastolic blood pressure minus 10 mm Hg
   C. Systolic blood pressure plus 10 mm Hg
   D. Systolic blood pressure minus 10 mm Hg

▓ ANSWERS WITH RATIONALES

1. The answer is **A**.[2]
   Although all modalities would provide heating for an increase in tissue extensibility, fluidotherapy and paraffin would allow increased exposure of irregular surfaces of fingers to heat over hot packs or heating pad. In addition, fluidotherapy is the only modality that allows the patient to exercise during the treatment for the optimal increase in ROM.

2. The answer is **D**.[2]
   A. When placing electrodes for motor stimulation, a common mistake is placing one electrode over a motor point and placing the other over a distal site on the extremity. The problem with this can be that the distal electrode is often placed away from the motor nerve region where the optimal response is obtained, rendering the stimulus less effective. Also, the distal electrode is often placed in a region where there is significantly less or no polarized muscle.
   B. Increasing the distance between the electrodes increases the depth of penetration. If the muscle or muscle group is very superficial, as in the wrist flexors, placing the electrodes too far apart can activate wrist extensors.

C. During muscle stimulation, if the patient's sensation goes straight from sensory to noxious, it is probably because one of the electrodes is not over an area of muscle tissue.

D. Motor points are where the greatest motor response is found for a given amount of stimulus. The other electrode should be placed over the muscle group rather than the tendon area.

3. The answer is **D**.
   A. Cervical traction is contraindicated in patients with severe rheumatoid arthritis due to possible ligament instability.[2]
   B. Ultrasound at these parameters would produce tissue heating, which is contraindicated in acute inflammation.[2]
   C. Hot packs would produce tissue heating, which is contraindicated in acute inflammation.[2]
   D. These symptoms are likely to respond to pain modulation via TENS.[3]

4. The answer is **B**.
   A. A mild burning sensation is a normal sensation during an ice massage and should pass quickly. A prolonged phase may result if the area covered is too large or if a hypersensitive response is imminent.[2]
   B. A treatment time of 5 to 10 minutes is generally sufficient for a 10 × 15 cm area.[2]
   C. Cold application over an area of a superficial peripheral nerve can lead to neuropraxia or axonotmesis. Numbness/tingling in the ring and little finger could indicate damage to the ulnar nerve.[2]
   D. A treatment time of 5 to 10 minutes is generally sufficient for a 10 × 15 cm area.[2]

5. The answer is **B**. More dense connective tissues absorb ultrasound better than less dense tissues such as muscle or fat. Therefore, ultrasound is more effective at heating denser tissues.[10]
   A. Attenuation of ultrasound in the blood is approximately 3%.
   B. Attenuation of ultrasound in fat is approximately 13%.
   C. Attenuation of ultrasound in muscle is approximately 24%.
   D. Attenuation of ultrasound tendon is approximately 59%, so of the choices, tendon tissue absorbs the highest percentage of heat.

6. The answer is **B**. Although studies suggest that pressure may not need to be that high, it is recommended that pressure not exceed patient diastolic blood pressure minus 10 mm Hg, as pressure higher than that will restrict venous return.[2]

CHECKLIST

It is expected that a student who has completed or nearly completed a PTA curriculum would know the mechanics of application of the various physical agents available.
When you complete this section, you should be able to:

❑ Determine the appropriate physical agents for patient application based on patient indications.
❑ Identify precautions and contraindications to the application of physical agents.
❑ Select appropriate parameters for the application of physical agents for a given patient.

REFERENCES

1. *Guide to Physical Therapist Practice.* 3d ed. Alexandria, VA: American Physical Therapy Association; 2014.
2. Belitsky RB, Odam SJ, Hubley-Kozey C. Evaluation of the effectiveness of wet ice, dry ice, and cryogen packs in reducing skin temperature. *Phys Ther.* 1987;67:1080-1084.
3. Oosterveld FGJ, Rasker JJ, Jacobs JWG, Overmars HJA. The effect of local heat and cold therapy on the intraarticular and skin surface temperature of the knee. *Arthritis Rheum.* 1992;35:146-151.
4. Travell JG, Simons DG. *Myofascial Pain and Dysfunction—The Trigger Point Manual.* Baltimore, MD: Williams & Wilkins; 1983.

5. Bell GW, Prentice WE. Infrared modalities. In: Prentice WE, ed. *Therapeutic Modalities for Allied Health Professionals.* New York, NY: McGraw-Hill; 1998:201-262.

6. Abramson DI, Tuck S, Lee SW, et al. Comparison of wet and dry heat in raising temperature of tissues. *Arch Phys Med Rehabil.* 1967;48:654.

7. Benson HAE, McElnay JC. Transmission of ultrasound energy through topical pharmaceutical products. *Physiotherapy.* 1988;74:587-589.

8. Cameron MH, Monroe LG. Relative transmission of ultrasound by media customarily used for phonophoresis. *Phys Ther.* 1992;72:142-148.

9. Reeves KD, Hassanein K. Randomized prospective double-blind placebo-controlled study of dextrose prolotherapy for knee osteoarthritis with or without ACL laxity. *Altern Ther Health Med.* 2000;6:68-74, 7-80.

10. Hakala RV. Prolotherapy (proliferation therapy) in the treatment of TMD. *Cranio.* 2005;23:283-288.

11. Kim SR, Stitik TP, Foye PM, Greenwald BD, Campagnolo DI. Critical review of prolotherapy for osteoarthritis, low back pain, and other musculoskeletal conditions: a physiatric perspective. *Am J Phys Med Rehabil.* 2004;83:379-389.

12. Britton KR. Is prolotherapy safe and effective for back pain? *Postgrad Med.* 2000;108:37-38.

13. Tanigawa MC. Comparison of hold-relax procedure and passive mobilization on increasing muscle length. *Phys Ther.* 1972;52:725-735.

14. Barak T, Rosen E, Sofer R. Mobility: passive orthopedic manual therapy. In: Gould J, Davies G, eds. *Orthopedic and Sports Physical Therapy.* St Louis, MO: CV Mosby; 1990.

15. Grieve GP. Manual mobilizing techniques in degenerative arthrosis of the hip. *Bull Orthop Section APTA.* 1977;2:7.

16. Yoder E. Physical therapy management of nonsurgical hip problems in adults. In: Echternach JL, ed. *Physical Therapy of the Hip.* New York, NY: Churchill Livingstone; 1990;103-137.

17. Wyke BD. The neurology of joints. *Ann R Coll Surg Engl.* 1967;41:25-50.

18. Freeman MAR, Wyke BD. An experimental study of articular neurology. *J Bone Joint Surg.* 1967;49B:185.

Equipment, Devices, and Technology

MARK DUTTON

OVERVIEW

Physical therapy has an extensive barrage of technology and equipment devices available. The rapid advances in technology benefit both clinicians and their clients. Technology ranges from exoskeletons that allow paraplegic clients to walk, monitoring devices that prevent individuals with Alzheimer from wandering out of their home, anatomy tables that replace cadavers, and equipment for biofeedback in the clinic ranging from pelvic floor contraction to balance and gait analysis. The clinician's responsibility is to keep up-to-date with any equipment and technology relevant to their clientele and provide appropriate referral or guidance to individuals seeking more information about specific types of technology.

▲ HIGH-YIELD TERMS

Adaptive device	An implement or equipment to increase the independence of a patient/client.
Assistive device	An implement or equipment to aid patients/clients in performing movements, tasks, or activities.

▪ EQUIPMENT

Definitions are as follows:

Adaptive devices: A variety of implements or equipment to increase the independence of patients/clients. Adaptive devices include the following:

- Environmental controls.
- Hospital beds.
- Raised toilet seats.
- Seating systems.

Assistive devices: A variety of implements or equipment to aid patients/clients in performing movements, tasks, or activities. Assistive devices include the following:

- Canes.
- Crutches.

- Long-handled reachers.
- Percussors and vibrators.
- Power devices.
- Static and dynamic splints.
- Walkers.
- Wheelchairs.

The clinician's role is to provide the most appropriate assistive device and then teach the patient to use it correctly. The assistive devices used for gait training are described in Chapter 5.

Protective devices:

- Cushions.
- Helmets.
- Protective taping.
- Restraints.

Personal protective equipment: See the section on Wheelchairs.

Supportive devices:

- Compression garments.
- Corsets.
- Elastic wraps.
- Mechanical ventilators.
- Neck collars.
- Serial casts.
- Slings.
- Supplemental oxygen.
- Supportive taping.

■ ASSISTIVE DEVICES

The clinician must always remember that several energy costs are associated with using various assistive devices (Table 5-10). The indications for using an assistive device include the following:

- Decreased ability to bear weight through the lower extremities.
- Muscle weakness or paralysis of the trunk or lower extremities.
- Decreased balance and proprioception in the upright posture.
- Joint instability and excessive skeletal loading.
- Fatigue or pain.

▲ HIGH-YIELD TERMS TO LEARN

Non–weight-bearing	A weight-bearing status used whenever a patient is not permitted to place any weight through the involved extremity.
Toe touch weight-bearing	A weight-bearing status used whenever a patient is not permitted to place any weight through the involved extremity but may place the toes on the ground to assist with balance.
Partial weight-bearing	A weight-bearing status used whenever a patient is only permitted to place a portion of their body weight through the involved extremity.

Assistive devices are often prescribed with an accompanying weight-bearing restriction. It must be remembered that most patients have difficulty replicating a prescribed weight-bearing restriction and will need constant reinforcing. Descriptions of the most common weight-bearing restrictions are presented here:

Non–weight-bearing (NWB): This restriction is used whenever a patient is not permitted to place any weight through the involved extremity or touch the ground or surface. The most common assistive devices used with this weight-bearing restriction include a standard walker or two crutches.

Toe touch weight-bearing (TTWB): This restriction is used whenever a patient is not permitted to place any weight through the involved extremity but may place the toes on the ground to assist with balance. The most common assistive devices used with this weight-bearing restriction include a standard walker or two crutches.

Partial weight-bearing (PWB): This restriction is used whenever a patient is permitted to put a particular amount of weight through the involved extremity. The amount of weight permitted is expressed as pounds of pressure or a percentage of the patient's total weight. This is the most difficult weight-bearing restriction to monitor as it is difficult to determine how much actual weight the patient is transferring through the involved foot during gait. A bathroom scale can be used to teach the patient. The most common assistive devices used with this weight-bearing restriction include a standard walker or two crutches.

Weight-bearing as tolerated (WBAT): This weight-bearing restriction allows the patient to determine the proper amount of weight-bearing using comfort as a guide. The amount of weight-bearing can range from minimal to full. An assistive device may or may not be required.

- Full weight-bearing (FWB): A patient can place full weight on the involved extremity. An assistive device is not required at this level but may be used to assist with balance.

Correct fitting for an assistive device is important for the patient's safety and allows for minimal energy expenditure. Once fitted, the clinician should ensure that the correct walking technique with the device is taught to the patient.

Parallel bars can provide maximum stability and security for patients during the beginning stages of ambulation or standing (see Chapter 5). The correct height for the bars should allow 20 to 25 degrees of elbow flexion while grasping the bars with the hands approximately 4 to 6 in in front of the body. The goal is to progress the patient out of the bars as quickly as possible to increase overall mobility and decrease dependence on the parallel bars.

There are three major categories of ambulatory assistive devices: canes, crutches, and walkers. Gait training using the various assistive devices is described in Chapter 5.

CANES

Canes are usually made out of wood, plastic, or aluminum (adjustable with a push pin lock). The function of a cane is to widen the base of support and improve balance. However, because canes provide minimal stability and support for patients during ambulation activities, they are not intended for restricted weight-bearing gaits. Patients are typically instructed to hold a cane in the hand opposite to the affected extremity. Using a cane in the contralateral hand widens the base of support and reduces the lateral shifting of the center of mass, helps preserve reciprocal motion and a more normal pathway for the center of gravity (COG),[1] and also helps to reduce forces. For example, using a cane can transmit 20% to 25% of body weight away from the involved lower extremity.[2,3]

A variety of cane types exist:

- Standard cane. A straight cane with a single contact point with the ground.
- Adjustable aluminum offset (J-shaped) or offset cane. This cane's design allows pressure to be borne over the cane's center, providing greater stability.
- Quad cane. This type of cane provides four points of contact with the ground. Any patient using this cane should be instructed to simultaneously place all four legs of the cane on the floor to obtain maximum stability. This cane provides a larger base of support (BOS) than a standard cane, increasing stability. However, depending on the specific design of

the cane, the pressure exerted by the patient's hand may not be centered over the cane and may result in patient complaints of instability.[4]

- A small-based quad cane is useful for stairs.
- A wide-based quad cane provides the largest BOS but cannot be used on stairs. Another disadvantage is that this type of cane warrants the use of a slower gait pattern—faster progressions often cause the cane to rock from the rear legs to the front legs.
- A rolling cane. This type provides a wide-wheeled base allowing uninterrupted forward progression. A pressure-sensitive brake is built into the handle and can be engaged using pressure from the palm. This cane allows weight to be continuously applied as the need to lift and place the cane forward is eliminated, allowing for a faster progression.

To measure the correct cane height, the cane is placed approximately 6 in from the lateral border of the patient's toes.[4] Two landmarks typically are used during measurement to obtain a correct fit for a cane[4]:

- Greater trochanter: The top of the cane should come to approximately the level of the greater trochanter.
- Angle at the elbow: The elbow should be flexed 20 to 30 degrees.

An alternative method involves standing the cane at the patient's side and then adjusting the handle to the wrist crease level at the ulnar styloid.

CRUTCHES

Crutches (regular or standard), typically made from wood or aluminum, provide an increased base of support, a moderate degree of lateral stability, increased mobility, and can be used with all levels of weight-bearing. However, crutches require a higher level of coordination than walkers, are awkward in small areas, and can cause pressure at the radial groove (spiral groove) of the humerus, creating potential damage to the radial nerve and adjacent vascular structures in the axilla.[4]

The correct height for axillary crutches includes positioning the crutches 6 in in front and 2 in lateral to the patient with the crutch height adjusted to be no greater than three finger widths from the axilla (the handgrip is adjusted to allow for approximately 20 to 30 degrees of elbow flexion). The crutch height can be adjusted by wing nuts (pushbutton locks on the aluminum crutches). Alternative methods of measurement include the following:

- In the standing position, one can subtract 16 in in the patient's height or measure from a point 2 in below the axilla to a point 6 in in front and 2 in lateral to the foot.
- With the patient supine, measure from the axilla to 6 to 8 in lateral to the heel.

Two other types of crutches are worth mentioning:

- Lofstrand (forearm): This type can be used for all weight-bearing levels, provide increased ease of movement, and allow the wearer to use their hands without dropping the crutches because of its forearm cuff. However, this type of crutch requires the highest level of coordination for proper use. Proper fit includes 20 to 25 degrees of elbow flexion while holding the handgrip with the crutches positioned 6 in in front and 2 in lateral to the patient. In addition, the arm cuff should be positioned 1 to 1.5 in below the olecranon process to not interfere with elbow flexion.
- Forearm platform: This allows weight-bearing on the forearm and is useful for patients who cannot bear weight through their hands. However, this type of crutch provides less lateral support owing to the absence of an axillary bar.

WALKERS

Walkers can be used with all weight-bearing restrictions and offer a large BOS and good anterior and lateral stability. Attachments include fold-down seats, a braking mechanism, platform attachments, wheel attachments, and carrying baskets. The correct height of the walker allows for 20 to 25 degrees of elbow flexion. Walkers are available with many variations, including the following:

- Folding (collapsible). This type facilitates mobility in the community and is easier to transport in cars.
- Rolling (wheeled). This design is available in either two wheels or four wheels, the latter of which requires a hand brake to provide added stability in stopping. The advantage of this type of walker is that it facilitates walking as a continuous movement sequence.
- Stair climbing. This type is fitted with two posterior extensions and additional handgrips off the rear legs for use on stairs.
- Reciprocal. This type is fitted with hinges that allow advancement of one side of the walker at a time, thereby facilitating a reciprocal gait pattern.
- Hemi. A hemi walker is modified for use with one hand only.

Before initiating instruction in gait patterns using a conventional walker, several points related to the use of the walker should be emphasized to the patient[4]:

- The walker should be picked up and placed on all four legs simultaneously to achieve maximum stability.
- The patient should be encouraged to hold their head up and to maintain good postural alignment.
- The patient should be cautioned not to step too close to the front crossbar to prevent falling.

■ WHEELCHAIRS

A wheelchair is a medical device that takes the form of a chair on wheels and is used by people for whom walking is difficult or impossible due to illness or disability. Wheelchairs are available in various sizes and styles, and wheelchair design continues to improve both in safety and construction. Whenever possible, every attempt should be made to reduce the amount of energy required for wheelchair propulsion.

▲ HIGH-YIELD TERMS TO LEARN

Seat depth	Measured from the user's posterior buttock, along the lateral thigh to the popliteal fold. Two inches are added to the measurement.
Seat width	Approximately 1 to 2 in wider than the width of the user's hip.
Footrest length	A measurement that ensures clearance of the footplates from the ground while maintaining the correct position of the user's hips and knees.
Wheelbase	The horizontal distance between the centers of the front and rear wheels of a wheelchair.
Physiatrist	A physician that specializes in physical medicine and rehabilitation (PM&R).

Wheelchairs can be grouped into several classes: indoor (small wheelbase to allow maneuvering in confined spaces, but lacks the ability or power to negotiate obstacles), indoor/outdoor (provides mobility for those who stay on finished services, such as sidewalks, driveways, and flooring), and active indoor/outdoor (provides the ability to travel long distances, move fast, and drive over unstructured environments such as grass, gravel, and uneven terrain).

Wheelchair fitting is highly individualized and requires a team effort between a physiatrist, neurologist or orthopedist, occupational or physical therapists, assistive technology and driver training specialist, and rehabilitation technology providers. When helping to choose a wheelchair, a few patient considerations must be made:

- Physical needs.
- Rental versus purchase.
- Seating system.

- Functional mobility.
- Physical abilities.
- Cognition.
- Coordination.
- Level of endurance.
- Manual versus power.

WHEELCHAIR MEASUREMENTS

To physically examine the patient for a wheelchair, the patient should be positioned supine on a firm surface. The range of available pelvic and hip movements related to spinal and pelvic alignment should be determined. The lower extremities must be well supported by the clinician, with the knee flexed to 95 to 100 degrees or as much as is needed to eliminate the influence of the hamstring muscle group. Range of motion (ROM) measurements should include hip flexion, abduction, adduction, internal and external rotation, and their effect on pelvic position and general body alignment. Once the ROM is documented, a linear measurement of seat depth should be determined. The standard wheelchair measurements are outlined in Table 8-1.

Once the supine examination is completed, the patient adopts a supported sitting position with the knees flexed to 100 degrees (or more) to eliminate the hamstring muscle group's influence.

TABLE 8-1 • Standard Wheelchair Measurements.		
Dimension	**Guidelines**	**Average Size**
Seat height/leg length	The measurement is taken from the user's heel to the popliteal fold. Two inches are added to this measurement to allow clearance of the footrest.	Adult: 20 in. Narrow adult: 20 in. Slim adult: 20 in. Hemi/low seat: 17.5 in. Junior: 18.5 in Child: 18.75 in. Tiny tot: 19.5 in.
Seat depth	The measurement is taken from the user's posterior buttock, along the lateral thigh to the popliteal fold. Approximately 2 in are subtracted from this measurement to avoid pressure from the seat's edge against the popliteal space.	Adult: 16 in. Narrow adult: 16 in. Slim adult: 16 in. Junior: 16 in. Child: 11.5 in. Tiny tot: 11.5 in.
Seat width	The measurement is taken of the widest aspect of the user's buttocks, hips, or thighs. Two inches are added to this measurement to provide space for bulky clothing, orthoses, or clearance of the trochanters from the armrest side panel.	Adult: 18 in. Narrow adult: 16 in. Slim adult: 14 in. Junior: 16 in. Child: 14 in. Tiny tot: 12 in.
Back height	The measurement is taken from the seat of the chair to the floor of the axilla with the user's shoulder flexed to 90°. Four inches are subtracted from this measurement to allow the final back height to be below the inferior angles of the scapulae. NB: This measurement will be affected if a seat cushion is to be used—the person should be measured while seated on the seat cushion, or the thickness of the cushion must be considered by adding that value to the actual measurement.	Adult: 16 to 16.5 in.
Armrest height	The measurement is taken from the seat of the chair to the olecranon process with the user's elbow flexed to 90°. One inch is added to this measurement. NB: This measurement will be affected if a seat cushion is to be used—the person should be measured while seated on the seat cushion, or the thickness of the cushion must be considered by adding that value to the actual measurement.	Adult: 9 in above the chair seat

Ideally, the seated examination should be done on a simulator, a chair specifically designed for planar seated examinations. However, if a simulator is not available, the measurement can be done on the map table with a thin front edge to allow 100 degrees of knee flexion.

WHEELCHAIR COMPONENTS

Frame

Whereas stainless steel used to be the only frame material available, wheelchair users today have their choice of stainless steel, chrome, aluminum, airplane aluminum, steel tubing, an alloy of chrome and lightweight materials, titanium, and other lightweight composite materials (sports chairs—accommodate a tucked position, include leg straps, slanted drive wheels, and small push rims). As a result, the ultralight wheelchair is the highest-quality chair designed specifically for active people. In general, the lighter the frame's weight, the greater the ease of use, but the lesser amount of structural strength provided. Therefore, the expected activity level and environment where the wheelchair will be used should be considered when deciding on frame construction.

The two most common types of frames currently available are as follows:

- Rigid frame: The frame remains in one piece, and the wheels are released for storage or travel.
- Facilitates stroke efficiency.
- Increases distance/stroke.
- Standard cross-brace frame: Enables the frame to collapse or fold for transport or storage.
- Facilitates mobility in the community.
- The wheelchair is folded by first raising the footplates and then pulling up on the handles (located on either side of the seat), rather than pulling up on the middle of the upholstery, the latter of which can tear the upholstery.

Anti-Tipping Device

These are posterior extensions attached to the low horizontal supports, which prevent the chair from tipping backward but limit the ability to go over curbs or doorsills. A similar device is the hill-holder, a mechanical brake that allows the chair to go forward but automatically applies the brake when the chair goes into reverse.

Upholstery

The upholstery for wheelchairs must be able to withstand daily use in all kinds of weather. Consequently, manufacturers provide various options to users, ranging from cloth to new synthetic fabrics to leather. Many manufacturers also offer a selection of upholstery colors, ranging from black to neon, to allow for individual selection and differing consumer tastes.

Seating System

Many standard wheelchairs come with a fabric or sling seat. The disadvantages of a sling seat are that the hips tend to slide forward, the thighs tend to adduct and internally rotate, and the patient sits asymmetrically, reinforcing a poor pelvic position. Because of these problems and the fact that seating must be customized individually, seating surfaces are often purchased separately from the wheelchairs themselves.

It is important when selecting a wheelchair or a seating system to ensure that the two components are compatible.

- Insert or contour seats: Fabricated from wood or plastic and padded with foam, these seats create a stable firm sitting surface, improved pelvic position (neutral), and reduce the tendency for the patient to slide forward or sit with a posterior pelvic tilt.
- Seat cushions: Function to distribute weight-bearing pressures, which help prevent decubitus ulcers in patients with decreased sensation, and prolong wheelchair sitting times.
- Pressure-relieving air cushion: These lightweight cushions accommodate moderate-to-severe postural deformity and improve pressure distribution. The disadvantages of

this type of cushion include the expense, the base may be unstable for some patients, and they require continuous maintenance.

- Pressure-relieving fluid/gel or combination cushion: These can be custom-molded, are designed to accommodate moderate-to-severe postural deformity, and are easy for caregivers to reposition the patient. The disadvantages are that they require some maintenance, are heavy, and are moderately expensive.
- Pressure-relieving contoured foam cushion: This type uses dense, layered foam. Is designed to accommodate moderate-to-severe postural deformity, and is easy for caregivers to reposition patient. The main disadvantage with this type is that they may interfere with slide board transfers.
- Suspension elements: Suspension elements reduce the negative effects of shock and vibration—extended exposure to the vibration sustained while propelling a wheelchair in communities may lead to discomfort and various harmful physiologic effects, such as chronic low back pain and disk degeneration.

Backrest

The standard height backrest provides support to the midscapula region. Several modifications can be made to suit the user:

- A lower back height may increase functional mobility—typically seen in sports chairs—but may also increase back strain.
- A high back height may be necessary for patients with poor trunk stability or with extensor spasms.
- Lateral trunk supports: These provide improved trunk alignment for patients with scoliosis or poor stability.
- Insert or contour backs: These improve trunk extension and overall upright alignment.

Brakes

Brakes are an important safety feature. Most brakes consist of a lever system with a cam or a ratchet. Extensions may be added to increase the ease of both locking and unlocking. When a wheelchair has a reclining back, an additional brake is necessary. Brakes must be engaged for all transfers in and out of the chair.

Wheels/Tires

Most wheelchairs use four wheels: two large wheels (standard spokes or spokeless) at the back (fitted with an outer rim that allows for hand grip and propulsion) and two smaller ones (casters) at the front. The tires used for the rear wheels may be narrow and hard rubber, pneumatic inflatable, semipneumatic, or radial tires. The pneumatic tires provide a smoother ride and increased shock absorption but require more maintenance than the solid ties. Mag wheels and off-road wheels also are options on some chairs. The standard size for the rear wheel is 24 in. Smaller and larger wheel sizes are available.

Most wheelchair wheels are fitted with an outer rim that enables the patient to propel himself or herself. For those patients with only one functional arm, two outer rims can be fitted on one wheel so that arm drive achieves both forward and backward propulsion. In addition, projections (vertical, oblique, or horizontal) may be attached to the rims to facilitate propulsion for patients who have a poor handgrip. However, the horizontal and oblique extensions add to the chair's overall width and reduce maneuverability.

Casters vary in size (ranging from 6 to 8 in in diameter) and composition (pneumatic, solid rubber, plastic, or a combination of these). In addition, caster locks can be added to facilitate wheelchair stability during transfers.

Leg Rests

Leg rests come in a variety of designs.

- Swing away: Detachable leg rests facilitate transfers and a front approach to the wheelchair when ambulating.

- Elevating: Most frequently necessary when the patient cannot flex the knee for postural support or when a dependent leg contributes to lower extremity edema. The leg rest's length can be adjusted to accommodate the full length of the patient's leg, and there is padded calf support. The leg rest's position is adjusted by pushing down on a lever on the side of the chair. Elevating leg rests can be released from the wheelchair or pivoted to one side during transfers. Elevated leg rests are contraindicated for patients with hypertonicity or adaptive shortening of the hamstrings.
- Fixed: As their name suggests, these leg rests are immovable.

Footrests

A footrest is standard equipment for a wheelchair. For rigid frame chairs, the footrests are usually incorporated into the chair's frame as part of the design. Cross-brace folding chairs often have footrests that swivel, flip up, and/or can be removed.

Footplates, which can be adjusted to accommodate the patient's foot, provide a resting base for the feet so that the feet are positioned in neutral with the knee flexed to 90 degrees.

Heel loops can be fitted to help maintain the foot position and prevent posterior sliding of the foot. Ankle and calf straps can be added to stabilize the feet onto the footplates. Toe loops may also be used when the patient has difficulty maintaining the foot on the footplate in a forward direction.

Armrests

Armrests are available in several styles, including desk length (to allow the user closer access to desks and tables) or full length, and both types may be flip-up, fixed, or detachable. The desk length design also allows the patient to remove and reverse the armrest so that the higher part is closer to the front edge to aid in pushing to standing. Wraparound (space saver) armrests reduce the overall width of the chair by 1.5 in. The height of the armrests can also be adjustable.

Armrests can also be fitted with upper extremity support surface trays or troughs, which can help a user with upper body balance difficulty or decreased upper extremity use.

Many lightweight manual chairs are designed without armrests, making it easier to roll up to a desk or table and perform transfers while also providing a streamlined look.

Seat Belts

Seat belts can be used for safety or positioning:

- Restraining belts are used to prevent patients from falling out of the wheelchair.
  - Seat belts can be fitted to grasp the pelvis at a 45-degree angle to the seat to help position the pelvis. The belt's position can also provide lateral or medial support at the hip and knee to maintain lower extremity alignment and/or control spasticity.

SPECIALIZED WHEELCHAIRS

Wheelchair designs can vary greatly to match the user's functional, posture support, environmental, and durability requirements.

Bariatric Wheelchairs

Bariatrics is the field of medicine that treats obese patients. This heavy-duty wheelchair has a seat width of up to 32 in and a weight limit of up to 1000 lb. A person may be referred to as a bariatric patient when they have a body mass index (BMI) equal to or greater than 30.

Pediatric Wheelchairs

Children with cerebral palsy, spina bifida, and osteogenesis imperfecta may be candidates for either a manual or power wheelchair, depending on their upper extremity strength, rate of fatigue, cognitive abilities, and family circumstances. Those with spinal muscular dystrophy, arthrogryposis, high-level spinal cord injuries, and progressively worsening Duchenne muscular dystrophy are typically immediate candidates for powered mobility. Key decisions concerning wheelchair design must be a team effort.

A pediatric wheelchair must have approximately 4 in of available space in the frame to accommodate the patient's growth. Also, the seating system should be flexible enough to accommodate tonal or postural changes. Examples of flexibility in the system involve the placement of laterals, which are often attached to tracks, or the backrest can include T-nuts placed throughout the back to allow easy hardware mounting. Pediatric chairs often employ linear seating systems (to accommodate the delicate balance between providing contours in the system and accommodating growth) versus molded seats, which are more difficult to increase in size. Similarly, a contoured backrest is more accommodating and provides more contact surface and thus more comfort. Caregivers should be made aware of all accessories, including head supports and upper chest supports, and their proper use.

The wheelchair team must always consider the aesthetic appeal of the wheelchair and, where possible, it should reflect individuality and personality. When deciding between a manual or power wheelchair, several considerations need to be made:

- Power chairs are more expensive than manual chairs. Power chairs have inherent safety concerns and create issues surrounding transportation and home accessibility.
- Manual wheelchairs are easier to transport and lift into a nonaccessible home.

Reclining wheelchairs

Reclining wheelchairs are designed with an extended back and typically have elevating leg rests. The angle of the back is adjusted by releasing knobs on the side of the wheelchair. A fitted head support is required on a reclining back wheelchair. A bar across the back of the reclining wheelchair provides support and stability. The purpose of the reclining wheelchair is to allow intermittent or constant reclined positioning. Reclining wheelchairs are indicated for patients who are unable to maintain an upright sitting position independently. The chairs can be either manually or electrically (if the patient cannot do active push-ups or pressure-relief maneuvers) controlled.

Hemi-Chair

This chair is designed to be low to the ground (seat height of approximately 17.5 in), allowing propulsion with the noninvolved upper and/or lower extremities.

Tilt in Space

This type of chair is designed to allow for a reclining position without losing the required 90 degrees of hip flexion and 90 degrees of knee flexion and is indicated for patients with extensor spasms that may throw the patient out of the chair or for pressure relief.

One-Arm Drive

These chairs are designed with the drive mechanisms located on one wheel, usually with two outer rims (or push lever). Thus, the patient can propel the wheelchair by pushing on either rim (or a lever) with one hand.

Amputee Chair

An amputee chair is a modified wheelchair where the drive wheels are placed posterior (approximately 2 in posterior) to the vertical back supports so that the BOS is lengthened and posterior stability is enhanced.

Powered Chairs

This design of chair utilizes a power source (battery) that propels the wheelchair. Microprocessors allow the control of the wheelchair to be adapted to various controls (joystick, head, and breath). This chair is usually prescribed for patients who are not capable of self-propulsion or have very low endurance. Recent changes in the power bases have allowed for such innovations as power seat functions (power tilt, recline, elevating leg rest, seat elevator) and control interfaces (mini joysticks, head controls). Power wheelchair bases can be classified in one of three categories, based on the drive wheel location relative to the system's COG:

- Rear-wheel drive: The drive wheels are located behind the user's COG, and the casters are located in the front, providing predictable drive characteristics and stability.
- Mid-wheel drive: The drive wheels are located below the user's COG and generally have a set of casters or anti-tippers on the front and rear of the drive wheels. The advantage of this system is a smaller turning radius. The disadvantage is a tendency to rock or pitch forward, especially with sudden stops or fast turns.
- Front-wheel drive: The drive wheels are located in front of the user's COG. This design provides stability and a tight turning radius, and the ability to climb obstacles or curbs more easily. However, one of the disadvantages is its rearward COG, making it difficult to drive in a straight line, especially on uneven surfaces.

WHEELCHAIR TRAINING

Several areas need to be addressed when training a patient to be as functionally independent as possible with a wheelchair.

Posture

The patient needs to maintain good posture in the wheelchair. He or she should be seated well back in the chair, with the lower extremities on the footrests or leg rests. The patient should be able to maintain a seated position when their balance is challenged.

Wheelchair Management

The various components of the wheelchair should be reviewed with the patient, and the patient should perform all of the necessary tasks while being supervised by the clinician. Wheelchair users are susceptible to muscle imbalances. Nearly every motion and repetitive motion is forward, stressing the shoulder flexors (pectoralis major and anterior deltoid) and shoulder internal rotators. These anterior muscles can become adaptively shortened, while the upper back muscles become weak and elongated. The typical posture of the wheelchair user has rounded shoulders with mild thoracic kyphosis and a forward head. This posture can result in impingement of the soft tissue structures of the subacromial space.

Wheelchair Mobility

Depending on their functional level, the patient is instructed on the following functions:

- Operate the wheel locks, foot supports, and armrests and use the mechanisms safely without tipping forward or sideways out of the chair seat.
- Transfer in and out of the chair with the least possible assistance. This may involve transfer training from the wheelchair to the car seat.
- Propel the wheelchair in all directions and around corners.
- Perform a wheelie. A wheelie is performed by balancing on the rear wheels of a wheelchair while the caster wheels are in the air. Wheelies are important for those patients who need to go up and down curbs independently when there are no curb ramps. Initially, the clinician must be positioned behind the chair and move with the chair, with the hands held beneath the wheelchair handles, ready to catch the wheelchair if it tilts too far backward. The patient should be taught how to tuck their head into the chest if they fall back to not hit the back of their head if they perform the maneuver without assistance. To perform a wheelie, the patient is asked to place their hands at 11:00 on the wheels, then lean forward and arch their back. Initially, the patient practices bouncing the body off the back of the chair and leaning back while holding the hands still—the front of the chair is raised by pushing backward on the back of the chair. Next, the patient practices until he or she can bounce the front end off the ground. Finally, by changing the COG (by pushing the chair forward while the body is going backward), the patient will achieve a point of equilibrium.

Once the patient can bounce the front end off the ground and find a point of equilibrium, they progress to reaching back and placing their hands at about 10:00 on the wheels. From this point, they lean forward, arch the back and then begin to push forward quickly while letting the body come back against the chair (when their back hits the chair, their hands should be in the 12:00 position). By continuing to lean back and pushing the chair forward, the front end should start to leave the ground, and by the time the hands get to the 2:00 position, the front end should feel weightless, as the chair balances on the rear axle. The patient will need to move the chair forward to maintain equilibrium if the front end begins to fall forward or backward if the chair begins to fall backward. This may be accomplished by sliding the hands back to about the 1:00 position without taking the hands off the wheels. Once the chair is up and balanced, the patient will need to keep just a fraction of weight on the front end so that if balance is lost, the chair will fall forward, not backward.

- "Pop a wheelie" and move forward and backward in the wheelie position. Once the patient is ready to try a wheelie independently, a good place to begin practicing is carpeting, grass, or sand.

■ PROTECTION AND SAFETY

An important role of the physical therapist assistant (PTA) is to maintain high protection and safety levels for themselves, their team members, and patients.

▲ HIGH-YIELD TERMS TO LEARN

Personal protective equipment (PPE)	Any equipment worn to minimize exposure to a variety of hazards, including infections.
Nosocomial infection	An infection that originates in a hospital or hospital-like setting.
Health care–associated infection (HAI)	An HAI refers to an infection acquired in any health care setting.
Contamination	Refers to any instance when an object, surface, or field comes into contact with anything that is not sterile.
Restraint	A physical or chemical measure used to keep someone or something under control or within limits.

PATIENT SAFETY AND EMERGENCIES

Within the medical profession, there will always be a potential for emergencies. Various patient populations have a higher risk of injury. These patient populations can include the cognitively impaired or the physically impaired. One example of a physically impaired patient is a bariatric patient. Any patient with the following medical conditions has a higher potential for impaired safety:

- Severe pain and discomfort.
- Joint replacements/instabilities.
- History of falls.
- Postural hypotension.
- Paralysis/paresis.
- Severe osteoporosis.
- Respiratory/cardiac problems.
- Amputations.
- Difficult weight-bearing status (NWB, TTWB).

Within an inpatient facility setting, the clinician's responsibility is to fully understand the various "codes" that may be announced that directly influence patient safety. On hearing the code alarms, the clinician should follow facility protocols to ensure patient and staff safety. These "codes" can include patient abduction, on-site threat, environmental threat, and individual patient emergencies. The appropriate and correct action is required in all cases to ensure patient and personal safety (Table 8-2).

TABLE 8-2 • Emergency Response.					
Location	**Policies**	**Obvious Injury**	**No Obvious Injury**	**Follow-up**	**Who to Contact**
Outpatient clinic	Follow clinic policy and procedures	Call 911 for medical support	Get patient up, take vital signs; if normal, continue with caution and patient consent	Continue to monitor the patient and only allow them to leave the clinic if you are sure they are stable and safe	Primary care physician Management of the facility
Home health setting	Follow agency policies and contact the agency immediately	Call 911 for medical support	Get patient up, take vital signs; if normal, continue with caution	Continue to monitor the patient throughout the session and do not leave the home until you are sure the patient is safe and stable and not alone	Home health agency Primary care physician Family as appropriate with patient consent
Inpatient setting	Follow facility protocols	Call nursing, emergency response team, and/or MD to the location	Call nursing and/or MD to the location Get patient up and continue per MD recommendations	Complete all facility paperwork and ensure that all appropriate follow-up calls will be made, or make them as needed	Ensure nursing has agreed to contact family and physician; otherwise, PT may be required to do so. Document all calls made.

Reproduced with permission from Burke-Doe A, Dutton M, eds. *National Physical Therapy Examination and Board Review.* 2019. Copyright © McGraw Hill LLC. All rights reserved. https://accessphysiotherapy.mhmedical.com.

FALLS AND FALL RISK

All patients should be evaluated for fall risk at every visit, particularly those over 65. In addition, the patient should be asked if they have experienced a fall since the previous visit, and the definition of a fall should also be clearly explained.

According to the World Health Organization, "A fall is defined as an event which results in a person coming to rest inadvertently on the ground or floor or other lower level." It does not have to result in injury, and many older adults will deny falling if they were not injured. Therefore, it is important to ensure that they understand what constitutes a fall and then determine if they have fallen.

Figure 8-1 shows protocols for a situation of a patient falling during therapy. No indication of guilt should be made during any family contact, facts should be reported, and the family should be referred to appropriate management for follow-up as needed. Everything from the fall to the follow-ups should be carefully and accurately documented immediately to ensure accurate and full recollection of the incident. If the incident was witnessed, be sure to get a statement from any witness.

Injuries from falls may range from minor injuries to more severe such as bone fractures or head injuries. The PTA should implement the physical therapist's selected interventions to address impairments of strength, ROM, gait, or balance. The patient's medical history and living environment should also be taken into consideration. Patients with a history of falls may become fearful of falling and may self-limit their activity. Fall risk factors include the following:

- Muscle weakness.
- Vision deficits.
- Decreased sensation.
- Balance impairments.
- Gait impairments and/or assistive device use.
- Multiple medications.
- Cognitive impairment.

Tests and measures that can be used to identify a fall risk include the following:

- Timed Up and Go (TUG).
- Tinetti Assessment Tool.

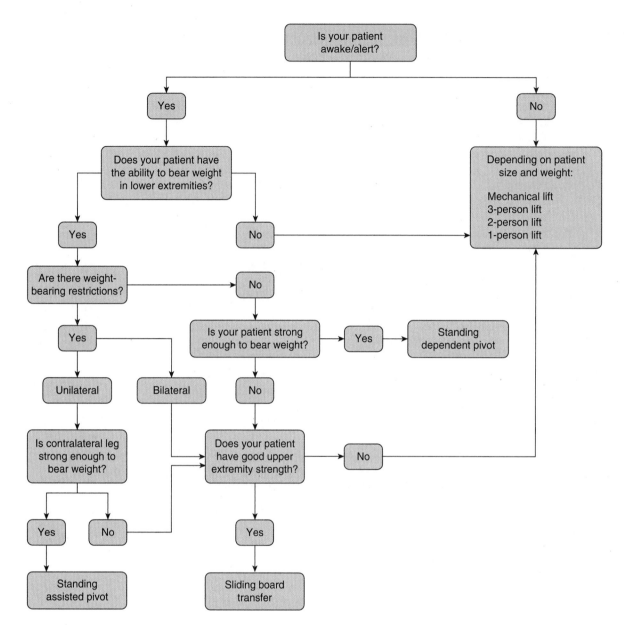

Figure 8-1. An algorithm for transfers. (Reproduced with permission from Prentice WE, Voight MI. *Techniques in Musculoskeletal Rehabilitation*. 2001. Copyright © McGraw-Hill LLC. All rights reserved.)

- Berg Balance Scale.
- Dynamic Gait Index (DGI).
- Functional Reach Test.
- 30-Second Chair Stand Test.

Fall prevention strategies include the following:

- Review of medications by doctor or pharmacist.
- Regular vision examinations.
- Appropriate footwear.
- Adequate lighting.
- Use a gait belt for transfers, gait activities, and balance training.
- Secure all lines, tubes, or cords, so they do not restrict or block mobility.
- Be sure the phone, TV remote, or call light are within the reach of the patient.
- Declutter by removing loose rugs or any items that may block the walking path.
- Install railings at stairs and grab bars by toilet/shower/tub.

STUDY PEARL
The PTA must ensure the patient has footwear that fits well and provides traction. The PTA must be sure non-slip socks or securely fitting shoes are applied before standing or walking and avoid footwear that may slide off the foot, has poor traction, or is ill-fitting.

RESTRAINTS

The Centers for Medicare and Medicaid Services (CMS) has very strict guidelines for using restraints in the skilled nursing arena. Each state has different interpretations of restraints, and local and state policies must be adhered to. The use of restraints is sometimes critical for patient safety; however, every effort must have been made and documented to try less restrictive measures. Physical restraint examples include leg restraints, vests, belts, lap cushions, and bed rails. Chemical restraints include any drug used for discipline or convenience that is not required to treat medical symptoms. Any inappropriate use of restraints, either chemical or physical, by a facility, caregiver, or family member, should be considered an act of abuse and be reported to the appropriate authorities using the correct policy per the facility, agency, or management guidelines. In many states, the failure of a clinician to report possible abuse is a criminal offense.

ENVIRONMENTAL FACTORS

The environment can be both beneficial and detrimental to the health of a patient. For example, a positive, well-lit, sunny, uncluttered setting can be positive and promote well-being. In contrast, a cluttered, dirty location can be hazardous for using assistive devices, can be unconducive to wound healing, and increase the risk of falls and medical complications. Therefore, it is the responsibility of all clinicians to ensure that their working environment is clean, the equipment is sanitized after each patient, and the equipment is safe, in good working order, and is regularly checked for damage. Any equipment suspected of improperly working should be tagged as *out of order*, and the appropriate repair technician contacted. In addition, routine calibration and safety checks should be conducted on equipment per state and certifying agencies. Most equipment is checked annually; however, it needs immediate recalibration if the equipment is not in operating order or damaged.

Patients admitted to the hospital or acute setting require interdisciplinary care with frequent special equipment, lines, or tubes to monitor status and improve body system function. Critical care units provide specialized high-level care to critically ill patients within the hospital setting. Physical therapy may help minimize the adverse effects of immobilization by performing functional activities per patient tolerance at various levels. The PTA must be prepared to handle equipment safely.

The PTA must maintain patient safety above all else. All monitors, lines, and tubes must be continuously monitored to prevent disruption or obstruction. Forward-thinking must be conducted to assemble all needed equipment components, assistive devices, etc, before starting treatment. The PTA should never leave a patient unguarded to retrieve an item and should constantly be monitoring any specialty equipment.

Contamination refers to any instance when an object, surface, or field comes into contact with anything not sterile. The most effective ways of preventing contamination and the spread of infection include effective personal and hand hygiene, effective cleaning and handling techniques, and the use of physical barriers. An example of a physical barrier is personal protective equipment (PPE).

In the home setting, the clinician should conduct a thorough examination of the home and make recommendations for the removal of hazards such as throw rugs, electrical cords, clutter, etc, but keeping in mind that in the home health setting, the clinician is a guest of the patient, so any recommendations should be made tactfully and carefully, and it is the choice of the patient whether or not to comply. Clear documentation of recommendations should be made to ensure that patient safety was considered.

BODY MECHANICS AND INJURY PREVENTION

The clinician is responsible for preventing injury to self and their patients and other staff within the facility. Therefore, the clinician will often be called on to demonstrate and train other departments about correct lifting and transfer techniques. Strong emphasis should be made at all times that using appropriate equipment, such as Hoyer lifts, techniques such as

STUDY PEARL

Common Critical Care Specialty Unit abbreviations include the following:

- ICU—intensive care unit.
- CCU—coronary care unit or critical care unit.
- MICU—medical intensive care unit.
- SICU—surgical intensive care unit.
- NICU—neurologic intensive care or neonatal intensive care unit.
- PACU—postanesthesia care unit.

STUDY PEARL

Nosocomial infections are those that originate or occur in a hospital or hospital-like setting. A health care–associated infection (HAI) refers to an infection acquired in any health care setting.

TABLE 8-3 • Body Mechanics General Guidelines.

- Think ahead—what equipment is needed? Do you have a clear path for movement?
- Position yourself close to the load
- Maintain a wide base of support (BOS)
- Keep a neutral spine by activating trunk stabilizing muscles
- Bend at hips and knees
- Maintain center of gravity (COG) within the BOS
- Keep load/object close to the body
- Push rather than pull
- Move in a slow, controlled manner
- Move feet or pivot rather than exert rotation on the spine or other joints
- Get assistance when needed, for example, if the load is a heavy or awkward shape to lift

two-person versus one-person, and lifting styles such as power lift or deep squat will prevent injuries, and even if these techniques take extra time or personnel, they should always be adhered to.

Lifting techniques such as the deep squat, power lift, straight-leg lift, golfers lift, and stoop lift should all be taught to other personnel and modeled by the physical therapy department members (Table 8-3). Transferring patients should always include appropriate use of a gait belt or equipment such as a Hoyer lift. Single or two or more person transfers should be correctly used depending on the patient's functional level. All staff within a facility should receive appropriate training with a reverse demonstration in the use of mechanical lifting devices. It is often the role of the physical therapy department to provide this training. Facility policies and procedures must be adhered to (see Figure 8-1). The PTA will carry out body mechanics and postural correction interventions with attention to various work environments (Table 8-4).

■ QUESTIONS

1. **A clinician arrives at a patient's home and finds the patient on the floor with an obvious injury to their right lower extremity. The caregiver is present but clearly distressed. Which of the following actions is most appropriate for the clinician to perform?**
   A. Get the patient off the floor and take vital signs.
   B. Call 911 and the home health agency for medical support.
   C. Call the home health agency and report the incident.
   D. Call 911 and leave the patient with the caregiver to wait for the paramedics.

2. **A clinician is working in a skilled nursing facility and has been informed that the patient has measles. Which of the following precautions are the minimum requirements for the therapist while working with this patient?**
   A. Personal mask at all times
   B. Mask if within 3 ft of the patient
   C. Gown, gloves, and mask at all times
   D. Gown if in direct contact with the patient

TABLE 8-4 • Work Environment Ergonomics (Dutton's Orthopaedic Examination).

- Head facing forward with a neutral spine
- Shoulders and arms relaxed with elbows bent approximately 90°
- Wrists and hands parallel to floor with neutral wrists; may use adjustable keyboard stand
- Trunk in neutral with level pelvis; lumbar support
- Seated with a supportive chair cushion and with knees at 90°, thighs and feet supported
- The monitor directly in front of chair 20-24 in away at a 10-15° downward viewing angle
- Task appropriate lighting
- Position change/breaks hourly
- Hands-free telephone

3. **A clinician is working with a patient with a long history of cardiac disease. The patient has recently had a pacemaker fitted and has been cleared for therapy to improve functional activity. Which of the following monitoring protocols is the most appropriate for the clinician to use with this patient?**
   A. Take pulse and respiratory rate regularly throughout the session.
   B. Continue working with the patient to 80% heart rate maximum.
   C. Do not exercise this patient as it is a contraindication.
   D. Exercise the patient using the rate of perceived exertion (RPE) scale to monitor exertion.

■ ANSWERS WITH RATIONALES

1. The answer is **B**. If a patient has an obvious injury, medical support is critical, and the clinician should call 911 but must also call the home health agency to report and complete paperwork as required. The patient and caregiver should not be left until after the paramedics have arrived.

2. The answer is **A**. Measles is an airborne infection, so a mask must be worn at all times when working with the patient. Gown and gloves are not required but can be used if the therapist or the facility requires them.

3. The answer is **D**. The pacemaker is designed to keep the patient's heart rate at a specific level regardless of exercise intensity, so monitoring pulse and aiming at 80% heart rate maximum is inappropriate. Instead, using the RPE scale is the safest way to exercise a patient with a fitted pacemaker.

■ PATIENT TRANSFERS

Depending on the clinical setting, a large portion of a PTA's day can be spent transferring patients to and from various surfaces. Although the PTA is less involved with patient transfers in an outpatient setting, many patient populations treated as outpatients (amputees, spinal cord, Parkinson, etc) require some form of transfer.

▲ HIGH-YIELD TERMS TO LEARN

Level of assistance	The amount of assistance that a patient needs to perform a functional task.
Contact guard	A level of assistance that requires a hand on the client.
Stand-by assist	A level of assistance that does not include any physical contact with the client.
Transfer/gait belt	An assistive device that can be used to help safely transfer a person from one surface or another or can be used during gait training.
Friction	The resistance that one surface or object encounters when moving over another and must be minimized during patient transfers.

TYPES OF TRANSFERS

The most common types of transfers encountered by the physical therapist include the following:

- Pulling a patient up the bed: The clinician and an assistant, standing on opposite sides of the bed, use a draw-sheet to slide the patient up in bed. The aim should be to decrease friction, reduce the stress on the lifter(s), and enhance patient comfort. The bed's head is lowered, and the bed height is adjusted to the shorter person's waist or hip level. The two lifters grasp the draw-sheet, palms up and elbows flexed, pointing one foot in the direction the patient is to be moved. The patient should be asked to bend their knees, push down with their feet, and pull up using a trapeze. The lifters lean in the direction of the move using the legs and body weight. On the count of three, the patient is lifted and pulled up the bed. This step is repeated as many times as needed.

- Out of bed to a wheelchair: The steps of the move are explained to the patient, and the patient is told that they can rest when they need to. The patient's ability to help is assessed, and the clinician determines whether further help will be necessary. A transfer belt is recommended to provide a firm handhold. That clinician positions and locks the wheelchair close to the bed and helps the patient turn over and sit on/scoot to the edge of the bed. The clinician places their arms around the patient's chest and clasps their hands behind the patient's back. Supporting the leg farther from the wheelchair between their legs, the clinician leans back, shifts his or her weight, and lifts. The patient pivots toward the chair (where possible) or is guided by the clinician. If the patient's legs are weak and appear to be buckling, the clinician can brace their knees against the patient's knees. Once correctly positioned, the patient bends toward the clinician, who bends their knees and lowers the patient into the back of the wheelchair.

- Level surfaces (bed to a gurney): The clinician and an assistant stand on opposite sides of the bed, with the clinician on the side of the transfer direction. A large plastic garbage bag is placed between the sheet and the draw-sheet, beneath one edge of the patient's torso. The patient's legs are moved closer to the edge of the bed. Grasping the draw-street on both sides of the bed, the clinician leans backward on a count of three and shifts their weight, sliding the patient to the edge of the bed, while the assistant holds the sheet keeping it from slipping. The bed is raised so that it is slightly higher than the gurney, and the head of the bed is lowered. The patient's legs are moved onto the gurney, and the assistant kneels on the bed. On the count of three, the clinician and assistant grasp the draw-sheet and slide the patient onto the gurney. This may take several attempts.

- Wheelchair to a toilet, tub seat: The wheelchair is positioned as close to the destination as possible. The clinician locks the wheelchair and fastens the transfer belt. The clinician helps the patient slide to the edge of the wheelchair and positions the patient's feet directly under their body. The clinician lifts the patient, grasping the back of the transfer belt, and helps the patient pivot around in front of the toilet, keeping the patient's knees between the clinician's legs. The patient grasps each safety rail as they are slowly and gently lowered down onto the toilet.

Dependent Transfers

See Table 8-5.

Assisted Transfers

See Table 8-6.

TABLE 8-5 • Dependent Transfers.	
Type of Transfer	**Description**
Three-person carry/lift	Used to transfer a patient from a stretcher to a bed or treatment plinth. Three clinicians carry the patient in a supine position; one clinician supports the head and upper trunk, the second clinician supports the trunk, and the third supports the lower extremities. The clinician at the head of the bed is usually the one to initiate commands. First, the clinicians flex their elbows and are positioned under the patient, and roll the patient on their side toward them. The clinicians then lift on command and move in a line to the destination surface, lower, and position the patient properly.
Two-person lift	Used to transfer a patient between two surfaces of different heights or when transferring a patient to the floor. Standing behind the patient, the first clinician should place their arms underneath the patient's axilla. Next, the clinician should grasp the patient's left forearm with their right hand and grasp the patient's right forearm with their left hand. The second clinician places one arm under the mid- to distal thighs, and the other arm is used to support the lower legs. The clinician at the head usually initiates the command to lift and transfer the patient out of the chair to the destination surface.

(Continued)

TABLE 8-5 • Dependent Transfers. (Continued)	
Type of Transfer	**Description**
Dependent squat pivot transfer	Used to transfer a patient who cannot stand independently but can bear some weight through the trunk and lower extremities. The clinician should position the patient at a 45° angle to the destination surface. The patient places the upper extremities on the clinician's shoulders but should not pull on the clinician's neck. The clinician should position the patient at the edge of the surface, hold the patient around the hips and under the buttocks, and block the patient's knees to avoid buckling while standing. The clinician should utilize momentum, straighten his or her legs, and raise the patient or allow the patient to remain in a squatting position. The clinician should then pivot and slowly lower the patient to the destination surface.
Hydraulic or mechanical lift	Used for transfers when a patient is obese, only one clinician is available to assist the transfer, the patient cannot help, or the patient has a weight-bearing restriction in both lower extremities. A body sling is required for the lift transfer. Two primary types of sling exist: • Full body: Covers the posterior surface of the patient from the shoulders to the back of the thighs/knees • Divided: Has divided legs that cross between the patient's legs and support them under the thighs. The hydraulic lift is locked in position before the transfer. The clinician positions the sling under the patient by rocking the patient from side to side and then attaching the S-ring to the lift's bars. The longer chain length is attached at the lower end of the sling to encourage a seated position. Once all the attachments are checked, the clinician pumps the device handle to elevate the patient. Once the patient is elevated, the clinician can navigate the lift and the patient to the destination surface. Once transferred, the chains should be removed, but the webbed sling should remain in place in preparation for the return transfer.

TABLE 8-6 • Assisted Transfers.	
Type of Transfer	**Description**
Sliding board	Used for a patient who has some sitting balance, some upper extremity strength, and who can adequately follow directions. Positioned at the edge of the wheelchair or bed, the patient leans to one side while placing one end of the sliding board sufficiently under the proximal thigh. The other end of the sliding board is positioned on the destination surface. The patient should not hold onto the sliding board's end to avoid pinching the fingers and should place the lead hand 4-6 in away from the sliding board. Both arms are used to initiate a push-up and scoot across the board while the clinician guards in front of the patient and assists as needed as the patient performs a series of push-ups across the board.
Stand pivot	Used when a patient can stand and bear weight through one or both of the lower extremities. The patient must possess functional balance and be able to pivot. Patients with unilateral weight-bearing restrictions or hemiplegia may utilize this transfer by leading with the uninvolved side. The transfer may also be used, leading with the involved side, for a patient post CVA. The patient is positioned at the edge of the wheelchair or bed to initiate the transfer. The clinician can help the patient keep their feet flat on the floor while bringing the head and trunk forward. The clinician assists the patient as needed with their feet and guards the patient through the transfer. The patient reaches back for the surface before they begin to sit down, and the clinician ensures a controlled descent of the patient to the destination surface.
Stand step	Used with a patient who has the necessary strength and balance to weight shift and can take a step during the transfer. The patient requires guidance or supervision from the clinician and performs the transfer similar to the stand pivot transfer, except the patient takes a step to maneuver and reposition their feet instead of using a pivot.
Push up (pop-over)	Use for a patient with good sitting balance who can lift buttocks clear of sitting surface (eg, a patient with a complete C7 level spinal cord injury can be independent with this transfer without a sliding board). It can also be used as a progression in transfer training from using a sliding board. The patient utilizes a head-hips relationship to complete the transfer—moving the head in one direction results in a hip movement in the opposite direction/toward the support surface being transferred to.

TABLE 8-7 • Levels of Physical Assistance.

Independent	The patient does not require any assistance to complete the task.
Supervision	The patient requires a clinician to observe throughout the completion of the task.
Contact guard	The patient requires the clinician to maintain contact with the patient to complete the task. A contact guard is usually needed to assist if there is a loss of balance.
Minimal assist	The patient requires 25% assist from the clinician to complete the task.
Moderate assist	The patient requires 50% assist from the clinician to complete the task.
Maximal assist	The patient requires 75% assist from the therapist to complete the task.
Dependent	The patient cannot participate, and the clinician provides all of the effort to perform the task.

Reproduced with permission from Dutton M. *McGraw-Hill's NPTE (National Physical Therapy Examination)*, 2nd ed. 2012. Copyright © McGraw Hill LLC. All rights reserved. https://accessphysiotherapy.mhmedical.com.

Before performing a transfer, the clinician should consider the following:

- The patient's level of cognition and mobility.
- How much assistance the clinician requires. When in doubt, a second person should be utilized.
- The appropriate equipment should be arranged before the transfer.
- Correct positioning of both the patient and the clinician. The clinician should maintain a large base of support and use proper body mechanics throughout the transfer.

It is important to communicate with the patient about the transfer details and their responsibility during the transfer. Verbal explanation and demonstration should be used to highlight the expectations and transfer sequence. If necessary, the patient should be instructed in the smaller transfer segments before performing the entire transfer. Commands and counts are used to synchronize those involved in the transfer, with the clinician at the head of the patient giving the commands during the transfer when more than one person is involved. Manual contacts can be used with the patient to direct their participation during the transfer.

LEVELS OF PHYSICAL ASSISTANCE

The various levels of physical assistance are outlined in Table 8-7.

REFERENCES

1. Baxter ML, Allington RO, Koepke GH. Weight-distribution variables in the use of crutches and canes. *Phys Ther*. 1969;49:360-365.
2. Jebsen RH. Use and abuse of ambulation aids. *JAMA*. 1967;199:5-10.
3. Kumar R, Roe MC, Scremin OU. Methods for estimating the proper length of a cane. *Arch Phys Med Rehabil*. 1995;76:1173-1175.
4. Schmitz TJ. Locomotor training. In: O'Sullivan SB, Schmitz TJ, eds. *Physical Rehabilitation*. 5th ed. Philadelphia, PA: FA Davis; 2007:523-560.

Other Systems

MARK DUTTON · CASSADY BARTLETT

OVERVIEW

This chapter will cover several topics, including the gastrointestinal, genitourinary, metabolic, and endocrine systems, and cover a few systematic issues, including cancer, obstetrics and gynecology, and psychiatric disorders. As a physical therapist assistant (PTA), these various systems are not within the scope of physical therapy in terms of diagnosis, but the PTA must be aware of all of the manifestations that dysfunction to any system can elicit. Also, the PTA must understand the impact on these conditions during exercise. Finally, understanding the physiology, pathology, and side effects of medications to treat these abnormalities is a prerequisite to determining the best treatment interventions, progression, and care.

As a typical patient will not be referred to physical therapy with a primary diagnosis of systemic involvement, the physical therapist's initial examination includes taking the individual's history, conducting a standardized system review, and performing selected tests and measures to identify existing movement-related disorders. During this examination, the physical therapist (PT) may receive information that points to systemic involvement that may or may not warrant referral for additional medical evaluation. In the vast majority of instances, the medical team will already be aware of such systemic involvement, but, on occasion, the patient may have one of these conditions that have remained undetected. Therefore, when reviewing a patient's medical chart, numerous tests and procedures are documented by the medical team that the PTA must be aware of.

STUDY PEARL

The PTA must have a working knowledge of the function, causes, signs, and symptoms of systemic involvement so that prompt action can be taken on behalf of the patient.

◼ GASTROINTESTINAL SYSTEM

The gastrointestinal (GI) tract serves to transport food and absorb nutrients to sustain life. The GI tract's main functions include the digestion of food, absorption of nutrients, and waste elimination. Pathologic conditions affecting the GI system, including malignancies, result from the impairment of these functions.

The anatomy of the GI system is shown in Figure 9-1. Table 9-1 summarizes the selected GI pathologies discussed in this chapter, and Table 9-2 identifies organs associated with abdominal quadrants.

STUDY PEARL

The GI system consists of three tracts:
- Upper: Consists of the mouth, esophagus, and stomach
- Lower: Consists of the small intestine (duodenum, jejunum, and ileum) and large intestine (cecum, colon, and rectum)

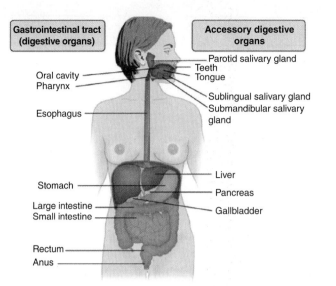

Gastrointestinal tract (digestive organs)

Accessory digestive organs

Parotid salivary gland
Teeth
Tongue
Oral cavity
Pharynx
Sublingual salivary gland
Submandibular salivary gland
Esophagus

Liver
Stomach
Pancreas
Large intestine
Gallbladder
Small intestine

Rectum
Anus

Figure 9-1. Gastrointestinal system. (Reproduced with permission from Ash R, Morton DA, Scott SA, eds. *The Big Picture: Histology*. 2013. Copyright © McGraw-Hill LLC. All rights reserved. https://accessbiomedicalscience.mhmedical.com.)

TABLE 9-1 • Selected Gastrointestinal Pathologies.
• Gastroesophageal reflux disease (GERD)
• Gastroenteritis
• Diverticular disease
• Appendicitis
• Pancreatitis
• Pancreatic cancer
• Crohn disease
• Colorectal cancer

Reproduced with permission from Burke-Doe A, Dutton M, eds. *National Physical Therapy Examination and Board Review*. 2019. Copyright © McGraw Hill LLC. All rights reserved. https://accessphysiotherapy.mhmedical.com.

TABLE 9-2 • Organs Associated with Abdominal Quadrants.	
Right Abdominal Quadrants	**Left Abdominal Quadrants**
Right Upper Quadrant (RUQ)	**Left Upper Quadrant (LUQ)**
RUQ extends from the median plane, superior to the transumbilical plane	*LUQ extends from the median plane, superior to the transumbilical plane*
• Liver	• Liver (left lobe)
• Gallbladder	• Pancreas (body and tail)
• Pancreas (head)	• Left suprarenal gland
• Right suprarenal gland	• Left kidney (upper lobe)
• Right kidney (upper lobe)	• Descending colon (proximal)
• Ascending colon (distal)	• Splenic flexure
• Hepatic flexure	• Transverse colon (distal)
• Transverse colon (proximal)	**Left Lower Quadrant (LLQ)**
Right Lower Quadrant (RLQ)	*LLQ extends from the median plane, inferior to the transumbilical plane*
RLQ extends from the median plane, inferior to the transumbilical plane	• Left kidney (lower lobe)
• Right kidney (lower lobe)	• Most of jejunum
• Cecum	• Descending colon
• Appendix	• Sigmoid colon
• Most of ileum	• Left uterine tube
• Ascending colon (proximal)	• Left ovary
• Right uterine tube	• Left ureter
• Right ovary	• Uterus (if enlarged)
• Right ureter	• Urinary bladder (if full)
• Uterus (if enlarged)	
• Urinary bladder (if full)	

Reproduced with permission from Hankin MH, Morse DE, Bennett-Clarke CA. *Clinical Anatomy: A Case Study Approach*. 2013. Copyright © McGraw-Hill LLC. All rights reserved. https://accessphysiotherapy.mhmedical.com.

▲ HIGH-YIELD TERMS

Gastroesophageal reflux disease (GERD)	A condition resulting from a weak lower esophageal sphincter that allows the stomach contents, including acidic digestive juices, to go back (reflux) into the esophagus.
Dysphagia	Difficulty swallowing.
Borborygmi	High-pitched bowel sounds that may be due to hyperactivity of the intestines.
Barrett esophagitis	A potentially serious complication (precancerous) of gastroesophageal reflux disease (GERD).
Esophageal achalasia	Condition in which the lower sphincter of the esophagus cannot relax properly, causing a functional obstruction resulting in dysphagia, regurgitation, and chest pain.
Diverticulosis versus diverticulitis	Diverticulosis is a benign condition in which the weakened areas in the lining of the mucosa of the colon balloon out. Diverticulitis refers to the inflammation and infection of the perforation of the diverticula.
Peritonitis	Inflammation of the peritoneum, the serous membrane, which lines part of the abdominal cavity and viscera. Peritonitis may result from infection (often due to rupture of a hollow organ as may occur in abdominal trauma or appendicitis) or from a noninfectious process.
Hiatal hernia	A congenital or acquired protrusion of the stomach upward through the diaphragm (rolling hiatal hernia), or displacement of both the stomach and gastroesophageal junction upward into the thorax (sliding hiatal hernia).
McBurney sign	Tenderness on palpation of the McBurney point (right side of the lower abdomen); a sign of appendicitis.
Steatorrhea	Fatty stools, which can be a sign of chronic pancreatitis.
Crohn disease	A chronic inflammatory disease that affects the distal portion of the ileum and the colon.
Rebound tenderness	Pain elicited during abdominal examination when the examiner removes pressure suddenly during palpation (pressure on the abdomen elicits less pain than releasing the pressure). This clinical sign (Blumberg sign) is associated with peritoneal inflammation (eg, peritonitis, appendicitis).

As GI problems can arise at any time, the PTA must be aware of the most common signs and symptoms associated with GI disease to take prompt action as necessary. These signs and symptoms include but are not limited to the following:

- Referred pain (eg, to the abdomen, shoulder, neck, sternum, scapula, back, pelvis, sacrum).
- Dysphagia (eg, difficulty swallowing).
- Odynophagia (eg, pain with swallowing).
- Acid reflux (eg, burning sensation).
- Early satiety (eg, full sensation with eating).
- Melena (eg, black stool).
- Symptoms during or after eating.
- Abdominal cramping.
- Bloody diarrhea.
- Increased urgency.
- Constipation.
- Weight loss.
- Nausea.
- Vomiting.
- Guarding (eg, muscle cramping).

GASTROESOPHAGEAL REFLUX DISEASE

Gastroesophageal reflux disease (GERD), considered to be the most common and most costly of all GI disorders, is the result of a weak lower esophageal sphincter (LES) that allows the stomach contents, including acidic digestive juices, to return (reflux) to the esophagus. Table 9-2 summarizes the causes of LES dysfunction. Repeated trauma to this area results in metaplasia, a change in the cellular type lining this structure, and dysplastic changes. Chronic GERD is a risk factor for adenocarcinoma.

STUDY PEARL

Malabsorption syndrome is a complex of disorders common in patients with cystic fibrosis, celiac disease, Crohn disease, chronic pancreatitis, and pernicious anemia. Problems with intestinal absorption of nutrients characterize the syndrome. The PTA must be aware of any signs and symptoms of:

- Anemia indicating an iron deficiency.
- Easy bruising and bleeding indicating a lack of vitamin K.
- Muscle weakness and fatigue indicating a lack of protein, iron, folic acid, and vitamin B.
- Bone loss, pain, and predisposition to develop fractures indicating a lack of calcium, phosphate, and vitamin D.
- Neuropathy including tetany and paresthesia indicating a lack of calcium, vitamin B and D, magnesium, and potassium.
- Muscle spasms indicating an electrolyte imbalance and lack of calcium.
- Generalized swelling indicating possible protein depletion.

The most common patient complaints include persistent heartburn (burning sensation in the chest) due to acid reflux, coughing, and dysphagia (difficulty swallowing). Sleep disturbance from coughing and heartburn at night can lead to fatigue and decreased functioning during the day.

PTAs should be aware of the side effects of the medications, such as headaches, constipation or diarrhea, dizziness, or abdominal pain. During the treatment sessions, the PTA should encourage positional changes from full supine to a more upright position using pillows or a wedge. Left sidelying is often preferred as right sidelying may promote acid flow into the esophagus. Finally, the PTA should avoid activities that promote the use of the Valsalva maneuver (forced expiration against a closed glottis).

GASTROENTERITIS

Gastroenteritis, a highly common and contagious condition, is intestinal lining inflammation due to viruses, bacteria, chemical toxins, or parasites. Table 9-3 shows the common organisms that cause gastroenteritis. Noroviruses are extremely contagious and are commonly transmitted through close contact or fecal–oral medium. For children, rotaviruses are the more common offending pathogen and follow the fecal–oral route of transmission. Dehydration often occurs with continuous diarrhea and vomiting. Children and the elderly are particularly susceptible to dehydration.

TABLE 9-3 • Common Organisms That Cause Gastroenteritis.
Viral, bacterial, and parasitic microorganisms most commonly cause gastroenteritis.
Viral (approximately 70% of cases of gastroenteritis) • Adenovirus • Coronavirus • Norovirus • Parvovirus • Rotavirus
Bacterial (15%-20% of cases of gastroenteritis) • *Bacillus cereus* • *Campylobacter jejuni* • *Clostridium difficile* • *Clostridium perfringens* • *Escherichia coli*—enterohemorrhagic O157:H7 • Enterotoxigenic, enteroadherent, enteroinvasive • *Listeria* • *Micobacterium avium-intracellulare*, immunocompromised • *Providencia* • *Salmonella* • *Shigella* • *Vibrio cholera* • *Vibrio parahaemolyticus* • *Vibrio vulnificus* • *Yersinia enterocolitica*
Parasitic (10%-15%) • *Amebiasis* • *Cryptosporidium* • *Cyclospora* • *Giardia lamblia*
Foodborne toxigenic diarrhea • Performed toxin: *Staphylococcus aureus*, *B. cereus* • Postcolonization: *V. cholera, C. perfringens, enterotoxigenic E. coli, Aeromonas*

The most common patient complaints are nausea, vomiting, and lower abdominal stomach pain and cramps.

PTAs must recognize signs and symptoms of dehydration (fainting, rapid heartbeat or breathing, dry skin, confusion, or irritability) and report these to a PT or a medical team member so the patient can be given immediate care. Also, the PTA should closely monitor patients taking nonsteroidal anti-inflammatory drugs (NSAIDs) long-term for reports of pain, bleeding in the stool, nausea, or vomiting. Signs of excess bleeding include fatigue, dizziness, pallor, and exercise intolerance.

STUDY PEARL
- Gastroenteritis is an inflammation of the stomach and intestines caused by an infection.
- Gastritis is inflammation of the stomach lining specifically and not always caused by infection.

ESOPHAGEAL ACHALASIA

Condition in which the lower sphincter of the esophagus cannot relax properly, causing a functional obstruction resulting in dysphagia, regurgitation, and chest pain. As the condition progresses, the esophagus will enlarge, resulting in an increased risk of aspiration pneumonia. In the absence of medical intervention, progressive weight loss will occur.

PTAs should be aware that patients with this condition may not be getting adequate nutrition and may demonstrate general weakness or muscle wasting.

DIVERTICULAR DISEASE

Diverticular disease is a generic term that describes the development of small bulges, sacs, or diverticula in the sigmoid colon wall. *Diverticulitis* refers to the inflammation and infection of the perforation of the diverticula. Complications may include abscess formation with peritonitis, rectal bleeding, the formation of a stricture (narrowing of the colon, causing difficulty in the passage of stool), or the formation of a fistula (a tunnel to the skin or another organ).

Most patients demonstrate no symptoms, but some may complain of lower abdominal pain and report rectal bleeding.

PTAs must be aware of this condition's signs and symptoms, including the referred pain patterns. Any suspicion should be reported to the PT or medical team member so the patient can be given appropriate care.

APPENDICITIS

Appendicitis refers to the inflammation of the appendix, a medical emergency requiring surgery to remove the inflamed appendix. If left untreated, the appendix could become obstructed and inflamed and could eventually burst, with the contents spreading to the abdominal cavity, which may cause peritonitis. The most common signs and symptoms include the following:

1. Positive McBurney sign (tenderness on palpation of McBurney point, located in the lower abdomen's right side, one-third of the distance between the anterior superior iliac spine and the navel). Coughing causes point tenderness at McBurney point.
2. Umbilical or upper abdominal pain that becomes sharp toward the right side of the lower abdomen.
3. Nausea and vomiting.
4. Fever.
5. Severe cramps.
6. Loss of appetite.
7. Abdominal distention.

PTAs must be aware of McBurney sign, which is a clinical indication of acute appendicitis with inflammation that is no longer limited to the appendix and is irritating the parietal peritoneum.

PANCREATITIS

Inflammation of the pancreas can be acute, with sudden onset and lasting for days, or chronic. Repeated occurrences of acute pancreatitis will damage the pancreas, causing scar tissue formation and affecting pancreatic function.

Patients with acute pancreatitis may complain of upper abdominal pain (it may also radiate to the back) that may be more severe after a meal. Patients may also suffer from nausea and vomiting.

PTAs must be aware of this condition's signs and symptoms, including the referred pain patterns. Any suspicion should be reported to the PT or medical team member so the patient can be given appropriate care.

PANCREATIC CANCER

Pancreatic cancer is an aggressive form of cancer, with the absence of significant symptoms until the later stages of the condition, when the bile ducts become obstructed or the malignancy is of significant size to press on neighboring structures. Risk factors include chronic pancreatitis, diabetes, smoking, obesity, old age, or pancreatic cancer history. The most common signs and symptoms include the following:

1. Upper abdominal pain with radiation to the low back (manifestation is dependent on the location of the malignancy).
2. Nausea and vomiting.
3. Fatigue.

Complications include weight loss, jaundice, pain, or bowel obstruction. PTAs must be aware of this condition's signs and symptoms, including the referred pain patterns. Any suspicion should be reported to the PT or medical team member so the patient can be given appropriate care.

CROHN DISEASE

Crohn disease is a chronic inflammatory disease affecting the ileum and the colon's distal portion and is often diagnosed as inflammatory bowel disease (IBD). Approximately 25% of people diagnosed with the condition have also been found to have arthritis or joint pain. The most common signs and symptoms include the following:

- Persistent diarrhea.
- Abdominal pain and cramps.
- Constipation.
- Rectal bleeding.
- Fever.
- Nausea.

PTAs need to be aware that patients diagnosed with Crohn disease could also present with arthralgias or arthritis, so it is very important to be aware of the potential musculoskeletal and nonmusculoskeletal causes of symptoms.

GASTRIC ULCER

A gastric ulcer (ulceration) is a lesion in the stomach's lining caused by acidic digestive juices. Ulcerations are often located in the stomach and duodenum. The most common causes of peptic ulcers include infection with the bacterium *Helicobacter pylori* and long-term use of aspirin and certain other pain medications. Stress and diets that include spicy foods do not cause peptic ulcers, but they can increase symptomology. The most common signs and symptoms include the following:

STUDY PEARL
Inflammatory bowel disease (IBD): Refers to two related chronic inflammatory intestinal disorders:
- Crohn disease.
- Ulcerative colitis.

Crohn disease can affect any part of the gastrointestinal tract, whereas ulcerative colitis is restricted to the colon and the rectum.

1. Burning stomach pain (stabbing pain in inferior sternum, left upper abdomen).
2. Heartburn.
3. Bloating.
4. Fatty food intolerance.
5. Left shoulder pain.
6. Nausea.
7. Hypoactive bowel sounds.
8. Internal bleeding.
9. Vomiting (coffee ground emesis is an indication of blood).
10. Melena (dark blood in stools, or stools that are black or tarry).
11. Guarding of the superior and anterolateral abdominal wall.
12. Epigastric and left upper quadrant tenderness during deep palpation.
13. Obstruction.
14. Infection.

> **STUDY PEARL**
> - Peptic refers to the digestive system. Peptic ulcers occur in the top of the small intestine—the duodenum.
> - Gastric refers to the stomach. Thus, gastric ulcers are found in the stomach lining.

PTAs must be aware of this condition's signs and symptoms, including the referred pain patterns. For example, pain from a gastric ulcer located on the stomach's posterior wall can radiate pain into the right shoulder. Any suspicion should be reported to the PT or medical team member so the patient can be given appropriate care.

COLORECTAL CANCER

Colorectal cancer, which often begins as a small, noncancerous growth (polyp) that forms in the rectum or colon's inner wall and becomes malignant over time, affects the large intestine. Patients with colon cancer are mostly asymptomatic in the early stages of the condition. The intensity of symptoms varies according to the size and location of the malignancy. Risk factors include old age, African American race, personal history of colorectal cancer and polyps, family history of colon cancer, sedentary lifestyle, obesity, and diabetes. When they appear, the most common signs and symptoms include the following:

1. Rectal bleeding.
2. Hemorrhoids.
3. Back pain that may radiate to the legs.
4. Constipation.
5. Diarrhea.
6. Nausea, vomiting.

PTAs must be aware of this condition's signs and symptoms, including the referred pain patterns. Any suspicion should be reported to the PT or medical team member so the patient can be given appropriate care.

■ QUESTIONS

1. **Which of the following conditions results from a weak esophageal sphincter that allows the stomach contents to go back into the esophagus?**
   A. Irritable esophageal syndrome (IES)
   B. Gastroesophageal reflux disease (GERD)
   C. Esophageal achalasia
   D. Diverticulosis

2. **Which is the most common symptom of GERD due to the reflux of stomach acid and contents into the esophagus?**
   A. Chest pain
   B. Abdominal pain
   C. Heartburn
   D. Dysphagia

3. **Which is the cause for the occurrence of esophageal achalasia?**
   A. Inability of the lower esophageal sphincter to relax
   B. Development of sacs in the lining of the esophagus
   C. Inflammation of the esophageal walls
   D. Abnormal distention of the esophageal tract

4. **Which of the following is a medical condition resulting from inflammation and infection in the weakened areas of the esophageal lining?**
   A. Diverticulosis
   B. Esophageal peritonitis
   C. Diverticulitis
   D. Gastroesophageal reflux disease

5. **Which of the following positive signs may be indicative of appendicitis?**
   A. Lhermitte sign
   B. Iliopsoas sign
   C. McBurney sign
   D. Thomas test

6. **Which of the following term indicates fatty stools, which could be due to decreased function of the pancreas?**
   A. Jaundice
   B. Steatorrhea
   C. Hematochezia
   D. Melena

7. **In cases of pancreatic cancer affecting the pancreatic head, the patient may complain of referred pain to which of the following areas?**
   A. Left shoulder
   B. Midscapular area
   C. Low back
   D. Epigastric and midthoracic regions

8. **Which of the following condition refers to the inflammatory disease affecting the distal portion of the ileum and the colon?**
   A. Crohn disease
   B. Irritable bowel syndrome
   C. Leaky gut syndrome
   D. Degenerative colitis

9. **Which is a major risk factor to consider in children and elderly individuals with vomiting and diarrhea due to gastroenteritis?**
   A. Orthostatic hypotension
   B. Tension headache
   C. Dehydration
   D. Dysphagia

■ ANSWERS WITH RATIONALES

1. The answer is **B**. GERD occurs when there is a backup (reflux) of stomach contents into the esophagus due to a weak esophageal sphincter.

2. The answer is **C**. Heartburn is caused by the backup of digestive acids and content into the esophagus.

3. The answer is **A**. In esophageal achalasia, the lower sphincter of the esophagus is unable to relax properly, causing a functional obstruction in the esophagus.

4. The answer is **C**. Diverticulitis is the inflammation and infection of perforations in the diverticula.

5. The answer is **C**. A positive McBurney test (tenderness to palpation of the McBurney point) may indicate appendicitis.

6. The answer is **B**. Steatorrhea refers to increased fatty content in the stool.

7. The answer is **D**. Cancer affecting the pancreatic head will likely refer pain in the epigastric and midthoracic regions. Cancer affecting the tail of the pancreas may refer pain in the left shoulder.

8. The answer is **A**. Crohn disease refers to the inflammatory disease affecting the distal portion of the ileum and the colon.

9. The answer is **C**. Dehydration is a risk factor in children and elderly who have vomiting and diarrhea due to gastroenteritis. Hospitalization may be necessary to replenish lost fluids and electrolytes.

■ GENITOURINARY SYSTEM

The genitourinary system comprises the organs and structures involved in reproduction and the formation and excretion of urine. This system performs important functions related to reproduction, maintaining a homeostatic environment, and eliminating the body's waste products. The kidneys regulate the water balance of the body through a combination of intrinsic and extrinsic mechanisms. The kidneys also regulate red blood cell production, metabolize hormones, and maintain the blood's acid-base balance. Figure 9-2A shows the female and Figure 9-2B shows male urinary systems. Table 9-4 shows the common signs and symptoms of urologic dysfunction, and Table 9-5 summarizes the conditions discussed in this chapter.

▲ HIGH-YIELD TERMS TO LEARN

Pyelonephritis	Infection affecting the kidneys.
Total body fluid	Intracellular fluid (ICF), the fluid found inside the cells, accounts for two-thirds of the total body fluid. Extracellular fluid (ECF), the fluid in the interstitial and intravascular compartments, comprises the remaining one-third of the body fluid.
Electrolytes	The ICF and ECF contain electrolytes (eg, sodium, calcium, potassium, magnesium, chloride, and bicarbonate) that separate into electrically charged particles called ions when dissolved in water, allowing them to conduct an electrical charge.
Acid-base balance	The normal function of body cells depends on the regulation of hydrogen ion concentration, so the levels remain within narrow limits to prevent acid-based imbalances—abnormalities of serum pH. Normal serum pH is 7.35 to 7.45 (slightly alkaline). Cell function is seriously undermined when the pH falls to 7.2 or lower or rises to 7.55 or higher.
Hematuria	Blood in the urine.
Nocturia	Increased or unusual need to urinate at night time.
Cystitis	Infection of the bladder.
Adjuvant therapy	Treatment that is given in addition to the main treatment. In cancer, these are interventions done after surgery (usually chemotherapy and/or radiation) to remove all malignancy and/or prevent reoccurrence.
Benign prostatic hyperplasia (BPH)	Enlargement of the prostate gland in men.
Prostate-specific antigen (PSA) test	A blood test that detects PSA in the blood. PSA levels increase when the prostate is enlarged.
Transurethral resection of the prostate (TURP)	A surgical procedure where an instrument is inserted in the urethra and most of the prostate is removed (the outer part is left).
Radical prostatectomy	Removal of the entire prostate gland and some surrounding tissues, including the seminal vesicles.

Androgen	Male hormone; increased levels of androgen may stimulate the growth of prostate cancer cells.
Urinary incontinence (UI)	An individual's inability to control the bladder, resulting in involuntary urine leakage.
Stress urinary incontinence (SUI)	Bladder leakage associated with exertion or physical activity.
Overactive bladder or urge incontinence	Results from the sudden contraction of the detrusor muscle causing a sudden and intense need to urinate that cannot be suppressed.
Kidney stone	Hard mineral and salt deposits that form inside the kidneys. Clinical manifestations include acute and unbearable pain (on the flank and upper outer abdominal quadrant) associated with urinary tract obstruction (renal colic), which usually occurs once the stone has moved out of the kidney into the ureter.
Dyspareunia	Pain during sexual intercourse.
Flatus	Gas or air in the gastrointestinal tract that is expelled through the anus.
Costovertebral angle	The angle formed on either side of the vertebral column between the last rib and the lumbar vertebrae. Tenderness in this region is indicative of renal disease.

As genitourinary problems can arise at any time, the PTA must be aware of the most common signs and symptoms associated with these problems to take prompt action as necessary. These signs and symptoms include, but are not limited to, the following:

- Urgency and increased frequency of urination.
- Dysuria.
- Pyuria.
- Hematuria.
- Foul-smelling urine.
- Positive urine culture.
- Low-grade systemic fever.
- Suprapubic tenderness.
- Dyspareunia.
- Stress incontinence.
- Changes in voiding.
- Nocturia.
- Pain (referred to the back flank).
- Dehydration.

KIDNEY FAILURE

Chronic kidney disease denotes the gradual decline in kidney function over time. In advanced stages of the condition, the body cannot eliminate dangerous waste products, causing toxicity. End-stage renal disease (ESRD) will necessitate dialysis and a kidney transplant. The most common signs and symptoms include the following:

1. Lethargy.
2. Edema of the extremities.
3. Weakness, excessive fatigue.
4. Congestive heart failure.
5. Increasing levels of urea in the blood, causing encephalopathy.
6. Muscle cramping.

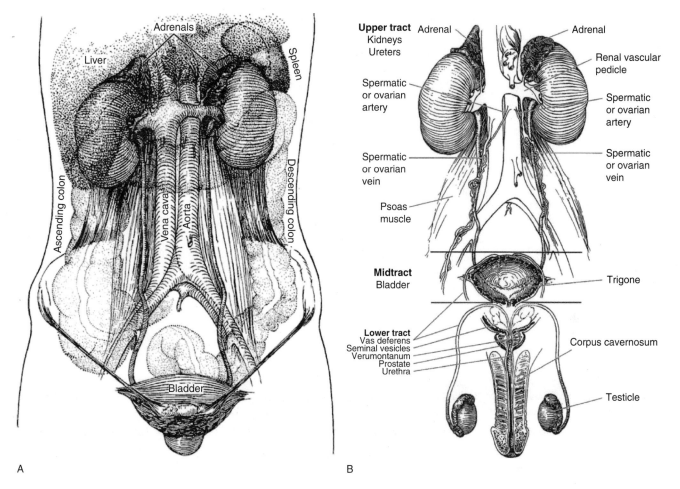

Figure 9-2. Female (A) and male (B) urinary system. (Reproduced with permission from McAninch JW, Lue TF, eds. *Smith & Tanagho's General Urology*, 18th ed. 2013. Copyright © McGraw Hill LLC. All rights reserved. https://accessmedicine.mhmedical.com)

TABLE 9-4 • Common Signs and Symptoms of Urologic Dysfunction.		
Sign or Symptom	**Description**	**Common Cause**
Dysuria	Pain and burning on urination	UTI
Frequency	An abnormally high amount of times that the patient needs to urinate	UTI, BPH, urologic obstruction, IC
Hesitancy	The interrupted flow of a urination	BPH
Urgency	A feeling that urination will occur imminently	UTI, BPH, IC

BPH, benign prostatic hyperplasia; IC, interstitial cystitis; UTI, urinary tract infection.

Reproduced with permission from Capriotti T, Frizzell JP. *Pathophysiology. Introductory Concepts and Clinical Perspectives.* 2016 © Copyright F.A. Davis. All rights reserved.

TABLE 9-5 • Selected Genitourinary Conditions.
• Kidney failure
• Urinary tract infection
• Interstitial cystitis
• Bladder cancer
• Benign prostatic hyperplasia
• Prostate cancer
• Urinary incontinence

Reproduced with permission from Burke-Doe A, Dutton M, eds. *National Physical Therapy Examination and Board Review.* 2019. Copyright © McGraw Hill LLC. All rights reserved. https://accessphysiotherapy.mhmedical.com.

From the PTA's perspective, some evidence suggests that exercise during hemodialysis sessions may help optimize function in people with ESRD undergoing dialysis. Therefore, exercise interventions should include strengthening and aerobic exercises.

URINARY TRACT INFECTION

An urinary tract infection (UTI), which can affect any part of the urinary system—kidneys, ureters, bladder, and urethra, is the most common disorder affecting the urogenital system.

UTI can be caused by offending bacteria, abnormal immune response reactions, drugs, radiation, or toxic substances (viruses, fungi, and parasites). Upper UTIs include the kidneys (pyelonephritis) or ureters, while lower UTIs involve the bladder (cystitis) or urethra (urethritis) and are more common in women than men.

Depending on the urogenital structures affected, patients with UTIs may complain of flank pain, ipsilateral shoulder pain, low back pain, or pelvic/lower abdominal pain. UTI is most common in women because the rectum is closer to the urethra in females, and *Escherichia coli* from the rectum can easily invade the female urogenital system. Table 9-6 summarizes abnormal laboratory findings that may be identified on urinalysis.

TABLE 9-6 • Abnormal Laboratory Findings on Urinalysis.

Urinalysis Finding	Description	Common Cause
Bacteriuria	Bacteria in the urine that can be visualized on microscopy	UTI or asymptomatic bacteriuria (ASB)
Bilirubinuria	Bilirubin in the urine	Liver disorders Excessive hemolysis
Crystalluria	Crystals or pieces of a kidney stone in the urine; commonly calcium or uric acid	Nephrolithiasis or urolithiasis
Glucosuria	Glucose in the urine	Uncontrolled diabetes mellitus (DM)
Hematuria	Blood in the urine	UTI Nephrolithiasis or urolithiasis Urologic malignancy
Ketonuria	Ketones in the urine	Fasting Starvation Uncontrolled DM
Leukocyte esterase	WBCs in the urine	UTI or ASB
Nitrites	Bacteria in the urine	UTI or ASB
Proteinuria (microalbuminuria)	A condition in which urine contains an abnormal amount of protein Normally urine should contain no more than 200 mg of protein per liter	Glomerular injury Kidney dysfunction caused by diabetes Kidney dysfunction caused by high blood pressure Inflammation of the kidney
Pyuria	WBCs (neutrophils) in the urine	UTI and ASB
Urinary casts	Cylindrical mucoprotein structures produced by the nephron tubules that appear in the urine Various casts found in urine sediment include hyaline, waxy, granular, fatty, crystal, RBC, WBC, bacterial, and epithelial	Nephrotic syndrome Dehydration Vigorous exercise Diuretics Tubular necrosis Autoimmune disorders Pyelonephritis Other kidney diseases

ASB, asymptomatic; DM, diabetes mellitus; UTI, urinary tract infection; WBC, white blood cell.

The most common signs and symptoms include the following:

1. Nocturia (increased or unusual need to urinate at night time).
2. Hematuria.
3. Burning sensation when urinating.
4. Fever, shaking, and chills.
5. Nausea and vomiting.
6. Pelvic/lower abdominal pain.
7. Frequent, painful urination.
8. Cloudy, bloody, dark, and/or foul-smelling urine.

The PTA needs to remember that upper UTI may result in complaints of flank and ipsilateral shoulder pain, while lower UTI may result in pelvic or lower abdominal pain, as these may mimic complaints of musculoskeletal pain. Any suspicion should be reported to the PT or medical team member so the patient can be given appropriate care.

INTERSTITIAL CYSTITIS

Interstitial cystitis, also known as painful bladder syndrome, is characterized by a feeling of fullness in the bladder, causing urgency and urination frequency. The condition is often diagnosed primarily by the symptoms. The most common signs and symptoms include the following:

1. Pelvic pain.
2. Perineal pain.
3. Dysuria.
4. Fullness of the bladder.

From the PTA's perspective, physical therapy may help alleviate symptoms in patients with interstitial cystitis, especially if there is an identified pelvic floor dysfunction. Specific interventions include manual therapy and soft tissue interventions, and also the use of physical and electrotherapeutic agents as appropriate.

BLADDER CANCER

Bladder cancer, which affects older adults and men, is the most common of all urinary tract cancers but highly treatable when diagnosed early. Cigarette smoking and environmental exposure are major risk factors in the development of bladder cancer. Signs and symptoms of bladder cancer are similar to UTI, which is the main reason for delayed diagnosis. The common signs and symptoms include the following:

1. Painless and intermittent hematuria (the main symptom).
2. Pelvic pain.
3. Frequent and painful urination.
4. Urge to urinate even if the bladder is not full.
5. Difficulty in urination.
6. Low back pain.

The PTA needs to provide interventions to optimize function in patients undergoing cancer treatment. Common residual impairments following cancer surgery, radiation, or chemotherapy include limitations in range of motion (ROM) and muscular weakness.

BENIGN PROSTATIC HYPERPLASIA

BPH refers to the enlargement of the prostate gland in men. The prostate's increased size can compress the urethra and obstruct urine flow, causing the urine to be retained in the bladder, resulting in overdistention, increased urination frequency, and increased

STUDY PEARL
- Myopathy and neuropathy.
The PTA must record the vital signs of a dialysis patient regularly during exercise. Care must be taken when taking blood pressure to avoid the dialysis shunts and avoid trauma to the peritoneal catheters.

STUDY PEARL
The genitourinary structures involved with urine excretion are as follows:
- Upper urinary tract: Kidney and ureters.
- Lower urinary tract: Bladder and urethra.

STUDY PEARL
- During pregnancy, the enlarging uterus can place pressure on the ureters, partially obstructing the normal downward flow of urine.
- Pregnancy also increases the risk of reflux of urine up the ureters by causing the ureters to dilate and reducing the muscle contractions that propel urine down the ureters into the bladder.

STUDY PEARL
Early detection and treatment of a UTI are important to prevent possible permanent structural damage.

STUDY PEARL
Interstitial cystitis can lead to scarring and stiffening of the bladder, decreased bladder capacity, glomerulations (pinpoint bleeding), and, rarely, ulcers in the bladder lining.

frequency of emptying the bladder, especially at night (nocturia). The blood test used to confirm an enlarged prostate is the prostate-specific antigen (PSA). The most common signs and symptoms include the following:

1. Problems with urination: Difficulty in the initiation, weak stream, dribbling, increased frequency and nocturia, inability to fully empty the bladder.
2. UTI.
3. Hematuria.

Complications arise due to obstruction of the urinary system caused by the enlarged prostate. These include urinary retention, UTIs, bladder stones, and bladder and kidney damage.

PTAs must be aware of the signs and symptoms of BPH and should alert the PT if a person presents with signs and symptoms of BPH.

PROSTATE CANCER

Prostate cancer is one of the most prevalent cancers in men. Patients are usually asymptomatic in the early stages of the disease but will start complaining of symptoms in the lower urinary tract, low back, hip, or lower extremity as the condition progresses. Risk factors include increasing age, African American men and Caribbean men of African heritage, family history of prostate cancer, and several inherited gene mutations. In addition, a digital rectal examination (DRE) may identify potential bumps or hard areas in the prostate that may be cancerous. The most common signs and symptoms include the following:

1. Problems with urination: Slow or weak stream, difficulty starting or stopping urination, nocturia, burning sensation when urinating.
2. Hematuria.
3. Blood in semen.
4. Erectile dysfunction.
5. Hip, back, or chest pain.
6. Loss of appetite, weight loss.
7. Nausea and vomiting.

PTAs need to provide interventions to optimize function in patients undergoing cancer treatment. Common residual impairments following cancer surgery (radical prostatectomy), radiation, or chemotherapy include limitations in ROM and muscular weakness.

URINARY INCONTINENCE

Urinary incontinence (UI), which ranges from leaking urine when coughing and sneezing to inability to get to the bathroom in time to urinate, refers to an individual's inability to control the bladder. Table 9-7 summarizes the types of incontinence.

The primary types of UI include the following:

1. Stress urinary incontinence (SUI) is bladder leakage associated with exertion or physical activity.
2. Overactive bladder, or urge incontinence, results from the sudden contraction of the detrusor muscle that causes a sudden and intense need to urinate that cannot be suppressed.
3. Overflow incontinence occurs when a person cannot empty the bladder, which in turn overflows and leaks out. The person does not have the sensation that the bladder is full or empty. This type is more common in men than women and can lead to a UTI when the urine pulls in the bladder, increasing its exposure to bacteria.
4. Functional incontinence refers to physical (lack of mobility, arthritis) or mental (dementia) impairments that cause the involuntary leakage of urine.

TABLE 9-7 • Types of Incontinence.

Type of Incontinence	Description
Stress incontinence	Involuntary leakage of urine as abdominal pressure rises, which typically occurs during coughing and sneezing. The leakage occurs because of either poor pelvic support or weakness in the urethral sphincter.
Urge incontinence also called overactive bladder (OAB)	Detrusor muscle overactivity is the cause of urine leakage. The cause is unclear, but IC is thought to be the etiology in some patients. The patient complains of feelings of urgency and frequency of urination many times a day.
Overflow incontinence	Chronic overdistention and urinary retention in the bladder result in overflow incontinence. BPH, which obstructs the urine outflow, is the most frequent cause in men. Failure of the detrusor muscle caused by damage of the pelvic spinal nerves can also cause this incontinence type.
Neurogenic bladder	This disorder results from an interruption of the sensory nerve fibers between the bladder and the spinal cord or the brain's afferent nerve tracts. Chronic overdistention of the bladder occurs.
Functional incontinence	Inability to hold urine is caused by CNS problems such as stroke, psychiatric disorders, prolonged immobility, dementia, or delirium.
Mixed incontinence	Combination of stress incontinence and OAB.

BPH, benign prostatic hyperplasia; CNS, central nervous system; IC, interstitial cystitis.

From the PTA's perspective, interventions aimed at the pelvic floor muscles may help individuals with urinary incontinence improve their bladder control. Specific exercises that target the pelvic floor musculature (primarily levator ani and urethral sphincter) are known as Kegel exercises.

■ QUESTIONS

1. **Which of the following is *false* regarding lower urinary tract infection?**
   A. The most common offending organism is bacterial—*Escherichia coli.*
   B. Females are more likely to have upper UTI than males.
   C. Patients with UTIs may complain of ipsilateral shoulder pain.
   D. Urinalysis can be used to detect the presence of infection.

2. **Nonmusculoskeletal flank pain is most associated with infection of which urogenital structure?**
   A. Kidney
   B. Bladder
   C. Urethra
   D. Testes/ovaries

3. **Nonmusculoskeletal low back or lower abdominal pain is most associated with infection of which urogenital structure?**
   A. Kidney
   B. Ureter
   C. Bladder
   D. Testes/ovaries

4. **A 75-year-old patient comes to physical therapy for balance and mobility exercises. He states that he has an enlarged prostate that causes difficulty in urination, made worse by his inability to ambulate to the bathroom quickly. An enlarged prostate is known by what other medical condition?**
   A. Nephrolithiasis
   B. Pyelonephritis
   C. Prostatitis
   D. Benign prostatic hyperplasia

STUDY PEARL
The PTA should educate a patient with UI to do the following:
- Avoid the Valsalva maneuver.
- Avoid activities that strain the pelvic floor and abdominal muscles.
- Preserve an acceptable skin condition by using adequate protection (diapers, underpads) and maintaining a toileting schedule.

5. **Which of the following blood tests can confirm the presence of an enlarged prostate?**
   A. Thyroid-stimulating hormone (TSH)
   B. Prostate-specific antigen (PSA)
   C. Bladder tumor-associated antigen (BTA)
   D. Microalbumin urine test (MUT)

6. **A PTA is reviewing the medical chart of a recently admitted patient to an acute care hospital due to multiple incidents of falls in the past 3 days. Upon review of the medical chart, the patient was noted to have an infection affecting the kidneys. The medical term to indicate this condition is**
   A. Glomerulonephritis
   B. Pyelonephritis
   C. Urethritis
   D. Cystitis

7. **A patient was referred to physical therapy for mobility and ambulation training following complete removal of the prostate gland due to prostate cancer. Which surgical procedure was performed on the patient?**
   A. Transurethral resection of the prostate (TURP)
   B. Transurethral needle ablation (TUNA)
   C. Radical prostatectomy
   D. Transurethral vaporization of the prostate

8. **A patient with urinary incontinence was referred to physical therapy for treatment. The patient reports being unable to empty his bladder completely, which in turn overflows and leaks out. What type of urinary incontinence does the patient have?**
   A. Stress urinary incontinence
   B. Overactive bladder
   C. Overflow incontinence
   D. Functional incontinence

9. **Which of the following types of stress incontinence is more common in men than women?**
   A. Stress urinary incontinence
   B. Overactive bladder
   C. Overflow incontinence
   D. Functional incontinence

10. **A PTA is treating a patient with urinary incontinence (UI). Which type of UI results in the bladder's incomplete emptying, resulting in a risk of urinary infection due to bacterial growth in the stagnant urine?**
    A. Stress urinary incontinence
    B. Overactive bladder
    C. Overflow incontinence
    D. Functional incontinence

■ ANSWERS WITH RATIONALES

1. **The answer is B.** Lower UTI is more common in females.

2. The answer is **A.** Flank pain that is nonmusculoskeletal and possibly urogenital in origin is likely caused by an upper urinary tract infection (kidney or ureter).

3. The answer is **C.** Nonmusculoskeletal low back or lower abdominal, but possibly urogenital in origin, is likely caused by an infection in the lower urinary tract (bladder or urethra).

4. The answer is **D.** Benign prostatic hyperplasia refers to a medical condition denoting an enlarged prostate.

5. The answer is **B**. Increased prostate-specific antigen (PSA) levels can indicate an enlarged prostate.

6. The answer is **B**. Pyelonephritis pertains to the infection affecting the kidneys.

7. The answer is **C**. Radical prostatectomy refers to the complete removal of the prostate gland.

8. The answer is **C**. Overflow incontinence refers to the inability to completely empty the bladder, which in turn overflows and leaks out. The person does not have the sensation that the bladder is full or empty.

9. The answer is **C**. Overflow incontinence occurs more in men than women.

10. The answer is **C**. In overflow incontinence, urine left in the bladder can be breeding grounds for bacteria that may cause urinary tract infections.

■ METABOLIC AND ENDOCRINE SYSTEMS

The endocrine and nervous systems work closely to coordinate various physiologic functions. The combined efforts regulate metabolism, water and salt balance, blood pressure, response to stress, and sexual reproduction. The endocrine system comprises cells, tissues, glands, and organs that produce and regulate signaling molecules called **hormones**. Hormones are released into the bloodstream, where they bind to receptors or target cells and regulate their activity to maintain homeostasis. The locations of selected endocrine glands and hormones released are shown in Figure 9-3. This system overlaps with the nervous system, and its responsibilities include regulating blood pressure, **metabolism**, growth and development, and reproduction. Hormone secretion is highly regulated by various mechanisms, including hormonal signals from the **hypothalamus** and the **pituitary gland** and **positive** and **negative feedback** from target cells.

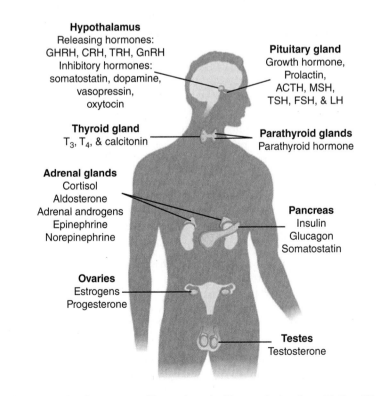

Figure 9-3. The endocrine system. (Reproduced with permission from Molina PE, ed. *Endocrine Physiology*, 5th ed. 2018. Copyright © McGraw Hill LLC. All rights reserved. https://accessmedicine.mhmedical.com.)

▲ HIGH-YIELD TERMS TO LEARN

Addison disease	A rare disease marked by deficient secretion of adrenocortical hormones (such as cortisol) that is characterized by fatigue, muscle weakness, weight loss, low blood pressure, irritability or depression, and brownish pigmentation of the skin, and is caused by progressive destruction of the adrenal glands (as by an autoimmune response or infection).
Addisonian crisis	Low levels of cortisol can cause weakness, fatigue, and low blood pressure. There may be more symptoms with untreated Addison disease or damaged adrenal glands due to severe stress, such as car accidents or infections. These symptoms may include sudden dizziness, vomiting, and loss of consciousness.
Aldosterone	A steroid hormone $C_{21}H_{28}O_5$ of the adrenal cortex that regulates the salt and water balance of the body.
Anabolism	The constructive part of metabolism responsible for macromolecular synthesis.
Androgens	A male sex hormone (as testosterone).
Buffalo torso	Extra fat around the torso; it is a symptom of Cushing syndrome.
Catabolism	Destructive metabolism involving the release of energy and resulting in the breakdown of complex materials within the organism.
Cretinism	A usually congenital abnormal condition marked by physical stunting and mental retardation caused by severe thyroid deficiency—also called *infantile myxedema*.
Cushing syndrome	An abnormal condition caused by excess levels of corticosteroids, especially cortisol, in the body due to either hyperfunction of the adrenal gland (as from adrenal adenoma or hypersecretion of adrenocorticotropic hormone (ACTH) by the pituitary gland) or to prolonged use of corticosteroid medications (as prednisone) and that is characterized by a variety of signs and symptoms including a change in appearance marked by moon face with plethora and truncal obesity, easy bruising, fatigue, muscle weakness, and hypertension.
Diabetes mellitus	A variable disorder of carbohydrate metabolism caused by a combination of hereditary and environmental factors and is usually characterized by inadequate secretion or utilization of insulin, excessive urine production, excessive amounts of sugar in the blood and urine, thirst, hunger, and weight loss.
Diabetic coma	A life-threatening diabetes complication that causes unconsciousness. In persons with diabetes, dangerously high blood sugar (hyperglycemia) or dangerously low blood sugar (hypoglycemia) can lead to a diabetic coma.
End-stage renal disease	The final stage of chronic kidney disease in which the kidneys no longer function adequately to meet the needs of daily life.
Exophthalmos	Abnormal protrusion of the eyeball.
Fragility fracture	Any fall from a standing height or less that results in a fracture.
Graves' disease	A common form of hyperthyroidism that is an autoimmune disease characterized by goiter, rapid and irregular heartbeat, weight loss, irritability, anxiety, and often a slight protrusion of the eyeballs—caused by the production of thyroid-stimulating immunoglobins (antibody) against the thyroid-stimulation hormone (TSH) receptor.
Glucocorticoids	Any of a group of corticosteroids (as cortisol or dexamethasone) that are involved, especially in carbohydrate, protein, and fat metabolism, that tend to increase liver glycogen and blood sugar by increasing gluconeogenesis, that are anti-inflammatory and immunosuppressive, and that are used widely in medicine (as in the alleviation of the symptoms of rheumatoid arthritis).

Goiter	An enlargement of the thyroid gland that often results from insufficient intake of iodine and is commonly visible as a swelling of the anterior part of the neck. Goiter is usually accompanied by hypothyroidism, and in other cases, is associated with hyperthyroidism, usually together with toxic symptoms and exophthalmos.
Hashimoto disease	Also known as chronic lymphocytic thyroiditis; an autoimmune disease in which the thyroid gland is gradually destroyed.
Hirsutism	Excessive growth of hair of normal or abnormal distribution.
Hormone	A product of living cells circulating in body fluids that produce a specific, often stimulatory, effect on cell activity, usually distant from its point of synthesis.
Hyperadrenalism	The presence of an excess of adrenal hormones (epinephrine) in the blood.
Hyperinsulinemia	The presence of excess insulin in the blood.
Hyperparathyroidism	An excess of parathyroid hormone in the body, resulting in calcium metabolism disturbance, increased serum calcium and decreased inorganic phosphorus, loss of calcium from bone, and renal damage, with frequent kidney stone formation.
Hyperthyroidism	Excessive functional activity of the thyroid gland; *also*, the resulting condition marked especially by increased metabolic rate, enlargement of the thyroid gland, rapid heart rate, and high blood pressure; also called *thyrotoxicosis*.
Hypoadrenalism	Abnormally decreased activity of the adrenal glands.
Hypothyroidism	Deficient activity of the thyroid gland; *also* a resultant bodily condition characterized by lowered metabolic rate and general loss of vigor.
Hypoparathyroidism	Deficiency of parathyroid hormone in the body; *also*, the resultant abnormal state marked by low serum calcium and a tendency to chronic tetany.
Hypothalamus	A basal part of the diencephalon lying beneath the thalamus on each side, forming the third ventricle floor and including vital autonomic regulatory centers (as in the control of food intake).
Insulin resistance	Reduced sensitivity to insulin by the body's insulin-dependent processes (as glucose uptake, lipolysis, and inhibition of glucose production by the liver) that results in decreased activity of these processes or an increase in insulin production or both, and that is typical of type 2 diabetes but often occurs in the absence of diabetes.
Ischemia	A deficient blood supply to a body part (the heart or brain) due to obstruction of arterial blood (as by the narrowing of arteries by spasm or disease).
Metabolic acidosis	An acidosis resulting from excess acid due to abnormal metabolism, excessive acid intake, renal retention, or excessive bicarbonate loss (as in diarrhea).
Metabolic syndrome	A syndrome marked by the presence of usually three or more of a group of factors (as high blood pressure, abdominal obesity, high triglyceride levels, low high-density lipoprotein [HDL] levels, and high fasting levels of blood sugar) that are linked to an increased risk of cardiovascular disease and type 2 diabetes—also called *insulin resistance syndrome*, *syndrome X*.
Metabolism	The sum of the buildup processes and destruction of protoplasm; specifically, the chemical changes in living cells by which energy is provided for vital processes and activities and new material is assimilated.
Mineralocorticoid	A corticosteroid (as aldosterone) that affects chiefly the electrolyte and fluid balance in the body.

Moon face	The full rounded facies characteristic, especially of Cushing syndrome, and typically associated with deposition of fat.
Myocardial infarction	An acute episode of coronary heart disease marked by the death or damage of heart muscle due to insufficient blood supply to the heart muscle, usually due to a coronary artery becoming blocked by a blood clot formed in response to a ruptured or torn fatty arterial deposit.
Myxedema	Severe hypothyroidism characterized by firm inelastic edema, dry skin and hair, and loss of mental and physical vigor.
Negative feedback	The feedback that tends to stabilize a process by reducing its rate or output when its effects are too great.
Osmotic diuresis	Increased urination due to the presence of certain substances in the fluid filtered by the kidneys. This fluid eventually becomes urine. These substances cause additional water to come into the urine, increasing its amount.
Osteoblast	A bone-forming cell.
Osteoclast	Any of the large multinucleate cells closely associated with areas of bone resorption (as in a fracture that is healing).
Osteomalacia	A disease of adults characterized by softening of the bones and is analogous to rickets in the young.
Osteoporosis	A condition that affects older women especially, characterized by decreased bone mass with decreased density and enlargement of bone spaces producing porosity and brittleness.
Periarthritis	Inflammation of the structures (as the muscles, tendons, and bursa of the shoulder) around a joint.
Pituitary	Relating to the pituitary gland. The pituitary gland produces hormones that control many functions of other endocrine glands.
Polydipsia	Excessive or abnormal thirst.
Polyphagia	Excessive appetite or eating.
Polyuria	Excessive secretion of urine.
Positive feedback	A process that occurs in a feedback loop in which the effects of a small disturbance on a system include an increase in the perturbation magnitude (childbirth, blood clotting).
Retinopathy	Any of various noninflammatory disorders of the retina, including some that cause blindness.
Rickets	A deficiency disease that affects the young during skeletal growth that is characterized especially by soft and deformed bones and is caused by failure to assimilate and use calcium and phosphorus, normally due to inadequate sunlight or vitamin D.
Stroke	Sudden impairment or loss of consciousness, sensation, and voluntary motion caused by rupture or obstruction (as by a clot) of a blood vessel supplying the brain and is accompanied by permanent damage of brain tissue.
Thyroid storm	A sudden life-threatening worsening of hyperthyroidism symptoms (high fever, tachycardia, weakness, or extreme restlessness) brought on by various causes (as infection, surgery, or stress).

A regulated cascade of events in the hypothalamus causes the initiation of synthesis, secretion, and biologic activity of most hormones, with some exceptions (pancreatic and adrenal medulla hormones). The hypothalamus and the pituitary in the brain control many other endocrine glands. The secretion of pituitary hormones is controlled by releasing factors or neurosecretory cells from the hypothalamus, giving rise to the **hypothalamic-pituitary axis** (Figure 9-4). A hormonal balance must be maintained within a narrow range because too little or too much of a hormone may produce profound changes in the body systemically, including abnormalities of the central nervous system, joints, and the integumentary,

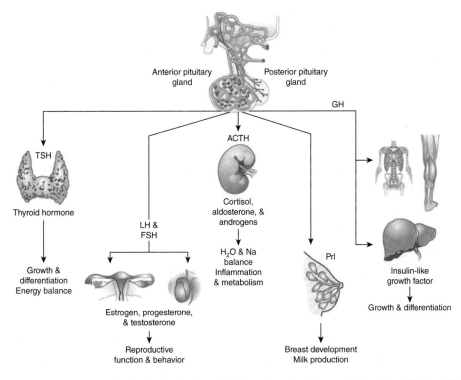

Anterior pituitary
gland

Posterior pituitary
gland

GH

TSH

ACTH

Thyroid hormone

Cortisol,
aldosterone, &
androgens

LH &
FSH

H_2O & Na
balance
Inflammation
& metabolism

Prl

Insulin-like
growth factor

Growth &
differentiation
Energy balance

Estrogen, progesterone,
& testosterone

Growth & differentiation

Reproductive
function & behavior

Breast development
Milk production

Figure 9-4. The hypothalamic-pituitary axis. (Reproduced with permission from Molina PE, ed. *Endocrine Physiology*, 5th ed. 2018. Copyright © McGraw Hill LLC. All rights reserved. https://accessmedicine.mhmedical.com.)

gastrointestinal, genitourinary, cardiopulmonary, and reproductive systems. Table 9-8 provides an overview of selected hormone systems and their most important actions.

The metabolic and neuroendocrine systems work together to maintain and control storage and mobilization of energy reserves required for cellular work for basic life functions (metabolism). Metabolism includes a range of biochemical processes within the cell and consists of building up cells/tissues (**anabolism**) and breaking down cells/tissues (**catabolism**). The basic functions of cellular metabolism are presented in Figure 9-5. Many of these functions require an energy source. Carbohydrates, fats, and proteins can be utilized by cells to synthesize adenosine triphosphate (ATP), which is used as an energy source for almost all cellular functions (metabolism). Hormones, digestion, exercise, and temperature alter cell function by altering enzyme activity and its metabolism. ATP energizes cellular synthesis and growth, muscle contraction, membrane transport, glandular secretion, nerve conduction, and active absorption. If greater amounts of energy are needed for cellular activities, it can be provided by oxidative aerobic metabolism and anaerobic breakdown of glucose. Alterations in metabolism can lead to bone, neuronal, and fluid and electrolyte disorders. Exercise can stimulate the release of several main hormones that will lead to muscle, fat, bone, and tissue responses outlined in Table 9-9.

During a physical therapy examination, the individual's history will be taken, a standardized systems review will be conducted, and selected tests and measures performed to identify potential and existing movement-related disorders. Tests and measures that may be relevant to endocrine and metabolic disorders include but are not limited to:

- Aerobic capacity and endurance (eg, osteoporosis, diabetes).
- Anthropometric characteristics (eg, weight gain, weight loss).
- Balance (eg, diabetes mellitus with peripheral neuropathy).
- Circulation (arterial, venous, lymphatic) (eg, diabetes).
- Cranial and nerve integrity (eg, Ménière disease, viral encephalitis).
- Joint integrity and mobility (eg, gout, osteoporosis).

TABLE 9-8 • Endocrine Hormones.

Location/ Endocrine Gland	Hormone(s)	Target Tissue/ Organ	Function
Pineal gland	Melatonin	Brain, other tissue	Circadian rhythm immune function antioxidant
Hypothalamus	Growth hormone-releasing hormone (GHRH), growth hormone inhibitor hormone (IH) (somatostatin), thyrotropin-releasing hormone (TRH), corticotropin-releasing hormone (CRH), gonadotropin-releasing hormone (GRH)	Anterior and posterior pituitary	Stimulation of hormones released from the posterior pituitary and hormones that regulate the anterior pituitary
Posterior pituitary	Antidiuretic hormone (ADH); also called vasopressin	Kidney	Increases water reabsorption by kidneys and causes vasoconstriction and increased blood pressure
	Oxytocin	Myoepithelial muscle of breast; uterus	Stimulates milk ejection from breasts and uterine contractions
Anterior pituitary	Growth hormone (GH)	Liver, bone, muscle, kidney, and others	Stimulates the liver to produce growth factors that stimulate bone and cartilage growth
	Thyroid-stimulating hormone (TSH)	Thyroid	Stimulates synthesis and secretion of thyroid hormones
	Adrenocorticotropic hormone (ACTH)	Adrenal cortex	Stimulates synthesis and secretion of adrenal cortical hormones
	Follicle-stimulating hormone (FSH)	Gonads	Causes growth of follicles in ovaries and sperm maturation in testes
	Luteinizing hormone (LH)		Stimulates testosterone synthesis in testes, stimulates ovulation, the formation of corpus luteum and estrogen, and progesterone synthesis in ovaries
	Prolactin	Breast	Stimulates mammary gland growth and milk production
Thyroid	Thyroxine (T_4) and triiodothyronine (T_3) Calcitonin	Most cells	Increases rate of chemical reaction in most cells, thus increasing metabolic rate Promotes deposition of calcium in bone and decreased extracellular fluid calcium ion concentration
Adrenal cortex	Cortisol Aldosterone		Multiple metabolic functions for controlling the metabolism of proteins, carbohydrates, and fats; also, anti-inflammatory effects Increased renal sodium reabsorption, potassium secretion, and hydrogen ion secretion
Adrenal medulla	Norepinephrine, epinephrine	Heart, lungs	Same effects as sympathetic stimulation
Pancreas	Insulin (beta cells) Glucagon (alpha cells)	Many cells	Promotes glucose entry into many cells; in this way, controls carbohydrate metabolism Increases the synthesis and release of glucose from the liver into the body fluids
Parathyroid	Parathyroid hormone (PTH)	Gut, kidneys, bone	Controls serum calcium ion concentration by increasing calcium absorption by the gut and kidneys and releasing calcium from bone

- Muscle performance (eg, diabetes).
- Neuromotor development and sensory processing (eg, fetal alcohol syndrome, lead poisoning).
- Pain (eg, osteoporosis, rheumatologic disease).
- Integumentary integrity (eg, diabetes, liver disease, kidney disease).

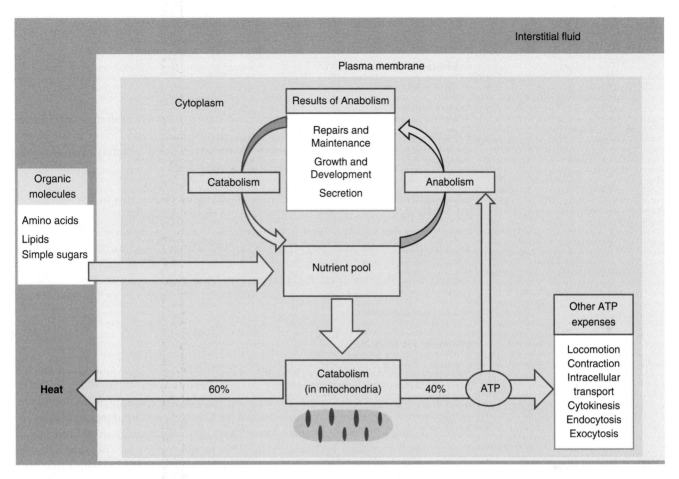

Figure 9-5. The basic functions of cellular metabolism. (Reproduced with permission from Burke-Doe A, Dutton M, eds. *National Physical Therapy Examination and Board Review*. 2019. Copyright © McGraw Hill LLC. All rights reserved. https://accessphysiotherapy .mhmedical.com.)

Hormone	Stimulant for Release	Target Tissue	Response
TABLE 9-9 • Hormones Released During Acute Exercise.			
Epinephrine	Moderate-to-intense exercise, stress, hypotension	Skeletal muscle	↑ Glycogenolysis (the breakdown of glycogen), vasoconstriction
Norepinephrine	Moderate-to-intense exercise, hypoglycemia	Adipose tissue, liver	↑ Lipolysis (the breakdown of fat), ↑ heart rate, ↑ glycogenolysis
Growth hormone (GH)	Exercise, hypoglycemia	Skeletal tissue, bone, adipose tissue, liver	Stimulation of growth, FFA mobilization, ↑ gluconeogenesis, ↓ glucose uptake
Testosterone	↑ FSH, ↑ LH, exercise, stress	Skeletal muscle, bone	Protein synthesis, sperm production, sex drive
Estrogen	↑ FSH, ↑ LH, light-to-moderate exercise	Skeletal muscle, adipose tissue	Inhibition of glucose uptake, fat deposition
Cortisol	↑ ACTH, intense, prolonged exercise	Skeletal muscle, adipose tissue, liver	↑ Gluconeogenesis, ↑ protein synthesis, ↓ glucose uptake
Insulin-like growth factor (IGF-1)	↑ GH	Almost all cells	Stimulation of growth

ACTH, adrenocorticotropic hormone; FFA, free fatty acid; FSH, follicle-stimulating hormone; GH, growth hormone; LH, luteinizing hormone.

Reproduced with permission from Burke-Doe A, Dutton M, eds. *National Physical Therapy Examination and Board Review*. 2019. Copyright © McGraw Hill LLC. All rights reserved. https://accessphysiotherapy.mhmedical.com.

The clinical manifestations of endocrine and metabolic disorders are as follows:

- Fatigue.
- Muscle weakness.
- Muscle and joint pain (occasionally).

These signs and symptoms may be early manifestations of pancreas dysfunction (diabetes mellitus), thyroid disease (hypothyroidism, hyperthyroidism, and Graves' disease), parathyroid disease (hypoparathyroidism, hyperparathyroidism), pituitary dysfunction, or adrenal dysfunction (Addison disease, Cushing syndrome).

PTAs can treat patients with metabolic and endocrine dysfunction as comorbidities or due to the pathology's clinical findings. Physical therapy addresses the various functional impairments that can be caused by metabolic and endocrine dysfunction, such as activity intolerance, weakness, atrophy, gait abnormalities, balance impairment, poor endurance, and weight gain. Activities may include strengthening, therapeutic exercise, balance training, functional training, energy conservation techniques, and activities of daily living (ADLs) training. What follows is an outline of the various dysfunctions and their common signs and symptoms.

HYPERTHYROIDISM

Hyperthyroidism (overactive thyroid; also called thyrotoxicosis) is a condition in which the thyroid gland is overactive and makes excessive amounts of thyroxine. When the thyroid gland is overactive, the body's metabolism speeds up, and patients experience nervousness, anxiety, weight loss, sweating, rapid heartbeat (tachycardia), and hand tremor (Table 9-10). **Graves' disease** is the most common form of hyperthyroidism and is an autoimmune disease in which antibodies form against the TSH receptor to induce continual activation. **Thyroid storm**, an acute episode of thyroid overactivity, is associated with inadequately treated hyperthyroidism and is characterized by high fever, severe tachycardia, delirium, dehydration, and extreme irritability. The most common signs and symptoms of hyperthyroidism include the following:

1. High state of excitability with nervousness or other psychic disorders.
2. Extreme fatigue but an inability to sleep.
3. Impaired cardiopulmonary function (increased heart and respiratory rates).

TABLE 9-10 • Key Features of Hyperthyroid and Hypothyroid.	
Hyperthyroid (Thyrotoxicosis)	**Hypothyroid**
Warm, moist skin due to capillary dilation	Pale, cool puffy yellowish skin, face, and hands Brittle hair and nails
Sweating, heat intolerance	The sensation of being cold
Tachycardia, increased stroke volume, cardiac output, and pulse pressure	Bradycardia, decreased stroke volume, cardiac output, and pulse pressure
Dyspnea, weakness of respiratory muscles, hypoventilation	Pleural effusions, hypoventilation, and CO_2 retention
Increased appetite	Reduced appetite
Nervousness, irritability, hyperkinesia, tremor	Lethargy, general slowing for mental processes, depression
Weakness, atrophy, increased deep tendon reflexes, periarthritis	Stiffness, decreased deep tendon reflexes, carpal tunnel syndrome, muscle, and joint edema
Menstrual irregularity, decreased fertility	Infertility, decreased libido, impotence, oligospermia
Weight loss	Weight gain
Reaction of upper lid with a wide stare, exophthalmos (Graves' disease)	Drooping eyelids

4. Intolerance of heat and increased sweating.
5. Hypermetabolism.
6. Mild to extreme weight loss (sometimes as much as 100 lb).
7. Varying degrees of diarrhea.
8. Muscle weakness (proximal).
9. Tremor of the hands.
10. **Exophthalmos.**
11. **Periarthritis.**
12. Osteoporosis.

HYPOTHYROIDISM

Hypothyroidism (underactive thyroid; also called myxedema) is a condition in which the thyroid gland does not produce enough thyroid hormones. Hypothyroidism is characterized by slowed metabolic rate, fatigue, extreme muscle sluggishness, and cardiac abnormalities (Table 9-10). Hypothyroidism is often initiated by autoimmunity against the thyroid gland, known as **Hashimoto disease**.

Cretinism is caused by extreme hypothyroid during fetal life, infancy, or childhood. This condition is characterized especially by failure of body growth and by intellectual disability.

The most common signs and symptoms of hypothyroidism are numerous and include the following:

1. Goiter (enlargement of the thyroid) can be caused by dietary iodide and iodine deficiency.
2. Fatigue.
3. Extreme somnolence, with sleeping up to 12 to 14 hours a day.
4. Extreme muscular sluggishness.
5. Cold sensitivity.
6. Slowed heart rate, decreased cardiac output, decreased blood volume.
7. Increased body weight.
8. Constipation.
9. Mental sluggishness.
10. Depression.
11. Failure of many trophic functions in the body (hair, skin).
12. Myxedema (edematous appearance throughout the body).
13. Cardiac abnormalities.
14. Poor circulation.
15. Atherosclerosis.
16. Joint edema.
17. Carpal tunnel syndrome.
18. Back pain.

ADDISON DISEASE

Hypoadrenalism (adrenal insufficiency)—insufficient production or release of glucocorticoids (cortisol), mineralocorticoids (aldosterone), and androgens (testosterone, estrogen). It is most frequently caused by the primary atrophy or injury of the adrenal cortices but can also have an autoimmune basis. These hormones have key roles in response to stress, electrolyte and fluid balance for maintenance of blood pressure, conversion of food to energy, and the inflammatory response. An acute form of the disease is called **Addisonian crisis**, in which patients have severe abdominal pain, back and leg pain, severe vomiting, and hypotension due to low levels of cortisol. The most common signs and symptoms include the following:

1. Muscle weakness.
2. Fatigue, decreased activity tolerance.
3. Poor endurance.
4. Loss of appetite, weight loss.
5. Hypoglycemia.
6. Hypotension.
7. Hyperpigmentation.
8. Metabolic derangement.
9. Pain (joints, lower back, leg).

The clinical setting should have carbohydrates available in case of a drop in blood sugar, the ability to monitor blood pressure, or response to treatment.

CUSHING SYNDROME

Hyperadrenalism is most common due to excess secretion of adrenocorticotropic hormone (ACTH) by the anterior pituitary, leading to excessive production and release of **glucocorticoids (cortisol)**, mineralocorticoids (**aldosterone**), and **androgens**. Hypersecretion can lead to Cushing syndrome with abnormalities ascribable to increased amounts of cortisol and androgens. Hypercortisolism can also occur with administering large amounts of glucocorticoids over prolonged periods for therapeutic purposes (such as chronic inflammation, eg, ulcerative colitis). A unique characterization of Cushing syndrome is the mobilization of fat from the lower part of the body, with deposition of the fat in the thoracic and upper abdominal regions (**buffalo torso**). Excess secretion of steroids also leads to an edematous appearance of the face (**moon face**), and the androgenic potency of some hormones can cause acne and **hirsutism** (excess growth of facial hair). The most common signs and symptoms include the following:

1. Fatigue.
2. Severe muscle weakness.
3. Paralysis.
4. Tendon rupture.
5. Excess body fat.
6. Round face (moon face).
7. Weight loss/gain.
8. Osteoporosis.
9. Hyperglycemia.
10. Diabetes.
11. Low back pain.
12. Cardiac abnormalities.
13. Gastrointestinal abnormalities.

The PTA must be aware that prolonged high-dose glucocorticoid therapy has many potential side effects that can impact physical therapy, including osteoporosis (glucocorticoids reduce bone formation and increase bone resorption), myopathy (glucocorticoids can have a direct catabolic effect on skeletal muscle), avascular necrosis, and some adverse systemic effects, including hypertension, and hyperglycemia.

DIABETES MELLITUS

Diabetes mellitus (DM) is a syndrome of impaired metabolism of carbohydrates, fat, and proteins caused by either a lack of insulin production by the pancreas or decreased tissue sensitivity to insulin. The pancreatic islets produce hormones that regulate blood glucose levels. The alpha cells produce glucagon, and the beta cells produce insulin.

The two general types of diabetes are type 1, caused by a lack of insulin secretion in the pancreas, and type 2, initially caused by decreased sensitivity of target tissues to insulin's metabolic effect. This reduced insulin sensitivity is often called **"insulin resistance."** **"Metabolic syndrome"**—a cluster of conditions including increased blood pressure, high blood sugar, excess body fat around the waist and abdomen, increased cholesterol and triglyceride levels, increasing the risk for heart disease, stroke, and diabetes—typically precedes type 2 diabetes.

Additionally, a third type of DM that can occur during pregnancy is **gestational diabetes** and affects approximately 5% of all pregnancies. Women who develop gestational diabetes are at an elevated risk of developing type 2 diabetes in the future. Consultation with the patient's treating physician or obstetrician-gynecologist (OB-GYN) should occur for management guidelines.

In all types of DM, the metabolism of all the main foodstuffs is altered. The basic effect of insulin lack, or insulin resistance, on glucose metabolism is to prevent efficient uptake and glucose utilization by most body cells. As a result, blood glucose concentration increases, cell utilization of glucose falls increasingly lower, and utilization of fats and proteins increases.

The two main manifestations of DM that can be seen in the clinic are hypoglycemia, which occurs when blood sugar levels are too low, and hyperglycemia, which occurs when blood sugar levels are too high. Each has its specific characteristics:

> *Hypoglycemia.* Signs of very low blood sugar levels (blood glucose < 60 mg/dL) may include light-headedness, drowsiness, trembling, anxiety, rapid heart rate, diaphoresis (sweating), seizures, and blurred vision.
>
> *Hyperglycemia.* Signs of very high blood sugar levels may include glycosuria (sugar in the urine), polyuria (frequent urination), and polydipsia (increased thirst). If hyperglycemia remains untreated, it may progress to ketoacidosis with the following symptoms: shortness of breath (dyspnea), fruity-smelling breath, nausea/vomiting, confusion, and dry mouth.

Physical therapy interventions may include therapeutic exercise, self-care management for skin integrity, peripheral neuropathy risk, stump care, prosthetic use, and generalized fitness for life. In addition, patients may require wound management.

PTAs educate the patient on diabetic foot care, control of risk factors (obesity, physical inactivity), and disease management while addressing functional impairments such as weakness, gait abnormalities, balance impairment, poor endurance, polyneuropathy, amputation, and wound healing. PTAs should instruct in moderate exercises with an adequate warm-up and cool-down while monitoring the patient's response closely (blood glucose uptake by the muscles increases during strenuous or prolonged exercises), as this relates to when and how the patient has taken their medication, if they have eaten, and their response to exercise. If blood glucose levels are high (at or near 250 mg/dL) or if blood glucose levels are poorly controlled, exercise is contraindicated. Episodes of hypoglycemia are a serious condition and may progress to syncope, cardiovascular shock, brain damage, coma, or death if left untreated.

HYPERPARATHYROIDISM

Hyperparathyroidism is an abnormality of the parathyroid gland leading to excess secretion of parathyroid hormone (PTH), which may be due to an impairment of the parathyroid (primary) or lack of vitamin D or chronic renal disease (secondary). Hyperparathyroidism causes extreme **osteoclastic** activity in the bones. This elevates the calcium ion concentration in the extracellular fluid while depressing phosphate ion concentration because of increased renal excretion of phosphate.

The most common signs and symptoms include the following:

1. Fatigue.
2. Depression.

STUDY PEARL

As exercise can produce hypoglycemia, several precautions need to be taken:

- The patient should eat at least 2 hours before exercise; as a precaution, the PTA or patient should have a carbohydrate snack readily available during exercise.
- Adequate hydration needs to be maintained both during and after the exercise session.
- The patient should not exercise when their blood glucose levels are high (at or near 250 mg/dL) or if their blood glucose levels are poorly controlled.
- The patient's glucose levels should be taken before and following exercise.

STUDY PEARL

Both hyperglycemia or hypoglycemia can lead to a diabetic coma, a life-threatening condition that requires swift action. Clinics should have carbohydrates available for low blood sugar.

⚠️ **YELLOW FLAG**

In the clinic, if you observe the patient having signs or symptoms of hypoglycemia, the patient may need to ingest a carbohydrate snack (orange juice, crackers, or candy). The American Diabetes Association recommends the "15-15 Rule." The patient should have 15 g of carbohydrate to raise blood sugar and recheck after 15 minutes. If their blood glucose is less than 70 mg/dL, then they should repeat.

- Patients with severe hypoglycemia issues may be prescribed the hormone glucagon (injectable or nasal spray).

🛑 **RED FLAG**

If the blood glucose levels are high (at or near 250 mg/dL) or if blood glucose levels are poorly controlled, exercise is contraindicated.

3. Forgetfulness.
4. Hypercalcemia.
5. Hypertension.
6. Depression of the central and peripheral nervous systems.
7. Muscle weakness (proximal).
8. Muscle spasms.
9. Poor endurance.
10. Constipation.
11. Abdominal pain.
12. Bone pain.
13. Arthralgias.
14. Gout.
15. Joint hypermobility.
16. Pathologic fractures.
17. Peptic ulcer, lack of appetite.
18. Kidney stones.
19. Depressed relaxation of the heart during diastole.

Patients with hyperparathyroidism may sustain pathologic and fragility fractures that will require physical therapy interventions for improved functional ability.

HYPOPARATHYROIDISM

Hypoparathyroidism occurs when the parathyroid does not secrete sufficient parathyroid hormone, leading to depressed calcium reabsorption from the bone and osteoclasts becoming almost inactive. As a result, the calcium level in body fluids decreases. Yet because calcium and phosphate are not being absorbed from the bone, the bone usually remains strong. When low calcium levels are reached, signs of muscle tetany develop. Laryngeal musculature is especially sensitive to low calcium levels, and spasms can lead to obstruction of respiration.

The most common signs and symptoms include the following:

1. Muscle weakness.
2. Neuroexcitability.
3. Muscle spasm.
4. Abdominal pain.
5. Breathing difficulties.
6. Cardiac abnormalities.
7. Dry, scaly skin.
8. Nausea, vomiting.
9. Constipation, diarrhea.
10. Irritability, depression, anxiety.

OSTEOPOROSIS

Osteoporosis is the most common bone disease in adults, especially with increased age. Osteoporosis is characterized by a decrease in bone mass, resulting in weak or brittle bones. Bones that are weakened come with an increased risk for fractures, including **fragility fractures** (fall from standing height that results in fracture). Osteoporosis can be a primary bone disorder or secondary to many other disorders. Primary osteoporosis occurs with increased age and after menopause in women. Secondary osteoporosis can be caused through dietary alterations, medications, endocrine dysfunction, and lifestyle choices (sedentary lifestyle, alcohol consumption, smoking). Osteoporosis can be contrasted with osteomalacia (bone softening), osteopenia (low bone mass), and osteopetrosis (increased bone density).

The most common signs and symptoms include the following:

1. Back pain due to vertebral compression fractures.
2. Loss of height.
3. Stooped or flex posture.
4. Bone fracture from a standing height or less.
5. Decreased physical activity.

PTAs will potentially treat osteoporosis patients to improve muscle strength, posture, the need for weight-bearing activities, balance activities, and pain management. Treatment may be after surgery for fractures or for prevention and wellness. PTAs address functional impairments such as weakness, atrophy, gait abnormalities, balance impairment, posture, and poor endurance. Physical therapy interventions should address the underlying findings from the physical therapy evaluation targeting movement abnormalities. Activities may include strengthening, therapeutic exercise, balance training, functional training, ADLs training, pain education, and the need for assistive devices and/or home modifications. Calcium intake and vitamin D in conjunction with exercise should be discussed.

■ QUESTIONS

1. **In Graves' disease, the cause of hyperthyroidism is the production of antibody that does which of the following?**
   A. Activates the pituitary thyrotropin-releasing hormone (TRH) receptor
   B. Activates the thyroid gland TSH receptor
   C. Activates thyroid hormone receptors in peripheral tissues
   D. Binds to thyroid gland thyroglobulin and accelerates the release of T_4 and T_3

2. **A PTA reviews the medical record of a 54-year-old woman who presented to the emergency room with tachycardia, shortness of breath, and chest pain. She reported shortness of breath and diarrhea for the last 2 days and is sweating and anxious. A TSH measurement reveals a value of less than 0.01 mIU/L (normal 0.4-4.0 mIU/L). The diagnosis of thyroid storm is made. Which of the following best describes thyroid storm?**
   A. A worsening of hypothyroidism symptoms
   B. A severe headache
   C. An autoimmune reaction to the thyroid
   D. A sudden life-threatening worsening of hyperthyroidism symptoms

3. **A PTA reviews the medical record of a 64-year-old woman who presented with complaints of fatigue, sluggishness, and weight gain. She reported needing to nap several times a day, which is unusual for her, and she complained of being cold and having difficulty with dry skin. What is the most likely diagnosis of her current condition?**
   A. Hyperthyroid
   B. Hypothyroid
   C. Hypoparathyroid
   D. Hyperparathyroid

4. **A PTA reviews the medical record of a 25-year-old woman who presented with insomnia and feared she might have "something wrong with [her] heart." She described her "heart jumping out of [her] chest," but felt healthy otherwise and reported she has lots of energy and had enjoyed her recent weight loss even though her appetite had increased. Which of the following is the most likely diagnosis?**
   A. Hyperthyroid
   B. Hypothyroid
   C. Hypoparathyroid
   D. Hyperparathyroid

5. A PTA reviews the medical record of a 36-year-old woman with ulcerative colitis who has required long-term treatment with pharmacologic doses of a glucocorticoid agonist. Which of the following is a toxic effect associated with long-term glucocorticoid treatment that would impact physical therapy?
   A. Fluid and electrolyte imbalance
   B. Adrenal gland neoplasm
   C. Hepatotoxicity
   D. Osteoporosis

6. A PTA reviews the medical record of a patient who presented to the emergency department with hypotension, tachycardia, and loss of consciousness. The family reported that the patient has a history of Addison disease and that the patient had severe abdominal pain with vomiting and leg and back pain over the last few days, which they thought was due to an infection. The patient is diagnosed with an Addisonian crisis. What is the hormone deficiency mostly likely to cause this crisis?
   A. ACTH
   B. Aldosterone
   C. Testosterone
   D. Cortisol

7. The pancreas is involved with the regulation of blood sugar. The alpha cells release_____, while the beta cells release _____.
   A. Cortisol; aldosterone
   B. Epinephrine; norepinephrine
   C. Glucagon; insulin
   D. Aldosterone; cortisol

8. The primary glucocorticoid produced by the adrenal cortex is _____, and the primary mineralocorticoid produced by the adrenal cortex is _____.
   A. Cortisol; aldosterone
   B. Progesterone; testosterone
   C. Estrogen; testosterone
   D. Testosterone; aldosterone

9. Upon entering a patient's room, a PTA notes that the patient presents what appears to be extra fat around the trunk (buffalo torso). What condition is associated with this symptom?
   A. Addison disease
   B. Graves' disease
   C. Hashimoto syndrome
   D. Cushing syndrome

10. Which of the following is a life-threatening complication due to severe hyperglycemia or hypoglycemia in patients with diabetes?
    A. Diabetic coma
    B. Hyperlipidemia
    C. Metabolic syndrome
    D. Polyneuropathy

■ ANSWERS WITH RATIONALES

1. The answer is **B**. The antibodies produced in Graves' disease activate thyroid gland TSH receptors.

2. The answer is **D**. A thyroid storm is a sudden life-threatening worsening of hyperthyroidism symptoms.

3. The answer is **B**. Patients with early hypothyroidism have clinical features of vague and ordinary fatigue, mild sensitivity to cold, mild weight gain, forgetfulness, depression, and dry skin and hair.

4. The answer is **A**. Patients with early hyperthyroidism have clinical features that include goiter, nervousness, heat intolerance, increased heart rate, tachycardia, tremors, and weight loss.

5. The answer is **D**. One of the adverse metabolic effects of long-term glucocorticoid therapy is a net loss of bone, resulting in osteoporosis.

6. The answer is **D**. Addisonian crisis is due to low cortisol levels, which cause weakness, fatigue, and low blood pressure. Symptoms may include sudden dizziness, vomiting, and loss of consciousness.

7. The answer is **C**. The pancreas is involved with the regulation of blood sugar. The alpha cells release glucagon, while the beta cells release insulin.

8. The answer is **A**. The primary glucocorticoid produced by the adrenal cortex is cortisol, and the primary mineralocorticoid produced by the adrenal cortex is aldosterone.

9. The answer is **D**. Buffalo torso is a typical symptom of Cushing syndrome.

10. The answer is **A**. Diabetic coma is a serious and life-threatening complication of diabetes.

■ ONCOLOGY

Oncology is the branch of medicine that deals with tumors, including the study of their development, diagnosis, treatment, and prevention. Cancer refers to many diseases characterized by uncontrolled cell growth and abnormal cell dispersion (Table 9-11). The cause of cancer varies and can include lifestyle factors (tobacco use, alcohol use, sexual and reproductive behavior), ethnicity (Black Americans are diagnosed with, and die, more often from, cancer than any other racial group in the United States[1-4]), genetic causes (prostate, breast, ovarian, and colon), dietary causes (obesity, high-fat diet, a diet low in vitamins A, C, E) and psychological causes (chronic stress). The causative agents are subdivided into two categories:

- Endogenous (genetic).
- Exogenous (environmental or external).

▲ HIGH-YIELD TERMS TO LEARN

Metastasis	The movement of cancer cells from one body part to another.
Biopsy	The surgical removal of a small section of a tumor. A needle biopsy uses a very fine needle, whereas a resection removes the whole tumor.
Tumor marker	A substance in the body that may indicate the presence of cancer.
Staging	A method to categorize cancer as to how far it has spread.
Remission	A state where the signs or symptoms of cancer are no longer present.
Palliative treatment	A treatment approach aimed at relieving symptoms and pain.
Total body irradiation	Radiation is applied to the whole body to destroy all malignant cells before a bone marrow transplant.
Chemotherapy	A form of drug treatment for cancer. Chemotherapy may be given intravenously, intramuscularly, orally, subcutaneously, intralesionally, intrathecally, and topically.
Neutropenia	A reduction in the levels of white blood cells.
Adjuvant treatment	An additional treatment provided with the primary treatment to enhance the effectiveness.
Brachytherapy	Internal radiation therapy that involves placing radioactive sources inside or adjacent to the tumor.
Intensity-modulated radiation therapy	A specialized form of external beam therapy that allows the radiation dose to be shaped to fit the size of the tumor

TABLE 9-11 • Oncologic Definitions.	
Term	**Definition**
Tumor/neoplasm	Abnormal growth of new tissues that serve no useful purpose and may harm the host organism by competing for blood supply and nutrients. These new growths may be benign or malignant.
Benign tumor	Localized, slow-growing, usually encapsulated; not invasive, but can become large enough to disband, compress, or obstruct normal tissues and impair normal body functions.
Malignant tumor	Invasive, rapid growth giving rise to metastasis; can be life-threatening.
Lymphoma	Malignancy originating in the lymphoid tissues, eg, Hodgkin disease, lymphatic leukemia.
Carcinoma	Originating in epithelial tissues, eg, skin, stomach, colon, breast, and rectum.
Sarcoma	Originating in connective and mesodermal tissues, eg, muscle, bone, fat.
Leukemias and myelomas	Involve the blood (unrestrained growth of leukocytes) and blood-forming organs (bone marrow).
Dysplasia	A general category suggesting cell disorganization in which an adult cell varies from its normal size, shape, or organization.
Differentiation	The process by which normal cells undergo physical and structural changes to form different tissues of the body.
Metaplasia	The first level of dysplasia. A reversible and benign but abnormal change in which one adult cell changes from one type to another.
Hyperplasia	An increase in the number of cells in a tissue, resulting in increased tissue mass.
Metastasis	Movement of cancer cells from one body part to another; spread is by lymphatic system or bloodstream.

After determining the type of cancer, the cancer is graded according to the degree of malignancy and differentiation of malignant cells. Staging is the process of describing the extent of disease at the time of diagnosis to aid in treatment planning, predict clinical outcome (prognosis), and compare different treatment approaches.

- Stage 0 (carcinoma in situ): The abnormal cells are found only in the first layer of the primary site's cells and do not invade the deeper tissues.
- Stage I: Cancer involves the primary site but has not spread to nearby tissues.
- Stage IA: A very small amount of cancer—visible under a microscope—is found deeper in the tissues.
- Stage IB: A larger amount of cancer is found in the tissues.
- Stage II: Cancer has metastasized to nearby areas but is still inside the primary site.
- Stage IIA: Cancer has metastasized beyond the primary site.
- Stage IIB: Cancer has metastasized to other tissue around the primary site.
- Stage III: Cancer has metastasized throughout the nearby area.
- Stage IV: Cancer has metastasized to other parts of the body.
- Stage IVA: Cancer has metastasized to organs close to the pelvic area.
- Stage IVB: Cancer has metastasized to distant organs, such as the lungs.

The signs and symptoms of cancer vary widely, but more commonly include the following:

- Unusual bleeding or discharge.
- A lump or thickening of any area, for example, breast.
- A sore that does not heal.
- A change in bladder or bowel habits.
- Hoarseness of voice or persistent cough.
- Indigestion or difficulty in swallowing.
- Unexplained weight loss.
- Night pain not related to movement.
- Change in the size or appearance of a wart or mole.

Prevention is the key with cancer:

- Primary prevention includes screening to identify high-risk people and reducing or eliminating modifiable risk factors (tobacco and alcohol use, diet). Also includes chemoprevention—the use of agents to prevent, inhibit, or reverse cancer (aspirin, lycopene, selenium).
- Secondary prevention is aimed at preventing morbidity and mortality by using drugs.
- Tertiary prevention manages symptoms, limits complications, and prevents disability.

From the PTA's perspective, the physical therapy intervention varies according to the patient's physical condition, cancer stage, and the cancer treatment the patient is undergoing. Functional deficits are often associated with cancer treatments. These deficits can be caused by the medications, the removal of a diseased organ or segmental bone, joint, or limb amputation. Consequently, patients undergoing cancer treatment may have limited motion, soreness, disuse atrophy, pain, fatigue, sensory loss, weakness, sleep disturbance, and lymphedema. Table 9-12[5] outlines the side effects of various cancer treatments. If the patient has undergone surgery, the PTA must be alert for any signs and symptoms of deep vein thrombosis and emboli.

As many of these patients have compromised immune systems, health care workers must be vigilant in the practice of standard precautions, especially proper hand washing and infection control principles. Some of the procedural interventions that may be used with this population include the following:

- Patient and family education on the expected goals, processes involved, and the expected intervention outcomes. The patient and family may require assistance with coping mechanisms and through the grieving process.

TABLE 9-12 • The Various Side Effects of Cancer Treatments.

Surgery	Radiation	Chemotherapy	Biotherapy	Hormonal Therapy
Fatigue	Fatigue	Fatigue	Fever	Hypertension
Disfigurement	Radiation sickness	Gastrointestinal effects	Chills	Steroid-induced diabetes
Loss of function	Immunosuppression	-- Anorexia	Nausea	Myopathy (steroid-induced)
Infection	Decreased platelets	-- Nausea	Vomiting	Weight gain
Increased pain	Decreased white blood cells	-- Vomiting	Anorexia	Hot flashes
Deformity	Infection	-- Diarrhea	Fluid retention	Impotence
Bleeding	Fibrosis	-- Constipation	Fatigue	Decreased libido
Scar tissue	Burns	Fluid/electrolyte imbalance from GI effects	CNS effects	Vaginal dryness
Fibrosis	Mucositis	Hepatotoxicity	Inflammatory reactions at injection sites	
	Diarrhea	Hemorrhage	Anemia	
	Edema	Bone marrow suppression	Leukopenia	
	Hair loss	Anemia	Altered taste sensation	
	Ulceration, delayed wound healing	Leukopenia (infection)		
	CNS/PNS effects	Thrombocytopenia		
	Malignancy	A decrease in bone density with ovarian failure		
		Muscle weakness		
		Skin rashes		
		Neuropathies		
		Hair loss		
		Sterilization		
		Stomatitis, mucositis		
		Sexual dysfunction		

CNS, central nervous system; GI, gastrointestinal; PNS, peripheral nervous system.

- Proper positioning to prevent or correct deformities, preserve integrity, and provide comfort.
- Edema control: Elevation of extremities, active ROM, massage.
- Pain control: Transcutaneous electrical nerve stimulation (TENS), massage.
- Maintaining or improving:
- Loss of ROM: Passive, active-assisted, active ROM exercises.
- Loss of muscle mass and strength within patient tolerance, weight-bearing limits, and prescribed guidelines.
- Activity tolerance and cardiovascular endurance.
- Independence with ADLs.

■ OBSTETRICS AND GYNECOLOGY

An obstetrician specializes in obstetrics, which is concerned with all aspects of pregnancy, from prenatal care to postnatal care. A gynecologist is a specialist concerned with the reproductive health of a woman. Many definitions are used in obstetrics to describe the number of pregnancies and deliveries and the stages of pregnancy, labor, and the postpartum phase (Table 9-13). The various physiologic changes that occur during pregnancy and the postpartum period within the various body systems are outlined in Table 9-14. Table 9-15 contains a partial list of symptoms during pregnancy that may mimic musculoskeletal dysfunction. Hypertensive disorders complicating pregnancy have been divided into five types (Table 9-16).

▲ HIGH-YIELD TERMS TO LEARN

Gestational hypertension	Hypertension that develops after week 20 in pregnancy but typically goes away after delivery.
Preeclampsia	A complication during pregnancy characterized by high blood pressure and signs of damage to another organ system, most often the liver and kidneys.
Eclampsia	A rare but serious condition where high blood pressure results in seizures during pregnancy.
Gestational diabetes	A form of diabetes that appears only during pregnancy.
Cerclage	A variety of procedures that use sutures or synthetic tape to reinforce the cervix.
Parturient	A woman in labor.
Amniocentesis	A procedure in which amniotic fluid is removed from the uterus for testing or treatment.
Supine hypotension	Decreased venous return is caused by a gravid uterus compressing the inferior vena cava when a pregnant woman is in a supine position. The symptoms (pallor, dizziness, low blood pressure, sweating, nausea, and increased heart rate) usually occur within 3 to 10 minutes after lying down but can be alleviated with a change of position (eg, sidelying)

STUDY PEARL
The PTA should be alert for any of the following signs and symptoms with exercise during pregnancy:
- Pain.
- Vaginal bleeding.
- Dizziness, feeling faint.
- Tachycardia.
- Dyspnea.
- Chest pain.
- Uterine contractions

Theoretically, because of the physiologic changes associated with pregnancy and the hemodynamic responses to exercise, some precautions should be observed during exercise. The contraindications and relative contraindications to exercise during pregnancy are listed in Table 9-17.

■ LYMPHATIC SYSTEM

The lymphatic system,[6-8] a unique system with a unique structure and function that works in conjunction with the immune, circulatory, and integumentary systems, facilitates the immune response to fight infection by destroying unwanted materials and mediating foreign organisms using macrophages and lymphocytes. Signs indicating presence of an infection would include swollen and tender lymph nodes.

TABLE 9-13 • Glossary of Obstetric Terminology.

Term	Definition
Active labor	The period after the latent (early) stage of labor when a woman is experiencing strong, regular contractions and her cervix continues to dilate from 4 cm until she is fully dilated (10 cm)
Apgar score	A test performed at 1 minute and 5 minutes after birth. 1-minute score: Determines how well the baby tolerated the birthing process 5-minute score: Assesses how well the newborn is adapting to their new environment The rating is based on a total score of 1 to 10, with 10 suggesting the healthiest infant
Expected date of delivery (EDD)	The date when the baby is due, sometimes called EDC (expected date of confinement)
Gestation/gestational age	Duration of the pregnancy, measured from the first day of the last menstrual period
Multigravida	A woman who has had more than one pregnancy, regardless of the outcome
Multipara	Also called a multip—a woman who has given birth at least once before
Primipara	Sometimes called the prim or primip—a woman giving birth for the first time.
Primigravida	A woman who is pregnant for the first time, regardless of the outcome
Postpartum	Relating to the period of a few days after birth
Postnatal	After the birth. Relates to the 28 days following giving birth
Term	The period at the end of a pregnancy (37-42 weeks) when a baby might be expected to be born. Preterm—born before 37 weeks of pregnancy
Trimesters	One-third of a pregnancy: first, 1-13 weeks; second, 14-17 weeks; third, 28-40 weeks
Postterm/postdates	Labor initiated after the 37th week of pregnancy but before the 42nd week

TABLE 9-14 • Changes Within the Body Systems That Occur With Pregnancy.

System	Changes	Implications
Endocrine	• The adrenal, thyroid, parathyroid, and pituitary glands enlarge • A female hormone (relaxin) is released that assists in the softening of the pubic symphysis so that during delivery, the female pelvis can stretch enough to allow birth	The release of relaxin results in: • Joint hypermobility, especially throughout the pelvic ring • Symphysis pubic dysfunction (SPD) • Sacroiliac joint dysfunction • Increased susceptibility to injury
Musculoskeletal	Weight gain (average is 20-30 lb)	• The abdominal muscles are stretched and weakened • The rib cage circumference increases • In advanced pregnancy, the patient develops a wider base of support and has increased difficulty with walking, stair climbing, and rapid changes in position
	Pelvic floor weakness can develop	May result in stress incontinence
	Postural changes related to the weight of growing breasts, and the uterus and fetus	A shift in the woman's center of gravity in an anterior and superior direction resulting in problems with balance
Neurologic	Nerve compression from fluid buildup	Involved structures include thoracic outlet, wrists, or groin (brachial plexus, median nerve, and lateral [femoral] cutaneous nerve of the thigh, respectively)
Gastrointestinal	High levels of certain hormones make it harder for the GI system to work efficiently	• Nausea and vomiting • A slowing of intestinal motility • The development of constipation, abdominal bloating, and hemorrhoids • Esophageal reflux • Heartburn (pyrosis)

(Continued)

TABLE 9-14 • Changes Within the Body Systems That Occur With Pregnancy. (*Continued*)

System	Changes	Implications
Respiratory	Weight gain and body shape changes cause the diaphragm to elevate	• A predominance of costal versus abdominal breathing • Mild increases in tidal volume and oxygen consumption • A compensated respiratory alkalosis • A low expiratory reserve volume
Cardiac	Primarily develop to meet the increased metabolic demands of the mother and fetus	• Increased blood volume • Increased plasma volume (40%-50%) • Increased cardiac output. During the first trimester, cardiac output is 30%-40% higher than in the nonpregnant state • Vascular tone is more dependent on sympathetic control than in the nonpregnant state so that hypotension develops more readily and more markedly
Metabolic	Primarily develop to meet the increased demand for tissue growth	• Insulin is elevated from plasma expansion, and blood glucose is reduced for a given insulin load • The metabolic rate increases during both exercise and pregnancy
Genitourinary	There are several anatomic and hormonal changes As the fetus grows, stress on the mother's bladder can occur	Higher risk for both lower and upper urinary tract infections and urinary incontinence

TABLE 9-15 • Symptoms That Can Mimic Musculoskeletal Conditions in Pregnancy.

Symptoms	Possible Medical Condition	Possible Musculoskeletal Dysfunction	Differentiating Tests or Measures
Calf, proximal thigh, or inguinal pain	Deep vein thrombosis	Gastroc-soleus sprain; radicular symptoms from nerve root impingement; compartment syndrome; pubic symphysis dysfunction	Duplex ultrasonography; positive Homan sign; assessment of response to treatment and provocation of pain by musculoskeletal examination of the pelvis and lower quadrant
Urinary incontinence	Urinary tract infection	Pelvic floor muscle dysfunction; cauda equina syndrome	Urinalysis; assessment of onset (acute or gradual) and aggravating factors
Lower abdominal pain	Abruption of the placenta; ectopic pregnancy	Pubic symphysis dysfunction (shears or separation)	Assessment of nature pain (constant or intermittent) and aggravating factors; provocation of pain by musculoskeletal assessment of the pelvis; diagnostic ultrasound
Low back pain or hip pain	Osteoporosis of pregnancy with or without fracture	Mechanical dysfunction of the low back or pelvic ring; disk disease; spondylolisthesis	Height assessment; pain pattern assessment; objective findings (provocation tests, palpatory findings, neurologic findings, end-feels)
Flank pain	Upper urinary tract infection (kidney)	Rib or thoracic spine dysfunction	Percussion over the ribs; assessment of response to treatment and provocation of pain by musculoskeletal examination of the thorax; fever assessment; urinalysis
Right upper quadrant/scapular pain	Gallstones	Shoulder girdle or thoracic spine/rib dysfunction	Diagnostic ultrasound; assessment of response to treatment and nature of symptoms (whether the pain is constant or provoked by activity)
Headache	Pregnancy-induced hypertension or preeclampsia	Upper cervical dysfunction or tension-type headache	Blood pressure assessment for hypertension; signs of recent onset of edema; provocation of headache by musculoskeletal assessment of the upper cervical spine

TABLE 9-16 • Summary of Types of Hypertension During Pregnancy.			
Disorder	**Definition**	**Diagnostic Criteria**	**Signs/Symptoms**
Gestational hypertension: Affects nulliparous women most often	Diagnosis made retrospectively when preeclampsia does not develop and blood pressure returns to normal by the 12th week postpartum	Blood pressure ≥ 140/90 mm Hg for the first time during pregnancy; no proteinuria; blood pressure returns to normal by 12 weeks postpartum	Epigastric pain, thrombocytopenia, headache
Preeclampsia	Pregnancy-specific syndrome of reduced organ perfusion from vasospasm and endothelial activation	Blood pressure ≥ 140/90 mm Hg after 20 weeks gestation; proteinuria: 300 mg or more of urinary protein in a 24-hour period or persistent 30 mg/dL in random urine samples	The more severe the hypertension or proteinuria, the more certain is the severity of preeclampsia; symptoms of eclampsia, such as headache, cerebral visual disturbance, and epigastric pain, can occur
Eclampsia	Seizures in a pregnant woman with preeclampsia not assigned to other causes	Grand mal seizures appearing before, during, or after labor; in nulliparas, seizures may develop 48 hours to 10 days after delivery	The mother may develop abruptio placentae, neurologic deficits, aspiration pneumonia, pulmonary edema, cardiopulmonary arrest, acute renal failure; maternal death
Superimposed preeclampsia on chronic hypertension	Chronic hypertensive disorders predispose the development of superimposed preeclampsia or eclampsia	New-onset proteinuria of ≥ 300 mg in 24 hours in hypertensive women; no proteinuria before 20 weeks gestation	The risk of abruptio placentae; fetus at risk for growth restriction and death
Chronic hypertension	Hypertension that persists longer than 12 weeks after delivery	Blood pressure ≥ 140/90 mm Hg before pregnancy; hypertension ≥ 140/90 mm Hg detected before 20 weeks' gestation; persistent hypertension long after delivery	Risk of abruptio placentae; fetus at risk for growth restriction and death; pulmonary edema; hypertensive encephalopathy; renal failure

Data from Boissonnault WG, ed. *Primary Care for the Physical Therapist: Examination and Triage.* 2005. © Copyright Elsevier Saunders. All rights reserved; American College of Obstetrics and Gynecology: Practice Bulletin 29: Chronic hypertension in pregnancy. *Obstet Gynecol.* 2001;98:177-185; Cunningham FG, Gant NF, Leveno KJ, et al. *Williams Obstetrics,* 21st ed. 2001. © Copyright McGraw Hill LLC. All rights reserved; and Livingston JC, Baha MS. Chronic hypertension in pregnancy. *Obstet Gynecol Clin North Am.* 2001;28:447-463.

TABLE 9-17 • Contraindications to Exercise During Pregnancy.	
Contraindications	Pregnancy-induced hypertension Preterm rupture of membranes Preterm labor during the prior or current pregnancy Incompetent cervix or cerclage (cervical stitch) placement Persistent second- or third-trimester bleeding Placenta previa Intrauterine growth retardation
Relative contraindications	Chronic hypertension Thyroid function abnormality Cardiac disease Vascular disease Pulmonary disease

STOP RED FLAG

Signs of infection may include enlarged lymph nodes or glands, fever, fatigue, and/or weight loss and should be communicated to the supervising PT immediately.

STOP RED FLAG

Application of blood pressure cuff, needle sticks/blood draws, intravenous lines (IV) should be avoided on the affected limb.

▲ HIGH-YIELD TERMS TO LEARN

Lymphocytes	White blood cells of immune cells made in the bone marrow and located in blood and lymph tissue.
Lymphadenopathy	An abnormal enlargement of the lymph nodes that may result from infection, autoimmune disorders, or malignancy. The inflamed nodules may be warm and tender but will remain mobile and soft, but malignant nodules are usually firm and not tender to the touch.
Stemmer sign	Completed during the physical examination by pinching the skin over the dorsal surface of the hand or foot. If the skin cannot be pinched, it is considered a positive finding associated with lymphedema.

Additionally, fluid movement by diffusion and filtration between the blood and interstitial tissue allows the removal of excess fluid, waste products, and protein molecules. Structures in the lymphatic system, including the lymph organs (tonsils, spleen, thymus), lymph nodes, lymph tissue, lymph fluid, and lymph vessels, are referred to as lymphatics and are found in varying layers from superficial to deep within the body (Figure 9-6). Lymph vessel structures consist of one-way valves that can collapse under less pressure than veins. Unlike venous return, lymph fluid is not normally adversely affected by gravity. However, in certain patients with comorbidities of chronic venous insufficiency or morbid obesity, you may see a collection of lymph fluid (most often in the lower extremities related to gravity).

Lymph fluid is absorbed at the capillary level then moves into smaller vessels known as *precollectors*, transitioning into larger *collector* vessels and eventually to the lymph nodes. After leaving the lymph nodes, the fluid will travel along larger trunks until it reaches one of two collecting ducts (thoracic duct or right lymphatic duct), and finally, the fluid will be directed into general circulation via the subclavian vein.[8] What follows is an outline of the various dysfunctions and their common signs and symptoms.

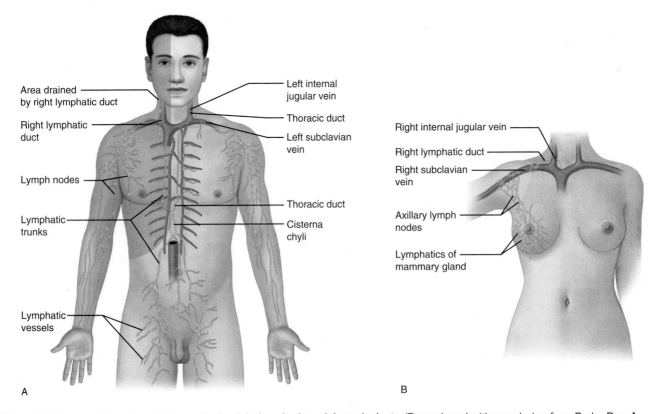

Figure 9-6. Lymphatic system drainage via the right lymphatic and thoracic ducts. (Reproduced with permission from Burke-Doe A, Dutton M, eds. *National Physical Therapy Examination and Board Review.* 2019. Copyright © McGraw Hill LLC. All rights reserved. https://accessphysiotherapy.mhmedical.com.)

LYMPHEDEMA

Clinical Significance

Lymphedema[6,9-12] occurs when an insufficiency or obstruction to the flow of lymph fluid causes an abnormal accumulation of fluid in the subcutaneous tissues. Lymphedema may lead to impaired chronic inflammation, skin conditions, and an increased risk of infection. There are two main types of lymphedema:

1. *Primary lymphedema*—A congenital or hereditary condition that causes an abnormal formation of lymph vessels or nodes. Congenital lymphedema often appears by the age of 2 years.
2. *Secondary lymphedema*—Condition occurs in response to an injury to the lymphatic system due to blockage, fibrosis, overload, or alteration from surgery or radiation.

Lymphedema follows a course of pathophysiology and is described by the International Society of Lymphology Staging System as follows[11]:

- Stage 0: No clinical edema observed, but lymph flow is impaired. Subtle symptoms or tissue changes may be present.
- Stage I: Early onset of swelling that is reversible with an elevation of the limb; pitting edema may be present.
- Stage II: Pitting edema with a consistent volume change, irreversible with elevation.
- Stage III: Pitting edema no longer occurs as skin changes show thickening, hyperpigmentation, fat deposits, and tissue fibrosis.

Clinical Findings, Secondary Effects, Complications

- Swelling distal or near the site of system impairment/blockage.
- Elevation does not usually resolve edema.
- Pitting edema in early stages, nonpitting edema in late stages as fibrotic changes occur.
- Discomfort, fatigue, pressure, tightness, or feeling of heaviness in the affected extremity.
- Fibrotic changes or discoloration.
- Decreased ROM.
- Impaired wound healing.
- Increased risk of infection.
- Numbness and/or tingling.

Diagnostic Tests and Measures

- Patient history.
- Physical examination.
- Girth measurements.
- Stemmer sign.
- Skin assessment.
- Lymphoscintigraphy—radioactive tracer used to provide images of the lymphatic system.
- Computed tomography (CT) scan.
- Magnetic resonance imaging (MRI).

Interventions/Treatment

Medical. In some cases, surgical reconstruction may be considered for primary lymphedema. In addition, patient education for skincare, infection recognition, avoidance of risk factors, and the recommendation of a healthy lifestyle with regular medical visits are necessary for managing this condition.

Pharmacologic.[10] Antibiotics may be used to treat cellulitis or lymphangitis that may occur along with lymphedema.

Physical Therapy. Treatment may vary depending on the etiology of the lymphedema and what stage of progression. Initially, the PT will interview the patient and then perform a physical examination consisting of ROM, strength, functional mobility, *Stemmer sign*, girth measurements (tape or volumetric), and skin assessment. The PTA must be aware of how to instruct the patient's activities to avoid exacerbating symptoms or require specialized skills to treat the unique presentation of the various pathologies. PTAs will potentially treat patients with lymphatic dysfunction as a comorbidity or due to the pathology itself. PTAs may assist in the implementation of interventions to facilitate mobility, strength, or endurance.

Currently recommended interventions surrounding *complete decongestive therapy* (CDT) require advanced expertise not taught at the entry-level professional educational program, so specialized training may be necessary to treat this patient population.[7] CDT involves two phases of treatment:

- Phase I aims to reduce symptoms with treatment methods, including manual lymphatic drainage (MLD), lymphedema bandaging, and exercise before advancing to a compression garment at the end of the phase.
- Phase II aims to establish a plan for self-management and maintenance of the condition. This phase incorporates skincare, daily compression garment donning, exercise, and bandaging/MLD as needed. An overview of the interventions and strategies is listed below.

Interventions

- *MLD*—Specialized gentle techniques[7,12] to address superficial lymph fluid circulation. MLD techniques may be used for other causes of edema beyond lymphedema. However, MLD is contraindicated in patients with cardiac, renal, or pulmonary edema to avoid overwhelming the respective system.
- *Elevation*—Elevating the extremities may provide resolution of early-stage mild swelling and is often temporary. The PTA may issue patient education on safe elevation and positioning.
- *Lymphedema multilayer bandaging*—Multiple layers of bandaging, including foam or padding and short-stretch bandages, are applied over the affected limb to provide a consistent external tissue pressure to assist in circulation, facilitate muscle pump, and localized pressure to soften fibrotic tissue.
- *Long-stretch and short-stretch bandages*—These bandages provide a supportive structure to the venous and lymphatic systems. Long-stretch bandages (such as an *ACE*) have more elastic fibers allowing for higher resting pressures and lower working pressures. Short-stretch bandages have more cotton fibers and stretch less, creating a low resting pressure and high working pressure. Short-stretch bandages are more appropriate for lymphedema as the application is more comfortable at rest while facilitating the muscle pump using inward pressure during activity by limiting the expansion of the contracted muscle. Specialized training is necessary for the application of short-stretch bandages to reduce or retain limb size.
- *Compression garments*—Compression garments may be utilized to manage scars, facilitate venous circulation, and prevent reoccurrences of edema. These garments are available in a variety of lengths, fabrics, and compression levels. Trained individuals should complete the selection and fitting of compression garments to be sure of an appropriate fit. Garments can be ordered by size or be custom-made. Patients should be encouraged to use the compression garments on a consistent and long-term basis.[13]
- *Limb containment systems*—These are quilted compression devices that may be used at night in place of bandaging.
- *Intermittent pneumatic compression (IPC)*—IPC pumps may be utilized to treat edema and lymphedema. Pressures must be kept low to avoid collapse of the lymph vessels, and blood pressure should be taken before application to determine safe pressure settings. IPC is contraindicated in patients with hypertension, acute inflammation, local infection, thrombus, cardiac or kidney dysfunction, lymph channel obstruction, and impaired cognition.

STUDY PEARL
The PTA should be aware that heat may exacerbate symptoms, so they must avoid applying heat packs or a hot tub. Additionally, prolonged sitting or standing may cause issues, and it is recommended that a compression garment is worn during air travel.

LYMPHANGITIS

Clinical Significance

Lymphangitis[6] occurs from an acute bacterial or fungal infection (most often streptococcal), affecting the arm or leg. The bacteria access the lymphatic system via a wound in the skin. As a result, the infection causes inflammation of the vessel walls and surrounding tissues.

Clinical Findings, Secondary Effects, Complications

- Fevers.
- Chills.
- Headache.
- Malaise.
- Cellulitis (skin infection).
- Leukocytosis.
- Throbbing pain.
- Warmth.

Diagnostic Tests and Measures

- Skin assessment for erythema often presents as streaking just below the skin surface.
- Temperature/presence of fever.
- Complete blood count (CBC).

Interventions/Treatment

Medical/Pharmacologic. Medical intervention to address the infection is treated with antibiotics, most commonly penicillin.

Physical Therapy. Moist heat packs, education on appropriate positioning to provide elevation of the limb, and careful evaluation of patient pain levels during exercise.

⚠ **YELLOW FLAG**

Lymphangitis may cause increased pain during exercise. Modification of activity to achieve no or minimal pain should be attempted.

🛑 **RED FLAG**

If the pain during exercise continues to be elevated, the PTA should stop the treatment and notify the supervising PT.

LIPEDEMA

Clinical Significance

Lipedema[6,10] can produce symmetrical swelling of both legs from the hips to the ankles with varying subcutaneous adipose tissue deposits but a lack of fat accumulation in the foot. Lipedema is not a pathology of the lymphatic system but is often confused with bilateral lower extremity lymphedema in its presentation. It occurs almost exclusively to women and is estimated to affect 11% of adult females.[6] Its stages of progression include the following:

- Stage I: Has soft tissue with palpable nodules present.
- Stage II: Presents with increased firmness of nodules, development of large fatty nodules, and pitting edema may be present.

Clinical Findings, Secondary Effects, Complications

- Fatty bulges on the medial thigh.
- Pitting edema.
- Hypersensitivity in anterior tibial region.
- Skin color changes.
- Decreased elasticity of epidermis/dermis.

Diagnostic Tests and Measures

- Physical examination (close attention to the symmetrical presentation).

Interventions/Treatment

Medical/Pharmacologic. No effective medical treatment is available, but there is an exploration into hormone therapy and liposuction. Regular activity and a healthy lifestyle are encouraged to avoid weight gain.

Physical Therapy. PTAs will potentially treat patients with lipedema as a comorbidity or due to the clinical findings of the pathology itself. It must be noted that exercise and diet cannot target the fatty accumulation areas, so the focus must be on a healthy lifestyle. Referral to a support group or other mental health counseling may be beneficial to maintain a positive mental perspective.

INFECTIOUS MONONUCLEOSIS

Clinical Significance

Infectious mononucleosis[6] is caused by the Epstein-Barr virus (EBV) when it enters the nose or mouth and targets the B lymphocytes. It will go through a 4- to 6-week incubation period, at which time it may cause enlargement of the spleen.

Clinical Findings, Secondary Effects, Complications

- Sore throat.
- Headache.
- Fever.
- Malaise.
- Fatigue lasting several weeks.
- Enlarged lymph nodes or spleen.
- Monocytes in blood.
- Complications: Hepatitis, ruptured spleen, airway obstruction due to enlarged lymph nodes, and meningitis.

Diagnostic Tests and Measures

- Heterophil antibody test (Monospot).
- EBV antibody testing.
- CBC.

Interventions/Treatment

Medical/Pharmacologic. The patient may be encouraged to rest and should regularly follow up with their treating physician as directed. Antivirals are generally not effective. Corticosteroids may be used for *lymphadenopathy* that may be obstructing the patient's airway.

Physical Therapy. Initially, any physical activity should be avoided until the treating physician has cleared the patient. Once cleared by the physician, low impact exercise with a gradual progression as the body heals should be prescribed.

STOP **RED FLAG**

Enlargement of the spleen may cause an increased risk of rupture, and physical therapy should be avoided for the first 3 to 4 weeks after diagnosis.

LYMPHOMAS (HODGKIN AND NON-HODGKIN)

Clinical Significance

Lymphoma[6,10] is a tumor grouping related to the lymphatic system but with close ties to leukemias. These malignant neoplasms cause a proliferation of the lymphocytes in the lymph nodes. There are two common types of lymphoma: Hodgkin and non-Hodgkin, which can be differentiated with a lymph node biopsy.

- **Hodgkin Disease/Hodgkin Lymphoma** usually involves a solitary neck lymph node and spreads to the lymph nodes and then organs.

- **Non-Hodgkin lymphoma** is more commonly occurring and has a similar clinical presentation to Hodgkin lymphomas with the expectation that non-Hodgkin lymphomas have multiple node involvement and a more disorganized pattern of metastasis.

Clinical Findings, Secondary Effects, Complications

- Lymph enlargement.
- Spleen enlargement.
- Anorexia.
- Anemia.
- Low-grade fever.
- Night sweats.
- Fatigue.
- Recurrent infections.

Diagnostic Tests and Measures

- Chest x-ray.
- Medical history.
- Physical examination.
- Lymph node biopsy.
- MRI.
- CT scan.
- Bone marrow biopsy (non-Hodgkin).

Interventions/Treatment

Medical/Pharmacologic. Both Hodgkin and non-Hodgkin lymphomas are treated primarily with radiation, chemotherapy, and surgery. However, due to the disorganized pattern of metastasis in non-Hodgkin lymphomas, it may be more difficult to localize the tumor for treatment.

Physical Therapy. The PTA will be involved with PT-selected interventions that focus on exercise and functional mobility training that provide a challenge level appropriate to the patient's level of recovery.

■ QUESTIONS

1. **A PTA notes pitting edema in the left lower extremity of their patient. However, upon an attempt to elevate the limb, the edema does not change. What stage of lymphedema would be suspected?**
   A. Stage 0
   B. Stage I
   C. Stage II
   D. Stage III

2. **A patient, status post left mastectomy, has increased edema in her left upper extremity. What tests and measure data collection could be conducted by the PTA to monitor progress for lymph fluid reduction?**
   A. CT scan
   B. Girth measurements
   C. Lymphoscintigraphy
   D. Physical examination

3. **A patient with recent lymphadenectomy to remove the lymph nodes for cancer treatment shows signs and symptoms of lymphedema. What type of lymphedema would this be categorized as?**
   A. Primary
   B. Secondary

> **STUDY PEARL**
> The PTA will need to monitor the patient's response during activities/exercise. Any vital signs and the patient's self-report on the Borg Rating of Perceived Exertion (RPE) to determine fatigue level should be documented.

C. Tertiary

D. Benign

4. **The evaluating PT has documented a positive Stemmer sign. What pathology is associated with this finding?**

A. Lymphedema

B. Lipedema

C. Lymphangitis

D. Lymphoma

5. **A patient presents with symmetrical bilateral pitting edema of the lower extremities that stops distally at the ankle, sparing the foot. Additionally, fatty nodules are noted upon palpation of the edematous area. Which of the following pathologies would these signs be characteristic of?**

A. Lymphedema

B. Lymphangitis

C. Lipedema

D. Lymphoma

ANSWERS WITH RATIONALES

1. The answer is **C**. Stage II would present as noticeable edema change, pitting edema, and elevation would have no effect. Stage 0 shows minimal observed changes, Stage I wound be reversed with an elevation of the limb, and Stage III would show fibrotic changes and no pitting edema in the late stage.

2. The answer is **B**. A PTA would perform girth measurements with either a tape measure or volumetric to provide objective data of lymph fluid fluctuation. A doctor and radiologist would perform a CT scan and lymphoscintigraphy while the PT would perform the physical examination during the physical therapy examination. Therefore, girth measurements are the only method within the scope of the PTA to collect data.

3. The answer is **B**. Secondary lymphedema results from a trauma or surgery causing the development of lymphedema. Primary lymphedema is a congenital condition often presenting by the age of 2 years.

4. The answer is **A**. A positive Stemmer sign consists of the inability to pinch the skin at the toe base, indicating an association with lymphedema.

5. The answer is **C**. Lipedema best fits the description as it has bilateral involvement but does not extend into the foot, causing the appearance of a flap of fatty, edematous tissue to extend at the ankle.

PSYCHOLOGICAL DISORDERS

Psychological disorders may present with mild-to-severe signs and symptoms. The factors related to each person's condition will affect how they interact with their social environment. Patients requiring physical therapy rehabilitation may have a psychiatric illness that will require the health care team to recognize and address appropriately to achieve the desired treatment outcomes. The treatment should be patient-centered, with the patient included in goal setting, high levels of engagement, motivation to participate, and education.[10] Table 9-18 outlines the more frequently encountered conditions.

SIGNS THAT PATIENT MAY NEED MENTAL HEALTH CONSULTATION

- Regression to a more immature pattern of function.[7,14]
- Disorientation.
- Delusional thinking.
- Inaccurate interpretation of the environment.
- Inappropriate affect.
- Hypovigilance or hypervigilance.

TABLE 9-18 • Psychological Disorders.

Affective	Generalized Anxiety	Personality	Somatoform	Substance Abuse-Related
Emotional disturbances of mood with periods of intense, unrealistic, extreme emotion that may be without cause. Occurs in children, adolescents, and adults.	Individuals experience fear and anxiety to the point of dysfunction and undue distress, which would then be considered maladaptive.	Disturbances show a pattern of behavior that is pervasive and enduring causing significant distress or impaired function.	Expression of mental phenomena as somatic (physical) symptoms. Symptoms may range from unconscious and nonvolitional to conscious and volitional.	Disorders involving drugs that activate the brain's reward system causing pleasure and a wide range of feelings. Substances may include tobacco, inhalants, opioids, sedatives, alcohol, stimulants, caffeine, etc.
Bipolar • Episodes of mania and depression • Episodes may alternate, or one may predominate • Unknown cause, but heredity may be a factor • Diagnosis based on history • Treatment: mood-stabilizing drugs and/or psychotherapy	**Anxiety Disorder** • Multiple worries that may shift over time • Worsens during stress • Many patients will have one or more comorbid psychiatric disorders • Anxiety attacks may include shortness of breath, heart palpitations, nausea, or dizziness	**Cluster A:** Odd and/or eccentric behavior • **Paranoid:** Mistrusting and suspicious • **Schizoid:** Disinterested in others • **Schizotypal:** Eccentric ideas or behaviors	**Somatic Symptom Disorder:** Persistent physical symptoms associated with maladaptive emotions or behaviors 1. **Conversion disorder:** Neurologic symptoms that may include paralysis, paresthesia, deafness, or blindness 2. **Illness anxiety disorder:** • (Previously hypochondriasis) • Fear will develop a serious disorder • Misinterpret minor symptoms to be more serious • May frequently examine themselves • Easily alarmed at new sensations	**Substance-Induced** • **Intoxication:** Specific to certain drug and reversible; may involve euphoria, cognitive or physical impairment, impaired judgment • **Withdrawal:** Behavior/symptoms that occur as a result • **Substance-induced mental disorders:** Mental alterations due to consumption or withdrawal that resemble other mental disorders (depression, psychosis, anxiety)
Depression • Depressed mood most of the day and lack of interest • Significant weight loss or gain • Insomnia or hypersomnia • Fatigue; loss of energy • Inability to think or concentrate • Recurrent thoughts of death/suicide	**Panic Attacks & Panic Disorder** • Sudden onset of a brief period of intense discomfort, anxiety, or fear • May have cognitive and/or somatic symptoms • May anticipate or worry about additional attacks	**Cluster B:** Dramatic, emotional, or erratic • **Antisocial:** Socially irresponsible, deceitful, manipulative for personal gain • **Borderline:** Intolerant of being alone, emotional dysregulation • **Narcissistic:** Fragile self-esteem, overt grandiosity	**Factitious Disorders** • Misrepresentation of signs or symptoms in the absence of external incentives • Previously referred to as Munchausen syndrome	**Substance-Use Disorders** • Pathologic pattern of behavior resulting from the continued use despite other problems linked to using the substance
Mania • Decreased need for sleep • Distractibility • Inflated self-esteem • The rapid flow of speech or talkativeness • Engage in impulsive or high-risk activities	**Posttraumatic Stress Disorder (PTSD)** • Reliving traumatic events in flashbacks or nightmares (combat, sexual abuse, etc) • Feelings of fear, helplessness, or horror • Negative emotions and distorted thoughts; may blame self	**Cluster C:** Appear anxious or fearful • **Avoidant:** Avoids contact; sensitive to rejection • **Dependent:** Submissive or need to be taken care of • **Obsessive-Compulsive:** Perfectionism, rigidity, and obstinacy	**Malingering** • Intentional fabricating of physical or psychological symptoms for external incentives	

Data from Merk Manual Professional Version. 2021. Copyright © Merck & Co., Inc. All rights reserved. https://www.merckmanuals.com; O'Sullivan SB, Schmitz TJ, Fulk GD. *Physical Rehabilitation*, 7th ed. 2019.

- Mood swings.
- Self-destructive behaviors.
- Normal behaviors acted to the extreme.
- Suicidal thoughts or noted sign of suicide risk.

SUBSTANCE ABUSE CONCERNS

- If the client is under the influence,[7] they may be inappropriate, argumentative, irritable, disinhibited, stubborn, illogical, or angry.
  - May disturb or be a danger to other clients and should be escorted from the treatment area.
  - May be a risk for falls and resulting injuries.
- Immediate referral needed when withdrawal signs noted (sweating, impaired sleep, shaking, anxiety, impaired judgment, slurred speech, fluctuating consciousness level).

IDENTIFYING AGITATION AND WAYS TO DE-ESCALATE

- Signs of agitation[14]: Clenched fists, pacing, angry facial expressions, grunting, groaning, swearing, tapping foot, throwing objects, or refusal to participate.
- How to de-escalate:
  - Identify the source of agitation or clarify reasons for anger.
  - Acknowledge the patient's concern or frustration in a nonaccusatory manner to establish trust.
  - Use a calm, low tone of voice and be respectful.
  - Do not force eye contact.
  - Set clear limits and an agreeable solution.
  - Avoid physical contact and use nonthreatening body language.
  - Maintain a safe distance.
  - Do not turn your back on the patient or allow them to block your exit.
  - If the patient becomes violent, remove all patients from the area, leave, and call for help.

> **STUDY PEARL**
> When the signs of substance abuse are noted, the PTA must notify the supervising PT or direct medical care team (nurses, doctors, etc) to determine the appropriate referral.

■ TIPS FOR PATIENT INVOLVEMENT IN THEIR REHAB

- Involve the patient as much as possible with goal setting, treatment planning, and ongoing evaluation.
- Clear communication using terms and language the patient understands.
- Speak respectfully and protect patient's dignity.
- Listen to patient's concerns in a nonjudgmental manner.
- Promote independence and self-reliance to engage patient in recovery.
- Encourage patient to provide feedback.
- As the therapist, be aware of your reaction to patients to avoid responding emotionally to the patient.

■ QUESTIONS

1. **The PTA is currently treating a patient who is 6 weeks status post a right total knee arthroplasty. The patient has had limited progress due to edema and elevated pain levels. In addition, the patient reports difficulty sleeping at night, disinterest in his previous hobbies, and a constant feeling of fatigue. What action should the PTA take?**
   A. The PTA should suspect anxiety disorder and provide frequent relaxation technique training.
   B. Notify the supervising PT of the potential need for referral due to concerns the patient shows signs of depression.
   C. Stop treatment immediately and call 911 for an immediate mental health consultation.
   D. Avoid lingering on the topic and move onto the next activity to redirect their thoughts.

2. **A PTA works with a nursing home resident with dementia when they observe the patient tapping his foot and clenching his fists. What would be the appropriate course of action for the PTA?**
   A. Recognize these as calming behaviors and encourage the patient to perform heel raises and handgrip strengthening to achieve calm.
   B. Note the patient is demonstrating signs of agitation. Use a calm, respectful, and low tone of voice to determine the cause of the agitation.
   C. Speak to the patient in an elevated volume and maintain eye contact at all times to achieve communication.
   D. End the session immediately and refer to the elevating PT for reexamination.

3. **During treatment in an outpatient gym, a patient becomes angry and violent, and begins throwing things at the wall. What is the best way to de-escalate or handle the situation?**
   A. Escort the patient to a private treatment room where you can close the door and discuss the issue privately.
   B. Maintain distance and remove any other patients in the area without turning their back to the patient. Call for help.
   C. Inform the patient you are done with treatment, turn and leave.
   D. Physically restrain the patient until they calm down.

4. **A patient presents to a treatment session with erratic behavior, rapid speech, and reports various high-risk activities they have taken part in. Which of the following psychiatric disorders would be suspected?**
   A. Anxiety attack
   B. Depression
   C. Paranoid personality disorder
   D. Mania

ANSWERS WITH RATIONALES

1. The answer is **B**. The PTA should recognize the signs and symptoms of depression, including insomnia, fatigue, loss of interest, and notify the supervising PT to determine if a mental health referral or recommendation for further support is needed. Signs and symptoms of anxiety attack would be increased respirations, palpitations, dizziness, or nausea. The therapist may want to engage in conversation to diffuse the anxiety or participate in a relaxing activity or guided imagery. If the patient verbalized or acted in a way that indicated they might be a risk to themselves or others, then a mental health professional or physician should be notified immediately, and the patient should not be left alone. Avoid being dismissive of the patient's report and provide motivation to continue.

2. The answer is **B**. Note the signs of agitation and determine the cause to remove or modify the agitating factor. Be respectful and clear in communication. Do not try to force the patient to maintain eye contact. Recognizing the signs of agitation before they escalate benefits both the patient and clinician.

3. The answer is **B**. Safety of the other patients and yourself would be the priority. Keeping the patient within site and exit calmly to call for help.

4. The answer is **D**. Mania is an affective disorder that affects mood with intense emotional changes. Anxiety attacks present with shortness of breath, palpitations, dizziness, or nausea. Paranoid personality disorder has characteristic distrust and paranoia. Finally, depression often has signs and symptoms of fatigue, disinterest, insomnia, and difficulty concentrating.

CHECKLIST

When you complete this chapter, you should be able to:
❑ Identify the structures comprising the genitourinary system.
❑ Identify specific clinical findings of selected pathologies affecting the genitourinary system.

❏ Identify pertinent diagnostic tests and measures to confirm the presence of selected genitourinary pathologies.

❏ Discuss pertinent medical imaging modalities to confirm the presence of selected genitourinary pathologies.

❏ Identify appropriate pharmacologic management of selected genitourinary conditions.

❏ List most common malignancies affecting the genitourinary system.

❏ Discuss the role of physical therapy in the medical management of selected genitourinary pathologies.

❏ Identify the main functions of the GI tract.

❏ List general classifications of signs and symptoms associated with GI disease.

❏ Identify the signs and symptoms of selected pathologies affecting the GI tract.

❏ Identify pertinent diagnostic tests and measures to confirm the presence of selected GI pathologies.

❏ Discuss pertinent medical imaging modalities to confirm the presence of selected GI pathologies.

❏ Recognize appropriate pharmacologic management of selected GI conditions.

❏ List the most common malignancies affecting the GI system.

❏ Discuss the role of physical therapy in the medical management of selected GI pathologies.

❏ Outline signs and symptoms of various endocrine pathologies.

❏ Compare hyperthyroidism and hypothyroidism.

❏ Compare hyperadrenalism and hypoadrenalism.

❏ Compare diabetes and metabolic syndrome.

❏ Describe the differences between hypoglycemia and hyperglycemia.

❏ List some of the lifestyle factors related to cancer.

❏ Describe the various stages of cancer.

❏ List some of the functional deficits associated with cancer treatments.

❏ List the most common complications associated with pregnancy.

❏ Describe some of the warning signs to be aware of when a pregnant patient is exercising.

❏ Outline signs and symptoms of selected lymphatic conditions.

❏ Identify clinical implications of lymphatic pathologies.

❏ Discuss the role of the PTA in the management of a patient with lymphatic pathology.

❏ Compare types of psychological disorders and their clinical significance.

❏ List the signs indicating a patient may need a referral for mental health consultation.

❏ Identify signs of agitation and strategies to de-escalate.

❏ List methods to improve patient participation in rehabilitation.

REFERENCES

1. Flenaugh EL, Henriques-Forsythe MN. Lung cancer disparities in African Americans: health versus health care. *Clin Chest Med*. 2006;27:431-439, vi.

2. Kendall J, Catts ZA, Kendall C, Jones L. African Americans' knowledge of cancer genetic counseling: an examination of information delivery. *Del Med J*. 2006;78:453-458.

3. O'Keefe SJ, Chung D, Mahmoud N, et al. Why do African Americans get more colon cancer than Native Africans? *J Nutr*. 2007;137:175S-182S.

4. Overmyer M. Search narrows for gene tied to prostate cancer in African-Americans. *RN*. 2007;70:suppl 2.

5. Goodman CC, Snyder TK. Oncology. In: Goodman CC, Boissonnault WG, Fuller KS, eds. *Pathology: Implications for the Physical Therapist*. 2nd ed. Philadelphia, PA: Saunders; 2003:236-263.

6. Moini J, Chaney C. *Introduction to Pathology for the Physical Therapist Assistant*. 2nd ed. Burlington, MA: Jones & Bartlett Learning; 2021.

7. O'Sullivan SB, Schmitz TJ, Fulk G. *Physical Rehabilitation*. 7th ed. Philadelphia, PA: FA Davis; 2019.

8. Sheir D, Butler J, Lemiw R. *Hole's Anatomy and Physiology*. 15th ed. New York, NY: McGraw-Hill; 2019.

9. Goss JA, Greene AK. Sensitivity and specificity of the Stemmer sign for lymphedema: a clinical lymphoscintigraphic study. *Plast Reconstr Surg Glob Open*. 2019;7:e2295.

10. Merck Manual Professional Edition. Available from: https://www.merckmanuals.com/professional. Accessed April 26, 2021.

11. National Lymphedema Network. Available from: https://lymphnet.org/. Accessed May 1, 2021.

12. Bjork R. The long and short of it: understanding compression bandaging. Available from: http://old.woundcareadvisor.com/. Accessed May 1, 2021.

13. Megens A, Harris SR. Physical therapist management of lymphedema following treatment for breast cancer: a critical review of its effectiveness. *Phys Ther*. 1998;78:1302-1311.

14. Safety JCQ. De-escalation in health care. Available from: https://www.jointcommission.org/-/media/tjc/documents/resources/workplace-violence/qs_deescalation_1_28_18_final.pdf?db-=web&hash=DD556FD4E3E4FA13B64E9A4BF4B5458A. Accessed April 24, 2021.

Non-Systems

CASSADY BARTLETT · JANICE LWIN

OVERVIEW

The non-systems portion of the examination covers those topics that do not fit into a particular category and include important areas that the physical therapist assistant (PTA) must be aware of to ensure patient safety.

■ EMERGENCY PREPAREDNESS

Every PTA's responsibility is to maintain current clinical prediction rule (CPR) certification and training and basic first aid knowledge. In all settings, the PTA should be aware of facility, agency, or management policies and protocols regarding disaster response and their role in the situation (Table 10-1). Within the home health setting, the PTA should be aware of the disaster levels of the patients and follow up after a natural disaster within the appropriate time frame. If a facility has to be evacuated, the PTA should assist as needed, providing the appropriate assistive device (AD) for ambulatory patients and coordinating with other interdisciplinary teams (IDTs) to provide oxygen and other medical support as appropriate.

CARDIAC EVENTS

All patients should be constantly monitored for their response to activity when participating in physical therapy. Exercise protocols, including maximum heart rates and response to activity, should be adhered to. In addition, patients on medications or pacemakers to control heart rate should be carefully monitored with rating of perceived exertion (RPE) scales to ensure they are not overdoing physical activity.

Any unexpected event, such as obvious bleeding, severe dyspnea, changes in pallor, or profuse sweating, should be acted upon in the same way as a fall (see Chapter 8). Facility protocols should be followed, and inpatient facilities should involve nursing and the MD, while outpatient and home health follow policies and determine whether to call 911 for additional medical support. In all cases, clear and accurate documentation of the event and the actions must be made immediately to ensure a timely and accurate recall of the situation.

TABLE 10-1 • Emergency Response.					
Location	**Policies**	**Obvious Injury**	**No Obvious Injury**	**Follow-up**	**Who to Contact**
Outpatient clinic	Follow clinic policy and procedures	Call 911 for medical support	Get patient up, take vital signs; if normal, continue with caution and patient consent	Continue to monitor the patient and only allow them to leave the clinic if you are sure they are stable and safe	Primary care physician Management of the facility
Home health setting	Follow agency policies and contact the agency immediately	Call 911 for medical support	Get patient up, take vital signs; if normal, continue with caution	Continue to monitor the patient throughout the session and do not leave the home until you are sure the patient is safe and stable and not alone	Home health agency Primary care physician Family as appropriate with patient consent
Inpatient setting	Follow facility protocols	Call nursing, emergency response team, and/ or MD to the location	Call nursing and/or MD to the location Get patient up and continue per MD recommendations	Complete all facility paperwork and ensure that all appropriate follow-up calls will be made, or make them as needed	Ensure nursing has agreed to contact family and physician; otherwise, the PT may be required to do so. Document all calls made.

Reproduced with permission from Burke-Doe A, Dutton M, eds. *National Physical Therapy Examination and Board Review.* 2019. Copyright © McGraw Hill LLC. All rights reserved. https://accessphysiotherapy.mhmedical.com.

■ INFECTION CONTROL

Infection control is a critical component of the health care industry. According to a World Health Organization report, health care–associated infections are a major public health problem because they can increase morbidity and mortality and burden the facility staff and patients. Most common infections include surgical incisions, gastrointestinal (GI) infections, respiratory and urinary tract infections. The very young, the very old, and those who are immunocompromised are at the greatest risk for infections.

The physical therapy department is a key area for infection risk due to high traffic and potential for cross-contamination. Therefore, the PTA must adhere to the standard and transmission-based precautions, including the use of personal protective equipment (PPE), hand hygiene, maintaining clean equipment, proper disposal of soiled linens, and biohazardous materials.

HAND HYGIENE

Hand hygiene is critical and should be performed before and after touching a patient or their surroundings, before a clean/aseptic procedure, after bodily fluid exposure risk, and hands should always be washed before the therapist consumes food or drink. Hand hygiene can be achieved through the application of hand sanitizer or accurate hand washing. Hand washing includes applying enough soap to cover surfaces followed by vigorous rubbing to cover all surfaces, including hands, fingers, and nails, before rinsing, which takes approximately 40 to 60 seconds. Alcohol-based hand sanitizer should be distributed over all hand surfaces until they feel dry, which should take approximately 20 to 30 seconds.

PRECAUTIONS FOR INFECTION CONTROL

Standard precautions are designed to minimize the spread of infection through careful hand hygiene, correct disposal of needles or sharps, use of protective clothing (gloves and gowns) if physical contact with the patient is anticipated, and careful disposal of soiled linens and waste from the patient.

Transmission-based precautions are more specific precautions designed for each of the different modes of infection transmission, contact, droplet, airborne, common vehicle, and vector-borne. Table 10-2 describes the minimal recommendations, but equipment such as

STUDY PEARL
When to wash your hands instead of using alcohol-based hand sanitizer?
- When hands are visibly soiled
- When working with a patient with known or suspected Infectious diarrhea, *Bacillus anthracis*, or *Clostridium difficile*
- After sneezing/blowing nose
- After using the restroom
- Before eating

TABLE 10-2 • Infection Control.

Mode of Infection	Example of Disease	Protective Equipment	Transportation Limitations
Contact	Skin, GI, or wound infection	Gown if in direct contact Gloves	Minimize transport out of the room
Droplet	Meningitis, influenza, pneumonia	Mask if within 3 ft of the patient Gown and gloves not required	Minimize transport, mask on the patient if leaving the room
Airborne	Measles, varicella, tuberculosis	Mask at all times (i.e. N-95 respirator) Gown and gloves not required	Minimize transport, mask on the patient if leaving the room
Common vehicle	Transmission by food, water, medication such as cholera	Depends on the infection At a minimum, standard precautions	Minimize transport
Vector	Transmission by mosquito, fly, rats, such as malaria	Depends on the infection At a minimum, standard precautions	

Reproduced with permission from Burke-Doe A, Dutton M, eds. *National Physical Therapy Examination and Board Review.* 2019. Copyright © McGraw Hill LLC. All rights reserved. https://accessphysiotherapy.mhmedical.com.

gloves can be added according to personal preference. It is also essential that all facility policies and procedures are followed.

COVID-19

According to the World Health Organization, a new coronavirus called SARS-CoV-2, commonly referred to as COVID-19, was discovered in late 2019 in Wuhan, China. A worldwide pandemic ensued with local, state, national, and international variations of mask mandates, school and business closures, and limitations to travel. This respiratory disease spread mainly person to person through respiratory droplets. People infected may have mild-to-severe symptoms, and others may be asymptomatic. The more severe illness risk fell upon adults age 65 years or older and people with underlying medical conditions. Specific precautions, including mask-wearing, maintaining 6-ft distance, and frequent hand washing, are recommended for the general public. Health care workers utilized standard and transmission-based precautions along with additional precautions to limit exposure (telehealth, limited occupancy/visitor policies, etc.). As science continues to collect data, there will likely be ongoing changes in recommendations for precautions, treatment, and vaccinations, requiring all health care workers to be aware of up-to-date policies and procedures.

■ ABUSE AND NEGLECT

Mandatory reporting procedures are in place at local, state, and federal levels to protect all of society but particularly the most vulnerable population, the young and the elderly. However, it is imperative to remember patients of all ages may experience various types of abuse (verbal, sexual, financial, domestic). Therefore, correct reporting of abuse, following facility protocols, and meeting local, state, and federal guidelines is critical. All abuse must be reported even if there is some level of doubt—that is for the authorities to determine. All facilities have abuse reporting policies that must be followed to meet the required standards.

Types of elder abuse include physical, financial, emotional/psychological, neglect, and sexual. These can occur within a facility setting, in the home, and the community. They can involve facility staff, family members, or strangers. Often clients will talk to the PTA during their treatment sessions, and careful note and follow-up must be made if there is a suspicion of abuse or neglect. In the home health setting, careful observation of the interactions between the patient and caregivers can sometimes reveal potential abuse. Signs of abuse, including withholding medication, not allowing visitors or phone calls, failure to provide adequate nutrition, or failure to provide support for activities of daily living, should be reported to the agency or facility management per policy.

Child abuse categories are similar to elder abuse and include neglect, physical, emotional, and sexual and can occur in any setting, typically occurring in combination rather than in isolation, and if observed or suspected, should be immediately reported per policy.

■ PATIENT CLIENT RIGHTS

AMERICANS WITH DISABILITIES ACT

The Americans with Disabilities Act (ADA) prohibits discrimination against those with disabilities concerning employment, transportation, public accommodation, communication, and government activities. The Office of Disability Employment Policy (ODEP) provides information and technical assistance on the ADA requirements but does not enforce any part of the law. However, all physical therapy clinics and all medical facilities must meet ADA standards, and the ODEP can assist with ensuring that these standards are met.

INDIVIDUALS WITH DISABILITIES EDUCATION ACT

The Individuals with Disabilities Education Act (IDEA) of 2004 and the resulting law ensures that children with disabilities receive the appropriate education provided by state and public agencies. The appropriate education includes early intervention, special education, and related services. Over 6.5 million infants, toddlers, children, and youths with a disability qualify under this act for special services.

HEALTH INSURANCE PORTABILITY AND ACCOUNTABILITY ACT

The Health Insurance Portability and Accountability Act (HIPAA) of 1996 ensures the protection of health information. The act sets standards for using and disclosing a person's health information, and failure to comply with the HIPAA rules is a federal offense. Privacy of health information includes discussing a patient with other people not authorized by the patient, including family members, leaving computers open and unmanned showing private health information, and talking about patients in an open area that can be overheard. In addition, the electronic transmission of medical information, including fax, scans, emails, and texts, is prohibited on open lines unless the information is encrypted. Any sharing of patient information should only be done with full awareness of the recipient and transmission mode. Employers must train all health care professionals on all aspects of the HIPAA and its implementation. If a violation of the HIPAA is suspected, it should immediately be reported to management per facility, agency, or corporate policy.

■ HUMAN RESOURCE LEGAL ISSUES

OCCUPATIONAL SAFETY AND HEALTH ADMINISTRATION

The Occupational Safety and Health Administration (OSHA) requires that all employers are responsible for providing a safe and healthful workplace under the laws of the US Department of Labor. To achieve this, employers must establish and enforce standards and provide training, education, and outreach assistance. The areas of consideration vary, depending on the type of work environment. For example, strict laws govern safety in agriculture, maritime work, construction, and the medical profession.

SEXUAL HARASSMENT

According to the US Equal Employment Opportunity Commission, it is unlawful for anyone, either applicant or employee, to be harassed in the workplace. Harassment includes sexual harassment, including unwelcome sexual advances, requests for sexual favors, or verbal or physical harassment of a sexual nature. Victims and harassers can be male or female and can be of the same sex. When frequent or severe enough to cause a hostile environment, or if it results in an adverse employment decision such as termination or demotion, it is illegal. Any suspicion of sexual harassment, whether personal or observed between others, should be reported per facility or management protocols.

■ DOCUMENTATION STANDARDS

The PTA is responsible for accurate and timely documentation of all occurrences, treatments, and incident reporting. Each arena, such as home health, inpatient, and outpatient, has unique aspects of documentation, and many corporations have additional documentation requirements for their employees.

The traditional SOAP note is still in use in many locations. In this style of documentation, the PTA uses the acronym for Subjective (information from the patient about their current state, how they feel, how things are going), Objective (documentation of tests, measures, and interventions), Assessment (the patient's response to treatment, including posttreatment measurements), and Plan (the thought process for the next patient–therapist interaction).

Health care settings are transitioning to electronic health records (EHRs) by the calendar year 2021 as CMS and the Office of the National Coordinator for Health Information Technology (ONC) have established this as criteria to be considered a meaningful user and avoid payment adjustments. These records often allow the PTA to access evaluations, laboratory results, etc, readily. However, it is illegal to access the medical record of personal family members and other individuals within the health setting unless the therapist is assigned to their care.

EHRs often have checkboxes with optional narrative sections. The PTA should always use the narrative sections to ensure adequate and individualized detail is provided in the documentation to provide an accurate picture of patient status and justify skilled physical therapy services. Litigation can take years, and a PTA facing an inquiry needs to utilize their documentation from the event to describe what occurred accurately. Falsification of medical records is illegal.

■ ROLES AND RESPONSIBILITIES OF THE INTERDISCIPLINARY HEALTH CARE TEAM

The appropriate delegation of work to support staff is highly regulated at the state level. Therefore, all practicing PTAs should be familiar with their state regulations concerning physical therapists, PTAs, PT technicians, and PT aides. For example, some states do not allow aides, while other states allow them but with varying levels of supervisory regulation.

The interdisciplinary team is an important component of any patient care, particularly in the inpatient setting. PTAs should learn the roles of the different professionals and communicate appropriately. These include but are not limited to the following:

- Occupational therapy.
- Speech and language therapy.
- Nursing.
- Social workers.
- Dietician.
- Orthotist and prosthetist.
- Physician, surgeon, primary care physician, nurse practitioner, physician's assistant.

Documentation of all patient-related discussions with any interdisciplinary team member must be completed, particularly when they relate to treatment intervention, such as changes in weight-bearing status, use of orthotics, and social setting changes that could affect discharge planning.

The American Physical Therapy Association (APTA) states the PT is responsible for the direction and supervision of the PTA by *general supervision*, which requires the PT to be available via telecommunication at all times. A student PT or student PTA must be supervised through *direct supervision* where the supervising therapist is physically present on-site and immediately available. *Direct personal supervision* also applies to the supervision of a physical therapy aide or when laws allow the PTA to be present and immediately available.

It is essential the PTA practice safely and legally, and the PT is responsible for the actions of the PTA during patient management. Therefore, the APTA has determined the initial specific skill set known as the APTA Minimum Required Skills of the PTA Graduates at Entry Level. Ultimately, it is the PTA's responsibility to know and understand the local, state, and federal laws and the conduct expected of a PTA.

Please see the following list of website references for a more detailed review of the content.

- American Physical Therapy Association.
  - https://www.apta.org/.
    - APTA Minimum Required Skills of PTA Graduates at Entry Level.
    - APTA Guide for Conduct of the PTA.
    - APTA Standards of Ethical Conduct for the PTA.
- National Institute of Health Patient's Bill of Rights.
  - https://clinicalcenter.nih.gov/participate/patientinfo/legal/bill_of_rights.html.

■ QUESTIONS

1. **A PTA arrives at a patient's home and finds the patient on the floor with an obvious injury to their right lower extremity. The caregiver is present but is evidently distressed. Which of the following actions is most appropriate for the therapist to perform?**
   A. Get the patient off the floor and take vital signs.
   B. Call 911 and the home health agency for medical support.
   C. Call the home health agency and report the incident.
   D. Call 911 and leave the patient with the caregiver to wait for the paramedics.

2. **A PTA is working in a skilled nursing facility and has been informed that the patient has measles. Which of the following precautions are the minimum requirements for the therapist while working with this patient?**
   A. Personal mask at all times.
   B. Mask if within 3 ft of the patient.
   C. Gown, gloves, and mask at all times.
   D. Gown if in direct contact with the patient.

3. **A PTA is working in the home of a patient with a long history of cardiac disease. The patient has recently had a pacemaker fitted and has been cleared for therapy to improve functional activity. Which of the following monitoring protocols is the most appropriate for the therapist to use with this patient?**
   A. Take pulse and respiratory rate regularly throughout the session.
   B. Continue working with the patient to 80% heart rate maximum.
   C. Do not exercise this patient as it is a contraindication.
   D. Exercise the patient using the rate of perceived exertion (RPE) scale to monitor exertion.

4. **A PTA works at a hospital their cousin has been admitted to. The cousin is very anxious to get the laboratory results back and asks the PTA to review the electronic health record to find out the results. What is the most appropriate response for the PTA?**
   A. Look at the chart and relay the laboratory results to assist the busy doctor.
   B. Ignore the patient and avoid addressing the question.
   C. Respectfully inform the patient that that would violate confidentiality rules, and they can only access the health record in order to provide care.
   D. State you cannot do so as it would violate the Americans with Disabilities Act (ADA).

5. **A PTA is treating a patient for an abnormal gait pattern. The patient asks the PTA if they can look at a wound on their heel and tell them what they should do about it. What would be the most appropriate response of the PTA?**
    A. Examine the wound and provide a dressing recommendation.
    B. Inform the patient that wound care is beyond the scope of physical therapy.
    C. Advise the patient to speak with the nurse next time she rounds.
    D. Explain to the patient the PT must be the one to perform the examination and evaluation and then establish a plan of care. Communicate the presence of the wound to nursing and the supervising PT.

■ ANSWERS WITH RATIONALES

1. The answer is **B**. If a patient has an obvious injury, medical support is critical, and the home health therapist should call 911 but must also call the home health agency to report and complete paperwork as required. The patient and caregiver should not be left until after the paramedics have arrived.

2. The answer is **A**. Measles is an airborne infection, so a mask must be worn at all times when working with the patient. Gown and gloves are not required but can be used if the therapist or the facility requires them.

3. The answer is **D**. The pacemaker is designed to keep the patient's heart rate at a specific level regardless of exercise intensity, so monitoring pulse and aiming at 80% heart rate maximum is inappropriate. Instead, using the RPE scale is the safest way to exercise a patient with a fitted pacemaker.

4. The answer is **C**. The patient should be addressed respectfully and explain this would be a misuse of the therapist's access to the electronic medical record (EMR). The therapist must only access health records necessary for patient care they are directly involved in providing.

5. The answer is **D**. The PTA cannot perform an examination or evaluation as this is the responsibility of the PT. Additionally, it would be imperative that a wound or change in status be communicated to the supervising PT and nursing staff.

■ TEACHING AND LEARNING

Education can be defined as any act or experience that has a formative effect on an individual's mind, character, or physical ability.

Learning refers to the ways people acquire, process, store, and apply new information. Learning is most effective when an individual is ready to learn, that is, when one wants to know something.

▲ HIGH-YIELD TERMS

Active learning	Having students engage in some activity forces them to reflect upon ideas and use those ideas. Requiring students to regularly assess their degree of understanding and skill at handling concepts or problems in a particular discipline. The attainment of knowledge by participating or contributing. The process of keeping students mentally, and often physically, active in their learning through activities that involve them in gathering information, thinking, and problem-solving.
Affective domain	Actions or behaviors controlled by feelings, attitudes, or values.
Cognitive domain	Actions or behaviors that are controlled by knowledge or understanding.
Decision-making	The reason that results in action.
Learning style	The preferred way in which a person absorbs, processes, comprehends, and retains knowledge.

Passive learning	A method of learning or instruction where students receive information from the instructor and internalize it, and where the learner receives no feedback from the instructor.
Problem-solving	Making, implementing, and evaluating decisions relating to some aspect of physical therapy.
Psychomotor domain	Manual or physical skills.
Reflection	The internal process of examining an experience that raises an issue of concern.
Sensory motor learning	Improvement, through practice, in the performance of sensory-guided motor behavior.
Teaching style	The general principles, pedagogy, and management strategies used for classroom instruction.

MOTIVATION

Motivation plays a critical role in the learning process, and success motivates more than failure (Table 10-3). Basic principles of motivation exist that apply to learning in any situation.

The environment can be used to focus the patient's attention on what needs to be learned. For example, interesting visual aids, such as booklets, posters, or practice equipment, motivate learners by capturing their attention and curiosity.

Incentives, including privileges and receiving praise from the educator, motivate learning. Both affiliation and approval are strong motivators.

Internal motivation is longer lasting and more self-directive than external motivation, which must be repeatedly reinforced by praise or concrete rewards.

MASLOW HIERARCHY OF NEEDS

Maslow hierarchy of needs is based on the concept that there is a hierarchy of biogenic and psychogenic needs that humans must progress through. Maslow hypothesizes that the higher needs in the hierarchy only come into focus once all the lower needs in the pyramid are mainly or entirely satisfied. Maslow hierarchy is often depicted as a pyramid consisting of five levels (Figure 10-1). The lower levels (physiologic and safety needs) are referred to as *deficiency needs*, while the top three levels (love/belonging, status, and self-actualization needs) are referred to as *being needs*. According to Maslow, for an individual to progress up the hierarchy to the *being needs*, the deficiency needs must be met. Growth forces (eg, personal growth, integration, and fulfillment) create upward movement in the hierarchy, whereas regressive forces (eg, sickness, discomfort, lack of security) push predominant needs further down the hierarchy.

DOMAINS OF LEARNING

Bloom[1] identified three domains of educational activities:

- **Cognitive:** Mental skills (knowledge).
  - Involves knowledge and the development of intellectual skills.
  - Includes the recall or recognition of specific facts, procedural patterns, and concepts that develop intellectual abilities and skills.
  - There are six major categories (degrees of difficulties) starting from the simplest behavior to the most complex, with the first one having to be mastered before the next one can take place (Table 10-4).
- **Affective:** Growth in feelings or emotional areas (attitude) (Table 10-5).
  - Includes how matters are dealt with from an emotional aspect.
  - Includes feelings, values, appreciation, enthusiasms, motivations, and attitudes.

TABLE 10-3 · Learning Theories.

Theory	Principle Elements	Strategies	Prominent Theorists	Clinical Application
Algo-heuristic	Identifying the mental processes (conscious and subconscious) that underlie expert learning, thinking, and performance in any area. All cognitive activities can be analyzed into operations of an algorithmic, semialgorithmic, heuristic, or semiheuristic nature. Teaching students how to discover processes is more valuable than providing them with already formulated processes.	Once discovered, the operations and their systems can serve as the basis for instructional strategies and methods.	L. Landa	Performing a task or solving a problem always requires a certain system of elementary knowledge units and operations.
Androgyny	Adults need to know why they need to learn something and experientially as they approach learning as problem-solving. Adults learn best when the topic is of immediate value.	There is a need to explain why specific things are being taught (eg, certain commands, functions, operations, etc). Learning activities should be in the context of common tasks to be performed instead of memorization. Instruction should consider the wide range of different backgrounds of learners; learning materials and activities should allow for different levels/types of previous experience with computers. Since adults are self-directed, instruction should allow learners to discover things for themselves, providing guidance and help when mistakes are made.	M. Knowles	Can be applied to any form of adult learning. Has been used extensively in the design of organizational training programs.
Adult learning	Integrates other theoretical frameworks for adult learning such as andragogy (Knowles), experiential learning (Rogers), and lifespan psychology. Consists of two classes of variables: personal characteristics (aging, life phases, and developmental stages) and situational characteristics (part-time vs full-time learning, and voluntary vs compulsory learning).	The three personal characteristics must be taken into consideration. Aging results in the deterioration of certain sensory motor abilities (eg, eyesight, hearing, reaction time) while intelligence abilities (eg, decision-making skills, reasoning, and vocabulary) tend to improve.	KP Cross	Adult learning programs should adapt to the aging limitations of the participants, while capitalizing on participants' experience. Adults should be challenged to move to increasingly advanced stages of personal development.
Behaviorist (stimulus-response theory)-operant conditioning	Learning is a function of a change in overt behavior. Changes in behavior result from an individual's response to events (stimuli) and their consequences that occur in the environment. The response of one behavior becomes the stimulus for the next response.	Positive reinforcement is used through the use of rewards that are meaningful to the individual. Timing of reinforcement. Continuous reinforcement: A behavior is reinforced every time it occurs. Partial reinforcement: A behavior is reinforced intermittently. Fixed interval: The time between the occurrences of each instance of reinforcement is fixed or set.	BF. Skinner, G. Watson	Limited clinical use: Behavior modification techniques may be used when working with adults with impaired or limited cognitive abilities or young children. Repetition is a necessary prerequisite for learning.

(Continued)

TABLE 10-3 • Learning Theories. (Continued)

Theory	Principle Elements	Strategies	Prominent Theorists	Clinical Application
Behaviorist (stimulus-response theory)-operant conditioning (cont.)	Learning occurs when an individual engages in specific behaviors to receive certain consequences (learned association). Behavior can be controlled or shaped by operant conditioning. Desired or correct behaviors are identified so that frequent and scheduled reinforcements (positive reinforcement) can be given to reinforce the desired behaviors. Negative behaviors are ignored (negative reinforcement) so that these behaviors become weakened to the point where they disappear (extinction).	Variable interval: The time between the occurrences of each instance of reinforcement varies around a constant average.		
Classical conditioning	First model of learning to be studied in psychology. Demonstrates the environment's control over behavior. Type of associative learning—relates the capacity of animals/humans to learn new stimuli and connect them to natural reflexes, allowing nonnatural cues to elicit a natural reflex. The conditioned stimulus, or conditional stimulus, is an initially neutral stimulus that elicits a response—known as a conditioned response—that is learned by the organism. Conditioned stimuli are associated psychologically with conditions such as anticipation, satisfaction (both immediate and prolonged), and fear. The relationship between the conditioned stimulus and conditioned response is known as the conditioned (or conditional) reflex. The process by which an individual learns to associate an unconditional stimulus with a conditional stimulus but receives no benefit from doing so.	Therapies associated with classical conditioning are aversion therapy, flooding, systematic desensitization, and implosion therapy. Much of what we like or dislike is a result of classical conditioning.	I. Pavlov, J.B. Watson	These techniques have been criticized for being unethical since they have the potential to cause trauma. Perhaps the strongest application of classical conditioning involves emotion. Common experience and careful research both confirm that human emotion conditions vary rapidly and easily, particularly when the emotion is intensely felt or negative in direction, it will condition quickly.
Cognitive dissonance	There is a tendency for individuals to seek consistency among their cognitions (ie, beliefs, opinions). When there is an inconsistency between attitudes or behaviors (dissonance), something must change to eliminate the dissonance. In the case of a discrepancy between attitudes and behavior, it is most likely that the attitude will change to accommodate the behavior.	There are three ways to eliminate dissonance: Reduce the importance of the dissonant beliefs. Add more consonant beliefs that outweigh the dissonant beliefs. Change the dissonant beliefs so that they are no longer inconsistent.	L. Festinger	Dissonance theory is especially relevant to decision-making and problem-solving.

Theory	Description	Theorist	Notes
Cognitive flexibility	Focuses on the nature of learning in complex and ill-structured domains. Emphasis is placed upon the presentation of information from multiple perspectives and use of many case studies that present diverse examples. Effective learning is context-dependent. Stresses the importance of constructed knowledge; learners must be given an opportunity to develop their own representations of information in order to properly learn.	Learning activities must provide multiple representations of content. Instructional materials should avoid oversimplifying the content domain and support context-dependent knowledge. Instruction should be case-based and emphasize knowledge construction, not transmission of information. Knowledge sources should be highly interconnected rather than compartmentalized.	R. Spiro, P. Feltovitch, R. Coulson	Limited: Cognitive flexibility theory is especially formulated to support the use of interactive technology.
Cognitive load	Learning happens best under conditions that are aligned with human cognitive architecture. The contents of long-term memory are sophisticated structures (schema) that permit us to perceive, think, and solve problems, rather than a group of rote-learned facts. Schemas are acquired over a lifetime of learning, and may have other schemas contained within themselves. The difference between an expert and a novice is that a novice hasn't acquired the schemas of an expert.	Change problem-solving methods to use goal-free problems or worked examples. Eliminate the working memory load associated with having to mentally integrate several sources of information by physically integrating those sources of information. Eliminate the working memory load associated with unnecessarily processing repetitive information by reducing redundancy. Increase working memory capacity by using auditory as well as visual information under conditions where both sources of information are essential (ie, nonredundant) to understanding.	J. Sweller	Cognitive load theory has many implications in the design of learning materials, such as handouts and home exercise programs.
Constructivist theory	Learning is an active process in which learners construct new ideas or concepts based on their current/past knowledge. Cognitive structure (ie, schema, mental models) provides meaning and organization to experiences and allows the individual to "go beyond the information given."	Instruction must be concerned with the experiences and contexts that make the student willing and able to learn (readiness). Instruction must be structured so that it can be easily grasped by the student (spiral organization). Instruction should be designed to facilitate extrapolation and/or fill in the gaps (going beyond the information given).	J. Bruner	Much of this theory is linked to child development.
Experiential learning	Two types of learning: Cognitive (meaningless)—academic knowledge such as learning vocabulary or multiplication tables. Experiential (significant)—applied knowledge such as personal change and growth.	Significant learning takes place when the subject matter is relevant to the personal interests of the student. Learning that is threatening to the self (eg, new attitudes or perspectives) is more easily assimilated when external threats are at a minimum. Learning proceeds faster when the threat to the self is low. Self-initiated learning is the most lasting and pervasive.	C. Rogers	Applies primarily to adult learners and adult learning.

(Continued)

TABLE 10-3 • Learning Theories. (Continued)

Theory	Principle Elements	Strategies	Prominent Theorists	Clinical Application
Genetic epistemology	Cognitive structures (ie, development stages) are patterns of physical or mental action that underlie specific acts of intelligence and correspond to stages of child development. There are four primary cognitive structures: Sensorimotor stage (0-2 years)—intelligence takes the form of motor actions. Preoperation period (3-7 years)—intelligence is intuitive in nature. Concrete operational stage (8-11 years)—cognition is logical but depends on concrete referents. Formal operations (12-15 years)—thinking involves abstractions.	Children will provide different explanations of reality at different stages of cognitive development. Cognitive development is facilitated by providing activities or situations that engage learners and require adaptation (ie, assimilation and accommodation). Learning materials and activities should involve the appropriate level of motor or mental operations for a child of given age; avoid asking students to perform tasks that are beyond their current cognitive capabilities. Use teaching methods that actively involve students and present challenges.	J. Piaget	The theory has been applied extensively to teaching practice and curriculum design in elementary education.
Modes of learning	Three modes of learning: Accretion: The addition of new knowledge to existing memory, the most common form of learning. Structuring: Involves the formation of new conceptual structures or schema. Tuning: The adjustment of knowledge to a specific task usually through practice, the slowest form of learning and accounts for expert performance.	Instruction must be designed to accommodate different modes of learning. Practice activities affect the refinement of skills but not necessarily the initial acquisition of knowledge.	D. Rumelhart, D. Norman	Multiple applications to physical therapy—general model for human learning.
Humanist	Emphasis placed on personal freedom, dignity of the individual, and the learner's needs and feelings during the learning process. The learner experiences unconditional positive regard, acceptance, and understanding. Promotes active rather than passive learning.	Teacher must function as a facilitator and resource finder. Learning must address relevant problems and issues.	A.H. Maslow	Used in clinical situations that emphasize self-discovery, self-appropriated learning, and experimental learning.
Social learning	The social learning theory emphasizes the importance of observing and modeling the behaviors, attitudes, and emotional reactions of others. Social learning theory explains human behavior in terms of continuous reciprocal interaction between cognitive, behavioral, and environmental influences.	The highest level of observational learning is achieved by first organizing and rehearsing the modeled behavior symbolically and then enacting it overtly. Coding modeled behavior into words, labels, or images results in better retention than simply observing. Individuals are more likely to adopt a modeled behavior if it results in outcomes they value, or if the model is similar to the observer and has admired status and the behavior has functional value.	A. Bandura	Applied extensively to the understanding of aggression and psychological disorders, particularly in the context of behavior modification.

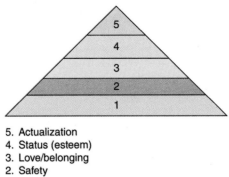

5. Actualization
4. Status (esteem)
3. Love/belonging
2. Safety
1. Physiologic (biological needs)

Figure 10-1. Maslow hierarchy of needs. (Reproduced with permission from Burke-Doe A, Dutton M, eds. *National Physical Therapy Examination and Board Review*. 2019. Copyright © McGraw Hill LLC. All rights reserved. https://accessphysiotherapy.mhmedical.com.)

- **Psychomotor:** Manual or physical aspects (skills).
  - Includes physical movement, coordination, and use of the motor skill areas.
  - Development of these skills requires practice and is measured in terms of speed, precision, distance, procedures, or techniques in execution.

The seven major categories of activities in the psychomotor domain are listed from the simplest to the most complex (Table 10-6).

DECISION-MAKING

Most theories accept the idea that decision-making consists of several steps or stages, such as recognition, formulation, the generation of alternatives, an information search, then selection, and action. Furthermore, it is well-recognized that routine cognitive processes

TABLE 10-4 • Cognitive Domain.	
Category	**Examples and Key Words**
Knowledge: Recall data or information.	Able to recite a poem; quote prices from memory. Key words: Defines, identifies, labels, lists, matches, names, outlines, recalls, recognizes, reproduces, selects
Comprehension: Understand the meaning, translation, interpolation, and interpretation of instructions and problems.	Able to rewrite a policy and procedures manual; can explain the steps for performing a complex task. Key words: Comprehends, distinguishes, estimates, explains, interprets, paraphrases, predicts, summarizes
Application: Use a concept in a new situation or unprompted use of an abstraction. Apply what was learned in the classroom to novel situations in the workplace.	Can use a manual to set up a video recorder, can apply the laws of statistics to evaluate a research study. Key words: Applies, computes, constructs, demonstrates, manipulates, modifies, operates, prepares, produces, relates, shows, solves
Analysis: Separate material or concepts into component parts so that its organizational structure may be understood. Distinguish between facts and inferences.	Can fix a piece of exercise equipment by using logical deduction; can gather information and select the required tasks for staff training. Key words: Analyzes, breaks down, compares, contrasts, differentiates, distinguishes, identifies, illustrates, infers, outlines, separates
Synthesis: Build a structure or pattern from diverse elements. Put parts together to form a whole, with emphasis on creating a new meaning or structure.	Can design or revise a process to perform a specific task, is able to integrate training from several sources to solve a problem. Key words: Categorizes, combines, compiles, composes, creates, devises, designs, generates, modifies, rearranges, reconstructs, reorganizes, summarizes
Evaluation: Make judgments about the value of ideas or materials.	Can select the most effective solution; hire the most qualified candidate; explain and justify a new budget. Key words: Appraises, compares, concludes, contrasts, critiques, discriminates, interprets, justifies, summarizes

TABLE 10-5 • Affective Domain: The Five Major Categories from the Simplest Behavior to the Most Complex.	
Category	**Example and Key Words**
Receiving phenomena: Awareness, willingness to hear, selected attention.	Able to listen to others with respect; listen for and remember the name of newly introduced people. Key words: Chooses, describes, follows, identifies, locates, names, points to, selects
Responding to phenomena: Active participation on the part of the learner. Attends and reacts to a particular phenomenon. Learning outcomes may emphasize compliance in responding, willingness to respond, or satisfaction in responding (motivation).	Is an active participant in staff discussions and is able to deliver an in-service presentation. Asks many questions about new ideas, concepts in order to fully understand them. Key words: Answers, assists, complies, conforms, discusses, labels, performs, practices, reads, recites, reports, tells, writes
Valuing: The worth or value a person attaches to a particular object, phenomenon, or behavior. This can range from simple acceptance to the more complex state of commitment.	Is sensitive toward individuals and various cultural differences. Informs management on matters that one feels strongly about. Key words: Completes, demonstrates, differentiates, initiates, invites, joins, justifies, proposes, reports, selects, shares
Organization: Organizes values into priorities by contrasting different values, resolving conflicts between them, and creating a unique value system. The emphasis is on comparing, relating, and synthesizing values.	Able to recognize the need for balance between freedom and responsible behavior. Accepts professional ethical standards. Prioritizes time effectively to meet the needs of the organization, family, and self. Key words: Adheres, alters, arranges, combines, compares, completes, defends, generalizes, identifies, integrates, modifies, organizes, relates, synthesizes
Internalizing values (characterization): Has a value system that controls their behavior. The behavior is pervasive, consistent, predictable, and most importantly, characteristic of the learner. Instructional objectives are concerned with the individual's general patterns of adjustment (personal, social, emotional).	Demonstrates self-reliance and can work independently, but also cooperates in group activities as a team player. Uses an objective approach in problem-solving. Values people for what they are, not how they look. Key words: Discriminates, displays, influences, listens, modifies, performs, proposes, qualifies, questions, revises, solves, verifies

such as memory, reasoning, and concept formation play a primary role in decision-making. In addition, decision-making behavior is affected (usually adversely) by anxiety and stress.

Clinical decision-making utilizes the clinician's knowledge and experience in collaboration with the patient, caregivers, and health care team to manage the multiple factors that may help or hinder the patient's progression. The evaluating physical therapist will integrate the ***patient/client management*** model upon start of care and determine the utilization of a PTA to deliver selected services. The PTA will follow the progression of this model under the supervision and direction of the evaluating PT. Throughout the course of care for each patient, the PTA will review all steps completed by the PT, participate in patient care, and communicate patient status to their supervising PT.

PROBLEM-SOLVING

Problem-solving skills appear to be related to many other aspects of cognition such as schema (the ability to remember similar problems), pattern recognition (recognizing familiar problem elements), and creativity (developing new solutions). The issue of transfer is highly relevant to problem-solving.

SENSORY MOTOR LEARNING

Motor skills can be classified as continuous (eg, tracking), discrete (eg, skills that have a definite beginning and end), or procedural (eg, typing). Behavioral psychology emphasizes using practice variables in sensory motor skills such as massed (concentrating the teaching or practice in a short period) versus spaced practice (distributing the teaching or practice over a longer period), part versus whole-task learning, and feedback/reinforcement schedules. Long-term retention of motor skills depends on regular practice. Learning

TABLE 10-6 • Psychomotor Domain.	
Category	**Examples and Key Words**
Perception: The ability to use sensory cues to guide motor activity.	Able to detect nonverbal communication cues; can estimate where a moving ball will land and can move to the correct location to catch the ball. Key words: Chooses, detects, differentiates, distinguishes, identifies, isolates, relates, selects
Set: Readiness to act—includes mental, physical, and emotional sets.	Knows and acts upon a sequence of steps in a construction process. Is able to recognize own abilities and limitations. Key words: Initiates, displays, explains, proceeds, reacts, states, volunteers
Guided response: The early stages in learning a complex skill that includes imitation and trial and error.	Can perform an exercise as demonstrated; follows instructions well. Key words: Copies, traces, follows, reproduce
Mechanism: This is the intermediate stage in learning a complex skill.	Can use a personal computer effectively; able to perform simple DIY projects at home; can drive a car. Key words: Assembles, calibrates, constructs, dismantles, fixes, manipulates, measures, mends, organizes
Complex overt response: The skillful performance of motor acts that involve complex movement patterns in a quick, accurate, and highly coordinated manner and with a minimum expenditure of energy.	Can parallel park a car into a tight spot. Displays skill and competence while playing sports. Key words: The same as for mechanism, except that the performance is quicker, better, more accurate, etc.
Adaptation: Skills are well developed and the individual can modify movement patterns to fit special requirements.	Responds effectively to unexpected experiences; able to modify instructions to meet the needs of the learners. Key words: Adapts, alters, changes, rearranges, reorganizes, revises, varies
Origination: Can create new movement patterns to fit a particular situation or specific problem.	Able to independently develop a new and comprehensive training program or exercise protocol. Key words: Arranges, builds, combines, composes, constructs, creates, designs, initiates

and retention of sensory motor skills are improved by the quantity and quality of feedback (knowledge of results) during training. Two ways in which learning/teaching of motor skills can be facilitated include the following:

- Slowing down the rate at which the information is presented.
- Reducing the amount of information that needs to be processed.

There is evidence that mental rehearsal, especially involving imagery, facilitates performance because it allows additional memory processing related to physical tasks (eg, schema formation) or because it maintains arousal or motivation for an activity.

LEARNING STYLES

There are several different theories regarding learning styles. However, it is not feasible to incorporate every learning theory into every session. One approach classifies learning styles as follows[2]:

- Accommodators. These learners look for the significance of the learning experience and enjoy being active participants in their learning, often asking many questions such as "What if?" and "Why not?"
- Divergers. These learners are motivated to discover the relevance of a given situation and prefer to have information presented to them in a detailed, systematic, and reasoned manner.
- Assimilators. These learners are motivated to answer the question, "What is there to know?" They like an accurate, organized delivery of information, and they tend to respect the expert's knowledge. These learners are perhaps less "instructor intensive" than some other learning styles. They will carefully follow prescribed exercises, provided a resource person is available and able to answer questions.

STUDY PEARL

Some form of guided learning seems most appropriate when high proficiency in a new skill is involved. On the other hand, if the task is to be recalled and transferred to a new situation, a problem-solving strategy may be better.

STUDY PEARL

Many forms of sensory motor behavior are learned by imitation, especially complex movements such as dance, singing, crafts, or manual therapy techniques.

- Convergers. These learners are motivated to discover the relevancy or "how" of a situation. The instructions given to this type of learner should be interactive, not passive.

Another series of learning styles that are used frequently were devised by Taylor,[3] who proposed three common learning styles:

- Visual. As the name suggests, the visual learner assimilates information by observation, using visual cues and information such as pictures, anatomic models, and physical demonstrations.
- Auditory. Auditory learners prefer to learn by having things explained to them verbally.
- Tactile. Tactile learners, who learn through touch and interaction, are the most difficult of the three groups to teach. Close supervision is required with this group until they have demonstrated to the clinician that they can perform the exercises correctly and independently. Proprioceptive neuromuscular facilitation (PNF) techniques, emphasizing physical and tactile cues, often work well with this group.

Other learner styles include the following:

Analytical learner. The analytical/objective learner processes information in a step-by-step order, objectively perceives information and can use facts and easily understand the relationships between them. This type of learner perceives information in an abstract, conceptual manner; information does not need to be related to personal experience. As this type of learner may have difficulty comprehending the big picture, a step-by-step learning process with some form of structure is recommended.

Intuitive/global learner. The intuitive/global learner processes all of the information at once and not in an ordered sequence. Global learners are spontaneous and intuitive, tend to learn in layers, absorb material almost randomly without seeing connections, and then suddenly "get it." The learning of this type reflects personal life experiences and is thus subjective. As this type of learner tries to relate the subject matter to things they already know, information needs to be presented interestingly using attractive materials.

REASONING: INDUCTIVE VERSUS DEDUCTIVE REASONING

Inductive and deductive reasoning are two methods of logic used to arrive at a conclusion based on information assumed to be true. Both are used in research to establish hypotheses.

- Deductive reasoning: Involves a hierarchy of statements or truths and arrives at a specific conclusion based on generalizations.
- Inductive reasoning: Essentially the opposite of deductive reasoning. It involves trying to create general principles by starting with many specific instances.
- Initiative: Active versus passive learning.
- Active/aggressive learner: Exhibits initiative, actively seeks information; may reach conclusions quickly before gathering information.
- Passive learner: Often exhibits little initiative; responds best to direct learning.

TEACHING STYLES

Bicknell-Holmes and Hoffman[4] describe a variety of teaching methods that correlate with most learning styles. These techniques involve active, or discovery, learning—the patient can actively participate in the learning process, which is in direct contrast with a teaching method such as lecturing, where the learner is a passive observer. Discovery learning has certain attributes:

- Emphasizes learning over content.
- Uses failure as an opportunity to learn.
- More is learned by doing than by watching.
- Involves patients in higher levels of cognitive processing.

Some of the methods of discovery learning include the following:

- Case-based learning: A fairly common active learning strategy in which the patient can participate in the decision-making or problem-solving process.
- Incidental learning: Learning is linked to game-like scenarios.
- Learning by exploring: A collection of questions and answers on a particular topic is organized into a system, and patients can explore the various topics at their own pace.
- Learning by reflection: A type of active learning that involves higher-level cognitive skills—patients are expected to model certain skills or concepts they have acquired through their instructor or another learning system.
- Simulation-based learning: The clinician creates an artificial environment where patients can practice skills or apply concepts they have learned without the pressure of a real-world situation.
- Real-life examples: Using real-life problems and examples in various scenarios (buying a house/car; using a bus schedule, etc).
- Relevant instruction: Instruction should be practical, and the examples and exercises should be important and meaningful to the patients because patients often need to know why they need to learn a particular skill or concept or how it will benefit them in their everyday lives.
- Humor: To help keep the patients engaged and interested and to make their sessions more enjoyable.

IMPROVING COMPLIANCE WITH LEARNING AND PARTICIPATION

Several factors have been outlined to improve compliance, including the following:

- Involving the patient in the intervention planning and goal setting.
- Realistic goal setting for both short- and long-term goals.
- Promoting high expectations regarding the outcome.
- Promoting perceived benefits.
- Projecting a positive attitude.
- Providing clear instructions and demonstrations with appropriate feedback.
- Keeping the exercises pain-free or with a low level of pain.
- Encouraging patient problem-solving.

COMMUNITY AND STAFF EDUCATION

When presenting community education programs or educating staff, the strengths and weaknesses of various teaching methods are outlined in Table 10-7.

USING VISUAL AIDS

Several guidelines when using visual aids are outlined in Table 10-8.

REFLECTION

Reflection is the internal process of examining an experience that raises concern to help refine our understanding of an experience, which may lead to changes in our perspectives. Literature suggests that expert clinicians routinely use the reflective process. In their study of expert clinicians, Jensen et al.[5] noted that the reflective process was a key factor that set expert clinicians apart from their peers. Reflection is integral to clinical decision-making (Table 10-9).

■ PATIENT/CLIENT MANAGEMENT

EXAMINATION

PT role: Collect subjective and objective data to identify impairments, activity limitations, and participation restrictions. During this ongoing process, the PT will perform reexaminations as needed to check progress, assess a change in status requiring modification of plan of care (POC), or discontinue services.

TABLE 10-7 • Teaching Methods.

Teaching Method	Strengths	Weaknesses	Preparation
Lecture	Presents factual material in a direct, logical manner Contains experience which inspires Useful for large groups	Experts are not always good teachers Audience is passive Learning is difficult to gauge Communication is one-way	Needs a clear introduction and summary Needs time and content limit to be effective Should include examples, anecdotes
Lecture with discussion	Involves audience, at least after the lecture An audience can question, clarify, and challenge	Time may limit the discussion period Quality is limited to the quality of questions and discussion	Requires that questions be prepared before discussion
Panel of experts	Allows experts to present different opinions Can provoke better discussion than a one-person discussion Frequent change of speakers keeps attention from lagging	Experts may not be good speakers Personalities may overshadow content Subject may not be in logical order	Facilitator coordinates focus of panel; introduces and summarizes Briefs panel
Brainstorming	Listening exercise that allows creative thinking for new ideas Encourages full participation because all ideas equally recorded Draws on group's knowledge and experience Spirit of congeniality is created One idea can spark off other ideas	Can be unfocused Needs to be limited to 5-7 minutes People may have difficulty getting away from known reality If not facilitated well, criticism and evaluation may occur	Facilitator selects issue Must have some ideas if group needs to be stimulated
Videotapes/slides	Entertaining way of teaching content (colorful) and raising issues Keeps group's attention Looks professional Stimulates discussion Demonstrates three-dimensional movement	Can raise too many issues to have a focused discussion Discussion may not have full participation Only as effective as the following discussion Can be expensive	Need to set up equipment Effective only if facilitator prepares questions to discuss after the show
Discussion	Pools ideas and experiences from group Effective after a presentation, film, or experience that needs to be analyzed Allows everyone to participate in an active process	Not practical with more than 20 people Few people can dominate Others may not participate Is time-consuming Can get off the track	Requires careful planning by a facilitator to guide discussion Requires question outline
Small group discussion	Allows participation of everyone People often more comfortable in small groups Can reach group consensus	Needs careful thought as to the purpose of group Groups may get sidetracked	Need to prepare specific tasks or questions for the group to answer
Role-playing	Introduces problem situation dramatically Provides an opportunity for people to assume roles of others and thus appreciate another point of view Allows for exploration of solutions Provides opportunity to practice skills	People may be too self-conscious Not appropriate for large groups People may feel threatened	Trainer has to define problem situation and roles clearly Trainer must give very clear instructions
Case studies	Develops analytic and problem-solving skills Allows for exploration of solutions for complex issues Allows patient to apply new knowledge and skills	People may not see relevance to own situation Insufficient information can lead to inappropriate results	Case must be clearly defined Case study must be prepared
Guest speaker	Personalizes topic Breaks down audience's stereotypes	May not be a good speaker	Contact speakers and coordinate Introduce speaker appropriately

TABLE 10-8 • Guidelines for the Use of Visual Aids.		
Overheads	**Flip Charts**	**Slides**
Use the most professional lettering available. Use transparencies of one color only and secure transparencies to cardboard frames (if available). Number each transparency. Before the session, check overheads for readability of type size by audience at far end of the room. Printing should be no smaller than 1/4" high. Information should be placed on the top two-thirds of the transparency. Be familiar with the operation of the projector and make sure projector works. Have extra bulbs available. While presenting, be certain neither you nor the projector blocks anyone's view. Use a pencil rather than a finger to note a detail on the transparency. If you have a list of points, black out all but the first point, then move the cover sheet one point at a time.	Choose a chart size that is appropriate for the design, your height, and the size of the audience. Draw the art to fit the vertical shape of the chart. Make the lettering dark enough and large enough to be read by everyone in the audience. During preparation, leave several blank pages between each written page to allow for corrections and additions. For the final presentation, remove all but one blank page at the beginning so that you can turn to that blank page when there is no relevant visual. Securely attach the chart to the easel and adjust the easel height for the presentation. When writing on the flip chart, don't speak to the chart.	Slides should be used instead of flip charts if the group is large. Design the visuals for continuous viewing and as notes. Maintain continuity—have all slides horizontal or vertical, not mixed. Allow sufficient production time. Place no more than 15 words per slide. Use black or blue background with bright colors. Check the position and order of the slide in the carousel or tray. Use a conventional pointer. Keep as many lights on as possible.

PTA role: Read and review the content of this evaluation and be aware of baseline data on initial examination and clinical implications. The PTA may assist in data collection for the PT to use in their evaluation process.

EVALUATION

PT role: Analyze the data collected during the examination to identify clinical problems, treatment priority, and make a clinical judgment to develop a diagnosis, prognosis, and plan of care. The PT must consider any comorbidities, barriers to treatment, and condition severity.

PTA role: Read and review the PT's interpretation of collected data and be prepared to perform ongoing data collection for assessment by the PT.

DIAGNOSIS AND PROGNOSIS

PT role: After evaluating collected data, the PT will determine a physical therapy diagnosis concerning impairment, activity limitation, and participation restrictions. The ***medical diagnosis*** is determined by the physician who identifies the illness, disorder, or pathology. In addition, the PT will determine the ***prognosis***, which will predict potential patient improvement and how long it will take.

PTA role: Be aware of both the medical and physical therapy diagnosis and the prognosis and clinical implications.

TABLE 10-9 • Different Types of Reflection.	
Element	**Definition**
Reflection-in-action	Analyzing the effectiveness of one's own cues and handling as well as patient performance and behaviors; decisions are made and interventions may be modified
Reflection-on-action	Thinking about clinician–patient interaction and performance once the treatment session is over
Reflection-for-action	Thinking about one's own prior experiences that lead to ways of thinking about clinical decision-making and professional practice that is broader than one-on-one practice

PLAN OF CARE

PT role: To develop an outline for the intended course of treatment, considering the patient's goals and the data collected to facilitate improved functional performance and/or societal interaction. The POC will include the *goals* (intended functional change), *outcomes* (actual functional achievement), prognosis, list of interventions to use, and the anticipated *discharge* (discontinuation of care).

PTA role: The PTA is responsible for reading and reviewing the entire POC to be aware of goals, what the PT has designated intervention categories, and staying within an updated plan of care.

INTERVENTIONS

PT and PTA roles: Actively participate in communication with patient/client/caregivers, coordinate care with patient/caregivers/other health care disciplines, and administer direct patient care through purposeful interactions according to the examination/evaluation/diagnosis/POC to meet set goals or outcome expectations. Treating therapists must be aware of any legal limitations to the scope of the PT or PTA skill set and modify interventions according to patient response/status to ensure patient safety.

OUTCOMES

PT and PTA roles: Ongoing data collection by the treating therapists is necessary to compare baseline status to posttreatment status to determine progress. The discharge occurs if one of three results occurs: the established goals/outcomes are met, there is a lack of progression, or no further benefit is evident. Additionally, the patient may decline or become physically, mentally, or financially unable to continue treatment. The documentation must include the patient's status, including met goals, the rationale for discharge, and any referrals or education. The PT will perform the discharge examination and evaluation, but the PTA may assist in data collection.

■ CULTURAL INFLUENCES

Clinicians must be sensitive to cultural issues in their interactions with patients. Cultural influences shape the framework within which people view the world, define and organize reality, and function in their everyday life. Individuals often group themselves based on cultural similarities, and as a result, form cultural groups. Cultural groups share behavioral patterns, symbols, values, beliefs, and other characteristics that distinguish them from other groups. Cultural differences are generally variations of differing emphasis or value placed on particular practices at the group level.

The PTA should be aware of potential differences and avoid forcing a patient to conform to different cultural beliefs. Being open to learning about the patient's values and attitudes and overcoming language barriers by using available resources such as interpreters or consultants can improve the quality of communication and build trust with the patient. In addition to language, cultures vary in their beliefs about societal roles, attitude toward health care, modesty, and how to offer the best care to loved ones. The PTA should be respectful and attempt to understand each cultural background to be aware of their comfort level.

■ RESEARCH AND EVIDENCE-BASED PRACTICE

EVIDENCE-BASED PRACTICE

Evidence-based medicine (EBM) is incorporated into physical therapy practice to continually utilize the most effective treatment techniques and approaches to therapy. Evidence-based practice (EBP) integrates the most current clinical research with clinical expertise and specific patient needs to determine best practice and decision-making for optimum patient outcomes.[6]

STUDY PEARL

The PTA may encounter a variety of clinical situations and must modify or coordinate appropriate care.

- Language barrier—use an interpreter for verbal communication and give home program instructions in their primary spoken language.
- Communication—acceptable eye contact or personal space may vary from culture to culture.
- Modesty—the patient may require the treating therapist to be of the opposite gender or require more draping to expose less skin.
- Societal roles—certain family members may be the primary decision-maker, and family education will be important to allow an informed decision.

The following components describe how EBP is incorporated into patient care to help clinicians select the most appropriate interventions for positive outcomes[7]:

1. **ASK** a clinically relevant question relating to physical therapy practice.
2. **SEARCH** the literature for current research and evidence to answer the question.
3. **APPRAISE** the evidence through critical analysis of validity, reliability, and applicability to the question.
4. **INTEGRATE** research findings with clinical expertise and specific patient needs.
5. **EVALUATE** the effectiveness of outcomes.
6. **DISSEMINATE** evidence to the physical therapy community and utilize it in practice.

LEVELS OF EVIDENCE

When using literature and research to support clinical decision-making for patient care, the clinician should consider the type of evidence utilized. When reviewing journal articles, a hierarchy of categories exists to rank research in terms of strength and quality of design, which will guide the clinician in the amount of confidence to incorporate the study results into sound clinical decision-making (Figure 10-2).[8]

Systematic Reviews

Existing literature is systematically reviewed to create a comprehensive summary of evidence discussing a specific clinical question.[9] The systematic review critically appraises research design, including methodology, validity, and findings.[9] This is the strongest level of evidence.

Meta-Analysis

Systematic reviews can further undergo statistical analysis of outcomes determined in the summary section of the article. This meta-analysis process integrates the results of the studies in the systematic review to strengthen the power of findings as it allows analysis of a larger sample size.[9] This is also the strongest level of evidence.

Randomized Control Trials. Experimental research assessing the effects of a specific variable on a population. This research has an independent variable (ie, an intervention) and a dependent variable (ie, the intervention outcomes). Subjects are randomly assigned to at least one experimental group or a control group. The **experimental group** receives the intervention while the **control group** does not. The **control group** may also receive a placebo or false treatment designed to simulate the actual intervention. The study aims to provide a nearly identical experience for both groups during the study. A **single-blind** study has either

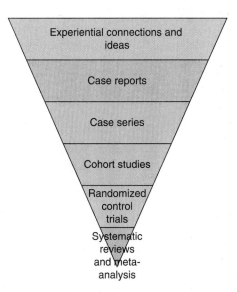

Figure 10-2. A diagrammatic representation of the different evidence levels.

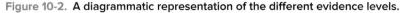

the researcher or subject blind, meaning the party is unaware of whether the experiment is being administered during the investigation. A ***double-blind*** study has both researcher and subject blind to who is receiving the experimental treatment. With the randomized assignment of variables, bias is minimized while the strength of results is increased.[9]

Cohort Studies

Subjects with a similar condition are followed over a long period in this longitudinal, observational study. This type of study can be done prospectively (in the future) or retrospectively (information from the past). Excessive length of study and introduction of other variables can negatively affect the strength of this type of study.[9]

Case Series

Compilation of multiple studies observing a similar case or variable.[10]

Case Report

Observation of an individual's response to treatment or condition. Case reports do not test hypotheses but may be useful in identifying a hypothesis or theory and inspiring additional research.[10]

ETHICS IN RESEARCH

When performing quality research, the subject's safety, well-being, and autonomy to participate must be protected. The following components are ethical considerations when conducting research using human subjects.

Human Subject

The cooperative participant in a study on whom research will be conducted. The researcher must ensure the subject is informed and willing to participate.

Informed Consent

Before beginning the research study, the subject is given a detailed summary of the study's investigation, methods and procedures, potential outcomes, and side effects (essentially the risks, benefits, and limitations). The subject can determine their desire to participate in the study based on the information presented and must be able to remove themselves from the study at any time.[9]

Confidentiality

Researchers have an ethical obligation to keep information revealed during the study private and not to disclose data, results, or other information except to authorized individuals.

Institutional Review Board

A group of scientists and non-scientists who ensure the rights and welfare of a subject participating in research is maintained. The Institutional Review Board (IRB) reviews a research proposal and determines approval.

RESEARCH PAPERS

Types of Research[10]

> ***Descriptive:*** Classification and understanding of clinical variables.
>
> ***Experimental:*** Determining cause-effect relationships between independent and dependent variables.
>
> ***Exploratory:*** Compares and examines a phenomenon and relationship to other relevant factors.

Components of A Research Paper[9]

Research papers have similar sections in the written document that helps standardize studies and literature. The sections are listed here in the order they tend to appear in research papers.

Abstract: A quick overview summary of the entire paper. Generally, one paragraph briefly introduces the topic and thesis, methods, results, and conclusion. Readers can gain a general understanding of the research from this section.

Introduction: Provides background to the research question and explains the purpose of the research. This section can include past research and support for the importance of the study. A thesis statement will also be included in this section.

Thesis: A statement often at the end of the introduction section that concisely states the study's main purpose. An *indirect thesis* generally describes the upcoming points of the paper (ie, three reasons why studying will help success on the NPTAE). A *direct thesis* points out the specific topics to be addressed in the paper (ie, studying hard, practice questions, and time management will promote success on the NPTAE).

Hypothesis: A proposition made to explain a phenomenon. A hypothesis is usually the spark for further research. A research paper may have either a thesis or a hypothesis statement.

- *Null hypothesis*: This claims there will be no statistical difference between variables in a study (ie, scapular stabilization exercises will not decrease the occurrence of rotator cuff injury in throwing athletes).
- *Alternative hypothesis*: This claims there *will* be a statistical difference in a variable based on the intervention (ie, the occurrence of rotator cuff injuries will decrease with the implementation of a specific scapular stabilizing exercise protocol).

Methods/Materials: A study's validity will be based on information in this section. This section must include a clear, concise outline of the research design, experimental variables (subjects, demographics, inclusion/exclusion criteria), study protocol, materials used, measurements, and calculations used.

Results: Statistical data analysis and comparisons are included in this section. Generally, raw results are presented here without much discussion or interpretation of data.

Discussion: This section provides a discussion of outcomes and interprets the findings based on the study results—it is a review of why the study was relevant, clinical comparisons or insights, and reintegration of introduction may be found in this section.

Conclusion: A summary of findings and significance toward clinical practice or research. Discussion of what was learned from this study, limitations, and suggestions for future studies.

DATA AND MEASUREMENT

Qualitative Data

Categorical data collected via surveys, interviews, or other interaction and study nonnumeric information such as hair color or food preference.

Quantitative Data

Numerical data collected and analyzed. These types of data represent a unique value for a data set, such as height or weight.

Levels of Measurement

Nominal scale: Variables classified into two or more mutually exclusive categories based on common characteristics (height, hair color).

Ordinal scale: Variables classified and ranked in order of sharing a common characteristic (grade point average [GPA], scores on a test).

Interval scale: Variables classified and ranked on predetermined intervals. There is no true zero for these values (temperature).

Ratio scale: Variables classified and ranked on common interval. There is a true zero for these values (goniometric measurement).

> **STUDY PEARL**
> When studies have a small subject pool, the strength of the study is weakened. The applicability of the study's results translating into a large population of people is also decreased. Studies should have a large subject size to ensure a significant population is represented.

Reliability

The ability for an instrument to consistently and accurately reproduce a measurement. **Threats to reliability** include random measurement errors or circumstances, such as blood pressure affected by anxiety, running speed affected by the ground surface.

> *Intrarater reliability:* Consistency of a measurement value to be repeated by the same person over time.[9]
>
> *Interrater reliability:* Consistency of a measurement value to be repeated by two or more persons over time.[9]
>
> *Test-retest reliability:* Consistency of a measurement value to be repeated on the same individual at separate time points.[9]

Validity

The degree to which an instrument accurately measures what it is intended to measure. Threats to validity include sampling bias by the researcher, failure to control subjects and variables, inaccuracy of the measurement instrument, pretest/ posttest influences, experimenter bias, the placebo effect (subjects receiving the placebo still have a positive outcome).

> *Content validity:* The degree to which an instrument measures the critical aspects of the variable being tested. Example: A questionnaire to assess balance should cover all aspects of balance.
>
> *Face validity:* An instrument measures what it is intended to measure. Example: A goniometer measures joint range of motion.
>
> *Construct validity:* The degree to which a test measures intangible factors such as thought process.
>
> *Internal validity:* The degree to which the dependent variable is affected by variations in the independent variable.
>
> *External validity:* The ability for results of a study to be extrapolated to a population outside the experimental design.
>
> *Concurrent validity:* Scores on two tests analyzing a similar factor, given at a similar time frame.
>
> *Predictive validity:* Scores from an instrument can be used to predict a future occurrence accurately. Example: High GRE scores predict future academic success.

Sensitivity

A test that correctly identifies every person in a study population who **has** the target disorder has a high sensitivity (1.0). A person who tests positive using a highly sensitive test is very likely to **have** the disorder tested. Therefore, anyone who tests *negative* when using a highly sensitive test will *not* have the disorder. The acronym "snOUT" is used because a sensitive test will help rule *out* a disorder when the test is negative.

Specificity

A test that correctly identifies every person in a study population that does **not** have the target disorder has a high specificity (1.0). A person who tests negative using a highly specific test is very likely **not** to have the disorder tested. Therefore, anyone who tests *positive* when using a highly specific test will **have** the disorder. The acronym "spIN" is used because a specific test will help rule *in* a disorder when the test is positive.

CLINICAL PREDICTION RULES

In physical therapy, clinical predication rules (CPRs) are often considered when determining best practice. CPRs are a cluster of findings that have statistically demonstrated a predictable outcome in determining a diagnosis. However, CPRs are often proven and disproven by researchers and clinicians; therefore, CPRs should be used as a guideline combined with clinical expertise to determine the most effective treatment for a patient.

NPTAE Practice Question

A PTA performs a goniometric measurement of a patient's shoulder flexion active range of motion. Which of the following characteristics describes the PTA's ability to reproduce the primary PT's measurements?
a. Specificity
b. Face validity
c. Intertester reliability
d. Intratester reliability

*Answer at the end of the chapter

CHECKLIST

When you complete this chapter, you should be able to:

❏ Compare and contrast various learning theories.

❏ Apply Maslow hierarchy of needs to patient performance.

❏ Use Bloom taxonomy to construct patient goals appropriate for their level of performance.

❏ Apply the concept of learning styles to improve patient education.

❏ Design appropriate visual aids for a given audience.

❏ Apply reflective elements to clinical practice.

❏ Define evidence-based practice.

❏ Describe the different levels of evidence.

❏ Outline the purpose of ethics in research.

❏ Describe the different components of a research paper.

❏ Discuss the differences between qualitative and quantitative data.

❏ Discuss the differences between sensitivity and specificity.

REFERENCES

1. Bloom BS. *Taxonomy of Educational Objectives, Handbook I: The Cognitive Domain*. New York, NY: David McKay Co Inc; 1956.

2. Litzinger ME, Osif B. Accommodating diverse learning styles: designing instruction for electronic information sources. In: Shirato L, ed. *What Is Good Instruction Now? Library Instruction for the 90s*. Ann Arbor, MI: Pierian Press; 1993:26-50.

3. Taylor JA. A practical tool for improved communications. Supervision. 1998;59:18-19.

4. Bicknell-Holmes T, Hoffman PS. Elicit, engage, experience, explore: discovery learning in library instruction. *Reference Services Review*. Emerald: Simmons College Library; 2000:313-322.

5. Jensen GM, Gywer J, Hack LM, Shepard KF. *Expertise in Physical Therapy*. 2nd ed. Boston, MA: Elsevier; 2006.

6. Sackett DL, Strauss SE, Richardson WS, et al. *Evidence Based Medicine: How to Practice and Teach EBM*. 2nd ed. Edinburgh, Scotland: Churchill Livingstone; 2000.

7. Lin SH, Murphy SL, Robinson JC. Facilitating evidence-based practice: process, strategies, and resources. *Am J Occup Ther*. 2010;64:164-171.

8. Bernadette MM. Integrating levels of evidence into clinical decision making. *Pediatr Nurs*. 2004;30:323-325.

9. Gresham B. *Concepts of Evidence Based Practice for the Physical Therapist Assistant*. Philadelphia, PA: FA Davis; 2016.

10. Portney L, Watkins M. *Foundations of Clinical Research: Applications to Practice*. 3rd ed. Hoboken, NJ: Prentice Hall; 2009.

∗Answer: c. Inter-tester reliability

Appendix A

The Shape, Resting Position, and Treatment Planes of the Joints

Mark Dutton

Joint	Convex Surface	Concave Surface	Resting Position	Treatment Plane and Relationship of the Osteokinematic Motion (OM) and Arthrokinematic Glide (AG)
Sternoclavicular	For elevation/depression, the sternum is concave, the clavicle is convex For protraction/retraction, the sternum is convex, the clavicle is concave		Arm resting by side	For elevation/depression the OM and AG are in opposite directions For protraction/retraction the OM and AG are in the same directions
Acromioclavicular	Clavicle	Acromion	Arm resting by side	OM and AG are in opposite directions
Glenohumeral	Humerus	Glenoid	55 degrees of abduction, 30 degrees of horizontal adduction	In scapular plane: OM and AG are in opposite directions
Humeroradial	Humerus	Radius	Elbow extended, forearm supinated	Perpendicular to long axis of radius: OM and AG are in the same directions
Humeroulnar	Humerus	Ulna	70 degrees of elbow flexion, 10 degrees of forearm supination	45 degrees to long axis of ulna: OM and AG are in the same directions
Radioulnar (proximal)	Radius	Ulna	70 degrees of elbow flexion, 35 degrees of forearm supination	Parallel to long axis of ulna: OM and AG are in the opposite directions
Radioulnar (distal)	Ulnar	Radius	Supinated 10	Parallel to long axis of radius: OM and AG are in the same directions
Radiocarpal	Proximal carpal bones	Radius	Line through radius and third metacarpal	Perpendicular to long axis of radius: OM and AG are in opposite directions
Intercarpal	Scaphoid	Trapezium and trapezoid	Midposition	Parallel to joint surfaces: OM and AG are in the same directions
Carpometacarpal joint of the thumb	For flexion/extension, the carpal is convex, the metacarpal is concave		Midposition	For flexion/extension: OM and AG are in the same directions
	For abduction/adduction the carpal is concave, the metacarpal is convex			For abduction/adduction: OM and AG are in opposite directions
Metacarpophalangeal (2-5)	Metacarpal	Proximal phalanx	Slight flexion	Parallel to joint: OM and AG are in the same directions

(Continued)

Joint	Convex Surface	Concave Surface	Resting Position	Treatment Plane and Relationship of the Osteokinematic Motion (OM) and Arthrokinematic Glide (AG)
Interphalangeal	Proximal phalanx	Distal phalanx	Slight flexion	Parallel to joint: OM and AG are in the same directions
Hip	Femur	Acetabulum	Hip flexed 30 degrees, abducted 30 degrees, slight external rotation	OM and AG are in opposite directions
Tibiofemoral	Femur	Tibia	Flexed 25 degrees	On surface of tibial plateau: OM and AG are in the same directions
Patellofemoral	Patella	Femur	Knee in full extension	Along femoral groove: OM and AG are in opposite directions
Talocrural	Talus	Mortise	Plantarflexed 10 degree	In the mortise in anterior/posterior direction: OM and AG are in opposite directions
Subtalar	Calcaneus	Talus	Subtalar neutral between inversion/ eversion	In talus, parallel to foot surface: OM and AG are in the same directions AG are in the same directions
Talonavicular	Talus	Navicular	Midposition	OM and AG are in the same directions
Calcaneocuboid	For flexion/extension the calcaneus is convex, the cuboid is concave For abduction/adduction, the calcaneus is concave, the cuboid is convex			For flexion/extension: OM and AG are in the same directions For abduction/adduction: OM and AG are in opposite directions
Metatarsophalangeal	Tarsal bone	Proximal phalanx	Slight extension	Parallel to joint: OM and AG are in the same directions
Interphalangeal	Proximal phalanx	Distal phalanx	Slight flexion	Parallel to joint: OM and AG are in the same directions

Reproduced with permission from Dutton M. *McGraw-Hill's NPTE (National Physical Therapy Examination)*, 2nd ed. 2012. Copyright © McGraw Hill LLC. All rights reserved. https://accessphysiotherapy.mhmedical.com.

Appendix B
Goniometric Techniques

Mark Dutton

Upper Extremity					
Joint	**Tested Motion/ Range (degrees)**	**Patient Position**	**Fulcrum/Axis**	**Stationary Arm**	**Moving Arm**
Shoulder	Flexion/0-170 to 180	Supine	Acromion process	Midaxillary line of the thorax	Lateral midline of the humerus using the lateral epicondyle of the humerus for reference
	Extension/0-50 to 60	Prone/supine with arm over edge	Acromion process	Midaxillary line of the thorax	Lateral midline of the humerus using the lateral epicondyle of the humerus for reference
	Abduction/0-170 to 180	Supine	Anterior aspect of the acromion process	Parallel to the midline of the anterior aspect of the sternum	Medial midline of the humerus
	Adduction (return from abduction)/180-0	Supine	Anterior aspect of the acromion process	Parallel to the midline of the anterior aspect of the sternum	Medial midline of the humerus
	Horizontal adduction/0-120	Seated	Superiorly on the acromion process of the scapula through the head of the humerus	Along the midline of the shoulder toward the neck	Along the midshaft of the humerus, in line with the lateral epicondyles of the humerus
	Horizontal abduction/0-120	Seated	Superiorly on the acromion process of the scapula through the head of the humerus	Aligned on the midline of the shoulder toward the neck	Along the midshaft of the humerus, in line with the lateral epicondyle of the humerus
	Internal rotation/ 0-60 to 100	Supine	Olecranon process	Parallel or perpendicular to the floor	Ulna using the olecranon process and ulnar styloid for reference
	External rotation/ 0-80 to 90	Supine	Olecranon process	Parallel or perpendicular to the floor	Ulna using the olecranon process and ulnar styloid for reference
Elbow	Flexion/0-145	Supine/seated	Lateral epicondyle of the humerus	Lateral midline of the humerus using the center of the acromion process for reference	Lateral midline of the radius using the radial head and radial styloid process for reference
	Extension/145-0	Supine/seated	Lateral epicondyle of the humerus	Lateral midline of the humerus using the center of the acromion process for reference	Lateral midline of the radius using the radial head and radial styloid process for reference

(Continued)

Upper Extremity *(Continued)*

Joint	Tested Motion/ Range (degrees)	Patient Position	Fulcrum/Axis	Stationary Arm	Moving Arm
Radioulnar	Pronation/0-90	Supine/seated	Lateral to the ulnar styloid process	Parallel to the anterior midline of the humerus	Posterior aspect of the forearm, just proximal to the styloid process of the radius and ulna
	Supination/0-90	Supine/seated	Medial to the ulnar styloid process	Parallel to the anterior midline of the humerus	Anterior aspect of the forearm, just proximal to the styloid process of the radius and ulna
Wrist	Flexion/0-90	Seated	Lateral aspect of the wrists over the triquetrum	Lateral midline of the ulna using the olecranon and ulnar styloid process for reference	Lateral midline of the fifth metacarpal
	Extension/0-70	Seated	Lateral aspect of the wrists over the triquetrum	Lateral midline of the ulna using the olecranon and ulnar styloid process for reference	Lateral midline of the fifth metacarpal
	Radial deviation/0-25	Seated	Over the middle of the posterior aspect of the wrist over the capitate	Posterior midline of the forearm using the lateral epicondyle of the humerus for reference	Posterior midline of the third metacarpal
	Ulnar deviation/0-35	Seated	Over the middle of the posterior aspect of the wrist over the capitate	Posterior midline of the forearm using the lateral epicondyle of the humerus for reference	Posterior midline of the third metacarpal
Thumb	Carpometacarpal flexion/0-15	Seated	Over the palmar aspect of the first carpometacarpal joint	Anterior midline of the radius using the anterior surface of the radial head and radial styloid process for reference	Anterior midline of the first metacarpal
	Carpometacarpal extension/0-70	Seated	Over the palmar aspect of the first carpometacarpal joint	Anterior midline of the radius using the anterior surface of the radial head and radial styloid process for reference	Anterior midline of the first metacarpal
	Carpometacarpal abduction/0-60	Seated	Over the lateral aspect of the radial styloid process	Lateral midline of the second metacarpal using the center of the second metacarpal or phalangeal joint for reference	Lateral midline of the first metacarpal using the center of the first metacarpal or phalangeal joint for reference
	Carpometacarpal adduction/60-0	Seated	Over the lateral aspect of the radial styloid process	Lateral midline of the second metacarpal using the center of the second metacarpal or phalangeal joint for reference	Lateral midline of the first metacarpal using the center of the first metacarpal or phalangeal joint for reference

(Continued)

Joint	Tested Motion/ Range (degrees)	Patient Position	Fulcrum/Axis	Stationary Arm	Moving Arm
	Metacarpophalangeal flexion/0-50	Seated	Over the posterior aspect of the metacarpophalangeal joint	Over the posterior midline shaft of the first metal bone	Over the posterior midline shaft of the proximal phalanx
	Metacarpophalangeal extension/0-10	Seated	Over the palmar aspect of the metacarpophalangeal joint	Aligned with the shaft of the first metacarpal on the palmar side	Along the palmar midline of the proximal phalanx of the thumb
	Interphalangeal flexion/0-80 to 90	Seated	Over the posterior surface of the interphalangeal joint	Along the posterior midline surface of the proximal phalanx	Along the posterior midline surface of the distal phalanx
	Interphalangeal extension/0-5	Seated	Over the interphalangeal joint on the palmar surface	Along the midline palmar surface of the proximal phalanx	On the palmar midline surface of the distal phalanx
Fingers	Metacarpophalangeal flexion/0-90	Seated	Over the posterior aspect of the metacarpophalangeal joint	Over the posterior midline of the metacarpal	Over the posterior midline of the proximal phalanx
	Metacarpophalangeal extension/0-30	Seated	Over the posterior aspect of the metacarpophalangeal joint	Over the posterior midline of the metacarpal	Over the posterior midline of the proximal phalanx
	Metacarpophalangeal abduction/0-20	Seated	Over the posterior aspect of the metacarpophalangeal joint	Over the posterior midline of the metacarpal	Over the posterior midline of the proximal phalanx
	Metacarpophalangeal adduction/0-20	Seated	Over the posterior aspect of the metacarpophalangeal joint	Over the posterior midline of the metacarpal	Over the posterior midline of the proximal phalanx
	Proximal interphalangeal flexion/0-120	Seated	Over the posterior aspect of the proximal interphalangeal joint	Over the posterior midline of the proximal phalanx	Over the posterior midline of the middle phalanx
	Proximal interphalangeal extension/0-10	Seated	Over the posterior aspect of the proximal interphalangeal joint	Over the posterior midline of the proximal phalanx	Over the posterior midline of the middle phalanx
	Distal interphalangeal flexion/0-80	Seated	Over the posterior aspect of the proximal interphalangeal joint	Over the posterior midline of the middle phalanx	Over the posterior midline of the distal phalanx
	Distal interphalangeal extension/0-10	Seated	Over the posterior aspect of the proximal interphalangeal joint	Over the posterior midline of the middle phalanx	Over the posterior midline of the distal phalanx

(Continued)

Lower Extremity					
Joint	**Tested Motion/ Range (degrees)**	**Patient Position**	**Fulcrum/Axis**	**Stationary Arm**	**Moving Arm**
Hip	Flexion/0-115 to 120	Supine	Over the lateral aspect of the hip joint using the greater trochanter of the femur reference	Lateral midline of the pelvis	Lateral midline of the femur using the lateral epicondyle for reference
	Extension/0-10 to 15	Prone/sideline	Over the lateral aspect of the hip joint using the greater trochanter of the femur reference	Lateral midline of the pelvis	Lateral midline of the femur using the lateral epicondyle for reference
	Abduction/0-45	Supine	Over the anterior superior iliac spine (ASIS) of the extremity being measured	Aligned with imaginary horizontal line extending from one ASIS to the other ASIS	Anterior midline of the femur using the midline of the patella for reference
	Adduction/ 0-20 to 30	Supine	Over the ASIS of the extremity being measured	Aligned with imaginary horizontal line extending from one ASIS to the other ASIS	Anterior midline of the femur using the midline of the patella for reference
	Internal rotation/0-30 to 45	Seated	Anterior aspect of the patella	Perpendicular to the floor or parallel to the supporting surface	Anterior midline of the lower leg using the crest of the tibia and a point midway between the two malleoli for reference
	External rotation/0-30 to 45	Seated	Anterior aspect of the patella	Perpendicular to the floor or parallel to the supporting surface	Anterior midline of the lower leg using the crest of the tibia and a point midway between the two malleoli for reference
Knee	Flexion/0-120 to 130	Prone/supine/ sidelying	Lateral epicondyle of the femur	Lateral midline of the femur using the greater trochanter for reference	Lateral midline of the fibula using the lateral malleolus and fibular head for reference
	Extension/0-15	Supine	Lateral epicondyle of the femur	Lateral midline of the femur using the greater trochanter for reference	Lateral midline of the fibula using the lateral malleolus and fibular head for reference

(Continued)

Joint	Tested Motion/ Range (degrees)	Patient Position	Fulcrum/Axis	Stationary Arm	Moving Arm
Talocrural	Dorsiflexion/0-20	Prone	Lateral aspect of the lateral malleolus	Lateral midline of the fibular using the head of the fibula for reference	Parallel to the lateral aspect of the fifth metatarsal
	Plantar flexion/0-50	Prone	Lateral aspect of the lateral malleolus	Lateral midline of the fibular using the head of the fibula for reference	Parallel to the lateral aspect of the fifth metatarsal
Hindfoot	Inversion/0-20	Prone	Posterior aspect of the ankle midway between the malleoli	Posterior midline of the lower leg	Posterior midline of the calcaneus
	Eversion/0-10	Prone	Posterior aspect of the ankle midway between the malleoli	Posterior midline of the lower leg	Posterior midline of the calcaneus
Transverse Tarsal	Inversion	Short-sitting	Anterior aspect of the ankle midway between the malleoli	Anterior midline of the lower leg using the tibial tuberosity for reference	Anterior midline of the second metatarsal
	Eversion	Short-sitting	Anterior aspect of the ankle midway between the malleoli	Anterior midline of the lower leg using the tibial tuberosity for reference	Anterior midline of the second metatarsal
First metatarsophalangeal	Flexion/0-45	Seated	Over the posterior aspect of the metatarsophalangeal	Over the posterior aspect of the shaft of the first metatarsal bone	Along the posterior surface of the shaft of the proximal phalanx
	Extension/0-70 to 90	Seated	Over the plantar surface of the first metatarsophalangeal joint	Over the plantar midline shaft of the first metatarsal bone	Along the plantar shaft of the proximal phalanx
Second to fifth metatarsophalangeal	Flexion/0-40	Seated	Over the posterior aspect of the metatarsophalangeal joints	Along the posterior midline longitudinal shaft of each metatarsal bone	Along the posterior midline longitudinal shaft of each proximal phalanx
	Extension/0-40	Seated	Over the plantar aspect of the metatarsophalangeal joints	Along the plantar midline longitudinal shaft of each metatarsal bone	Along the plantar midline aspect of the shaft of the proximal phalanx of each digit
First interphalangeal	Flexion/0-90	Seated	Over the posterior aspect of the distal interphalangeal joint	Along the posterior midline shaft of the middle phalange	Along the posterior midline shaft of the distal phalange
	Extension/minimal	Seated	Over the plantar aspect of the interphalangeal joint	Over the plantar midline shaft of the proximal phalange	Over the plantar midline shaft of the distal phalanx

(Continued)

Lower Extremity (*Continued*)					
Joint	**Tested Motion/ Range (degrees)**	**Patient Position**	**Fulcrum/Axis**	**Stationary Arm**	**Moving Arm**
Second to fifth proximal interpha-langeal joint	Flexion/0-35	Seated	Over the posterior aspect of the proxi-mal interphalangeal joint	Over the posterior midline shaft of the proximal phalanges	Over the posterior midline shaft of the middle phalanges of the other toes
	Extension/minimal	Seated	Over the plantar aspect of the inter-phalangeal joints	Over the plantar midline shaft of the proximal phalanges	Over the plantar midline shaft of the middle phalanges of the other toes
Second to fifth distal interphalan-geal joint	Flexion/0-60	Seated	Over the posterior aspect of the distal interphalangeal joints	Along the posterior midline shaft of the middle phalanges	Along the posterior midline shaft of the distal phalanges
	Extension/0-30	Seated	Over the posterior aspect of the distal interphalangeal joint	Along the posterior midline shaft of the middle phalanges	Along the posterior midline shaft of the distal phalanges

Appendix C

Spinal Nerves and Plexuses

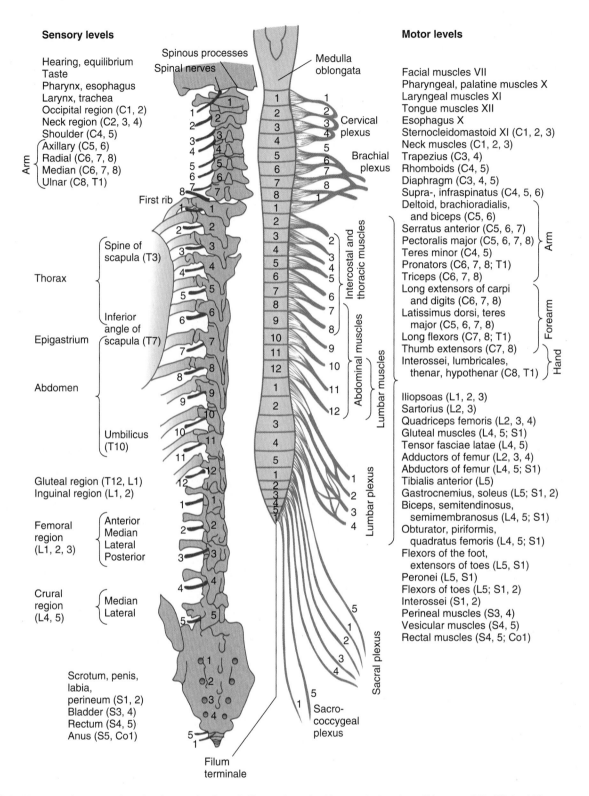

Figure C-1. **Motor and sensory levels of the spinal cord.** (Reproduced with permission from Waxman SG. *Clinical Neuroanatomy*, 27th ed. 2013. Copyright © McGraw Hill LLC. All rights reserved.)

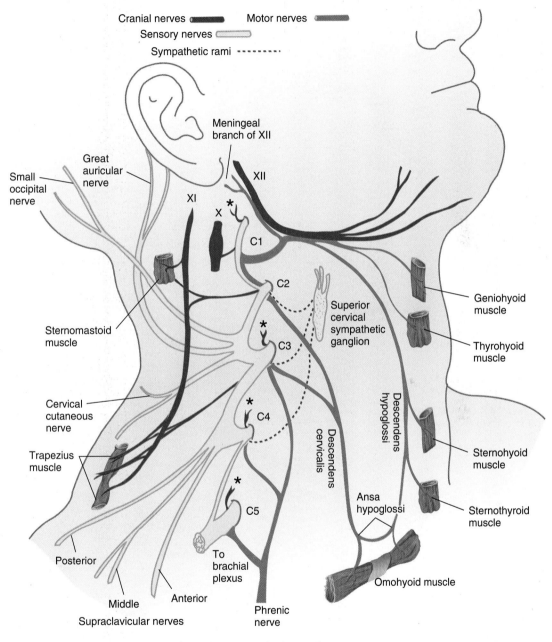

Figure C-2. The cervical plexus. (Reproduced with permission from Waxman SG. *Clinical Neuroanatomy*, 27th ed. 2013. Copyright © McGraw Hill LLC. All rights reserved.)

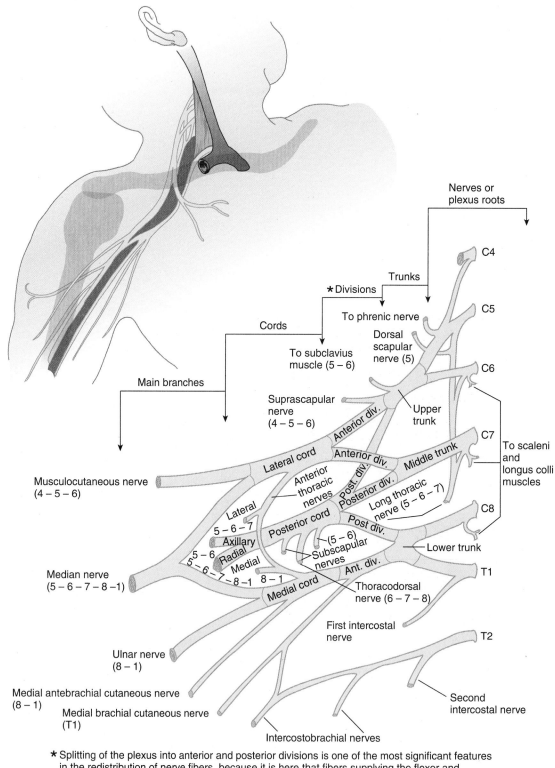

Nerves or plexus roots

C4

Trunks

★Divisions

To phrenic nerve

C5

Cords

Dorsal scapular nerve (5)

To subclavius muscle (5 – 6)

Upper trunk

C6

Main branches

Suprascapular nerve (4 – 5 – 6)

Anterior div.

Anterior div.

Middle trunk

C7

To scaleni and longus colli muscles

Lateral cord

Musculocutaneous nerve (4 – 5 – 6)

Anterior thoracic nerves

Post. div.

Posterior div.

Long thoracic nerve (5 – 6 – 7)

Lateral
5 – 6 – 7

Posterior cord

Post div.

C8

Axillary

Radial

5 – 6

Medial

5 – 6 – 7 – 8 – 1

(5 – 6)
Subscapular nerves

Lower trunk

Median nerve (5 – 6 – 7 – 8 – 1)

8 – 1

Ant. div.

T1

Medial cord

Thoracodorsal nerve (6 – 7 – 8)

First intercostal nerve

T2

Ulnar nerve (8 – 1)

Medial antebrachial cutaneous nerve (8 – 1)

Medial brachial cutaneous nerve (T1)

Second intercostal nerve

Intercostobrachial nerves

★ Splitting of the plexus into anterior and posterior divisions is one of the most significant features in the redistribution of nerve fibers, because it is here that fibers supplying the flexor and extensor groups of muscles of the upper extremity are separated. Similar splitting is noted in the lumbar and sacral plexuses for the supply of muscles of the lower extremity.

Figure C-3. **The brachial plexus.** (Reproduced with permission from Waxman SG. *Clinical Neuroanatomy*, 27th ed. 2013. Copyright © McGraw Hill LLC. All rights reserved.)

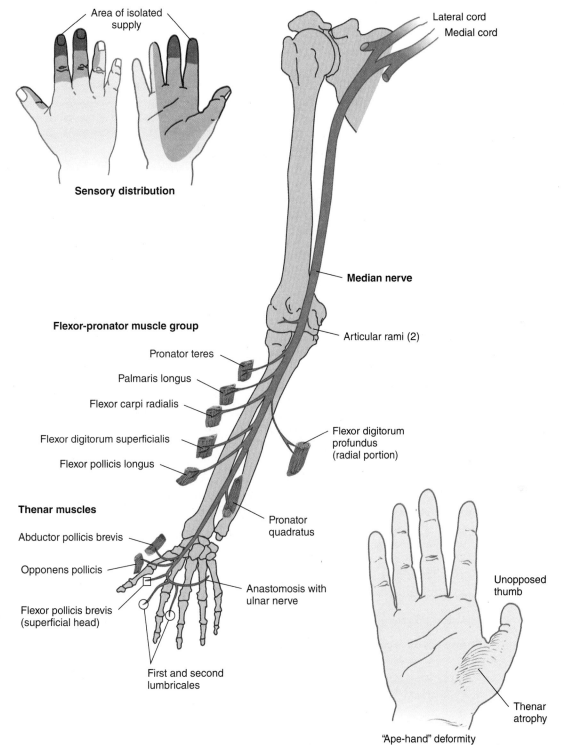

Sensory distribution

Area of isolated supply

Lateral cord
Medial cord

Median nerve

Articular rami (2)

Flexor-pronator muscle group

Pronator teres

Palmaris longus

Flexor carpi radialis

Flexor digitorum superficialis

Flexor pollicis longus

Flexor digitorum profundus (radial portion)

Thenar muscles

Abductor pollicis brevis

Opponens pollicis

Flexor pollicis brevis (superficial head)

Pronator quadratus

Anastomosis with ulnar nerve

First and second lumbricales

Unopposed thumb

Thenar atrophy

"Ape-hand" deformity in median nerve lesion

Figure C-4. The median nerve (C6-C8; T1). (Reproduced with permission from Waxman SG. *Clinical Neuroanatomy*, 27th ed. 2013. Copyright © McGraw Hill LLC. All rights reserved.)

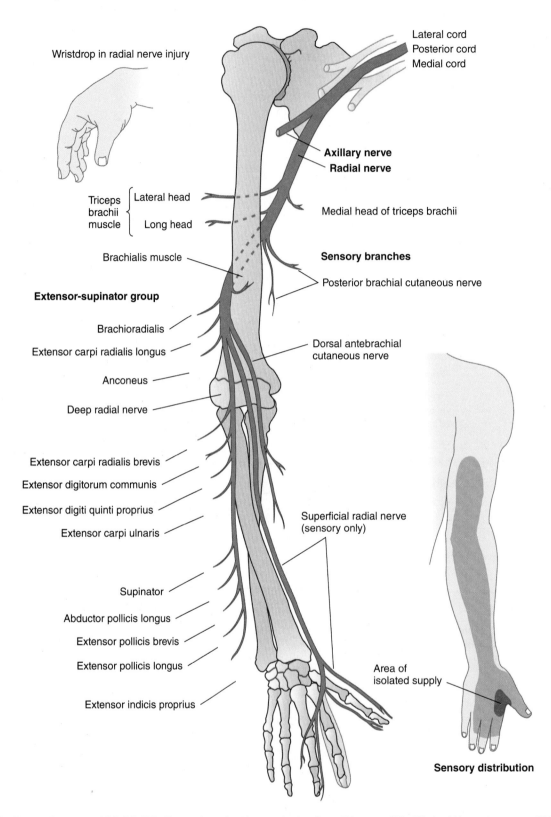

Wristdrop in radial nerve injury

Lateral cord
Posterior cord
Medial cord

Axillary nerve
Radial nerve

Triceps brachii muscle { Lateral head / Long head }

Medial head of triceps brachii

Sensory branches

Brachialis muscle

Extensor-supinator group

Posterior brachial cutaneous nerve

Brachioradialis

Extensor carpi radialis longus

Anconeus

Deep radial nerve

Dorsal antebrachial cutaneous nerve

Extensor carpi radialis brevis

Extensor digitorum communis

Extensor digiti quinti proprius

Extensor carpi ulnaris

Superficial radial nerve (sensory only)

Supinator

Abductor pollicis longus

Extensor pollicis brevis

Extensor pollicis longus

Area of isolated supply

Extensor indicis proprius

Sensory distribution

Figure C-5. **The radial nerve (C6-C8; T1).** (Reproduced with permission from Waxman SG. *Clinical Neuroanatomy*, 27th ed. 2013. Copyright © McGraw Hill LLC. All rights reserved.)

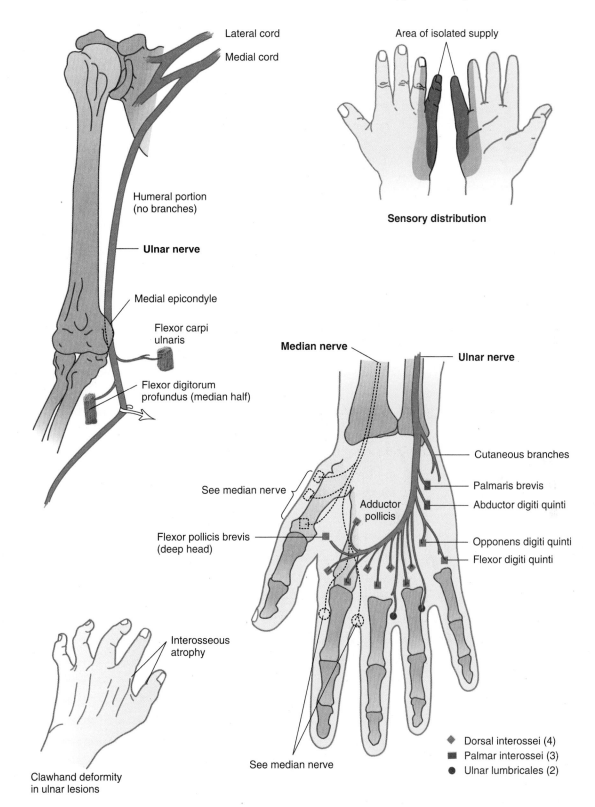

Lateral cord
Medial cord

Area of isolated supply

Sensory distribution

Humeral portion
(no branches)

Ulnar nerve

Medial epicondyle

Flexor carpi
ulnaris

Flexor digitorum
profundus (median half)

Median nerve

Ulnar nerve

See median nerve

Cutaneous branches

Palmaris brevis

Abductor digiti quinti

Adductor
pollicis

Flexor pollicis brevis
(deep head)

Opponens digiti quinti

Flexor digiti quinti

Interosseous
atrophy

♦ Dorsal interossei (4)
■ Palmar interossei (3)
● Ulnar lumbricales (2)

See median nerve

Clawhand deformity
in ulnar lesions

Figure C-6. The ulnar nerve (C8, T1). (Reproduced with permission from Waxman SG. *Clinical Neuroanatomy*, 27th ed. 2013. Copyright © McGraw Hill LLC. All rights reserved.)

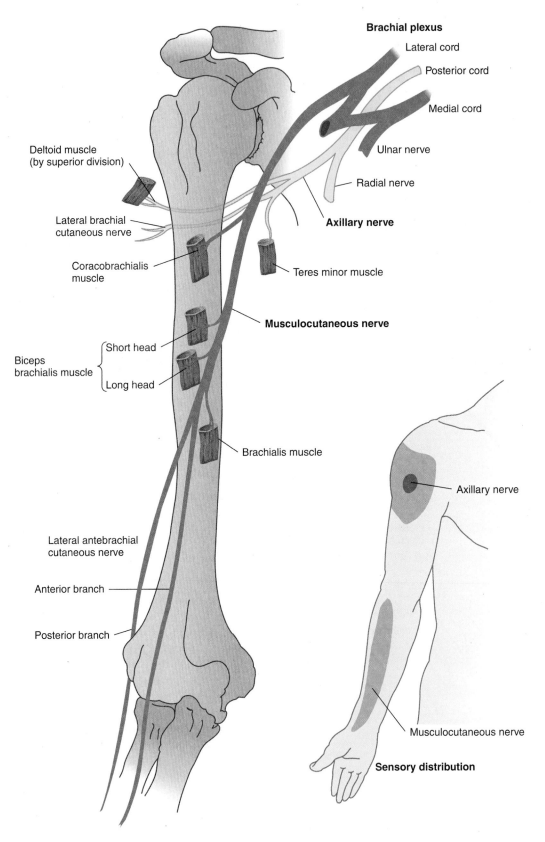

Figure C-7. Musculocutaneous (C5, C6) and axillary (C5, C6) nerves. (Reproduced with permission from Waxman SG. *Clinical Neuroanatomy*, 27th ed. 2013. Copyright © McGraw Hill LLC. All rights reserved.)

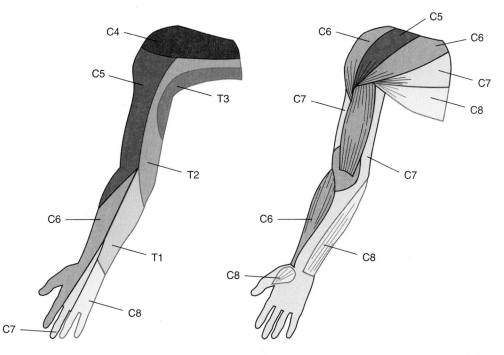

Figure C-8. **Segmental innervation of the right upper extremity, anterior view.** (Reproduced with permission from Waxman SG. *Clinical Neuroanatomy*, 27th ed. 2013. Copyright © McGraw Hill LLC. All rights reserved.)

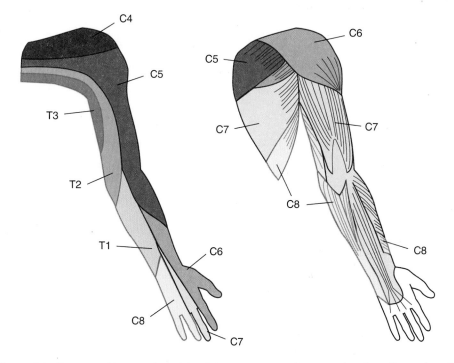

Figure C-9. **Segmental innervation of the right upper extremity, posterior view.** (Reproduced with permission from Waxman SG. *Clinical Neuroanatomy*, 27th ed. 2013. Copyright © McGraw Hill LLC. All rights reserved.)

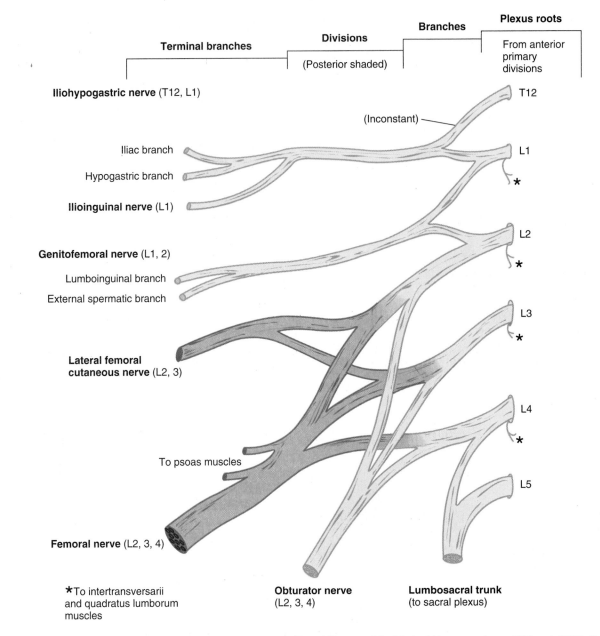

Figure C-10. The lumbar plexus. (Reproduced with permission from Waxman SG. *Clinical Neuroanatomy*, 27th ed. 2013. Copyright © McGraw Hill LLC. All rights reserved.)

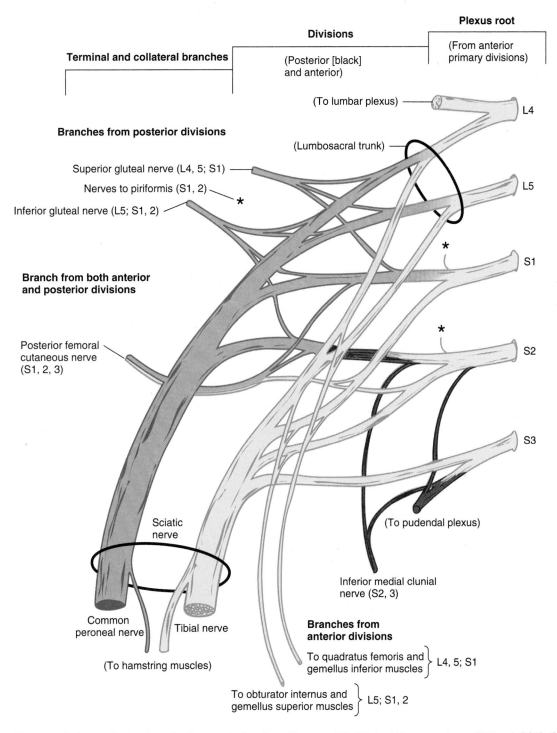

Plexus root

Divisions

(From anterior primary divisions)

Terminal and collateral branches

(Posterior [black] and anterior)

L4

(To lumbar plexus)

Branches from posterior divisions

(Lumbosacral trunk)

Superior gluteal nerve (L4, 5; S1)

L5

Nerves to piriformis (S1, 2)   *

Inferior gluteal nerve (L5; S1, 2)

*

S1

Branch from both anterior and posterior divisions

*

S2

Posterior femoral cutaneous nerve (S1, 2, 3)

S3

(To pudendal plexus)

Sciatic nerve

Inferior medial clunial nerve (S2, 3)

Common peroneal nerve   Tibial nerve

Branches from anterior divisions

(To hamstring muscles)

To quadratus femoris and gemellus inferior muscles } L4, 5; S1

To obturator internus and gemellus superior muscles } L5; S1, 2

Figure C-11. The sacral plexus. (Reproduced with permission from Waxman SG. *Clinical Neuroanatomy*, 27th ed. 2013. Copyright © McGraw Hill LLC. All rights reserved.)

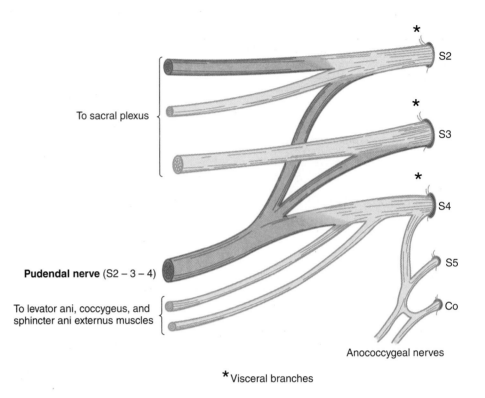

To sacral plexus

* S2

* S3

* S4

S5

Co

Pudendal nerve (S2 – 3 – 4)

To levator ani, coccygeus, and
sphincter ani externus muscles

Anococcygeal nerves

*Visceral branches

Figure C-12. **The pudendal and coccygeal plexuses.** (Reproduced with permission from
Waxman SG. *Clinical Neuroanatomy*, 27th ed. 2013. Copyright © McGraw Hill LLC. All rights
reserved.)

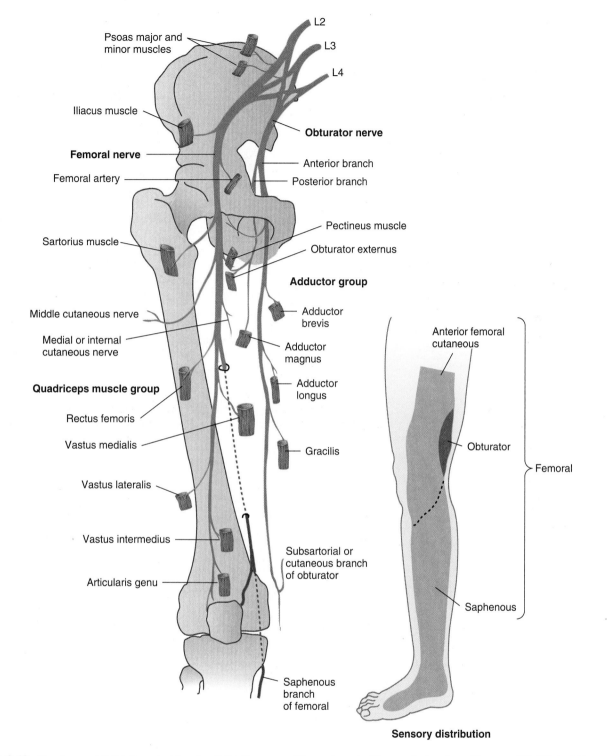

Figure C-13. **The femoral (L2-L4) and obturator (L2-L4) nerves.** (Reproduced with permission from Waxman SG. *Clinical Neuro-anatomy*, 27th ed. 2013. Copyright © McGraw Hill LLC. All rights reserved.)

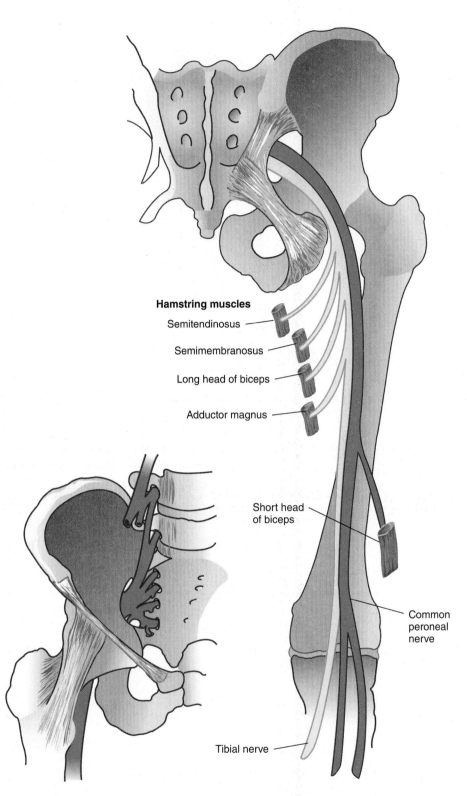

Figure C-14. The sciatic nerve (L4, L5; S1-S3). (Reproduced with permission from Waxman SG. *Clinical Neuroanatomy*, 27th ed. 2013. Copyright © McGraw Hill LLC. All rights reserved.)

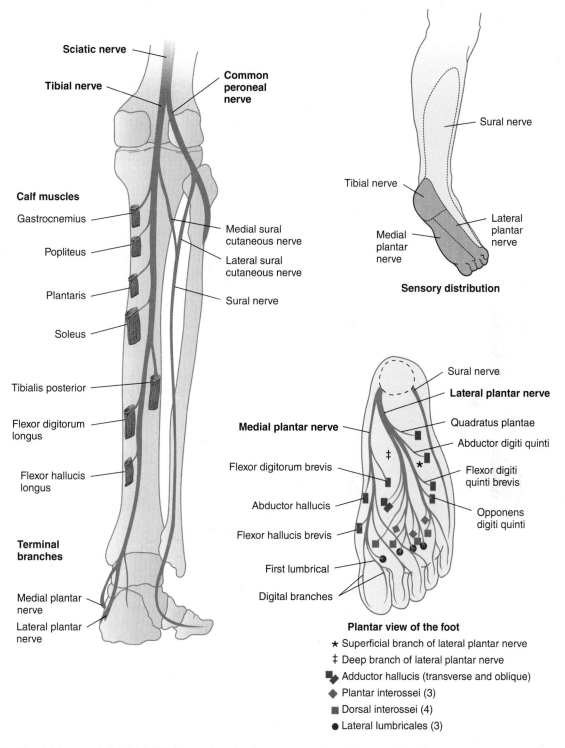

Sciatic nerve

Tibial nerve

Common peroneal nerve

Sural nerve

Calf muscles

Gastrocnemius

Tibial nerve

Popliteus

Medial sural cutaneous nerve

Lateral plantar nerve

Plantaris

Lateral sural cutaneous nerve

Medial plantar nerve

Soleus

Sural nerve

Sensory distribution

Tibialis posterior

Sural nerve

Flexor digitorum longus

Lateral plantar nerve

Flexor hallucis longus

Medial plantar nerve

Quadratus plantae

Abductor digiti quinti

Flexor digitorum brevis

Flexor digiti quinti brevis

Abductor hallucis

Opponens digiti quinti

Flexor hallucis brevis

Terminal branches

First lumbrical

Medial plantar nerve

Digital branches

Lateral plantar nerve

Plantar view of the foot

★ Superficial branch of lateral plantar nerve

‡ Deep branch of lateral plantar nerve

◼ Adductor hallucis (transverse and oblique)

◆ Plantar interossei (3)

▪ Dorsal interossei (4)

● Lateral lumbricales (3)

Figure C-15. The tibial nerve (L4, L5; S1-S3). (Reproduced with permission from Waxman SG. *Clinical Neuroanatomy*, 27th ed. 2013. Copyright © McGraw Hill LLC. All rights reserved.)

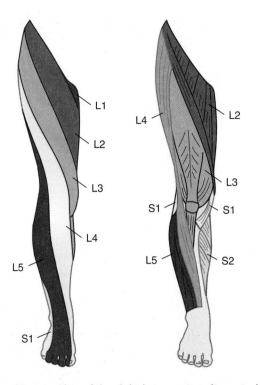

Figure C-16. **Segmental innervation of the right lower extremity, anterior view. Note the similarity between dermatomes (on left) and myotomes (on right).** (Reproduced with permission from Waxman SG. *Clinical Neuroanatomy*, 27th ed. 2013. Copyright © McGraw Hill LLC. All rights reserved.)

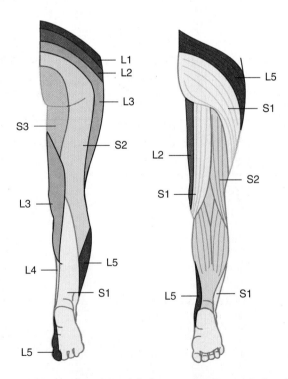

Figure C-17. **Segmental innervation of the right lower extremity, posterior view.** (Reproduced with permission from Waxman SG. *Clinical Neuroanatomy*, 27th ed. 2013. Copyright © McGraw Hill LLC. All rights reserved.)

Appendix D
Pharmacology Overview

Annie Burke-Doe

Pharmacology is the study of how drugs (chemicals) affect the physiology of the body. Physical therapists and physical therapist assistants have direct contact with patients taking medication to impact response to exercise and movement. Most of your patients will be taking medication related to their condition, and it is important to understand how drugs will impact the patient and physical therapy treatment. Patients today have access to prescribed medications and over-the-counter (OTC) formulations such as herbs, vitamins, and tinctures. The benefits of both OTC and prescribed medications are varied, but a key point is a need for health care professionals to understand the benefits, side effects, signs, and symptoms of medications working correctly or when they are not. This section will provide a general overview of the basic principles of pharmacology.

▲ HIGH-YIELD TERMS

Agonist	A compound that binds to a receptor and produces a biological response.
Antagonist	Blocks or reverses the effect of an agonist—they have no effect on their own.
Absorption	A process involving the movement of a substance from its side of administration across one or more body membranes. A drug may be absorbed locally or produce a biological effect at a distant site.
Bioavailability	Refers to how completely the system absorbs a particular drug and is available to produce a response.
Distribution	The process by which drugs are transported after they have been absorbed or administered directly into the bloodstream.
Excretion	The process by which drugs are removed from the body through urine, exhalation, sweat, saliva, bile, feces, and tears.
Efficacy	The maximal response a drug can produce.
First-pass effect	The liver is a metabolic machine and often inactivates drugs on their way from the GI tract to the body, called the first-pass effect.
Metabolism	The process where the drugs are made less or more active.
Partial agonist	Produces the biological response but cannot produce 100% of the biological response even at very high doses.
Pharmacokinetics	The effects of the body on drugs are related to four processes: absorption, distribution, metabolism, and excretion.
Pharmacodynamics	The drug's action on the body, such as the mechanism of action or how the drug exerts its effects.
Potency	A measure of the dose that is required to produce a response.
Receptor	A specialized target macromolecule that binds a drug and mediates its pharmacologic action.
Topical drug	A topical drug is applied locally to the skin and membranous linings of the eyes, ears, nose, respiratory tract, urinary tract, vagina, and rectum.
Volume distribution	The volume of plasma, or fluid, in which the drug is dissolved, indicates the extent of distribution of that drug.

TABLE D-1 · General Routes of Drug Administration.		
Route	**Characteristics**	**Bioavailability (%)**
Enteral		
Oral (PO)	Most convenient First-pass effect may be significant	5 to < 100
Sublingual/buccal	Avoids first-pass effect	75 to < 100
Rectal (PR)	Less first-pass effect than oral	30 to < 100
Parenteral		
Intravenous (IV)	Most rapid onset	100 (by definition)
Intramuscular (IM)	Large volumes up to 5 mL often feasible May be painful	75 to ≤ 100
Subcutaneous (SC)	Smaller volumes than IM May be painful	75 to ≤ 100
Inhalation	Often a very rapid onset	5 to < 100
Transdermal	Usually very slow absorption	80 to ≤ 100

Data from Jobst EE, Panus PC, Kruidering-Hall M. *Pharmacology for the Physical Therapist*, 2nd ed. 2020. Copyright © McGraw Hill LLC. All rights reserved. https://accessphysiotherapy.mhmedical.com.

Drugs are commonly organized in two major ways by their therapeutic effect and pharmacologic classification. The therapeutic effect classifies a medication by its clinical action using biochemical and physiologic principles—"a drug used for high blood pressure," "a drug used for pain." Pharmacologic classification addresses how the medication produces its effects within the body. For example, *diuretics* lower blood pressure by lowering plasma volume, and *calcium channel blockers* treat hypertension by limiting the force of contraction. Drugs have more than one name, a *generic* name assigned by the US Adopted Name Council, and a *trade* name assigned by the company making the drug. One example is penicillin (generic name) and Amoxil (trade name).

There are three general routes of drug administration (Table D-1):

Topical—delivered locally to the skin and associate membranes.
Enteral—delivered orally or via nasogastric or gastrostomy tubes.
Parenteral—delivered by routes other than oral or topical.

Not all drugs affect all patients the same way due to many factors, including age, hydration level, body mass, and genetics, as examples. To understand the impact of a drug on a patient, you must understand concepts from two important pharmacology principles: **pharmacokinetics** and **pharmacodynamics** (Figure D-1).

Pharmacokinetics describes the effects of the body on drugs. For example, absorption, distribution, metabolism, and excretion (Figure D-2). **Absorption** involves the movement of a drug from its site of administration. A drug may be absorbed locally or produce a biological effect at a distant site. Once the drug is in the system, it must be dissolved before it can be absorbed. The rate and extent of absorption are determined by the chemical characteristics of the drug, the dosage form (eg, tablet, solution), and gastric emptying. Solutions have the fastest rate of absorption, and time-released medications have the slowest. **Bioavailability** refers to how completely a particular drug is absorbed by the system and is available to act. **Distribution** begins after the drug is absorbed into the bloodstream or tissue. The drug is transported through the blood to a specific target site. The drug will be distributed to other parts of the body as well.

The *volume of distribution* is the volume of plasma, or fluid, in which the drug is dissolved and indicates the extent of distribution of that drug. A drug's *efficacy* is its ability to produce a specific therapeutic effect once it reaches a particular receptor site in a target tissue.

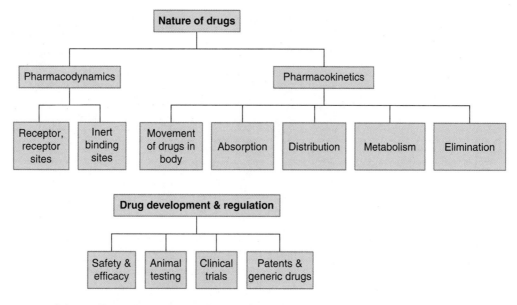

Figure D-1. The nature of drugs. (Reproduced with permission from Katzung BG, Kruidering-Hall M, Trevor AJ, eds. *Katzung & Trevor's Pharmacology: Examination & Board Review*, 12th ed. 2019. Copyright © McGraw-Hill LLC. All rights reserved. https://accesspharmacy.mhmedical.com.)

Potency is the dose of the drug required to produce a desired therapeutic effect across many membranes before reaching the target. **Metabolism** of a drug is the process where the drugs are made less or more active. The metabolic process takes place in the liver and, to a lesser extent, in organs such as the kidneys and cells of the gastrointestinal tract. The **first-pass effect** is an important phenomenon where drugs are absorbed across the intestinal wall and enter blood vessels to be carried to the liver. Next, the liver metabolizes the drugs into a less active form, distributed to the rest of the body. The last step in pharmacokinetics is the **excretion** of a drug or its metabolites. Excretion is when drugs are removed from the body through urine, exhalation, sweat, saliva, bile, feces, and tears. These pathways are used to eliminate drugs and their metabolites. The main organ involved in excretion is the kidney. The rate of elimination from the body and the **half-life** characteristics influence a drug's effectiveness. A drug's half-life is defined as the amount of time required for the plasma drug level to be reduced by one-half. For most drugs, the half-life is measured in hours, but it is measured in minutes or days for some. Knowing the half-life of a drug is essential in determining how often and in what dosage drugs must be administered to achieve and maintain therapeutic concentration levels.

Pharmacodynamics denotes the drug's action on the body, such as the mechanism of action and therapeutic and toxic effects. Successful drug therapy depends on the effectiveness of these responses. Drugs will activate specific receptors to produce a biological response. A drug receptor is a specialized target macromolecule that binds a drug and mediates its pharmacologic action. These receptors may be enzymes, nucleic acids, or specialized membrane-bound proteins located on the plasma membrane, or they may be found in the cytoplasm (Figure D-3). A customary way to present the relationship between the drug concentration and the biological response is with a dose-response curve (Figure D-4).

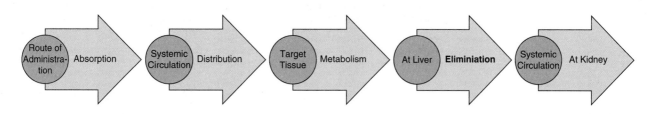

Figure D-2. Pharmacokinetics.

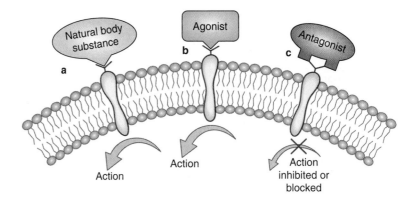

Figure D-3. Cell membrane receptors.

An **agonist** is a compound that binds to a receptor and produces a biological response. A partial agonist produces the biological response but cannot produce 100% of the biological response even at very high doses (Figure D-5). When comparing the differences between drugs, the terms **efficacy** and **potency** are often used. Efficacy is the maximal response a drug can produce. Potency is a measure of the dose that is required to produce a response. **Antagonists** block or reverse the effect of an agonist. The binding of an antagonist to a receptor does not produce a biological effect. Therefore, the antagonist can block the effect of an agonist, or it can reverse the effect of an agonist. An example of an antagonist is naloxone, an opioid antagonist. Naloxone has no effect of its own but will completely reverse the effects of any opioid agonist administered and is used when a person overdoses.

More drugs are being administered to the consumer than ever before. Therefore, physical therapists and physical therapy assistants need to have a thorough knowledge of pharmacology to assist patients with education, management, and enforcement of drug laws. More specifically, we need to understand pharmacology in the contest of exercise. In general, exercise decreases a drug's absorption after oral administration, whereas exercise increases absorption after intramuscular or subcutaneous administration because of an increased blood flow in the muscle. Thus, exercise influences the amount of a drug that reaches a

STUDY PEARL
Throughout the appropriate chapters, you will find tables that describe common medications for treating disease and symptoms of the disease.

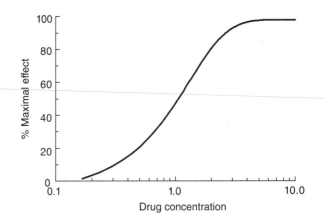

Figure D-4. In a concentration-response curve, the concentration of the drug is plotted against the percent maximal effect. Notice that the drug concentration is plotted on a log scale. In this graph, the drug is a full agonist—the effect reaches 100% of the maximum possible. (Reproduced with permission from Stringer JL. *Basic Concepts in Pharmacology: What You Need to Know for Each Drug Class*, 5th ed. 2017. Copyright © McGraw Hill LLC. All rights reserved. https://accesspharmacy.mhmedical.com.)

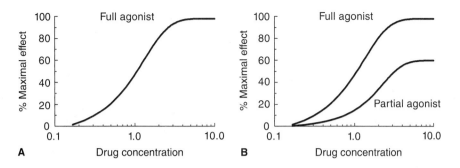

Figure D-5. In A, the concentration-response curve for a full agonist is presented. The drug can produce a maximal effect. In B, the concentration-response curve for a partial agonist is also shown. In this case, the partial agonist is able to produce only 60% of the maximal response. (Reproduced with permission from Stringer JL. *Basic Concepts in Pharmacology: What You Need to Know for Each Drug Class*, 5th ed. 2017. Copyright © McGraw Hill LLC. All rights reserved. https://accesspharmacy.mhmedical.com.)

TABLE D-2 • List of Drug Classifications and Definitions.	
Analgesics	**Pain-relieving drugs**
Anesthetics	Agents that produce local or general numbness to touch, pain, or stimulation.
Antacids	Substances that neutralize acidity; commonly used in the digestive tract.
Antibiotics	Drugs that kill bacteria or inhibit their growth.
Anticholinergics	Drugs that block the action of the neurotransmitter acetylcholine in the brain.
Anticoagulants	Agents that prevent the coagulation of blood.
Anticonvulsants	Drugs used in the treatment of seizures.
Antidepressants	Drugs used for the treatment of depression.
Antidotes	Substances that prevent or counteract the action of a poison.
Antifungals	Drugs that kill fungi or inhibit their growth.
Antihistamines	Class of drugs used to treat allergic reactions.
Antihypertensives	Drugs used to treat hypertension (high blood pressure).
Anti-inflammatories	Drugs that reduce and/or control inflammation.
Antipruritics	Agents that relieve itching.
Antipsychotics	Drugs used to manage psychosis (delusions, hallucinations, disordered thought).
Antipyretics	Drugs that reduce body temperature.
Antiseptics	Agents that kill bacteria or inhibit their growth and can be applied to living tissue.
Antispasmodics	Agents that relieve muscle spasm.
Antitussives	Agents that inhibit or prevent coughing.
Astringents	Agents that cause contraction or puckering action.
Anxiolytics	Drugs that inhibit anxiety.
Bacteriostatics and fungistatics	Agents that retard or inhibit the growth of bacteria and fungi, respectively.
Bronchodilators	Drugs used to relax and dilate the airways in the lungs.
Carminatives	Agents that relieve flatulence (caused by gases) in the intestinal tract.
Cathartics	Agents used to evacuate substances from the bowels; active purgatives.
Caustics	Burning agents, capable of destroying living tissue.
Chemotherapeutics	Drugs used in the treatment of cancer.

(Continued)

TABLE D-2 • List of Drug Classifications and Definitions. (*Continued*)	
Analgesics	**Pain-relieving drugs**
Counterirritants	Agents applied locally to produce an inflammatory reaction for the relief of a deeper inflammation.
Decongestants	Drugs used to relieve nasal congestion in the upper respiratory tract.
Depressants	Agents that diminish body functions or nerve activity.
Disinfectants	Agents that kill or inhibit the growth of microorganisms; should be applied only to nonliving materials.
Diuretics	Agents that increase the excretion of urine.
Emetics	Agents that cause vomiting.
Expectorants	Agents that increase airway secretions to enhance the clearance of mucus.
Hemostatics	Substances that either slow down or stop bleeding.
Hormonal contraceptives	Birth control drugs that act on the endocrine system.
Irritants	Agents that irritate.
Narcotics	Drugs that produce analgesic and hypnotic effects.
Sedatives	Agents that relieve anxiety.
Skeletal muscle relaxants	Drugs that depress neural activity within skeletal muscles.
Stimulants	Agents that excite the central nervous system.
Suppressants	Agents that reduce or control appetite.
Vasoconstrictors and vasodilators	Drugs that constrict and dilate blood vessels, respectively.

receptor site that significantly affects the pharmacodynamic activity of the drug. Whether your patient is taking traditional medications that are synthetically produced in a laboratory, or biologics naturally produced in the body (hormones, vaccines) or natural alternative products (herbs, extracts, vitamins), understanding drug classes (Table D-2), indications for use, and adverse effects will assist your patients in understanding the benefits and risk of taking medications.

Exam 1

QUESTION 1
You are treating a patient who is 3 days post-op right medial meniscus repair. Which treatment goal would be most important to achieve during this period?
  A. Normalize gait
  B. Increase isolated quadriceps strength
  C. Increase knee flexion range of motion
  D. Control swelling

Rationale: D

QUESTION 2
Which of the following conditions would benefit from exercises emphasizing spinal flexion?
  A. Vertebral body fracture
  B. Lumbar zygapophyseal dysfunction
  C. Herniated L4-L5 intervertebral disk
  D. Spinal foramen stenosis

Rationale: D

QUESTION 3
You are treating a patient with an acute herniated L4-L5 disk. The patient injured his back 2 days ago. Which modality would be the least appropriate at this stage?
  A. Transcutaneous electrical stimulation (TENS)
  B. Cold pack applied to the low back
  C. Mechanical traction
  D. Electrical stimulation

Rationale: C

QUESTION 4
You are treating a patient with a left rotator cuff tear in the critical zone, which is an area very susceptible to a tear. It is called the critical zone because the area is known for which of the following?
  A. Hypertrophy
  B. Hypervascularity
  C. Hypovascularity
  D. Atrophy

Rationale: C

QUESTION 5
You are treating a patient with a scaphoid fracture. Which anatomic area of the hand would you expect to be tender?
  A. Hypothenar eminence
  B. Anatomic snuff box
  C. The no-man zone
  D. Palmar fascia

Rationale: B

QUESTION 6
During the normal gait cycle, which muscle would *NOT* play a concentric role during toe-off (preswing)?
  A. Flexor hallucis longus
  B. Plantaris
  C. Tibialis anterior
  D. Gastrocnemius

Rationale: C

QUESTION 7
You are treating a patient who fractured the distal humerus and subsequently suffered vascular compromise to the brachial artery. Which of the following complication did this patient have?
  A. Volkmann ischemic contracture
  B. Shoulder hand syndrome
  C. Dupuytren contracture
  D. Radial head fracture

Rationale: A

QUESTION 8
You are treating a patient with patellofemoral dysfunction. The treatment plan is for the patient to receive only closed-chain kinematic exercises. Of the following exercises, which would be appropriate to start with this patient?
  A. Knee extensions on an exercise machine
  B. Wall slides
  C. Short-arc quads
  D. Isokinetic exercises with extension blocked at minus 10 degrees

Rationale: B

QUESTION 9
You are treating a patient with carpal tunnel syndrome. You would expect the patient to report tingling in all the areas on the hand *EXCEPT* which of the following?
  A. Index finger
  B. Radial aspect of the palm
  C. Fifth digit
  D. Middle finger

Rationale: C

QUESTION 10
You are treating a patient at a nursing home who has cognitive deficits. Which cognitive condition has memory loss as the first noticeable sign and is classified into four stages: preclinical, mild, moderate, and severe?
  A. Lou Gehrig disease
  B. Parkinson disease
  C. Alzheimer disease
  D. Huntington chorea disease

Rationale: C

QUESTION 11
You are treating a person with quadriplegia who has the potential for developing a pressure ulcer. The favorite position of a patient with quadriplegia is sidelying. Which of the following areas of this patient's body would be the *LEAST* susceptible to pressure ulcers?
  A. Medial malleoli
  B. Scapulae
  C. Lateral malleoli
  D. None of the above

Rationale: B. The scapulae are the only bony prominences (areas where bones are close to the skin surface) listed that are not susceptible to pressure in sidelying

QUESTION 12
If a patient is able to stand safely while unsupported with the eyes closed for 10 seconds, he would receive a score of_____ on the Berg Balance Scale.
A. 2
B. 4
C. 6
D. 8

Rationale: B. Being able to stand for 10 seconds safely with the eyes closed scores 4 points on the Berg Balance Scale

QUESTION 13
You are measuring the strength of a patient's wrist extensors using manual muscle testing (MMT). As the patient cannot hold the test position against gravity, you decide to place the forearm in an antigravity position. Which of the following would be the best position in which to place the patient's forearm?
A. Supinated
B. Neutral
C. Pronated
D. None of the above

Rationale: B

QUESTION 14
During a review of the plan of care (POC) before seeing a patient, you note that the patient recently underwent a Lisfranc amputation. This amputation involves which of the following?
A. Amputation of the foot through the tarsometatarsal joint
B. Resection of the third, fourth, fifth metatarsals, and digits
C. The disarticulation of all five metatarsals and the digits
D. None of the above

Rationale: A Lisfranc (midfoot) amputation involves amputation of the foot at the tarsometatarsal joint. An amputation at this level preserves the dorsiflexors and plantarflexors

QUESTION 15
Which of the following best describes the wound healing technique that uses controlled subatmospheric pressure to remove excess wound fluid from the extravascular space?
A. Hyperbaric oxygen
B. Intermittent pneumatic compression
C. Psoralen plus ultraviolet A irradiation (PUVA) theory
D. Vacuum-assisted closure

Rationale: D. Vacuum-assisted closure is a noninvasive, negative pressure healing technique used to treat a wide range of chronic, nonhealing wounds and is particularly useful in treating deep cavitating wounds

QUESTION 16
You are treating a 56-year-old man with a deep thigh bruise and knee pain from a fall 1 week ago. Which of the following is a complication associated with a deep thigh bruise?
A. Myositis ossificans
B. Vitamin D deficiency
C. Vitamin E deficiency
D. Vitamin C deficiency

Rationale: A. Myositis ossificans (MO) is an uncommon injury that can occur as a result of blunt force trauma to large muscle bellies such as the quadriceps or biceps

QUESTION 17

You are about to treat a patient in the coronary care unit diagnosed with congestive heart failure (CHF). All of the following are *NOT* characteristics of CHF, *EXCEPT*:
  A. Markedly decreased exercise tolerance
  B. Decrease diastolic blood pressure during exercise
  C. Increased alertness
  D. All of the above are not characteristics of CHF

Rationale: A. Of those listed, only a marked decrease in exercise tolerance is suggestive of CHF. There would be a decrease in systolic blood pressure during exercise, not diastolic blood pressure, and decreased alertness/difficulty concentrating

QUESTION 18

You have just instructed a patient in the D_2 proprioceptive neuromuscular facilitation (PNF) technique for the upper extremity. Later in the session, you are watching the patient and note that the patient begins with shoulder flexion, abduction, elbow extension, and forearm pronation before moving into shoulder flexion, shoulder abduction, elbow extension, and forearm supination. This patient is demonstrating which of the following?
  A. The correct technique
  B. The incorrect technique at the elbow
  C. The incorrect technique at the forearm
  D. The incorrect technique at the shoulder

Rationale: C. The forearm should be pronated

QUESTION 19

You are reviewing a patient's medical history and note the following findings: (1) insufficient production and release of adrenal hormones, (2) excessive fatigue, (3) low blood pressure, and (4) hyperpigmentation. What do you expect is the patient's diagnosis?
  A. Thyroid hyperfunction
  B. Adrenal gland hypofunction
  C. Adrenal gland hyperfunction
  D. Thyroid hypofunction

Rationale: B. These are all characteristic findings of adrenal gland hypofunction or Addison disease

QUESTION 20

While reviewing a patient's medical records, you note that the patient has a diagnosis of Cushing syndrome. All of the following are true statements about Cushing syndrome, *EXCEPT*:
  A. It is the result of extended exposure to high levels of cortisol.
  B. It is caused by a pituitary dysfunction.
  C. A common symptom is facial cachexia.
  D. It is most often seen in ages 25 to 40.

Rationale: C. Cushing syndrome results in fatty deposits in the face that cause a moon-shaped appearance

QUESTION 21

You are doing a clinical rotation in the neurology department of a local hospital. You are about to treat a patient with a diagnosis of peripheral neuropathy. All of the following are true statements about peripheral neuropathy, *EXCEPT*:
  A. The symptoms can range from mild to disabling.
  B. The neuropathy can affect the motor, sensory, and autonomic nerves.
  C. Genetically caused polyneuropathies are common.
  D. It can be diagnosed using nerve conduction velocity (NCV) tests and/or electromyography (EMG).

Rationale: C. Genetically caused polyneuropathies are rare

QUESTION 22
Your supervising physical therapist has delegated a patient with elbow dysfunction. On reviewing the patient's notes, you note that the therapist had recorded the left elbow range of motion as -10-0-150 degrees. From this measurement, you can assume that the patient's total available range of motion at the left elbow is which of the following?
  A. 160 degrees
  B. 140 degrees
  C. 150 degrees
  D. 130 degrees

Rationale: A. The available range of motion is 10 degrees + 150 degrees—160 degrees

QUESTION 23
You are reviewing a patient's medical history and note that the patient has a history of hemorrhagic disorders. All of the following test results are likely to be listed in the patient's chart, *EXCEPT*:
  A. Tourniquet test
  B. Prothrombin time
  C. Ischemia modified albumin
  D. Partial thromboplastin

Rationale: C. The ischemia-modified albumin test is used to assess for cardiac ischemia

QUESTION 24
You have been treating a patient who recently had a cast removed from the knee. As part of tracking the patient's progress, you measure the patient's knee range of motion and find that the range of motion for flexion begins at 10 degrees and ends at 80 degrees. How should you document the patient's knee range of motion?
  A. -10-0-80
  B. 10-0-80
  C. 10-80
  D. All would be appropriate to use

Rationale: C. This is the only one that would be appropriate

QUESTION 25
You are about to treat a patient with a recent onset of amyotrophic lateral sclerosis (ALS). All the following are characteristic signs and symptoms in the early stages of ALS, *EXCEPT*:
  A. Generally painless progressive muscle weakness
  B. Abnormal fatigue of the arms
  C. Occasional tripping and clumsiness
  D. All of the above are characteristic signs and symptoms in the early stages of ALS

Rationale: D. Although not all people with ALS experience the same initial signs and symptoms, the ones listed here are the most common

QUESTION 26
You are reviewing the supervising physical therapist's intervention plan for a patient with amyotrophic lateral sclerosis (ALS). What type of exercise would you expect to see?
  A. Mild-to-moderate endurance training
  B. Postural control exercises
  C. Intensive strengthening exercises
  D. All of the above are recommended

Rationale: A. Aerobic exercise at a mild-to-moderate intensity is recommended. Intensive strengthening is contraindicated to avoid fatiguing the person as this exacerbates their symptoms. Although postural control exercises will not harm, the clinician should focus on flexibility and range of motion exercises with this population

QUESTION 27

You are about to treat a patient who has agnosia as one of his symptoms following a stroke. Agnosia is characterized by a difficulty in which of the following?

A. Swallowing

B. Understanding speech

C. Recognizing the shapes of an object or face

D. Controlling bowel and bladder function

Rationale: C. Although patients with agnosia can often perceive shapes of an object or face, they cannot recall what the object is used for or whether a face is familiar or not

QUESTION 28

You are about to treat a patient recovering from a C5-C6 spinal cord injury (SCI). Which of the following upper extremity motions are you expecting to have normal strength?

A. Shoulder extension

B. Elbow flexion

C. Shoulder abduction

D. B and C

Rationale: D. The biceps and deltoid should be functioning normally

QUESTION 29

You are about to treat a patient with Parkinson disease. Which of the following is *NOT* a true statement about Parkinson disease?

A. It is a progressive nervous system disorder that disturbs movement.

B. It commonly causes stiffness or slowing of movement.

C. It produces a scissoring gait pattern.

D. It is characterized by difficulty with facial expressions.

Rationale: C. The festinating gait pattern is characteristic of Parkinson disease, not a scissoring gait pattern, which is primarily associated with spastic cerebral palsy

QUESTION 30

You are about to treat a patient with Parkinson disease. All of the following are valid statements about Parkinson disease, *EXCEPT*:

A. It is a progressive degenerative disorder of the central nervous system, particularly the substantia nigra.

B. It is often characterized by bradykinesia, difficulty with walking, and a resting tremor.

C. It is associated with dementia in the advanced stages of the disease.

D. It is no longer incurable.

Rationale: D. There is currently no cure for Parkinson disease. Instead, treatment aims to improve the symptoms

QUESTION 31

While performing a joint mobilization at a patient's radiocarpal joint, you note a decrease in the anterior (palmar) glide of the carpals on the radius compared to the other wrist. Which associated active wrist motion would you also expect to be decreased?

A. Wrist flexion

B. Wrist extension

C. Radial deviation

D. Ulnar deviation

Rationale: B. A decreased anterior glide indicates that there is a loss in wrist extension

QUESTION 32

You are reviewing lung volumes before seeing a patient with lung pathology. Which two lung volumes make up the functional residual capacity (FRC)?

A. Inspiratory reserve volume (IRV) plus expiratory reserve volume (ERV)

B. Tidal volume (TV) plus residual volume (RV)

C. ERV plus RV

D. IRV plus TV

Rationale: C. FRC is the sum of ERV plus RV

QUESTION 33

You are reviewing the medical chart of a patient you are about to treat who is diagnosed with ankylosing spondylitis (AS). Which of the following findings would you NOT expect to see?

A. Presence of the *HLA-B27* gene

B. High levels of C-reactive protein

C. The presence of antinuclear antibodies (ANA)

D. A decrease in serum creatinine (SCr) levels

Rationale: D. SCr levels assess for kidney function. All of the other findings are common with AS

QUESTION 34

You have been asked to provide patient education to an individual with insulin-dependent diabetes. The focus of patient education is on foot care. Which of the following would be the MOST effective method to teach the patient?

A. Inform the patient that no infections will occur if your directions are followed, then demonstrate the procedures

B. Have the patient demonstrate a foot inspection, and then provide feedback on the patient's performance

C. Observe the patient performing a foot inspection while cautioning him/her about how poor foot inspections can lead to amputations

D. Describe a foot inspection and have the patient demonstrate

Rationale: B. An effective foot inspection requires psychomotor skills and strategic planning, both of which can be enhanced by practicing and receiving feedback

QUESTION 35

Your department supervisor has asked you to design a utilization and peer review for the department. Which of the following categories use a utilization and peer review?

A. Policy and procedure

B. Quality improvement

C. Financial audit

D. Performance evaluation

Rationale: B. The written plan for continuous improvement of quality of care includes a continuing review and appraisal of the physical therapy services provided

QUESTION 36

You are collaborating with your supervising physical therapist on a research study, and she wants to know the difference between the median and the mean indicates. The difference between the median and the mean indicates which of the following?

A. That the two measures should be averaged

B. The value of the Z-score

C. That the distribution is skewed

D. The value of the standard deviation score

Rationale: C. If the median and mean are not of equal value, the distribution is skewed such that if the median is of a higher value than the mean, the distribution is skewed to the left, but if it is lower, it is skewed to the right.

QUESTION 37

You are reviewing a patient's chart and see that the supervising physical therapist used the van Gelderen bicycle test. What is the van Gelderen bicycle test?

A. It is a test designed to stress the lower extremity vascular system without causing any foraminal stenosis.

B. It is a test designed to stress the cardiovascular system in a non–weight-bearing position.

C. It is a test used by professional cyclists to determine their cadence.

D. None of the above. There is no such test.

Rationale: A. The test is used to differentiate between a diagnosis of intermittent vascular claudication and intermittent neurogenic claudication

QUESTION 38

You have been asked to provide patient education to a patient who recently underwent a transfemoral amputation. What positioning of the hip should you emphasize to the patient?

A. To position the hip in flexion and abduction

B. To position the hip in extension and adduction

C. To position the hip in adduction and external rotation

D. To position the hip in flexion and internal rotation

Rationale: B. As the residual limb following a transfemoral amputation tends to develop contractures in the hip flexors and abductors, the patient must regularly position the hip in extension and adduction

QUESTION 39

You are about to treat a 14-year-old adolescent boy with Duchenne muscular dystrophy. You would not expect to find all of the following, *EXCEPT*:

A. Waddling gait

B. Small calf muscles

C. Normal growth milestones

D. No difficulty with sit to stand

Rationale: A. The common characteristics of Duchenne muscle dystrophy include a waddling gait, large calf muscles, delayed growth, difficulty rising from a lying or sitting position, frequent falls, walking on the toes, muscle pain and stiffness, and learning difficulties

QUESTION 40

You are reviewing a patient's chart and note that the patient demonstrated many pathologic reflexes. All the following are pathologic reflexes, *EXCEPT*:

A. Tromner

B. Jendrassik

C. Oppenheim

D. Chaddock

Rationale: D. The Jendrassik is a maneuver used to distract a patient while performing a muscle stretch reflex. The Tromner sign is elicited by supporting the patient's proximal phalanx of the middle finger and then flicking its distal phalanx upward. Oppenheim sign is great toe dorsiflexion elicited by applying an irritation downward of the medial side of the tibia. Chaddock sign is present when stroking of the lateral malleolus causes extension of the great toe

QUESTION 41

As part of recording a patient's progress, you perform resisted hip flexion with the patient in the sitting position and note that the patient demonstrates external rotation with abduction of the thigh as your resistance is applied. Which of the following muscle is likely substituting?

A. Tensor fascia latae

B. Iliopsoas

C. Sartorius
D. Adductor magnus

Rationale: C. The sartorius flexes, externally rotates, and abducts the hip joint

QUESTION 42
You are reviewing a patient's chart who has a diagnosis of medial elbow tendinopathy. All the following are special tests you would expect to see in the supervising physical therapist's examination, *EXCEPT*:
  A. Reverse Cozen test
  B. Maudsley test
  C. Polk test
  D. None of the above

Rationale: B. Maudsley test is used to help confirm a diagnosis of lateral elbow tendinopathy

QUESTION 43
You receive a phone call from a patient's father requesting a copy of the patient's medical record. What should be your response?
  A. Allow the request.
  B. Inform the father that the request for a copy must be made in writing to the insurer.
  C. Inform the father that the medical record is the property of the hospital and can only be released with written authorization from the patient.
  D. Inform the father that the medical record can only be released with written authorization from the patient's physician.

Rationale: C. Unless restricted by state or federal law or regulation, a hospital shall furnish to a patient or a patient's representative parts of the hospital record upon request in writing by the patient or their representative.
Roach WH. *Medical Records and the Law.* 4th ed. Sudbury, MA: Jones & Bartlett; 2006:111-114

QUESTION 44
You are treating a female teenager with a posterior cruciate ligament (PCL) tear diagnosis. All of the following are true statements regarding the PCL, *EXCEPT*:
  A. The PCL is larger and stronger than the anterior cruciate ligament (ACL).
  B. PCL injuries are less common than ACL injuries.
  C. Most individuals hear a popping sensation in the knee with a PCL injury.
  D. The PCL functions to resist the tibia moving posteriorly to the femur.

Rationale: C. Hearing a popping in the knee is more common with an injury to the ACL. All of the other statements are true

QUESTION 45
While reviewing a patient's chart, you note that the patient is recently diagnosed with deep venous thrombophlebitis, for which he was prescribed heparin. Which of the following is the primary function of heparin?
  A. To act as a blood thinner
  B. To act as an anticoagulant
  C. To act by decreasing systolic blood pressure
  D. To act by increasing cardiac contractility

Rationale: B. Heparin is an anticoagulant used to retard the ability of the body to form blood clots. Although heparin is often referred to as a "blood thinner" by the layperson, it does not thin the blood.

QUESTION 46

You are supervising a group exercise class in which a 56-year-old man with a history of limited physical activity and angina pectoris is participating. You begin to suspect the patient is experiencing an episode of unstable angina because of which of the following signs?

A. A slightly delayed cessation of pain following the administration of nitroglycerin.

B. Angina that increases in intensity and is unresponsive to decreased activity or rest.

C. The anginal pain responds quickly to a decrease in activity or rest.

D. Evidence of arrhythmias that increase in frequency, especially atrial arrhythmias.

Rationale: B. While stable angina occurs predictably and responds positively to a decrease in activity and the administration of nitroglycerin, unstable angina can occur at rest or with exertion

QUESTION 47

You are about to treat a 60-year-old man with a history of cardiovascular disease. Which of the following is a leading cause of sudden cardiac death in individuals with cardiovascular disease?

A. Cardiac ischemia

B. Cardiac arrhythmias

C. Cardiac infarction

D. Cardiac failure

Rationale: B. Ventricular fibrillation and ventricular tachycardia lead to an abrupt halt to cardiac output

QUESTION 48

You are monitoring a patient while she exercises as part of her cardiac rehabilitation program. Which of the following signs or symptoms would cause you to stop the patient from exercising further?

A. The patient complains of mild angina.

B. There is a plateau or slight decrease in the patient's diastolic blood pressure.

C. There is a drop of 5 mm Hg in the patient's systolic blood pressure.

D. The patient complains of increased dizziness.

Rationale: D. Any signs or symptoms of nervous system involvement (eg, ataxia, dizziness, or near-syncope) are absolute contraindications to continuing with the exercise. The other signs or symptoms listed are relative contraindications to continuing with the exercise

QUESTION 49

You are performing a chart review on a patient who was admitted to the hospital with breathing difficulties. The chart review indicates that the patient has a pectus carinatum. Which of the following best describes this condition?

A. A cone-shaped appearance of the rib cage

B. An anterior protrusion of the sternum and chest

C. Paradoxical movement of the rib cage during inspiration and expiration

D. A posterior indentation of the sternum and chest

Rationale: B. Pectus carinatum results in an anterior protrusion of the sternum and chest

QUESTION 50

The next patient on your schedule has a diagnosis of Boutonnière deformity. In which position would you expect to find the proximal interphalangeal (PIP) joint and the distal interphalangeal (DIP) joint of the involved finger?

A. PIP flexion and DIP flexion

B. PIP extension and DIP extension

C. PIP extension and DIP flexion

D. PIP flexion and DIP extension

Rationale: D. The Boutonnière deformity is characterized by flexion of the PIP joint and extension of the DIP joint

QUESTION 51

You are reviewing the surface anatomy of the hand and wrist before treating a patient with a carpal fracture. Which of the following carpal bones would not be found in the proximal road?

A. Lunate
B. Capitate
C. Scaphoid
D. Triquetrum

Rationale: B. The proximal row of carpal bones consists of the scaphoid, lunate, triquetrum, and pisiform

QUESTION 52

You are reviewing the surface anatomy of the hand and wrist with your student. Which of the following is not part of the triangular fibrocartilage complex (TFC) of the wrist?

A. Ulnar collateral ligament
B. Ulnar articular cartilage
C. Radial collateral ligament
D. Posterior radioulnar ligament

Rationale: C. The radial collateral ligament is not considered part of the triangular fibrocartilage complex

QUESTION 53

You are reviewing the surface anatomy of the foot and ankle with your student. Which of the following articulates with the second cuneiform?

A. Navicular
B. Talus
C. Cuboid
D. Calcaneus

Rationale: A. The second cuneiform articulates with the navicular

QUESTION 54

You are setting up a patient to perform joint mobilizations on the proximal radioulnar joint. How would you position the elbow and forearm to place the joint in its open-packed position?

A. 70 degrees flexion, 35 degrees supination
B. 10 degrees flexion, 10 degrees pronation
C. 45 degrees flexion, 20 degrees supination
D. 20 degrees flexion, 45 degrees supination

Rationale: A. 70 degrees flexion, 35 degrees supination is the open-packed position for the proximal radioulnar joint

QUESTION 55

You are working with a patient who fatigues easily but needs to improve ballistic movements. Which of the following is the best exercise approach for this patient?

A. Low-intensity workouts for long durations to help develop slow-twitch fibers
B. Low-intensity workouts for short durations to help develop slow-twitch fibers
C. High-intensity workouts for long durations to help develop fast- and slow-twitch fibers
D. High-intensity workouts for short durations to help develop fast-twitch fibers

Rationale: D. High-intensity exercises develop fast-twitch fibers, which are needed for ballistic movements

QUESTION 56

You are gait training a patient to use a reciprocating gait orthosis (RGO) with a walker. Which of the following is the correct sequence?

A. Shift the weight onto one leg and swing the other leg through while leaning on the walker.

B. Shift the weight onto the walker, extend the upper trunk, and swing both legs forward together to approach the walker.

C. Shift the weight onto the walker and one leg, extend the upper trunk and swing the other leg through.

D. Shift the weight onto the walker, flex the upper trunk, and move both legs forward together to approach the walker.

Rationale: C. This is the correct sequence

QUESTION 57

You are reviewing the surface anatomy of the wrist and hand. Which of the following structures does not pass through the anatomic snuff box?

A. Extensor pollicis brevis

B. Abductor pollicis brevis

C. Abductor pollicis longus

D. Extensor pollicis longus

Rationale: C. The abductor pollicis longus does not pass through the anatomic snuff box

QUESTION 58

You are treating a patient who sustained a left tibial fracture. In today's session, you will teach the patient how to use crutches using a four-point gait pattern. Which of the following describes this pattern?

A. (R) crutch, (L) foot, (L) crutch, (R) foot

B. (L) crutch, (R) foot, (R) foot, (L) crutch

C. (R) crutch, (R) foot, (L) crutch, (L) foot

D. (L) crutch, (R) foot, (R) crutch, (L) foot

Rationale: D. With the four-point gait pattern, the crutch moves with the uninvolved leg

QUESTION 59

You are reviewing the various muscles of the wrist and hand. Which of the following is the primary extensor of the metacarpophalangeal (MCP) joints of the hand?

A. Extensor carpi radialis longus (ECRL)

B. Extensor digitorum communis (EDC)

C. Extensor carpi ulnaris

D. None of the above

Rationale: B. The extracellular matrix (ECM) extends the MCP and carpometacarpal (CMC) articulations

QUESTION 60

You are examining a patient's wrist and measuring the range of motion for radial deviation using a goniometer. You align the proximal arm with the forearm and the distal arm with the third metacarpal. What structure should be used as the goniometer's fulcrum point?

A. Scaphoid

B. Pisiform

C. Capitate

D. Lunate

Rationale: C. The capitate should be used as the fulcrum

QUESTION 61

You are reviewing a patient's medical record and see that the patient has a history of Heberden nodes. Which of the following conditions are associated with Heberden nodes?

A. Rheumatoid arthritis

B. Osteoarthritis

C. Ankylosing spondylitis

D. Osteoporosis

Rationale: B. Heberden nodes, bony enlargements of the distal interphalangeal (DIP) joints are associated with osteoarthritis

QUESTION 62

You are performing manual muscle testing on a patient who recently sustained a spinal cord injury. Which nerve segment primarily innervates the long toe extensors?

A. L2

B. L3

C. L4

D. L5

Rationale: D. The L5 spinal cord segment innervates the long toe extensors

QUESTION 63

You are watching your supervising physical therapist performing a cranial nerve (CN) test on a patient. The patient demonstrates ipsilateral wasting of the tongue and deviation of the tongue during protrusion. Which cranial nerve is involved?

A. IX

B. X

C. XI

D. XII

Rationale: D. Cranial nerve XII (hypoglossal) supplies motor innervation to the tongue, innervating the ipsilateral side of the tongue

QUESTION 64

You are reviewing a patient's medical record before performing a treatment. You note in the medication section that the patient has been prescribed tissue plasminogen activator (tPA). What is this medication commonly used to treat?

A. Multiple sclerosis

B. Traumatic brain injury

C. Hemorrhagic stroke

D. Ischemic stroke

Rationale: D. tPA, which increases blood flow, is commonly given following the immediate onset of an ischemic stroke but is, therefore, contraindicated in cases of hemorrhagic stroke

QUESTION 65

You are reviewing the various body systems. Which of the following structures make up the integumentary system?

A. The dermis, hypodermis, and subcutaneous tissue

B. The skin, hair, nails, mucous membrane, circulation, and related sensory structures

C. The dermis, epidermis, and subcutaneous tissue

D. The skin, hair, nails, and teeth

Rationale: B. All of the other options (except for the teeth, which are part of the skeletal system) are only some of the parts of the integumentary system

QUESTION 66

You are reviewing a patient's medical chart and note that the patient has cellulitis. Which of the following would be the best definition of cellulitis?

A. The presence of dried fragments of sloughed dead epidermis

B. Inflammation of the dermis

C. An infection of the dermis and subcutaneous tissue

D. The presence of a dermal or subcutaneous solid and elevated lesion

Rationale: C. Cellulitis is an infection of the dermis and subcutaneous tissue

QUESTION 67
You are discussing the role of the pancreas in diabetes mellitus with your student. Which of the following is a correct statement about the alpha and beta cells of the pancreas?
- A. The alpha cells release aldosterone, and the beta cells release cortisol.
- B. The alpha cells release glucagon, and the beta cells release insulin.
- C. The alpha cells release epinephrine, and the beta cells release norepinephrine.
- D. The alpha cells release cortisol, and the beta cells release aldosterone.

Rationale: B. The pancreas, through a balanced release of glucagon and insulin, is involved with the regulation of blood sugar

QUESTION 68
You are about to apply a low-level laser to a patient for treatment. What must you ensure before you begin the treatment?
- A. Whether the patient wants to wear protective goggles.
- B. You and the patient are wearing goggles.
- C. The patient is wearing goggles.
- D. You are wearing goggles.

Rationale: B. Both the patient and the therapist need to be wearing goggles to prevent retinal damage

QUESTION 69
You are about to use electrical stimulation to increase active dorsiflexion during the swing phase of gait. Which of the following electrode placements would be the most appropriate to use?
- A. Posterior tibialis muscle belly
- B. Anterior tibialis muscle belly and fibularis (peroneal) nerve
- C. Fibularis longus and brevis muscle bellies
- D. Gastrocnemius and anterior tibialis muscle bellies

Rationale: B. This placement would allow the foot to be balanced between inversion and eversion

QUESTION 70
You are about to apply iontophoresis to a patient. Which of the following equations should be used to determine the correct dosage?
- A. Dosage = current × frequency
- B. Dosage = voltage × duration
- C. Dosage = current × duration
- D. Dosage = voltage × frequency

Rationale: C. This is the correct formula to determine the dosage

QUESTION 71
You are outlining the different scales of measurement to your student. Diagnosis, blood type, and race are examples of which of the following scales of measurement?
- A. Ratio
- B. Ordinal
- C. Nominal
- D. Interval

Rationale: C. On a nominal scale, objects or people are assigned to categories according to some criteria or code

QUESTION 72
You are discussing statistics with your student with an emphasis on sampling. Which of the following sampling methods would be considered probability sampling?
- A. Quota sampling
- B. Cluster sampling
- C. Convenience sampling
- D. None of the above

Rationale: B. The other two are examples of nonprobability sampling

QUESTION 73
You are discussing the various types of study designs with your student. Which of the following study designs is most used for cross-cultural studies?
A. Experimental
B. Comparative
C. Case study
D. Longitudinal

Rationale: C. This type of study design commonly involves a comparison of cultural traits across a timeframe

QUESTION 74
A patient has a rotator cuff tear, and you are performing a manual muscle test (MMT) on their shoulder. The patient has a palpable muscle contraction, but no joint motion occurs. In this situation, what MMT test grade would you give the patient?
A. Trace (1)
B. Zero (0)
C. Trace minus (1−)
D. Poor minus (2−)

Rationale: A. This grade indicates that no visible movement of the tested body part is detected except a slight contraction

QUESTION 75
Which medical field is concerned with weight loss causes, issues and prevention, and the treatment of obesity?
A. Endocrinology
B. Internal medicine
C. Bariatrics
D. Obstetrics

Rationale: C

QUESTION 76
You instruct a patient who has a left ankle injury and is partial weight-bearing with axillary crutches to ascend a curb. For this activity, where should you stand relative to the patient?
A. In front of the patient
B. To the left of the patient
C. To the right of the patient
D. Behind the patient

Rationale: B. When assisting a patient with ambulation, you should stand on the involved side

QUESTION 77
You perform static balance activities with a patient, and he can stand on both feet without assistance. Of the choices below, which added activity would *NOT* be more challenging?
A. Standing on one foot
B. Standing on a foam mat
C. Sitting in a straight-back chair with no armrests
D. Standing with the eyes closed

Rationale: C

QUESTION 78
What is the amount of blood pumped by the heart per beat called?
A. Cardiac output
B. Stroke volume
C. Tidal volume
D. Ejection volume

Rationale: B. Stroke volume is the amount of blood pumped by the heart's left ventricle in one contraction. Cardiac output is the volume of blood being pumped by the heart in a minute

QUESTION 79
Which of the following choices is *NOT* a modifiable risk factor for obesity?
  A. Inactivity
  B. Family history
  C. Diet
  D. Stress

Rationale: B

QUESTION 80
Which of the following would *NOT* found in the objective section of a SOAP note?
  A. The patient's vital signs
  B. Description of the patient's present treatment
  C. Discussion of the patient's past medical history
  D. The patient's range of motion measurements

Rationale: C

QUESTION 81
You are treating a patient exhibiting postural tremors, cogwheel and lead pipe rigidity, postural instability, and bradykinesia. These are all signs of which of the following?
  A. Parkinson disease
  B. Lou Gehrig disease
  C. Cerebellar disease
  D. Raynaud disease

Rationale: A

QUESTION 82
You are treating a patient with C5 quadriplegia who is susceptible to pressure sores at an inpatient facility. How often should the patient be turned to prevent a pressure sore from developing?
  A. Every 30 minutes
  B. Every 60 minutes
  C. Every 120 minutes
  D. Every 180 minutes

Rationale: C

QUESTION 83
You are palpating the elbow of a patient with the diagnosis of lateral elbow tendinopathy (LET). After palpating the lateral epicondyle, you move distally and cross the joint line. If you continue distally, what would be the next bony landmark you would palpate?
  A. Medial epicondyle
  B. Olecranon process
  C. Radial head
  D. Lateral supracondylar ridge

Rationale: C

QUESTION 84
You are about to measure a patient's walking endurance using the 6-minute walk test (6MWT). Which of the following are *NOT* true statements about the 6MWT?
  A. The score of the test is the distance a patient walks in 6 minutes.
  B. An assistive device can be used but must be documented.
  C. When the patient takes a standing rest, the stopwatch is stopped during the length of the rest period.
  D. The patient may take as many standing rests as they like.

Rationale: C. The patient can take a standing rest, but the stopwatch is not stopped—the time continues throughout.

QUESTION 85
You are treating a patient with a diagnosis of osteoporosis. Which of the following types of exercises should be avoided with this patient?
  A. Weight-bearing exercises
  B. Lumbar extension exercises
  C. Lumbar flexion exercises
  D. All of the above

Rationale: C. Lumbar flexion exercises can produce excessive strain on the lumbar spine and increase the potential for compression fractures

QUESTION 86
You are performing gait training on stairs with a patient status post transfemoral amputation. In which of the following locations should you stand when the patient is ascending the stairs?
  A. On the involved side
  B. On the uninvolved side
  C. Behind, and more on the involved side
  D. In front, and more on the uninvolved side

Rationale: C. When a patient is ascending the stairs, the clinician needs to be behind the patient and slightly more toward the involved side as the involved side is likely to be weaker

QUESTION 87
You are instructing a patient on how to ascend stairs using crutches. The patient has physician orders for partial weight-bearing. Which of the following is the correct sequence?
  A. Uninvolved leg first, then involved leg, then crutches
  B. Crutches up first, then the uninvolved leg, then the involved leg
  C. Crutches up first, then the involved leg, then the uninvolved leg
  D. Involved leg first, then the uninvolved leg, then the crutches

Rationale: A. This is the correct sequence

QUESTION 88
You instruct a non–weight-bearing patient on using a standard walker and a three-point gait pattern (step to). Which of the following would be the correct gait pattern to teach?
  A. Walker first, then the uninvolved leg, and then the involved leg up to and not past the involved leg
  B. Uninvolved leg first, then the walker, and then the involved leg up to and not past the uninvolved leg
  C. Walker first, then the involved leg, and then the uninvolved leg up to and not past the involved leg
  D. None of the above

Rationale: C. The correct sequence is always the assistive device first, then the involved leg, and then the uninvolved leg

QUESTION 89
You are discussing with your student the advantages and disadvantages of the various assistive devices for long-term use. When comparing Lofstrand crutches to axillary crutches, which of the following benefits are the most accurate?
  A. Lofstrand crutches are more aesthetically pleasing for the patient.
  B. Lofstrand crutches are more durable.
  C. There is a decreased risk of brachial plexus injury when using Lofstrand crutches.
  D. All of the above

Rationale: C. Of those benefits listed, the most accurate is that Lofstrand crutches decrease the risk of brachial plexus injury when compared to axillary crutches

QUESTION 90

You are teaching a caregiver how to use a wheelchair in the community for their client. How would you teach the caregiver to move a wheelchair down a curb when there is no ramp available?

A. With the patient strapped in, and the patient facing forward, lower the caster wheels off the curb and then the large wheels.

B. With the patient facing backward, lower the large wheels off the curb and then tip the chair back enough to clear the caster wheels.

C. With the patient facing forward, tip the wheelchair back so that the caster wheels are in the air, and then lower the chair of the curb.

D. All of the above would be appropriate methods.

Rationale: B. The safest way is for the caregiver to have the patient facing backward and lower both back wheels together before tipping the chair enough to clear the small caster wheels. Any method that has the patient facing forward increases the risk of the wheelchair tipping forward.

QUESTION 91

You are reviewing a hospital's policy about the various restraint levels. Which of the following scenarios would most likely be considered a form of restraining a patient?

A. Applying a seat belt to a wheelchair that the patient can voluntarily take off

B. A family member allowing a patient to use a prescribed sleeping medication

C. Allowing a family member to use a gait belt to tie around the patient and the chair to improve trunk positioning

D. Asking a patient to self-apply a seat belt when using a powered wheelchair

Rationale: C. Although the family member is trying to help the patient, this scenario would be considered a restraint as the patient cannot get out of the chair voluntarily

QUESTION 92

You are training a physical therapy aide on how to wash their hands in between patients correctly. What is the minimum length of time that the aide should use the application of soap on their hands?

A. 5 to 10 seconds

B. 10 to 15 seconds

C. 15 to 30 seconds

D. 30 to 45 seconds

Rationale: C. The recommended time for the application of soap during hand washing is 15 to 30 seconds.

QUESTION 93

You are teaching a caregiver how to use a wheelchair in the community for their client. How would you teach the caregiver to move a wheelchair up onto a curb when there is no ramp available?

A. With the patient facing forward, raise the caster wheels onto the curb and then the large wheels.

B. With the patient facing backward, tilt the chair back and pull the large wheels onto the curb and then the caster wheels.

C. With the patient facing forward, approach the curb at a diagonal angle and then raise the caster wheel closest to the curb onto the curb and then the large wheel on the same side. Then, the other caster wheel is moved onto the curb, followed by the other large wheel.

D. With the patient facing backward, approach the curb at a diagonal angle, and then raise the nearest large wheel onto the curb and then the caster wheel on the same side. Then, the other large wheel is moved onto the curb, followed by the other castor wheel.

Rationale: A. This would be the safest method. Depending on the patient's ability, the patient could assist the caregiver by leaning forward and placing his/her hands on the hand rims where the most force can be applied and then pushing the wheels forward as the caregiver lifts the wheelchair. Approaching the curb with the patient facing backward requires more effort from the caregiver and risks the patient falling backward onto their head if the caregiver releases their grip

QUESTION 94
You are discussing the various types of safe lifting techniques with a physical therapy aide. Which of the following lifting techniques would be the most appropriate to lift a light object off the floor?
  A. Straight-leg lift
  B. Golfer's lift (extending a straight leg behind)
  C. No specific technique as the object is light
  D. Power lift using a wide stance

Rationale: B. The golfer's lift is the most appropriate for small, light objects

QUESTION 95
You are presenting an in-house in-service to the department's support personnel about COVID-19. All the following are true statements, *EXCEPT*:
  A. The virus that causes COVID-19 is in a family of viruses called Coronaviridae.
  B. Most people who get COVID-19 have mild or moderate symptoms and can recover with supportive care.
  C. The prolonged use of medical masks, when properly worn, causes CO_2 intoxication and/or oxygen deficiency.
  D. The COVID-19 virus can spread quicker in hot and humid climates.

Rationale: C. When properly worn, the prolonged use of medical masks *DOES NOT* cause CO_2 intoxication nor oxygen deficiency

QUESTION 96
You are about to apply intermittent pneumatic compression to a patient. Which of the following settings concerning inflation pressure is generally recommended when applying intermittent pneumatic compression?
  A. Inflation pressure should not exceed the patient's systolic blood pressure minus 10 mm Hg.
  B. Inflation pressure should not exceed the patient's diastolic blood pressure plus 10 mm Hg.
  C. Inflation pressure should not exceed the patient's systolic blood pressure plus 10 mm Hg.
  D. Inflation pressure should not exceed the patient's diastolic blood pressure minus 10 mm Hg.

Rationale: D. Studies suggest that a pressure higher than a patient's diastolic blood pressure minus 10 mm Hg will restrict venous return

QUESTION 97
You are working in a local skilled nursing facility and, while reviewing a patient's chart, you note that the patient has measles. Which of the following would be the minimum precautions that you should take while working with this patient?
  A. Wear a gown, gloves, and mask at all times.
  B. Wear a personal mask if working within 3 ft of the patient.
  C. Wear a gown if in direct contact with the patient.
  D. Wear a personal mask at all times.

Rationale: D. Measles is an airborne infection, so a mask must be worn at all times while working with the patient. Depending on the facility's requirements, a gown and gloves may also be required.

QUESTION 98

You are involved with an academic study examining the effect of ultrasound intensities on patients' pain level with lateral elbow tendinopathy. In this study, "pain level" is which of the following types of variable?

A. Dependent variable
B. Independent variable
C. Categorical variable
D. Continuous variable

Rationale: A. A dependent variable is the variable being tested and measured—in this case, "pain level"

QUESTION 99

You review the various types of validity in statistics. What type of validity is being used when comparing the relationship between goniometric measurement results and radiographic measurement results when the latter's validity is known?

A. Concurrent validity
B. Content validity
C. Construct validity
D. None of the above

Rationale: A. Concurrent validity measures how well a new test (goniometry) compares to a well-established test (radiographic measurement)

QUESTION 100

You are discussing with your supervising physical therapist the various terms and definitions used with outcome measures. Which of the following definitions best describes the most common threshold for meaningful change used to determine if a treatment has been beneficial to a patient?

A. Standard deviation (SD)
B. Minimal detectable difference (MDD)
C. Minimal clinical important difference (MCID)
D. None of the above

Rationale: C. The minimal clinically important difference (MCID), or minimal important difference (MID), is the smallest change in a treatment outcome that a patient would identify as important

QUESTION 101

You are about to treat a patient who has been experiencing delirium, according to the medical chart. Which of the following would you expect to see with this patient?

A. Impaired consciousness and a highly variable mood
B. Impaired consciousness and a normal attention span
C. Impaired consciousness and a depressed mood
D. Highly variable levels of consciousness and a short attention span

Rationale: D. This is the typical finding with delirium. Impaired consciousness is associated more with dementia

QUESTION 102

You are reviewing a patient's chart and note that the patient has a diagnosis of Duchenne muscular dystrophy (DMD). All of the following are true statements, *EXCEPT*:

A. DMD is a genetic disorder characterized by progressive muscle degeneration and weakness.
B. DMD is one of four conditions known as dystrophinopathies.
C. Gowers sign, a characteristic of DMD, compensates for proximal contractures.
D. DMD results from alterations of a protein called dystrophin.

Rationale: C. Gowers sign compensates for the proximal weakness

QUESTION 103
You are treating a patient with a diagnosis of fibromyalgia at your aquatic therapy center. The physical therapist examination reveals that the patient is moderately deconditioned due to months of inactivity resulting from a mild myocardial infarction 2 years ago. What are the expected effects of hydrostatic pressure exerted by the water on this patient?
  A. To increase resistance as the speed of active movement increases
  B. To increase cardiovascular demands both at rest and with exercise
  C. To assist in venous return and reduce effusion
  D. All of the above

Rationale: C. According to Pascal law (a pressure change in one part is transmitted without loss to every portion of the fluid), as the depth of immersion increases, so does hydrostatic pressure. This increased pressure works to limit effusion and assist venous return

QUESTION 104
While performing gait training, you note that the patient walks with a significant posterior trunk lean as he takes full weight on his left leg. Upon questioning, the patient reports difficulty walking up ramps. Which of the following would be the best intervention to recommend to the physical therapist?
  A. Core strengthening
  B. Strengthening of the hip extensors
  C. Stretching of the lumbar extensors
  D. All of the above

Rationale: B. A posterior trunk lean during gait, particularly at initial contact, is commonly referred to as gluteus maximus gait as it highlights the weakness of the hip extensors

QUESTION 105
You are treating a 78-year-old patient to enhance balance and gait. During the discussion, the patient reports mistaking images directly in front of him, especially in bright light. Further questioning reveals that the patient can locate items in his environment with his peripheral vision when walking but that his reading has become more difficult. Which of the following conditions do you expect the patient may have?
  A. Cataracts
  B. Homonymous hemianopsia
  C. Glaucoma
  D. None of the above

Rationale: A. With cataracts, central vision is lost first, then peripheral. With glaucoma, the opposite is true—loss of peripheral vision first, then central. Homonymous hemianopsia is associated with a cerebrovascular accident (CVA).

QUESTION 106
Your supervising physical therapist is discussing the results of a study that she and her colleague completed. The study looked at the effectiveness of transcutaneous electrical nerve stimulation (TENS) and massage in treating patients with pain, and the pain instrument they used had a possible score of 50, with 50 being the worst pain. The data analysis revealed that the TENS group had a mean score of 34 with a standard deviation of 1.0, while the massage group had a mean of 36 with a standard deviation of 6.0. Based on these results, what conclusion could one make?
  A. The spread of scores with the massage group has a greater variability.
  B. TENS has a greater effect on pain relief than massage.
  C. Massage has a greater effect on pain relief than TENS.
  D. The spread of scores with the TENS group has greater variability.

Rationale: A. The massage group has a standard deviation of 6.0, indicating that this treatment produces more variability than the TENS. None of the other conclusions can be determined based on the data presented.

QUESTION 107

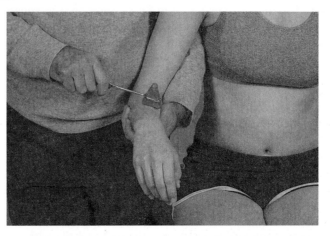

The clinician in the photograph is testing which muscle stretch reflex?
A. Biceps
B. Brachialis
C. Brachioradialis
D. None of the above

Rationale: C. The muscle stretch reflex being tested is the brachioradialis

QUESTION 108
You are about to treat a patient with a diagnosis of status post anterior dislocation of the left shoulder. Which of the following findings would you expect to see in the physical therapist's examination findings?
A. Weak biceps brachii
B. Weak deltoids
C. Weak rhomboids
D. Weak subscapularis

Rationale: B. The axillary nerve, which innervates the deltoids and the teres minor, is often injured during an anterior-inferior dislocation at the glenohumeral joint. An axillary nerve injury would not impact all of the other choices

QUESTION 109
You are reviewing a patient's chart before performing the initial examination. The patient's physician wants the patient to get out of bed today. The patient has a diagnosis of congestive heart failure and has been prescribed diuretics and calcium channel blockers. Which of the following potential side effects of these medications should you be alert for when getting the patient out of bed?
A. Decreased electrolyte levels resulting in increased arrhythmias
B. Dizziness and orthostatic hypotension
C. Extreme fatigue
D. Unstable blood pressure

Rationale: B. Dizziness and orthostatic hypotension are well documented side effects that diuretics or calcium channel blockers can cause

QUESTION 110
In this model of the hand, which joint is being mobilized by the clinician?

Reproduced with permission from Dutton M. *Dutton's Orthopaedic Examination, Evaluation, and Intervention*, 4th ed. 2017. © Copyright McGraw Hill LLC. All rights reserved. https://accessphysiotherapy.mhmedical.com.

A. Triquetrum-hamate
B. Capitate-hamate
C. Capitate-lunate
D. Capitate-scaphoid

Rationale: B. It is the capitate-hamate joint that is being mobilized

QUESTION 111
You are treating a patient who is recovering from a right transtibial amputation. During one of your sessions, the patient complains of numbness and tingling in the posterior aspect of his right foot and big toe. Although you suspect the possibility of phantom symptoms, you decide to check whether the residual limb wrapping might be causing the symptoms before talking to the supervising physical therapist. Which of the following nerves could be compromised by the wrapping and caused the patient's symptoms?

A. Common fibular (peroneal) nerve
B. Tibial nerve
C. Sural nerve
D. None of the above

Rationale: A. The distribution of the patient's symptoms closely relates to the sensation provided by the superficial fibular (peroneal) nerve, a branch of the common fibular (peroneal) nerve

QUESTION 112
You want to determine the accuracy of two types of wrist heart rate monitors used in your department during exercise. The correlational analysis measured the strength of the relationship between the two types of monitors during a treadmill exercise and found that the measured heart rates of both had a correlation of 0.88 at high levels of exercise but only 0.67 at low levels of exercise. The results of this study suggest which of the following?

A. Both devices are accurate at all exercise levels.
B. The accuracy of the measurements increases at higher exercise levels.
C. The accuracy of the measurements decreases at higher exercise levels.
D. Both devices are only moderately accurate.

Rationale: B. The analysis revealed that the correlation between the two heart rate monitors was high when the exercise levels were high (0.88) but only moderate (0.67) at low exercise levels

QUESTION 113
You are discussing the release of medical information to third parties with your supervising physical therapist. In which of the following scenarios is it illegal to release patient information without obtaining the patient's consent?
A. The insurance company that is paying for the patient's treatment.
B. The patient's employer when the condition is work-related.
C. The referring physician.
D. All of the above are legal.

Rationale: B. Only the patient's payer, or those individuals involved in the care of the patient (a legal guardian or power of attorney), has a legal right to information regarding a patient's care without obtaining the patient's consent for releasing information

QUESTION 114
A patient recovering from a stroke has a family member come to his treatment session to be instructed on a stand pivot transfer. Which of the following would be the best way to teach the family member?
A. Demonstrate the transfer with the patient and then have the family member perform the transfer on you.
B. Demonstrate the transfer with the family member as the patient.
C. Demonstrate the transfer on the family member and then on the patient.
D. Demonstrate the transfer with the patient and then have the family member practice with the patient.

Rationale: D. The best, and safest, method would be to demonstrate the transfer with the patient at the correct speed and then provide feedback to the family member as he/she practices with the patient

QUESTION 115
You are treating a patient who has a diagnosis of left hemiplegia with the patient's wife in attendance. During the session, you notice that the patient can recognize his wife when she talks to him but cannot recognize the face of one of his adult children when they arrive late for the session. Which of the following would be the *MOST* likely explanation for this behavior?
A. Alzheimer
B. Dementia
C. Prosopagnosia
D. Ideational apraxia

Rationale: C. The most likely explanation would be prosopagnosia, an inability to recognize human faces, despite the normal functioning of the eyes and optic tracts. In this case, the patient was able to recognize his wife by her voice

QUESTION 116
You treat a patient with quadriceps weakness (4-/5) who has reported difficulty descending stairs. Functional quad strengthening is written in the plan of care (POC). Which of the following would be the best method to regain functional strength in the quadriceps?
A. Partial wall squats progressing to lunges
B. Short arc quads
C. Isokinetic knee extensions
D. Multiple-angle isometric exercises performed maximally

Rationale: A. The best choice in terms of functional carryover would be to use closed kinetic chain exercises such as partial wall squats progressing to lunges as they will help develop stability and balance

QUESTION 117
You are working on increasing a patient's pelvic/lower back mobility using a therapy ball. Which of the following therapy ball movements could you incorporate to improve lower abdominal control?
A. Backward movement to produce posterior tilting of the pelvis
B. Forward movement to produce anterior tilting of the pelvis

C. Forward movement to produce posterior tilting of the pelvis
D. Backward movement to produce anterior tilting of the pelvis

Rationale: C. Posterior tilting of the pelvis, by contracting the lower abdominals, can be achieved using a forward movement of the therapy ball

QUESTION 118
You are reviewing a patient's medical chart before treating them for the first time. According to the chart, the patient has demonstrated impairment of light touch and pain and temperature sensation of the face. Without reading any more from the chart, which of the following structures would you expect to be involved?
A. Cranial nerve VII
B. Cranial nerve VI
C. Cranial nerve IV
D. Cranial nerve V

Rationale: D. The sensory areas of the face are controlled largely by cranial nerve V.

QUESTION 119
You have been asked to interview a physical therapy aide candidate for an open position in your department. Which of the following should you avoid discussing?
A. Your company's health insurance benefits
B. The potential work schedule
C. The candidate's marital status
D. None of the above

Rationale: C. It is illegal to ask a potential candidate about their marital status

QUESTION 120
You are discussing with your supervising physical therapist about the various types of wheelchairs available for patients with a spinal cord injury (SCI). What is the main purpose of a tilt-in-space wheelchair?
A. To facilitate handgrip and propulsion
B. To improve positioning for pressure relief and/or postural hypotension
C. To improve lower extremity positioning
D. To improve the patient's ability to transfer independently

Rationale: B. A tilt-in-space wheelchair is used for high-level SCIs to decrease pressure and shear forces, manage postural hypotension, control edema, and facilitate feeding and respiratory functions

QUESTION 121
You are treating a patient with a right CVA that has left her hemiparetic on the left side. At her current stage of healing, the patient is demonstrating strong and dominant hemiplegic synergies in the leg. Which of the following activities would *NOT* help lessen the synergies?
A. Rolling from the hooklying position using the lower extremity D1 flexion proprioceptive neuromuscular facilitation (PNF) pattern
B. Weight shifts in kneeling
C. Assuming the bridging position
D. Foot tapping in a seated position

Rationale: D. Lower extremity synergies can be grouped into extension synergies (internal rotation, adduction, and extension of the hip; extension of the knee; and extension and inversion of the ankle) and flexion synergies (external rotation, abduction, and flexion of the hip; flexion of the knee; and flexion and eversion of the ankle). Treatment strategies to interrupt the synergies include repetitive practice (e.g., massed practice) or activities such as kneeling, bridging, and rolling.

QUESTION 122

You are discussing Medicare reimbursement criteria with a home health care physical therapist. Which of the following does not apply in determining homebound status according to Medicare?

A. An individual needs the help of another person to leave the home.

B. An individual needs the help of medical equipment such as crutches, walker, or wheelchair to leave the home.

C. An individual is dependent on others for all transportation needs.

D. An individual's physician believes that the health or illness could get worse if the individual leaves the home.

Rationale: C. Being dependent on others for transportation does not meet the homebound criteria according to Medicare

QUESTION 123

You are observing a physical therapist performing an examination technique. First, the patient is asked to assume a long-sitting position, and the head is turned slightly to one side. The therapist then quickly moves the patient backward so that the head is extended over the end of the table, approximately 30 degrees below the horizontal. Which of the following examination techniques is the therapist using?

A. Epley maneuver

B. Rotenberg maneuver

C. Dix Hallpike test

D. None of the above

Rationale: C. The therapist performs the Dix Hallpike test, which is used to help detect benign paroxysmal positional vertigo (BPPV)

QUESTION 124

You are reviewing the medical chart of a patient with a spinal cord injury. A note in the chart recently entered by the physician indicates that the patient has contracted a respiratory infection. Which of the following patients would be most susceptible to this condition?

A. A patient with a cauda equina lesion

B. A patient with anterior cord syndrome

C. A patient with a complete C4 tetraplegia

D. A patient with posterior cord syndrome

Rationale: C. Of the patient listed, the patient with complete C4 tetraplegia would be the most compromised due to the level of the lesion as he/she may not be able to breathe on his or her own and/or cough independently

QUESTION 125

You are providing preoperative instruction for a 65-year-old patient scheduled for a total knee replacement. During the treatment session, the patient expresses a fear of dying during the surgery. Which of the following would be your most appropriate response to the patient?

A. You will be back to your family before you know it.

B. The surgeon is very experienced.

C. Surgery can be a very worrying experience.

D. These types of surgeries are very common.

Rationale: C. This would be the most empathetic response

QUESTION 126

You are discussing the various terms and units used when discussing electrical stimulation with your supervising physical therapist. What is the standard unit of measure when measuring the phase charge of a monophasic waveform?

A. Ampere

B. Ohm

C. Watt

D. Coulomb

Rationale: D. The phase charge, represented by the area under a single-phase waveform, is measured using the coulomb.

QUESTION 127

You are discussing with your supervising physical therapist about the various types of muscle contractions. What type of muscle contraction occurs in the hip extensors when an individual moves from standing to sitting?

A. Eccentric

B. Concentric

C. Isotonic

D. Isokinetic

Rationale: A. The hip extensors (gluteus maximus and the hamstrings) function eccentrically when an individual moves from standing to sitting

QUESTION 128

You are about to perform a series of manual muscle tests for a patient's trapezius muscle. In which of the following positions should the patient be in to test the left lower trapezius muscle?

A. Right sidelying

B. Left sidelying

C. Prone

D. Supine

Rationale: C. According to Kendall, to test the lower trapezius, the patient should be positioned in prone with the shoulder abducted greater than 120 degrees, and pressure should be applied against the forearm in a direction toward the floor

QUESTION 129

You are working to improve functional tasks with a patient who has right hemiplegia. You ask the patient to brush his teeth but notice that the patient puts the toothpaste directly in his hair instead of the toothbrush. How would you document this finding?

A. Constructional apraxia

B. Ideational apraxia

C. Conceptual apraxia

D. Ideomotor apraxia

Rationale: B. A patient with ideational apraxia finds it difficult to follow a sequence of movements, such as getting dressed, brushing teeth, or bathing.

QUESTION 130

You are about to instruct a patient with a transfemoral amputation in residual limb wrapping. Which of the following bandages would be the most appropriate?

A. Two-inch

B. Four-inch

C. Six-inch

D. Eight-inch

Rationale: C. The 6-in wrap would be the most appropriate as it adequately covers the larger surface area of the residual limb in a patient with a transfemoral amputation

QUESTION 131

You are performing a quantitative gait analysis. If you measure the number of steps taken by the patient in a 30-second period, which of the following are you measuring?

A. Velocity

B. Cadence

C. Acceleration

D. Distance

Rationale: B. Cadence is defined as the number of steps taken by a person per unit of time

QUESTION 132
You are discussing with your supervising physical therapist about the various types of intravenous (IV) lines and monitors encountered in a hospital setting. What is the primary purpose of an arterial line?
A. To measure pulmonary artery pressure
B. To measure right arterial pressure
C. To measure blood pressure
D. To measure heart rate and oxygen saturation

Rationale: C. An arterial line (also referred to as an art-line or a-line) is a thin catheter inserted into an artery to monitor blood pressure directly and obtain samples for arterial blood gas analysis

QUESTION 133
You decide to use proprioceptive neuromuscular facilitation (PNF) techniques to improve a patient's bed mobility skills. What would be your initial command if you are using rhythmic initiation (RI) to assist the patient in learning to roll from supine to prone?
A. "Help me roll you over."
B. "Stop me from rolling you over."
C. "Slowly rollover by yourself?"
D. "Relax, and let me move you."

Rationale: D. RI begins with the clinician passively moving the patient. This is usually followed by active-assisted movement, active movement, and finally, resisted movement

QUESTION 134
You decide to use the proprioceptive neuromuscular facilitation (PNF) technique of hold-relax (H-R) to increase a patient's shoulder range of motion. Which type of contraction is used at the endpoint of the patient's available range of motion?
A. Eccentric
B. Isometric
C. Concentric
D. Isokinetic

Rationale: B. The H-R technique uses an isometric contraction at the end of the patient's available range of motion. The patient is then instructed to relax as the clinician moves the extremity into the newly gained range.

QUESTION 135
You are providing gait training to a patient with hemiplegia. The patient has been ambulating with an ankle-foot orthosis (AFO), but today you notice that the patient's involved foot frequently catches the ground during the initial swing phase of gait. Which of the following muscles should be the focus of a strengthening program to treat this problem effectively?
A. Hamstrings
B. Iliopsoas/rectus femoris
C. Gluteus maximus
D. Gluteus medius

Rationale: B. The muscles involved with foot clearance during the initial swing phase of the dorsiflexors and the hip flexors. In the absence of the dorsiflexors, the hip flexors have to be strengthened to allow for foot clearance

QUESTION 136
You decide to use the D1 extension proprioceptive neuromuscular facilitation (PNF) technique to improve a patient's wrist extension. If you resist the patient's elbow extension to help improve the ability of the patient to extend the wrist, which of the following is this an example of?
A. Quick stretch
B. Reciprocal inhibition

C. Irradiation
D. a. and b

Rationale: C. The principle behind irradiation occurs when the strong component of a pattern results in irradiation, or overflow, of impulses from the stronger muscle group to the weaker muscle group

QUESTION 137
You are treating a patient who has suffered a CVA 3 weeks ago using the Brunnstrom method. According to Brunnstrom, if the patient is beginning to show the ability to produce movement patterns outside of limb synergies, in which stage of recovery is the patient?
A. Stage 2
B. Stage 3
C. Stage 4
D. Stage 5

Rationale: C. According to Brunnstrom stages of recovery, individuals showing the ability to produce movement patterns outside of limb synergies fall into stage 4.

QUESTION 138
You are working with the patient to improve their bed mobility. Which of the following exercises would be the most beneficial for increasing hip stability?
A. Trunk rotations in the hooklying position
B. Straight-leg raises
C. Bridging
D. None of the above

Rationale: C. Bridging exercises increase the strength of the low back muscles and the hip extensors

QUESTION 139
You are discussing with your supervising physical therapist about obtaining subjective information from the patient emphasizing the need to avoid leading questions. Which of the following questions would not be considered to be leading?
A. Is your pain worse in the morning?
B. Does your pain decrease with rest?
C. Does walking alter your pain in any way?
D. Does the pain get worse when you bend your elbow?

Rationale: C. This type of question avoids putting words in a patient's mouth

QUESTION 140
You are treating a patient who recently underwent a total knee replacement and has difficulty achieving the last 10 degrees of knee extension. You want to use a joint mobilization technique. Which of the following mobilization techniques could be used to help achieve the last 10 degrees of extension?
A. A posterior glide of the tibia on the femur
B. An inferior glide of the patella
C. An anterior glide of the tibia on the femur
D. A medial glide of the patella

Rationale: C. Based on the shape of the articulating surfaces, an anterior glide of the concave tibial plateau on the convex femur could be used to help achieve the last 10 degrees of knee extension

QUESTION 141

You are reviewing a patient's chart, and you note that the patient is taking a drug via enteral administration. Which of the following is an example of enteral administration?

A. Injection
B. Oral
C. Inhalation
D. Topical

Rationale: B. Enteral administration involves the esophagus, stomach, and small and large intestines (ie, the gastrointestinal [GI] tract). Other examples of enteral administration include sublingual (dissolving the drug under the tongue) and rectal.

QUESTION 142

You are reevaluating the strength of a patient with a C6 spinal cord injury using manual muscle testing. Which of the following muscles would not be innervated based on the patient's level of injury?

A. Subclavius
B. Brachialis
C. Triceps
D. Teres minor

Rationale: C. The triceps muscle is innervated by the radial nerve (C7-C8).

QUESTION 143

You are discussing with your supervising physical therapist about the various functions of the naturally occurring chemicals in the body. Which of the following chemicals is stimulated to act as a vasoconstrictor by a decrease in arterial pressure?

A. Angiotensin
B. Epinephrine
C. Norepinephrine
D. Histamine

Rationale: A. Angiotensin is a protein hormone that causes blood vessels to constrict to maintain blood pressure and fluid balance

QUESTION 144

You are reviewing the chart of a patient who is on a waiting list for a heart transplant. The patient recently received a right ventricular assistive device (RVAD) due to persistent ventricular failure. In which two structures would the tubes for this device be located?

A. Right atrium and pulmonary artery
B. Left atrium and pulmonary artery
C. Right atrium and aorta
D. Left atrium and aorta

Rationale: A. An RVAD functions to pump blood from the right atrium (or right ventricle), where one of the tubes is located, into the pulmonary artery, where the other two was located

QUESTION 145

You are discussing the brachial plexus with your supervising physical therapist. Which of the following muscles would not be involved with an injury to the posterior cord of the brachial plexus?

A. Infraspinatus
B. Latissimus dorsi
C. Teres major
D. Subscapularis

Rationale: A. The infraspinatus muscle is innervated by the suprascapular nerve (C4-C6) that extends from the superior trunk of the brachial plexus

QUESTION 146
You discuss the various support structures of the knee joint complex and their respective functions with your supervising physical therapist. Which of the following does not serve as a secondary restraint to the posterior cruciate ligament (PCL)?
   A.   Medial collateral ligament (MCL)
   B.   Popliteus tendon
   C.   Lateral collateral ligament (LCL)
   D.   Iliotibial band (ITB)

Rationale: D. The iliotibial band serves as a secondary restraint to the anterior cruciate ligament (ACL), not the PCL.

QUESTION 147
You are working through a strengthening program with a patient rehabilitating from an anterior shoulder dislocation. Which of the following muscle groups should be emphasized?
   A.   The adductors and internal rotators
   B.   The abductors and internal rotators
   C.   The adductors and external rotators
   D.   The abductors and external rotators

Rationale: A. The internal rotators and adductors provide support for the anterior joint capsule

QUESTION 148
You are working in a sterile environment and wearing sterile protective clothing. Which of the following areas of the protective clothing would not be considered sterile even before coming in contact with a nonsterile object?
   A.   The front of the gown above waist level
   B.   The front of the gown below waist level
   C.   The sleeves of the gown
   D.   Either glove

Rationale: B. The front of the gown below the waist level is considered nonsterile due to the probability of incidental contact

QUESTION 149
You are critically analyzing a recently published research study with your supervising physical therapist. Which of the following types of sampling procedures would result in the greatest degree of sampling error?
   A.   Stratified random sample
   B.   Cluster sample
   C.   Systematic sample
   D.   Simple random sample

Rationale: B. With cluster sampling, the researcher divides the population into separate groups, called clusters. Then, a simple random sample of clusters is selected from the population. However, since the technique requires two or more samples to be drawn, sampling error is increased.

QUESTION 150
You are applying transcutaneous electrical neuromuscular stimulation (TENS) on a patient for pain modulation. Which of the following set of parameters best describes conventional TENS?
   A.   50-100 pps, short phase duration, low intensity
   B.   100-150 pps, short phase duration, high intensity
   C.   150-200 pps, long phase duration, low intensity
   D.   200-250 pps, short phase duration, high intensity

Rationale: A. These are the correct parameters for conventional TENS, which delivers sensory level stimulation

QUESTION 151

You are calculating a patient's heart rate by counting the number of QRS complexes in a 6-second electrocardiogram strip. Assuming that there are eight QRS complexes in the strip, the patient's heart rate should be recorded as which of the following?

A. 40 beats/min
B. 60 beats/min
C. 80 beats/min
D. 100 beats/min

Rationale: C. The heart rate is calculated by multiplying the number of QRS complexes in a 6-second interval by 10

QUESTION 152

You are treating an 11-month-old with cerebral palsy who consistently demonstrates an abnormal persistence of the positive support reflex. As your treatment progresses, which of the following would this abnormal persistence most likely interfere with?

A. Supine activities
B. Sitting activities
C. Standing activities
D. Prone on elbow activities

Rationale: C. The positive support reflex, which normally integrates at 2 months of age, promotes extension of the lower extremities and trunk with weight-bearing through the balls of the feet

QUESTION 153

You are supervising a patient while they perform a D1 extension pattern for the upper extremity. Which of the following are the prime movers of the scapula during this pattern?

A. Levator scapulae, rhomboids, and pectoralis minor
B. Pectoralis major and pectoralis minor
C. Trapezius and middle deltoid
D. Pectoralis major, serratus anterior, and anterior deltoid

Rationale: A. The D1 extension pattern involves scapular depression (pectoralis minor), adduction (rhomboids), and downward rotation (pectoralis minor, rhomboids, and levator scapulae)

QUESTION 154

You are reviewing a patient's medical chart. The patient has been diagnosed with cerebellar degeneration. Which of the following clinical findings would you not expect to find in the patient's medical record?

A. Dysmetria
B. Dysdiadochokinesia
C. Nystagmus
D. Athetosis

Rationale: D. Athetosis, usually caused by a lesion to the basal ganglia, is characterized by slow, involuntary, convoluted, writhing movements of the fingers, hands, toes, feet, and in some cases, the arms, legs, neck, and tongue.

QUESTION 155

You are performing gentle strengthening exercises with a patient status post CVA positioned in supine. You notice that as you resist adduction of the uninvolved leg, the involved leg begins to adduct. What is the correct name for this phenomenon?

A. Angelman phenomenon
B. Raimiste phenomenon
C. Behçet phenomenon
D. None of the above

Rationale: B. Raimiste phenomenon refers to a hemiplegia reaction in which resistance to hip adduction (or abduction) in the uninvolved extremity evokes the same motion in the involved extremity

QUESTION 156
You are reviewing the laboratory report of an adult male. Which of the following would be considered a normal hemoglobin value?
A. 10 g/dL
B. 15 g/dL
C. 20 g/dL
D. 25 g/dL

Rationale: B. Normal results for an adult male are 13.8 to 17.2 g/dL

QUESTION 157
You are about to treat a patient in isolation. Which of the following is the correct order of application for protective clothing?
A. Gloves, then gown, then mask
B. Gloves, then mask, then gown
C. Mask, then gown, then gloves
D. Gown, then gloves, then mask

Rationale: C. Although the order of application of the gown and mask may vary, gloves must be the last item to be applied

QUESTION 158
You discuss the passive restraints around the elbow with your supervising physical therapist. Which ligament is typically involved with medial instability of the elbow?
A. Lateral (radial) collateral
B. Medial (ulnar) collateral
C. Annular
D. Olecranon

Rationale: B. As its name suggests, the medial (ulnar) collateral resists medial angulation of the ulna on the humerus

QUESTION 159
You are reviewing a research study that examined elbow extension range of motion 2 weeks following arthroscopic surgery. Assuming a normal distribution, what percentage of patients participating in the study would you expect to achieve a goniometric measurement value between the mean and one standard deviation above the mean?
A. 28%
B. 34%
C. 44%
D. 68%

Rationale: B. In a normal distribution, 68% of the population will fall between plus one and minus one standard deviation units, which means that 34% would fall between the mean and one standard deviation above the mean

QUESTION 160
You are reviewing the carpal bones of the wrist and hand with your supervising physical therapist. Which of the following would not be in the distal row of carpal bones?
A. Trapezoid
B. Lunate
C. Trapezium
D. Hamate

Rationale: B. The distal row of carpal bones consists of the trapezium, trapezoid, capitate, and hamate

QUESTION 161

You are providing gait training to a 22-year-old woman with a non–weight-bearing status on the left lower extremity. Which of the following would be the most appropriate gait pattern for this patient?

A. Swing to
B. Two-point
C. Three-point
D. Four-point

Rationale: C. The three-point gait pattern is used when a patient can bear weight on one lower extremity but is non–weight-bearing on the other

QUESTION 162

You are observing a colleague perform a manual muscle test on a patient. Your colleague applies resistance toward plantarflexion and eversion. Which of the following muscles is your colleague testing?

A. Tibialis posterior
B. Fibularis longus
C. Fibularis brevis
D. Tibialis anterior

Rationale: D. The tibialis anterior functions to dorsiflex the ankle joint and assists with inversion of the foot

QUESTION 163

After you have instructed a patient to pull the bar down behind their head when performing a lat pulldown, the patient asks you the difference between pulling the bar down behind the head and pulling the bar down in front of the head. Which of the following muscles are emphasized when pulling the bar down behind the head?

A. The middle trapezius and teres minor
B. The biceps and pectoralis major
C. The rhomboids and pectoralis major
D. The middle trapezius and rhomboids

Rationale: D. Both the middle trapezius and rhomboids act as strong adductors of the scapula, and adduction of the scapula is required to complete the pulldown exercise with the bar pulldown behind the patient's head

QUESTION 164

You are setting up a patient on electrical stimulation for muscle reeducation. Which of the following is the most appropriate on:off time ratio?

A. 1:5
B. 5:1
C. 1:15
D. 15:1

Rationale: A. A duty cycle of 1:5 prevents premature muscle fatigue while also allowing for adequate periods of muscle stimulation

QUESTION 165

You are reviewing the medical chart of a 6-year-old child and note that the child has a lengthy medical history that includes a selective dorsal rhizotomy. Which of the following medical conditions is typically associated with this surgical procedure?

A. Spina bifida
B. Duchenne muscular dystrophy
C. Cerebral palsy
D. Down syndrome

Rationale: C. A selective dorsal rhizotomy is a procedure used to help reduce spasticity in children with cerebral palsy

QUESTION 166

You are observing a patient referred to your outpatient department with a previous history of anterior compartment syndrome. During the examination by the physical therapist, the patient demonstrates an inability to dorsiflex the foot and a mild sensory disturbance between the first and second toes. Which of the following nerves is most likely involved with this patient?

A. Tibial nerve
B. Lateral plantar nerve
C. Deep fibular nerve
D. Medial plantar nerve

Rationale: C. Anterior compartment syndrome often affects the deep fibular nerve

QUESTION 167

You are reviewing a patient's chart before an initial examination, and you note that the laboratory testing reveals a markedly high platelet count. In which of the following conditions is a markedly high platelet count typically found?

A. Metabolic alkalosis
B. Chronic obstructive pulmonary disease
C. Liver disease
D. Malignancy

Rationale: D. A markedly high platelet count (thrombocytosis) is a manifestation of an occult neoplasm

QUESTION 168

You are observing a colleague perform an anterior glide of the distal tibiofibular articulation. Which of the following motions would this type of mobilization technique improve?

A. Subtalar eversion
B. Subtalar inversion
C. Talocrural dorsiflexion
D. Talocrural plantarflexion

Rationale: C. The concave articulation of the distal tibiofibular joint moves anteriorly over the convex talus during ankle dorsiflexion

QUESTION 169

A patient you have been treating informs you that he has been taking corticosteroid medication for an unrelated condition. Which of the following is a common side effect of prolonged corticosteroid use?

A. Tachycardia
B. Bradycardia
C. Arrhythmias
D. Increased blood pressure

Rationale: A. Prolonged corticosteroid use can result in hypertension

QUESTION 170

You are reviewing the laboratory section of a 25-year-old man's medical chart. Which value would be considered within normal limits for oxygen saturation?

A. 88%
B. 92%
C. 94%
D. 96%

Rationale: D. Normal ranges for oxygen saturation correspond to 95% to 98%

QUESTION 171

If you assess a patient's heart rate by measuring it for 30 beats and find the time to be 22 seconds, which of the following should be recorded as the patient's heart rate?
A. 72 beats/min
B. 78 beats/min
C. 82 beats/min
D. 86 beats/min

Rationale: C. Although a rather complicated method, if there are 30 beats in 22 seconds, then there are 1.36 beats/s, which, when multiplied by 60 seconds, results in a value of 81.6 beats/min

QUESTION 172

You measure the blood pressure of a 1-month-old infant. Which of the following would be the most typical measurement based on the patient's age?
A. 65/40 mm Hg
B. 75/40 mm Hg
C. 85/60 mm Hg
D. 95/70 mm Hg

Rationale: C. A newborn's blood pressure typically ranges from 70 to 90/45 to 65 mm Hg

QUESTION 173

You observe a physical therapist perform a cognitive assessment by asking a patient to count from 0 to 25 using increments of five. Which of the following types of cognitive function does this task most accurately assess?
A. Memory
B. Attention
C. Decision-making
D. Perception

Rationale: B. This type of task assesses the ability of the patient to concentrate

QUESTION 174

You have just completed reviewing the medical chart of a patient status-post a left hemisphere stroke. As you enter the patient's room, which of the following patient behaviors would you *NOT* expect to see with this patient?
A. Difficulty with mathematical reasoning and judgment
B. Difficulty processing information in a sequential linear manner
C. Difficulty with language production
D. Difficulty with the sequencing of movements

Rationale: A. Except for difficulty with mathematical reasoning and judgment, this patient is likely to demonstrate all of the other behaviors

QUESTION 175

You are discussing the various catheters and monitors encountered in a hospital setting with your supervising physical therapist. Which of the following catheters is inserted into the internal jugular vein and then travels through the superior vena cava into the right atrium to permit removal of blood samples, administration of medication, and the monitoring of central venous pressure?
A. Swan–Ganz catheter
B. Hickman catheter
C. Central venous pressure catheter
D. None of the above

Rationale: B. The description is of a Hickman catheter

QUESTION 176
You are discussing the various planes of the body with your supervising physical therapist. Which of the following planes is being utilized when a patient is performing shoulder internal and external rotation exercises using elastic tubing when positioned in standing with their arm positioned at the side and the elbow in 90 degrees of flexion?
A. Sagittal
B. Coronal
C. Transverse
D. Frontal

Rationale: C. The transverse plane divides the body into upper and lower portions. Therefore, the patient exercise is performed in the transverse plane around a vertical axis

QUESTION 177
While you are treating a patient at bedside, you notice that a line from an IV has become tangled around the patient's bed rail. Before adjusting the IV, which of the following methods of medical asepsis would be indicated?
A. Don gloves
B. Don gloves and a gown
C. Don gloves, gown, and mask
D. No medical a sepsis is required

Rationale: C. The IV line can be repositioned using direct hand contact

QUESTION 178
While talking to a patient who was involved in a serious motor vehicle accident, she reports to you that she is currently taking Dilaudid. Which of the following side effects is most pertinent when taking his medication?
A. Dependency
B. Hypertension
C. Tachycardia
D. Peripheral neuropathy

Rationale: A. Medications such as Dilaudid (and Demerol) are potent opioid analgesics and can result in physical dependence with inappropriate utilization

QUESTION 179
You are reviewing the medical chart of a patient diagnosed with left-sided heart failure. Which of the following findings is not typically associated with this condition?
A. Muscular weakness
B. Dependent edema
C. Chronic and persistent cough
D. Pulmonary edema

Rationale: B. Dependent edema is a characteristic of right-sided heart failure

QUESTION 180
You are attempting to examine the relationship between scores on a functional independence measure (FIM) and the Barthel index, whose validity is known. Which type of validity does this describe?
A. Content validity
B. Concurrent validity
C. Face validity
D. Predictive validity

Rationale: B. Concurrent validity is demonstrated when a test correlates well with a measure that has previously been validated

QUESTION 181
You have been treating a patient who is recovering from a traumatic brain injury for several days. You notice today that the patient has become lethargic since being placed on phenobarbital. Which of the following is the primary purpose of this medication?
A. To reduce spasticity
B. To decrease agitation
C. To prevent seizures
D. To treat depression

Rationale: C. Phenobarbital is a barbiturate prescribed to prevent adult seizures by slowing brain and nervous system activity

QUESTION 182
You are setting up a patient for electrical stimulation to help increase the strength of a patient's quadriceps. What is the most appropriate on:off time ratio for muscle strengthening?
A. 1:3
B. 1:5
C. 5:1
D. A and B

Rationale: D. These are both the correct on:off time ratio to be used with muscle strengthening

QUESTION 183
You are reviewing wrist and hand anatomy with your supervising physical therapist. Which of the following carpal bones does *NOT* articulate with the lunate?
A. Capitate
B. Trapezium
C. Triquetrum
D. Scaphoid

Rationale: B. The trapezium, located in the distal carpal row on the radial side, does not articulate with the lunate

QUESTION 184
You are about to administer iontophoresis over the anterior surface of the patient's elbow. To avoid skin irritation by keeping the current density low, which of the following parameters should be used?
A. An electrode with an area of 12 cm^2 and current amplitude of 4 mA
B. An electrode with an area of 6 cm^2 and current amplitude of 3 mA
C. An electrode with an area of 4 cm^2 and current amplitude of 4 mA
D. An electrode with an area of 4 cm^2 and current amplitude of 3 mA

Rationale: A. Current density can be calculated by dividing the current amplitude by the electrode size (4 mA/12cm^2 = 0.33 mA/cm^2)

QUESTION 185
The patient has been referred to physical therapy for instruction in an exercise program. Which of the following conditions is *NOT* an absolute contraindication to exercise training?
A. Deep venous thrombosis
B. Acute myocarditis
C. Hypertrophic cardiomyopathy
D. None of the above

Rationale: C. Hypertrophic cardiomyopathy is only considered to be a relative contraindication to exercise testing

QUESTION 186
You are discussing the various axes of the body with your student. Which of the following axes is being utilized when a patient performs hip abduction and adduction when positioned in standing?
A. Vertical
B. Coronal
C. Anterior-posterior
D. Longitudinal

Rationale: C. Hip abduction and adduction typically occur in a frontal plane around an anterior-posterior axis

QUESTION 187
You have been applying pulsed wave ultrasound to a patient's anterior thigh at 1.4 W/cm^2 for 6 minutes that used a 2-millisecond on-time and 8-millisecond off-time for one pulse wave. Which of the following would be the correct duty cycle to document?
A. 10%
B. 15%
C. 20%
D. 25%

Rationale: C. Duty cycle is defined as the ratio of the on-time to the total time so, in this case, the duty cycle = 2 milliseconds/(2 milliseconds + 8 milliseconds) = 0.20(100) = 20%

QUESTION 188
In a hospital setting, a patient refuses to participate in the physical therapy session. The physical therapist assistant explains the benefits of participating in the therapy session, but the patient does not reconsider and refuses treatment. Of the following statements, which is the *most appropriate* action to be taken by the assistant?
A. Insist the patient to participate in the therapy session.
B. Inform the physician who referred the patient for therapy treatment.
C. Document the refusal in the medical record explaining the refusal.
D. Communicate the event with the supervising therapist and schedule the patient with another staff member for a future visit.

Rationale: C. The most appropriate next step is to document the refusal and the reason for refusal. After documentation has been completed, further communication can be made to the supervising therapist and medical team as needed

QUESTION 189
A patient suffered a cerebrovascular accident (CVA) of the left hemisphere. Which of the following transfer training techniques is *best* to use with this patient?
A. Utilize tactile and visual cues through demonstration to assist with patient comprehension
B. Manual assistance with placement of the left-side extremities
C. Verbal cues to assure proper hand placement
D. Sequential tactile cues during motor planning activities

Rationale: D. The best answer is the use of sequential tactile cues. The CVA patient with a left-hemispherical lesion is likely to suffer disorganization, difficulty processing verbal cues and commands, and has difficulty with planning and sequencing movements (O'Sullivan, 2019)

QUESTION 190
You are scheduled to work with a person currently staying on an inpatient rehabilitation unit. The patient was previously on a respiratory mechanical ventilator for 3 weeks and continues to have hypotonicity and dynamic balance impairments. Symptoms are improving overall. All medical history for this patient is consistent with which of the following diagnoses?
  A. Guillain–Barré syndrome (GBS)
  B. Multiple sclerosis
  C. Parkinson disease
  D. Amyotrophic lateral sclerosis

Rationale: A. GBS is the most consistent diagnosis. GBS symptoms involve hypotonicity, history of respiratory ventilation, but approximately 95% of GBS patients have normal functional mobility after their symptoms subside

QUESTION 191
An acute care nurse provides a medical status update to the physical therapist assistant scheduled to treat a patient currently being seen for a viral infection, decreasing blood oxygen saturation, and increasing paralysis of the extremities. Which of the following laboratory studies will help rule out a diagnosis for this patient?
  A. Spinal tap
  B. Nerve conduction study
  C. Antibody blood titer
  D. Electromyography

Rationale: A. Guillain–Barré syndrome (GBS) can be difficult to diagnose in the earliest stages, and signs and GBS can be similar to other neurologic disorders. After physical examination, the physician will recommend a spinal tap laboratory test to determine a consistent change that commonly occurs in GBS patients (MayoClinic, 2021).

QUESTION 192
A patient with multiple sclerosis exhibits 3/5 strength of the iliopsoas bilateral, 2/5 quadriceps strength bilateral, and 2/5 anterior tibialis strength bilateral. Which of the following activities would be the most difficult to perform?
  A. Bilateral bridging
  B. Unilateral bridging
  C. Unilateral straight-leg raises
  D. Rolling from supine to sidelying

Rationale: B. The muscle grades indicate the patient has greater strength proximally more than distally in the lower extremities. All activities are focused on hip strength in consideration with unilateral bridging being the most difficult to perform

QUESTION 193
You are working with a patient who begins to complain of feeling dizzy and states the room is spinning. You can suspect the patient may have which of the following diagnoses?
  A. Dysmetria
  B. Vertigo
  C. Dysdiadochokinesia
  D. Oscillopsia

Rationale: B. The patient complains of symptoms consistent with benign paroxysmal positional vertigo (BPPV). BPPV is an official diagnosis made after a patient first complains of dizziness and "spinning rooms." The term vertigo can be defined as dizziness. BPPV provides a diagnosis and reason causing the dizziness

QUESTION 194

You are working with a patient who exhibits muscle tension, decreased joint sense, and proprioception deficits. You can suspect the patient has an injury to which of the following spinal cord tracts?

A. Spinoreticular
B. Vestibulospinal
C. Spinocerebellar
D. Corticospinal

Rationale: D. The corticospinal tract is a primary motor pathway, descending motor tract. This tract helps with the control of discrete and skillful movements of the extremities

QUESTION 195

You are instructing a patient who suffered a Brown-Sequard spinal cord injury to roll from supine to sidelying. The rolling should be initiated with movement toward which direction?

A. Toward the weaker side
B. Toward the stronger side
C. Push up on elbows from supine and push over to a sidelying position in either direction
D. Have the patient put their hands behind the head to give momentum and roll toward the easier side

Rationale: A. Brown-Sequard spinal cord injured patients lose motor function, proprioception, and vibration on the same side of the body as the cord injury. Therefore, rolling techniques are more effective when rolling from the strong side toward the weaker or paralyzed side. The momentum of the rolling from the stronger side to the weaker side will help achieve the transition and movement (O'Sullivan, 2019)

QUESTION 196

You are attempting to assess the integrity of the L4 spinal level. Which deep tendon reflex would provide you with the most useful information?

A. Patellar
B. Lateral hamstrings
C. Achilles tendon
D. Medial hamstrings

Rationale: A. The L4 spinal nerve root level innervates the quads and portions of the patellar and tibialis anterior. The patellar tendon reflex associates with the L4 spinal nerve root level. The patellar tendon deep tendon reflex reaction indicates innervation of the quadriceps muscle group and patellar region

QUESTION 197

You are reviewing the plan of care (POC) in preparation to treat a client in an outpatient setting. The client was in a car accident 21 days ago and suffered a cervical fracture with incomplete spinal cord damage. The POC identifies a strengthening, balance, and endurance program. You can anticipate the patient will most likely be using which type of stabilizing orthotic at this stage of recovery?

A. Minerva brace
B. Thoracolumbar corset
C. Halo orthosis attached to a thoracic body jacket
D. Body jacket

Rationale: A. The Minerva brace is a supportive brace for both the cervical spine and thoracic spine, limiting motion in both areas. The Minerva brace is noninvasive and appropriate for the patient in the subacute stages of healing (O'Sullivan, 2019)

QUESTION 198

You are working with a patient who suffered a traumatic brain injury 4 weeks ago. Supine posturing exhibits increased trunk and lower extremity extension and upper extremity flexion. Which of the following techniques will be the most beneficial to decrease hypertonicity?

  A. Approximation through the upper extremities with all joints in extension
  B. D2 flexion PNF pattern of the upper extremity in a sidelying position
  C. D1 Flexion PNF pattern of the upper extremity in a sidelying position
  D. Asymmetrical reverse lifting pattern of the upper extremity

Rationale: A. Approximation is an initial step to help relax muscle tone and encourage the extension of the upper extremity joints. Approximation will initiate increased joint mobility and progression to joint stabilization while in an optimal position (Martin, 2021).

QUESTION 199

A patient is suffering from a left visual field cut after being diagnosed with a tumor of the right optic tract. Which of the following diagnoses best identifies the patient's optical deficits?

  A. Homonymous hemianopsia
  B. Contralateral homonymous hemianopsia
  C. Ipsilateral hemianopsia
  D. Complete blindness

Rationale: B. If both fields are affected, the answer would be homonymous hemianopsia indicating the involvement of both tracts. A lesion of a single tract will affect the vision on the opposite side, leading to the answer of contralateral homonymous hemianopsia

QUESTION 200

You are seeing a patient diagnosed with a cerebrovascular accident for inpatient rehabilitation. During static seated balance activities, the patient exhibits hypertonicity toward the hemiplegic side, limiting controlled mobility. Which of the following techniques will best alleviate the patient's symptoms?

  A. Pelvic extension and trunk extension of the hemiplegic side
  B. Thoracolumbar rotation toward the hemiplegic side
  C. Scapular mobilizations on the hemiplegic side
  D. The use of a long warm arm upper extremity splint

Rationale: A. Although a warm air splint would help with hypertonicity, having the patient actively move into a trunk and pelvic extension will provide thalamic activity and decrease the pushing toward the hemiplegic side

Exam 2

QUESTION 1

During a neurologic screening for a patient who suffered an ischemic cerebral vascular accident, you note the patient has abarognosis. You can suspect the patient experienced ischemia in which lobe of the brain?

A. Right parietal
B. Left frontal
C. Occipital
D. Parieto-occipital

Rationale: A. Barognosis is the ability to identify and differentiate between the weight of objects when holding them or lifting them; abarognosis is the inability to differentiate the weight of objects. Barognosis and other perceptual evaluation occurs in the right parietal lobe primarily (O'Sullivan, 2019)

QUESTION 2

You are working with a patient whose goal is to reduce "freezing" episodes. The patient also has complaints of hallucinations and occasional gastrointestinal changes. You can expect the patient is taking which of the following medications?

A. Tegretol
B. Baclofen
C. Lisinopril
D. Sinemet

Rationale: D. Sinemet is the "gold" standard medication used with a patient with freezing episodes with Parkinson disease. Tegretol does help with tonic spasms yet more commonly used with patients with multiple sclerosis (Martin, 2021) (O'Sullivan, 2019)

QUESTION 3

You are treating a patient with a history of lower extremity lymphedema who has left knee pain after a fall. Upon initiating the treatment session, the patient reports she feels her lymphedema has progressed and her compression garment is no longer fitting. She asks you to wrap her left leg with compression wraps to control the edema. The evaluating PT has no inclusion of lymphatic treatment in the initial evaluation or plan of care, and you have no additional training in lymphedema treatment. What action would be most appropriate for you to take?

A. You should wrap the lower extremity with long-stretch compression bandages to facilitate reduction of edema and advise the patient to wear until bedtime and then remove
B. You should notify the supervising PT and refer the patient back to the PT for evaluation of lymphatic symptoms before initiating any treatment for the lymphedema
C. You should recommend the patient continue with the use of her compression garment and apply a neoprene sleeve over the top for added compression
D. You should perform manual lymphatic drainage (MLD)

Rationale: B. The PTA should be referred back to the PT for assessment before performing any lymphedema treatment as it was not addressed in the initial evaluation. The other answers are incorrect because the PT needs to assess the patient to determine the plan of care and appropriate interventions to be performed by an appropriately trained individual

QUESTION 4

A patient with a history of lymphedema reports a concern that her lymphedema is progressing. The swelling is no longer resolved with elevation, pitting edema is present, and palpable fibrosis is noted. What stage of lymphedema would be suspected based on these findings?

A. Stage 0
B. Stage I
C. Stage II
D. Stage III

Rationale: C. Stage II will present with pitting edema with developing scar tissue/fibrosis; elevation of the limb has no significant effect on reversing edema; irreversible changes (Moini and Chaney, 2021)

QUESTION 5

You are providing therapeutic exercise instruction to a patient before the PT performs manual lymphatic drainage to the right lower extremity. You note the involved limb presents with a small wound on the lower lateral leg with a red-streaked discoloration. When you ask the patient how they feel, they admit not feeling well and feel they have a fever. What is the most appropriate next course of action for you to take?

A. Continue with the current plan of care for exercises and notify the PT before beginning manual lymphatic drainage
B. Hold treatment and consult immediately with the supervising PT
C. Increase the warm-up time and modify the exercise to a lower resistance level
D. Continue with the current plan of care with no changes

Rationale: B. Due to the presence of cardinal signs of infection with erythema and fever indicating a possible acute infection, most likely lymphangitis or cellulitis, the treatment should be halted until the PT can evaluate. The patient will likely require referral to their primary health provider for antibiotic treatment

QUESTION 6

You are working in an outpatient setting and are currently treating a patient with a history of left upper extremity lymphedema and hypertension. Before initiation of aerobic exercise, blood pressure readings are to be taken. Please select the most appropriate method to obtain these vital signs for this patient.

A. You should take blood pressure on the left upper extremity brachial artery via sphygmomanometer before, during, and after activity to monitor patient tolerance.
B. You should take blood pressure on the left radial artery via wrist blood pressure cuff before, during, and after activity to monitor patient tolerance.
C. You should take blood pressure on the right radial artery via sphygmomanometer during and after activity to monitor patient tolerance.
D. You should take blood pressure on the right brachial artery via a sphygmomanometer before, during, and after activity to monitor patient tolerance.

Rationale: D. BP is normally taken at the left brachial artery via a sphygmomanometer; however, to avoid an exacerbation of the condition with a patient with a history of lecture with minor patient lymphedema, the reading should be taken on the other arm

QUESTION 7

For a patient who is status post a right mastectomy due to breast cancer, which of the following would be the correct type of lymphedema to document?

A. Primary
B. Secondary
C. Congenital
D. Lipedema

Rationale: B. Secondary lymphedema results from injury (eg, surgery, radiation) to the lymphedema structures. Primary lymphedema has an idiopathic cause; it can be congenital or hereditary with abnormal lymphedema structure. Lipedema is not a form of lymphedema

QUESTION 8

You treat a patient with a history of Stage I bilateral lymphedema for balance training after an ankle sprain. Which of the following activities would be the *MOST* appropriate intervention for this patient?

A. Focus on long periods of standing balance activities without sitting breaks to increase standing endurance

B. Applying a moist heat pack to increase blood circulation and decrease pain post-balance activities

C. Performing strengthening exercise only while sitting on the edge of the bed with the legs dangling to allow full range of motion

D. Performing strengthening and balance activities with alternating sitting and standing positions

Rationale: D. The PTA should avoid prolonged periods of sitting and standing so alternating positions allow an increased variety of functional positions and challenges while lowering the risk of obstruction to lymphatic flow by remaining stationary or in a dependent position

QUESTION 9

You are treating a patient in the acute setting who has been on long-term prednisone treatment. The patient is observed to have a "moon face," muscle weakness, hypertension, and bruises easily. What condition corresponds with these signs?

A. Addisonian disease

B. Cushing syndrome

C. Cretinism

D. Graves disease

Rationale: B. Cushing syndrome results in excess corticosteroid levels due to a hyperactive adrenal gland, or prolonged corticosteroid use (prednisone) with signs/symptoms of the moon face, truncal obesity, easily bruised, fatigue, muscle weakness, and hypertension. Addison disease is a rare disease with signs/symptoms of muscle weakness, fatigue, low blood pressure, irritability, brownish pigmentation of the skin. Graves disease is a form of hyperthyroidism and is an autoimmune disease, while cretinism is usually a congenital abnormality and leads to thyroid deficiency

QUESTION 10

You are treating a patient with a history of hypoadrenalism. Which of the following disturbances may be present clinically due to this condition?

A. Loss of proteins may lead to fatigue, weakness, and risk of tendon rupture

B. Deposits of fat localized in the lower extremities

C. Hypoglycemia

D. Overproduction of collagen-building scar tissue

Rationale: A. Loss of protein may lead to poor muscle development, fatigue, and increased risk of tendon rupture. Fat deposits would most likely be localized in the trunk and upper abdominal regions, and there would be reduced collagen production due to the loss of protein. Finally, hyperglycemia is more likely to occur

QUESTION 11

You are treating a patient diagnosed with metabolic syndrome who presents with an "apple-shaped" torso. What other conditions is this patient at an elevated risk of developing?

A. Diabetes mellitus

B. Graves disease

C. Addison disease

D. Cushing syndrome

Rationale: A. Metabolic syndrome is also known as insulin resistance syndrome and often precedes diabetes mellitus. Patients tend to have an "apple shape" due to excess fat accumulation in the abdomen. Graves disease is more associated with weight loss rather than fat accumulation. Addison disease and Cushing syndrome are both hypoadrenalism conditions

QUESTION 12

You are treating a patient with a history of metabolic syndrome for general deconditioning. What vital signs would be *MOST* imperative to monitor, knowing the associated complications of this condition?

A. Oxygen saturation
B. Respiration rate
C. Blood pressure
D. Temperature

Rationale: C. Metabolic syndrome has a high risk for complications of hypertension and stroke. Blood pressure would be imperative to monitor for this progression. However, all vital signs are significant data to determine patient activity tolerance

QUESTION 13

You are progressing a patient through an exercise program for strengthening. The patient reports weight loss, polydipsia, and polyuria over the past several months. He is concerned that his eyesight is changing. What is the *MOST* appropriate immediate action the PTA should take?

A. Increase the warm-up and cool-down time and increase the frequency of rest breaks for water consumption due to concerns of dehydration.
B. Discharge the patient and referred the patient immediately back to their primary physician to rule out a cancer diagnosis.
C. Notify the supervising PT that the patient demonstrates symptoms of diabetes mellitus and refer the patient to their primary care physician for diagnostic testing while continuing treatment with the patient, monitoring symptoms, and making treatment modifications based on patient tolerance.
D. Advise the patient that they have developed diabetes and should follow up with their primary care physician.

Rationale: C. The evaluating PT should be notified of the potential need for additional assessment and referral to the primary care physician for diagnosis. The adjustments to the warm-up and cooldown time and the increased frequency of water breaks are appropriate, but the patient must be referred back to their primary care physician. There is no need to discharge the patient as the patient may still benefit from skilled PT once the appropriate diagnosis has been made. Finally, it is beyond the scope of the PTA to make diagnostic statements.

QUESTION 14

You are providing physical therapy services for appropriate core stability to a pregnant patient. The patient reports she has recently been diagnosed with gestational diabetes. What clinical significance do you need to consider during treatment?

A. The potential for a decrease in blood glucose levels with exercise
B. Extended cooldown. To normalize body temperature
C. Provide a carbohydrate snack at each session
D. Elevated blood glucose levels during activity

Rationale: A. Gestational diabetes can occur during pregnancy and may place the patient at the same risk of hypoglycemia due to decreased blood glucose with activity in type I or II DM. The other choices of adequate warm-up and cooldown times and the provision of a carbohydrate snack would also be appropriate but are not as important. Finally, exercise causes a reduction in blood glucose levels, which is why it is an effective tool (along with diet) to assist in the management of diabetes

QUESTION 15

You are working with a patient with bipolar depression. The patient's nurse informs you that the patient is in the manic phase today. What characteristics should you be prepared to encounter during this phase?

A. The patient to act erratically, highly distractible, and to communicate with rapid speech
B. The patient to show disinterest in therapy and poor concentration

C. The patient to report very low energy and the urge to sleep most of the day

D. The patient reports feeling guilty and requiring a lot of attention

Rationale: A. The manic phase usually involves rapid speech, erratic behavior, high self-esteem, highly distracted, but has a decreased need for food or sleep (Moini and Chaney, 2021). Bipolar depression involves either periods of depression and mania or can have unipolar mania, which does not have periods of depression

QUESTION 16

During an early morning treatment of an elderly nursing home resident, you notice that the patient avoids eye contact, pulls at his hair, swears, and taps his foot. What are these signs indicative of, and what is the best way to handle the situation?

A. Hearing loss; maintain eye contact at all times, speak loudly and firmly

B. Agitation; speak calmly and respectfully to the patient to determine the cause of the agitation

C. Sundowning; move the patient to a quiet room with few distractions and resume treatment

D. Low-vision; adjust the lighting, and provide more auditory cues and instruction

Rationale: B. Early recognition of these signs of agitation will help de-escalate situations and potentially avoid increasing anger or violence. Speak in a low, calm voice, show respect to the patient while trying to determine what the cause of agitation is so it can be removed. As its name suggests, sundowning usually occurs at dusk/evening

QUESTION 17

You are working with a very anxious patient who is concerned about whether she can return to her job. After discussing potential discharge, the patient reports feeling nauseated, light-headed, and cannot catch her breath. What situation should be recognized by you, and what is the most appropriate response?

A. The patient is having a heart attack and should be transported to the ER immediately.

B. The patient is having an anxiety attack or something more serious; assess vital signs and work to have the patient remain calm with deep breathing and relaxation techniques as well as notifying the supervising PT.

C. The patient is most likely hypoglycemic; blood glucose levels should be taken and a carbohydrate snack given.

D. The patient may be experiencing a deep vein thrombosis (DVT); treatment should be terminated, and the patient should be allowed to leave.

Rationale: B. An assessment of vital signs would be imperative to determine the seriousness of the condition. As the patient is anxious, attempting to keep the patient calm using a relaxation technique could be used to see if that improved her symptoms. Anxiety attacks may present with dizziness, nausea, palpitations, and shortness of breath (Mayo Clinic, 2018). If vital signs are not within range or symptoms escalate, emergency help should be summoned

QUESTION 18

During a treatment session, a patient reports having nightmares about the traumatic car accident that caused her injuries. The patient also reports she has a great deal of fear, preventing her from driving herself to treatment, and blames herself for her difficulty in progressing. What potential condition could she be experiencing?

A. Depression

B. Paranoid personality disorder

C. Posttraumatic stress disorder (PTSD)

D. Malingering

Rationale: C. PTSD falls under generalized anxiety disorders. However, it often relates to reliving a traumatic event through flashbacks or nightmares and may have feelings of fear and blame themselves (Barnhill, 2020). A patient exhibiting mental health concerns and significant changes in behavior should be reported to evaluating PT and referred to an appropriately trained health care provider.

QUESTION 19
You are performing drainage of a leg wound. The wound appears to have drainage that is opaque, yellow in color, and is a thin, watery consistency. Which of the following would be the most appropriate way to document wound exudate type?
A. Sanguinous
B. Serosanguinous
C. Seropurulent
D. Purulent

Rationale: C. The description of this drainage indicates seropurulent—the serous portion represents the thin, watery, and the purulent portion of the term represents the opaque yellowish color. Sanguinous is typically red, thin, and watery—the red or brown coloration is due to the presence of blood. Serosanguinous is typically light red or pink with a thin watery consistency, and purulent drainage tends to be of a thick consistency of yellow or green color, indicating infection

QUESTION 20
You are performing a wound dressing change and note purulent exudate of moderate amount with an odor. What would be the most appropriate conclusion for you to make about the status of this wound?
A. Lack of blood flow
B. Infection
C. Compartment syndrome
D. Normal wound healing

Rationale: B. Purulent exudate is generally an indication of infection

QUESTION 21
A wound is observed to have necrotic tissue with firm, crusted tissue strongly attached to the wound base. It is black and firmly adherent. What would be the most appropriate terminology to describe this?
A. Granulation tissue
B. Slough
C. Eschar
D. Nonviable

Rationale: C. Eschar, often black or brown, may be soft or crusty but is usually firmly attached. Granulation tissue is usually red and beefy, indicating a sign of wound healing. Slough is usually yellow and may vary between nonadherent and adherent and can be stringy or mutinous, while nonviable tissue is typically white or gray, occurring at the wound opening

QUESTION 22
A patient is noted to have a skin rash with blisters located within the T4 dermatome distribution. The blisters appear to have a mild exudate, and the patient reports them to be very painful. What would be your most appropriate action?
A. Continue with the treatment per the plan of care and keep the blisters covered with a shirt or gown.
B. Utilize standard precautions to avoid direct contact and notify the supervising PT.
C. Recommend the patient to see their primary care physician and ask for an oral antiviral medication.
D. Order a viral culture and Tzanck smear.

Rationale: B. Utilize standard precautions to avoid direct contact with vesicular fluid from blisters as it may cause varicella in a susceptible person. The primary care physician may order viral cultures or a Tzanck smear to confirm the diagnosis, and the supervising PT may need to determine if any reassessment is necessary due to a change in condition

QUESTION 23

In reviewing the chart before treating a patient's burns, you note that the PT documented the total body surface area (TBSA). Which of the following methods are commonly used to determine the extent of injured tissue using TBSA for burn patients?

A. Bates-Jensen assessment tool
B. Rule of nines
C. Complete blood count (CBC)
D. Tzanck smear

Rationale: B. The rule of nines is a generalized method to determine the TBSA for adults. Charts of varying detail depict the percentage for body regions to estimate the surface area injured

QUESTION 24

You are seeing a patient with a diagnosis of dermatitis. What would be the most appropriate pharmaceutical treatment that you would likely see in the patient's chart?

A. Anti-inflammatory corticosteroid cream
B. Antimicrobial silver sulfadiazine (Silvadene)
C. Antibiotic (amoxicillin)
D. Lidocaine for pain relief

Rationale: A. An anti-inflammatory corticosteroid cream is the most likely as it aims to control inflammation

QUESTION 25

While inspecting a patient's scar, you note that it is white, flat, and flexible. Which of the following statements best describes this type of scar?

A. It indicates early healing and signifies chronic inflammation.
B. It indicates later tissue healing and signifies a mature scar.
C. It indicates evidence of hypertrophic scarring.
D. It indicates keloid scarring.

Rationale: B. As a scar matures later in the healing process, it becomes paler in color and flattens out

QUESTION 26

The supervising PT has instructed the wound dressing to be an occlusive or semi-occlusive dressing to cover a wound with 50% black eschar. What is the advantage of using this dressing with this type of wound?

A. It traps in bacteria or pathogens so they can be contained to the wound.
B. It allows drainage of the wound to keep it from becoming macerated.
C. It contains moisture and allows the body's enzymes to soften the eschar.
D. It primarily provides mechanical debridement due to its adhesive nature.

Rationale: C. An occlusive dressing is designed to contain the fluid allowing for softening of the eschar and autolytic debridement to occur. An occlusive dressing may not be appropriate for a highly exudating wound as it may macerate the healthy tissue and lead to more loss of healthy tissue. Frequent dressing changes and wound cleansing would facilitate the reduction of bacteria burden on the wound

QUESTION 27

A patient presents with a wound located along the lateral malleoli surrounded by dry skin. Upon skin inspection, you note the skin is cool and pale and lacks hair growth. Based on these characteristics, which wound type best fits this description?

A. Arterial
B. Neuropathic
C. Venous
D. Traumatic

Rationale: A. Due to arterial insufficiency and a lack of oxygen-rich blood to the area, an arterial would tend to present with dry, cool, pale skin that may lack hair growth. Additionally, arterial wounds tend to be located laterally on the ankle and foot

QUESTION 28

You perform passive range of motion (PROM) on a patient's upper extremity who sustained a burn over 30% of their total body surface area (TBSA) 8 weeks ago. During the session, you note a significant decrease in ROM, and the patient is complaining of a point tender area in the biceps/brachialis region. Which common complication of a burn injury would be the concern with these symptoms?

A. Heterotopic ossification
B. Heterotrophic scarring
C. Infection
D. Neuropathy

Rationale: A. Heterotopic ossification often presents as a potential complication after suffering burns. A common location for this condition is the biceps/brachialis region

QUESTION 29

You are about to perform gait training with a patient who has an indwelling catheter. How should you handle the catheter to allow the activity?

A. Attach or carry the catheter below the bladder level and safely secure the tubing to avoid stepping on or compressing it.
B. Call nursing to remove the catheter for the duration of the physical therapy treatment.
C. You should not perform gait training with a patient who has an indwelling catheter.
D. Secure the catheter to the bed and only ambulate the distance allowed by the tubing

Rationale: A. The catheter should be secured below bladder level with care to avoid compression of the tube or to cause a tripping hazard

QUESTION 30

You have been instructed to use a pulse oximeter on a patient during an activity to monitor oxygen saturation. The patient is noted to have lower than expected values based on their presentation. What measure would be the best to ensure the reading is accurate?

A. Instruct the patient to perform pursed-lip breathing while using the pulse oximeter.
B. Switch to using a sphygmomanometer to measure the patient's blood pressure.
C. Check the patient is not wearing nail polish or switch to an alternate finger.
D. Notify the nurse immediately so the level can be checked.

Rationale: C. Pulse oximeters can provide low values if nail polish obscures the sensor. The nail polish would need to be removed. Alternatively, the PTA may try another finger to determine if a more accurate reading matches the patient's presentation. If the patient demonstrated dyspnea/shortness of breath, the patient should be seated, educated on breathing techniques, and the PTA should be called for immediate assistance if the patient continued to decline

QUESTION 31

You are treating a patient who has an intracranial pressure (ICP) monitor fitted. Which of the following activities would be the most appropriate to perform for this patient?

A. Isometric abdominal and lower extremity exercises
B. AROM hip flexion to 120 degrees and extension to 10 degrees
C. Practice performing the Valsalva maneuver to increase intra-abdominal stability
D. Gentle range of motion to tolerance for the lower extremities with hip flexion limited to 90 degrees

Rationale: D. When working with a patient with an ICP placement, the following activities are contraindicated: avoid raising/lowering bed, isometric exercises, Valsalva maneuver, hip flexion greater than 90 degrees, neck flexion, prone position, or patient's head greater than 15 degrees below horizontal

QUESTION 32

Upon initiating a treatment session for a nursing home resident, you note that the patient is extremely lethargic and cannot follow commands consistently. All vital signs are within normal limits, but you feel that the change in cognitive status warrants you communicating your concern with the nursing staff. The nursing staff informs you that

the patient was sedated as he was repeatedly yelling and crying, and the nursing staff was having difficulty keeping him calm. Which of the following could be occurring?
  A. Inappropriate use of a physical restraint
  B. Inappropriate use of a chemical restraint
  C. Appropriate use of a physical restraint
  D. Appropriate use of a chemical restraint

Rationale: B. Per CMS guidelines, the patient is inappropriately chemically restrained. Restraints should only be used to maintain the safety of patients. The patient may need further redirection or attention to determine the cause of distress rather than sedation out of convenience. All restraints should be appropriately documented and abide by the policy, or it may be considered abuse

QUESTION 33
Your supervising PT has documented that a patient has a high likelihood of meeting her goal to return to her previous functional level of full ROM and 5/5 strength. The PT has established the treatment to include therapeutic exercise, manual techniques, ultrasound, ice packs, moist heat packs, and e-stim to occur two times per week × 4 weeks. What portion of the patient management model would this represent?
  A. Diagnosis and plan of care (POC)
  B. Examination
  C. Prognosis and plan of care (POC)
  D. Intervention

Rationale: C. The prognosis is the determination of the patient's likelihood to meet the set goals, and the plan of care is the outline of the intervention list to be incorporated to meet those set goals

QUESTION 34
Which of the following would be the *LEAST* effective method to foster adherence to an exercise program?
  A. Not addressing difficulties and barriers
  B. Pointing out exercise-related progress
  C. Explaining the rationale and importance of each exercise and functional activity
  D. Encouraging patient input on the nature and scope of the program

Rationale: A. It is important to address all difficulties and barriers to an exercise program appropriately. The other answers are examples of how to foster adherence to an exercise program effectively.

QUESTION 35
You are about to talk to a group of senior citizens about Alzheimer disease. Which stage of the disease is most likely demonstrated by a patient with obvious spatial-visual deficits and moderate gait abnormalities?
  A. Early stage
  B. Intermediate stage
  C. Late stage
  D. Advanced stage

Rationale: B. Spatial-visual deficits and moderate gait abnormalities tend to occur in the intermediate stage

QUESTION 36
You are about to treat a patient who has been experiencing delirium, according to the medical chart. Which of the following would you expect to see with this patient?
  A. Impaired consciousness and a highly variable mood
  B. Impaired consciousness and a normal attention span
  C. Impaired consciousness and a depressed mood
  D. Highly variable levels of consciousness and a short attention span

Rationale: D. This is the typical finding with delirium. Impaired consciousness is associated more with dementia

QUESTION 37

You are reviewing a patient's chart and note that the patient has a diagnosis of Duchenne muscular dystrophy (DMD). All of the following are true statements, *EXCEPT*:

- A. DMD is a genetic disorder characterized by progressive muscle degeneration and weakness.
- B. DMD is one of four conditions known as dystrophinopathies.
- C. Gowers sign, a characteristic of DMD, compensates for proximal contractures.
- D. DMD results from alterations of a protein called dystrophin.

Rationale: C. Gowers sign compensates for the proximal weakness

QUESTION 38

You are treating a patient with a diagnosis of fibromyalgia at your aquatic therapy center with a prescription for progressive aquatic therapy. The patient is moderately deconditioned due to months of inactivity resulting from a mild myocardial infarction 2 years ago. What are the expected effects of hydrostatic pressure exerted by the water on this patient?

- A. To increase resistance as the speed of active movement increases
- B. To increase cardiovascular demands both at rest and with exercise
- C. To assist in venous return and reduce effusion
- D. All of the above

Rationale: C. According to Pascal law (a pressure change in one part is transmitted without loss to every portion of the fluid), as the depth of immersion increases, so does hydrostatic pressure. This increased pressure works to limit effusion and assist venous return

QUESTION 39

You treat a patient who has developed a thick eschar secondary to a severe (full-thickness) burn. Which of the following topical agents would be the most effective in controlling any potential infection?

- A. Amphotericin B
- B. Silver sulfadiazine
- C. Silver nitrate
- D. Sulfamylon (mafenide acetate)

Rationale: D. Sulfamylon diffuses freely into the eschar and is highly effective against gram-negative organisms, including pseudomonal species. Amphotericin B is an antifungal agent. Silver sulfadiazine and silver nitrate have poor eschar penetration

QUESTION 40

You are treating a 78-year-old patient to enhance balance and gait. During the discussion, the patient reports mistaking images directly in front of him, especially in bright light. Further questioning reveals that the patient can locate items in his environment with his peripheral vision when walking but that his reading has become more difficult. Which of the following conditions do you expect the patient may have?

- A. Cataracts
- B. Homonymous hemianopsia
- C. Glaucoma
- D. None of the above

Rationale: A. With cataracts, central vision is lost first, then peripheral. With glaucoma, the opposite is true—loss of peripheral vision first, then central. Homonymous hemianopsia is associated with a cerebrovascular accident (CVA)

QUESTION 41

Your student is discussing the results of a study that she and her colleague completed. The study looked at the effectiveness of transcutaneous electrical nerve stimulation

(TENS) and massage in treating patients with pain, and the pain instrument they used had a possible score of 50, with 50 being the worst pain. The data analysis revealed that the TENS group had a mean score of 34 with a standard deviation of 1.0, while the massage group had a mean of 36 with a standard deviation of 6.0. Based on these results, what conclusion could one make?

A. The spread of scores with the massage group has a greater variability.
B. TENS has a greater effect on pain relief than massage.
C. Massage has a greater effect on pain relief than TENS.
D. The spread of scores with the TENS group has greater variability.

Rationale: A. The massage group has a standard deviation of 6.0, indicating that this treatment produces more variability than the massage treatment. None of the other conclusions can be determined based on the data presented

QUESTION 42

In discussion with your student, you address the impact a cerebrovascular accident (CVA) can have on a patient's motor learning strategies. For example, a patient with left hemiplegia would be *LEAST* likely to respond in therapy to which of the following?

A. A simplification of the environment, including the removal of all clutter
B. Extensive use of demonstrations and gestures
C. An extensive use of verbal cues
D. All of the answers are correct

Rationale: C. An individual with left hemiplegia typically demonstrates visuospatial perceptual deficits and would therefore not respond well to the use of demonstrations and gestures

QUESTION 43

You want to design a study to see whether a joint mobilization of the cervical spine improves neck range of motion that lasts longer than 20 minutes. In this study, the range of motion would be which of the following?

A. Dependent variable
B. Independent variable
C. Control variable
D. None of the above

Rationale: A. The dependent variable is the change of difference in behavior (in this example, neck range of motion) resulting from the intervention (joint mobilization—independent variable)

QUESTION 44

A 33-year-old patient you have been treating for low back pain reports waking up with a left-sided facial droop—absent brow furrowing, weak eye closure, drooping of the mouth angle, and an inability to smile or control the left-sided muscles of the face. There is no other evidence of neurologic injury, but the patient does report experiencing earache in the left ear during the previous 2 days. You suspect Bell palsy, which the supervising PT can confirm by examining which of the following?

A. The patient's corneal reflex
B. The ability of the patient to protrude the tongue
C. The ability of the patient to taste over the anterior tongue and to puff the cheeks
D. The patient's hearing

Rationale: C. Bell palsy affects the facial nerve (CN VII), which controls the muscles of facial expression and the ability to taste over the anterior aspect of the tongue

QUESTION 45
Which of the following methods would be the most appropriate to measure wheelchair seat back height?
A. Seat platform to the superior portion of the axilla and subtract 5 inches
B. Seat platform to the base of the axilla and subtract 3 inches
C. Seat platform to the acromion process and subtract 5 inches
D. Seat platform to the base of the axilla and subtract 4 inches

Rationale: D. This is the most appropriate method

QUESTION 46
When checking vitals signs prior to treatment, the PTA measures the following: heart is at 58 beats per minute; respiratory rate is 7 breaths per minute; blood pressure is 125/75 mmHg; and the oral temperature is 98.8 degrees F. Which vital sign presents the greatest concern at this time??
A. Respiratory rate
B. Heart rate
C. Blood pressure
D. Temperature

Rationale: A. A normal range of breaths per minute is 12-16

QUESTION 47
1. A PTA takes a pulse oximetry level on a patient who completed 12 minutes of bicycle riding at a moderate resistance and gets a pulse oxygenation value of 85%. What does this value represent?
A. Inadequate arterial blood oxygen saturation
B. Adequate arterial blood oxygen saturation.
C. Inadequate systolic oxygen saturation.
D. Adequate systolic oxygen saturation.

Rationale: A. A normal blood saturation level should be 90 percent or greater

QUESTION 48
An 80 year old patient is ambulating with a walker and is ready for discharge from physical therapy. Which of the following BEST describes the amount of assistance the PTA would give to this modified independent person?
A. Minimal assistance with a gait belt
B. Standby assist with a gait belt
C. Contact guard without a gait belt
D. No assistance

Rationale: D. Based on this patient's level of independence, no assistance would be required

QUESTION 49
Which of the following measurements is the appropriate height for wheelchair foot plates from the ground?
A. Approximately half an inch.
B. Approximately 1 inch.
C. Approximately 1 1/2 inches.
D. Approximately 2 inches.

Rationale: D. 2 inches from the ground is the appropriate height for wheelchair foot plates

QUESTION 50
Which of the following measurements would be the most appropriate for the seat depth of a wheelchair?
A. Posterior lateral buttock to the popliteal fossa and subtract 2 inches
B. Posterior lateral buttock to the popliteal fossa and add 2 inches
C. Posterior lateral buttock to the popliteal fossa
D. Greater trochanter to the popliteal fossa and subtract 2 inches

Rationale: A. These are the correct landmarks to measure for the most appropriate seat depth

QUESTION 51
which of the following tests would be the most appropriate to perform to assess circulatory changes in a patient?
  A. Skin assessment
  B. Nail blanch test
  C. Tugor test
  D. Two-point discrimination

Rationale: B. The nail blanch test would be the most appropriate

QUESTION 52
Upon assessing the blood pressure during an exercise session, the PTA determines systolic blood pressure increased. How would the PTA interpret this finding?
  A. Hypertensive
  B. Hypotensive
  C. Abnormal response
  D. Normal response

Rationale: D. An increase in systolic blood pressure during exercise is a normal response

QUESTION 53
You are providing gait training for a patient with Parkinson disease. The patient is demonstrating a propulsive gait, with the steps becoming faster and shorter. Which of the following could you use to help correct this problem?
  A. A toe wedge
  B. A heel wedge
  C. Floor markers to increase stride length
  D. A metronome to increase cadence

Rationale: A. The toe wedge would help to displace the patient's center of gravity posteriorly. Increasing the stride length or the cadence would only serve to worsen the problem

QUESTION 54
You are treating a patient who recently sustained a traumatic brain injury (TBI). During the treatment, you note the ptosis and meiosis of the left eye with loss of facial sweating. Which of the following would you suspect is causing this?
  A. Trigeminal neuralgia
  B. Autonomic dysreflexia
  C. Horner syndrome
  D. None of the above

Rationale: C. Horner syndrome, caused by damage to the sympathetic nerves of the face, is a rare condition characterized by meiosis (constriction of the pupil), ptosis (drooping of the upper eyelid), and anhidrosis (absence of sweating of the face)

QUESTION 55
As a PTA you are performing a sensation test. You ask your patient to close his eyes, you then proceed to flex and extend his elbow. You follow it up with asking the patient to replicate the movement you just performed. This is known as?
  A. Monofilament
  B. Two-point discrimination
  C. Kinesthesia
  D. Proprioception

Rationale: C. Kinesthesia is the ability to recognize movement

QUESTION 56

As part of her coursework, your student has to perform a clinical study. The student wants to make sure she has included everything on her informed consent form. Which of the following would not be essential on a valid informed consent form?

A. A clear description of the purpose of the study and the procedures to be used
B. All the foreseeable risks and discomforts that can be anticipated
C. The potential benefits of participating in the study
D. A statement ensuring the participants' commitment for the duration of the study

Rationale: D. Each participant must be aware that they can refuse to participate and withdraw from a study at any time

QUESTION 57

You are discussing with your student about the various types of wheelchairs available for patients with a spinal cord injury (SCI). What is the main purpose of a tilt-in-space wheelchair?

A. To facilitate handgrip and propulsion
B. To improve positioning for pressure relief and/or postural hypotension
C. To improve lower extremity positioning
D. To improve the patient's ability to transfer independently

Rationale: B. A tilt-in-space wheelchair is used for high-level SCIs to decrease pressure and shear forces, manage postural hypotension, control edema, and facilitate feeding and respiratory functions

QUESTION 58

You are treating a patient with a right cardiovascular accident (CVA) that has left her hemiparetic on the left side. At her current stage of healing, the patient is demonstrating strong and dominant hemiplegic synergies in the leg. Which of the following activities would NOT help lessen the synergies?

A. Rolling from the hooklying position using the lower extremity D1 flexion proprioceptive neuromuscular facilitation (PNF) pattern
B. Weight shifts in kneeling
C. Assuming the bridging position
D. Foot tapping in a seated position

Rationale: D. Lower extremity synergies can be grouped into extension synergies (internal rotation, adduction, and extension of the hip; extension of the knee; and extension and inversion of the ankle) and flexion synergies (external rotation, abduction, and flexion of the hip; flexion of the knee; and flexion and eversion of the ankle). Treatment strategies to interrupt the synergies include repetitive practice (eg, massed practice) or kneeling, bridging, and rolling activities

QUESTION 59

You are discussing Medicare reimbursement criteria with a home health physical therapist. Which of the following does not apply in determining homebound status according to Medicare?

A. An individual needs the help of another person to leave the home.
B. An individual needs the help of medical equipment such as crutches, walker, or wheelchair to leave the home.
C. An individual is dependent on others for all transportation needs.
D. An individual's physician believes that the health or illness could get worse if the individual leaves the home.

Rationale: C. Being dependent on others for transportation does not meet the homebound criteria according to Medicare

QUESTION 60
You are observing the supervising physical therapist perform an examination technique. The patient is asked to assume a long-sitting position, and the head is turned slightly to one side. The therapist then quickly moves the patient backward so that the head is extended over the end of the table, approximately 30 degrees below the horizontal. Which of the following examination techniques is the therapist using?
  A. Epley maneuver
  B. Rotenberg maneuver
  C. Dix Hallpike test
  D. None of the above

Rationale: C. The therapist performs the Dix Hallpike test, which is used to help detect benign paroxysmal positional vertigo (BPPV)

QUESTION 61
You review the medical chart of a patient who sustained cerebral thrombosis 3 days ago. The chart indicates that the patient exhibits nystagmus, vertigo, nausea, dysphagia, ipsilateral Horner syndrome, decreased pain and temperature sensation of the ipsilateral face, and contralateral loss of pain and temperature sensation of the body. In your opinion, where is the most likely site of thrombosis?
  A. Internal carotid artery
  B. Posterior inferior cerebellar artery
  C. Posterior cerebral artery
  D. None of the above

Rationale: B. The patient has the characteristic signs and symptoms of Wallenberg (lateral medullary) syndrome, which results from infarction of the posterior inferior cerebellar artery

QUESTION 62
At what level should the handgrip of a walker be placed?
  A. The patient's fingertips
  B. The patient's waist
  C. The patient olecranon process
  D. The patient's wrist crease

Rationale: D. The most appropriate level would be the patient's wrist crease

QUESTION 63
You are providing preoperative instruction for a 65-year-old patient scheduled for a total knee replacement. During the treatment session, the patient expresses a fear of dying during the surgery. Which of the following would be your most appropriate response to the patient?
  A. You will be back to your family before you know it.
  B. The surgeon is very experienced.
  C. Surgery can be a very worrying experience.
  D. These types of surgeries are very common.

Rationale: C. This would be the most empathetic response

QUESTION 64
You are discussing with your student about the various terms and units used when discussing electrical stimulation. What is the standard unit of measure when measuring the phase charge of a monophasic waveform?
  A. Ampere
  B. Ohm
  C. Watt
  D. Coulomb

Rationale: D. The phase charge, represented by the area under a single-phase waveform, is measured using the coulomb

QUESTION 65
You receive a phone call from a 24-year-old patient's stepfather requesting a copy of the patient's medical record. What should be your response?
    A. Allow the request.
    B. Inform the stepfather that the request for a copy must be made in writing to the insurance company.
    C. Inform the stepfather that the medical record is the property of the hospital and can only be released with written authorization from the patient.
    D. Inform the stepfather that the medical record can only be released with written authorization from the patient's physician.

Rationale: C. Unless restricted by state or federal law or regulation, a hospital shall furnish parts of the hospital record to a patient or a patient's representative upon request in writing by the patient or their representative
Roach WH. *Medical Records and the Law*. 4th ed. Sudbury, MA: Jones & Bartlett; 2006:111-114

QUESTION 66
You are discussing with your student about the various types of muscle contractions. What type of muscle contraction occurs in the hip extensors when moving from standing to sitting?
    A. Eccentric
    B. Concentric
    C. Isotonic
    D. Isokinetic

Rationale: A. The hip extensors (gluteus maximus and the hamstrings) function eccentrically when moving from standing to sitting

QUESTION 67
A second-degree quadriceps strain is described by which of the following statements?
    A. A full tear across the muscle belly with a significant decrease in motion and pain
    B. A minimal loss of strength and range of motion (ROM) with local tenderness
    C. No pain with movement but restrictions with activity and motion
    D. Pain with activity and decreased ROM and function

Rationale: D. This is the definition of a second-degree strain

Grade 1 muscle strain is overstretching of fibers and small tears with some tenderness and pain but no limitation in motion or strength

Grade 2 muscle strain is a partial tear with tenderness and pain, which results in some limitation in ROM and strength

Grade 3 muscle strain is a full tear of the muscle with pain and significant loss of motion and strength

QUESTION 68
Your patient has a diagnosis of Osgood-Schlatter disease. Which of the following activities should you avoid during treatment?
    A. Overhead press, biceps curl, and pull up
    B. Step-ups, straight-leg raises, and calf raises
    C. Jumping, descending stairs, squats
    D. Push-ups, bent over rows, tricep press

Rationale: C. All of these activities could exacerbate Osgood-Schlatter disease. Osgood-Schlatter disease is characterized by possible avulsion fracture and pain at the tibial tuberosity due to overcontraction of the quadriceps. Using the quadriceps with functional activities such as jumping, squatting, and stairs can increase pain

QUESTION 69
A joint mobilization that involves a large amplitude oscillation from the middle to the end range of joint motion is described as which of the following grades of oscillation?
    A. Grade I

B. Grade II

C. Grade III

D. Grade IV

Rationale: C. A grade III mobilization involves a large amplitude oscillation from the middle to the end range of joint motion

QUESTION 70

Which of the following interventions would be the *MOST* appropriate to treat a patient with Morton neuroma?

A. A foam pad just proximal to the metatarsal heads

B. A tension band just distal to the lateral epicondyles

C. A shoe cutout medial to the first metatarsophalangeal joint

D. A shock-absorbing insole

Rationale: A. A foam pad just proximal to the metatarsal heads would relieve stress from the area of the neuroma. Morton or interdigital neuroma is characterized by enlargement or irritation of the interdigital nerve, typically between the metatarsal heads. Weight-bearing and compression of the forefoot increase pain. Treatment may include a metatarsal pad placed proximal to the metatarsal heads to decrease weight-bearing across the affected region

QUESTION 71

A patient is having difficulty performing great toe extension while walking. Which of the following joint mobilization techniques would be most *SPECIFIC* for this patient's dysfunction while stabilizing the proximal joint?

A. Anterior glide of the metatarsophalangeal joint

B. Posterior glide at the metatarsophalangeal joint

C. Distraction at the metatarsophalangeal joint

D. Rotation of the metatarsophalangeal joint

Rationale: A. Based on the convex-concave principles of joint mobilization, an anterior glide of the metatarsophalangeal joint would help increase great toe extension

QUESTION 72

A patient suffered a fracture at the fibular head. Weakness in which of the following motions might indicate injury to the common fibular (peroneal) nerve?

A. Ankle dorsiflexion and inversion

B. Knee flexion

C. Ankle plantarflexion and inversion

D. Knee extension

Rationale: A. The common fibular nerve, which wraps around the fibular head, innervates the muscles that produce ankle dorsiflexion and inversion

QUESTION 73

Which of the following findings is the *MOST* consistent with a gastrocnemius strain?

A. Pain with active ankle plantarflexion, pain with passive ankle dorsiflexion, tenderness along the posterior lower leg

B. Pain with active ankle dorsiflexion, pain with passive ankle plantarflexion, tenderness along the posterior lower leg

C. Pain with active ankle plantarflexion, pain with passive ankle dorsiflexion, tenderness along the anterior lower leg

D. Pain with active ankle dorsiflexion, pain with passive ankle dorsiflexion, tenderness along the posterior lower leg

Rationale: A. The gastrocnemius, located in the posterior lower leg, is primarily an ankle plantarflexor, so there would be pain with active ankle plantarflexion and passive ankle dorsiflexion when the gastrocnemius is put on stretch

QUESTION 74

A patient with lateral cutaneous nerve of the thigh (femoral cutaneous nerve) irritation would benefit from which of the following instructions?

A. Stretch out the hip flexors
B. Wear loose-fitting pants
C. Strengthen the knee extensors
D. Foam roll over the greater trochanter

Rationale: B. Meralgia paresthetica involves entrapment of the lateral femoral cutaneous nerve along the anterior thigh. Numbness, tingling, and burning in the outer thigh can result when this nerve is entrapped due to tight clothing, pregnancy, belts, girdles, obesity

QUESTION 75

A patient with patellofemoral syndrome (PFS) should avoid which of the following activities during exercise treatment due to increased compressive forces at the tibiofemoral joint?

A. Transfers from sitting to standing
B. Inclined walking on a treadmill
C. Squats to end range
D. Straight-leg raises

Rationale: C. Although partial squats can be used during the rehabilitation of PFS, deeper squats impose significant compressive forces through the patellofemoral joint

QUESTION 76

A patient suffered a fracture at the fibular head and damaged the nerve that runs in this region. Which of the following motion would you expect to be affected by this injury?

A. Ankle dorsiflexion
B. Great toe flexion
C. Ankle plantarflexion
D. Abduction of the great toe

Rationale: A. The deep fibular (peroneal) nerve innervates the musculature of the anterior compartment and is responsible for the dorsiflexion of the foot and toes. A common result of damage to the deep peroneal nerve is drop foot, in which there is a loss of the capacity to dorsiflex the foot

QUESTION 77

A tear to which of the following portions of the meniscus has the MOST potential for healing?

A. Outer one-third
B. Middle one-third
C. Inner one-third
D. Blood flow is limited throughout the meniscus

Rationale: A. The outer one-third of a meniscus has the most potential for healing due to its blood supply

QUESTION 78

Following a total hip arthroplasty, a patient exhibits warmth, redness, and pain in the calf region. Which of the following actions would be the MOST appropriate for the PTA to take?

A. Cease treatment and then apply cryotherapy for 10 minutes before reassessing.
B. Continue treatment but monitor the patient closely for any increase in symptoms.
C. Continue treatment as this is a typical side effect following a total knee arthroplasty.
D. Cease treatment and refer immediately to a physician.

Rationale: D. Deep vein thrombosis or DVT is a risk factor following surgery, especially total joint arthroplasty. Hallmark signs of DVT are extremity swelling, calf tenderness, and cramping, especially with weight-bearing, warmth, tachycardia, inflammation. DVT is a medical emergency; therefore, treatment should be ceased, and referral to a physician made

QUESTION 79

A patient with plantar fasciitis and excessive forefoot pronation would benefit MOST from which of the following interventions?
   A. Strengthening of the flexor digitorum longus muscle
   B. Stretching to the anterior tibialis muscle
   C. Placement of a metatarsal pad
   D. A heel cushion

Rationale: A. Interventions to treat plantar fasciitis include stretching or soft tissue to the gastrocsoleus complex, stretching of the plantar fascia into great toe extension, strengthening of the foot intrinsic muscles and posterior tibialis

QUESTION 80

Which of the following joint mobilization techniques would be the most appropriate to improve a lack of knee extension?
   A. Posterior glide of the tibia on the femur
   B. Anterior glide of the femur on the tibia
   C. Inferior glide of the patella
   D. Anterior glide of the tibia on the femur

Rationale: D. Based on the convex-concave rule, an anterior glide of the tibia on the femur would help improve knee extension

QUESTION 81

An inversion injury of the ankle is likely to sprain which of the following ligaments?
   A. Deltoid
   B. Posterior tibiofibular
   C. Anterior talofibular
   D. Tibiocalcaneal

Rationale: C. The anterior talofibular ligament is the most commonly sprained ligament with an inversion injury of the ankle—60% to 70% of lateral (inversion) ankle sprain injuries (Dutton, p. 698)

QUESTION 82

A patient with a history of femoral anteversion would be expected to present with which of the following conditions?
   A. Limited hip internal rotation and excessive hip external rotation
   B. Excessive hip abduction and limited hip adduction
   C. Limited hip external rotation and excessive hip internal rotation
   D. Excessive hip adduction and limited hip abduction

Rationale: C. Femoral anteversion is greater than 15 degrees of femoral torsion and is characterized by limited hip external rotation and increased hip internal rotation. The patient often has a "toe-in" posture in standing

QUESTION 83

Which of the following interventions would be the MOST important to prevent a repeat injury in a patient with a history of recurrent lateral ankle sprains?
   A. Strengthening of the quadriceps and hamstrings
   B. Enhancing balance and proprioception
   C. Stretching the gastrocnemius and anterior tibialis
   D. Restoring normal talocrural joint mobility

Rationale: B. The most important intervention to decrease instances of recurrent ankle sprain and injury would be to enhance balance and proprioception

QUESTION 84

A patient with a diagnosis of trochanteric bursitis would complain of tenderness to palpation in which of the following regions?

A. Deep to the buttocks
B. Anterior aspect of the iliac crest
C. Lateral proximal thigh
D. Gluteal fold

Rationale: C. The trochanteric bursa is located on the lateral proximal thigh

QUESTION 85

A patient limited in external hip rotation would benefit from which of the following joint mobilization techniques of the femur?

A. Inferior glide
B. Medial glide
C. Anterior glide
D. Posterior glide

Rationale: C. Based on the convex-concave rule, an anterior glide of the femur would help restore external rotation of the hip

QUESTION 86

Which of the following treatment techniques is the *MOST* appropriate for a patient suffering from a herniated disk?

A. Prone alternating upper/lower extremity lifts
B. Standing forward trunk flexion
C. Seated marching with leg weights
D. Supine marching

Rationale: A. Of the possibilities given, prone alternating upper/lower extremity lifts would be the most appropriate. A patient with a disk herniation usually has increased pain with spinal flexion and decreased pain with spinal extension. Exercises for a patient with a disk herniation would include positions of extension and avoid exercises in a spinal flexed posture

QUESTION 87

Weakness in which of the following muscles would hinder a patient's ability for inspiration?

A. External obliques
B. Internal obliques
C. Diaphragm
D. Rectus abdominis

Rationale: C. The diaphragm is the main muscle of quiet inspiration

QUESTION 88

Your patient has an L3 nerve root compression. Which of the following phases of gait would be the *MOST* dysfunctional due to this condition?

A. Loading response
B. Midswing
C. Midstance
D. Terminal swing

Rationale: D. The quadriceps muscle group, served by the L3-L4 nerve, contracts immediately before the heel hits the ground to keep the knee bent and prevent the knee from buckling when the foot hits the ground

QUESTION 89

Which of the following regions would have decreased sensation for a patient with an L5-S1 intervertebral disk herniation?

A. Medial knee
B. Medial lower leg

C. Lateral lower leg
D. Lateral aspect of the fifth toe

Rationale: C. An L5-S1 disk herniation would affect the L5 nerve root. The dermatome for L5 is the lateral lower leg and dorsum of the foot, which would have decreased sensation

QUESTION 90
A patient has a C7-C8 disk herniation. Where would you test for dermatomal involvement of the affected nerve root with this level of herniation?
A. Middle finger
B. Lateral upper arm
C. Thumb
D. Little finger

Rationale: D. A C7-C8 disk herniation would affect the C8 dermatome, which is located at the fourth and fifth digits of the hand

QUESTION 91
A physical therapy research study states that participants who demonstrate an inability to flex the knee greater than 90 degrees and report more than 5/10 pain cannot participate in the study. This involves which of the following components of research?
A. Randomization
B. Subject demographics
C. Inclusion criteria
D. Exclusion criteria

Rationale: D. Exclusion criteria are part of sample selection for research to minimize bias. This includes those characteristics that would be excluded from the research if a participant were to have them

QUESTION 92
A patient with a cervicogenic headache due to forward head posture and rounded shoulders would most benefit from which of the following interventions?
A. Strengthening of the scapular retractors
B. Stretching of the scapular retractors
C. Strengthening of the shoulder adductors
D. Stretching of the neck flexors

Rationale: A. Forward head posture is often associated with cervicogenic headaches and is characterized by weakness in deep cervical neck flexors and forward flexion of the cervical spine. Strengthening the deep neck flexors is an appropriate intervention to improve posture and decrease contributing factors to the cervicogenic headache

QUESTION 93
Validity in research refers to which of the following terms?
A. The extent to which an assessment tool measures what it claims to measure
B. The ability for a test to correctly identify those with the disease
C. The extent to which an assessment tool produces stable, consistent results
D. The ability for a test to correctly identify those without the disease

Rationale: A. Validity is defined as the relation to a test to describe whether the test measures what it is supposed to measure

QUESTION 94
Which of the following factors can be harmful to the validity of research?
A. A large sample size
B. Financial support from a stakeholder in the research
C. Strict exclusion criteria
D. A diverse population of participants

Rationale: B. Minimizing risk of bias in research includes a large sample size, blinding or masking with research, utilizing more than one group, having consistent, strict inclusion/exclusion criteria for research participants, and diversifying the research population

QUESTION 95

A patient has decreased sensation along the medial aspect of the knee. Which of the following dermatomes is likely involved?

  A. L3

  B. L4

  C. L5

  D. S1

Rationale: A. The L3 dermatome runs along the medial aspect of the knee

QUESTION 96

Which of the following muscles may supplement the diaphragm if it becomes ineffective?

  A. Middle trapezius

  B. Sternocleidomastoid

  C. Rectus abdominis

  D. Internal obliques

Rationale: B. The sternocleidomastoid, pectoralis major and minor, as well as the serratus posterior and anterior are active during forced inspiration

QUESTION 97

A patient with temporomandibular joint dysfunction would be expected to have clicking in which of the following regions?

  A. Superior to the zygomatic arch

  B. Along the inferior angle of the mandible

  C. Anterior to the ear

  D. Sublingual

Rationale: C. Clicking of the temporomandibular joint would be felt anterior to the ear due to its location

QUESTION 98

A patient with a facet capsular entrapment at C6-C7 on the left would have *MOST* difficulty with which of the following movements?

  A. Right rotation

  B. Left rotation

  C. Right side-bending

  D. Forward flexion

Rationale: B. Any motion that introduces extension at the left C6-C7 joint would create difficulty. Another motion that would be difficult is left side-bending

QUESTION 99

Which of the following interventions should you avoid when treating a patient with lumbar spinal stenosis?

  A. Prone alternating upper/lower extremity lifts

  B. Supine alternating knee to chest

  C. Quadruped alternating upper/lower extremity extension

  D. Seated bicep curls

Rationale: A. Flexion of the spine will increase the diameter of the spinal canal and decrease pain and pressure due to spinal stenosis or narrowing. Flexed postures are preferred for exercise as extension of the spine will further narrow the canal and increase pain

QUESTION 100

A nerve entrapment at L5-S1 would result in decreased sensation in which of the following areas?

  A. Medial knee

  B. Medial lower leg

C. Lateral lower leg

D. Lateral aspect of the fifth toe

Rationale: C. The L5-S1 dermatome runs along the lateral aspect of the lower leg

QUESTION 101

A patient with a rib hump on the right with lumbar flexion likely has which of the following conditions?

A. Dowager hump

B. Left rotoscoliosis

C. Right rotoscoliosis

D. Adaptive shortening of the right intercostal muscles

Rationale: C. With rotoscoliosis, a rib hump will appear on the side of convexity. A right lumbar convexity will be associated with left lumbar side-bending and compensatory right thoracic rotation to keep the eyes forward. As a result, forward flexion of the spine will result in a rib hump on the right (Dutton, p. 408)

QUESTION 102

The patient is having difficulty with expiration. Which of the following muscles could be strengthened to improve forced expiration?

A. External intercostals

B. Transversus abdominis

C. Diaphragm

D. Scalenes

Rationale: B. Muscles of forced expiration include the transverse abdominis, rectus abdominis, obliques, and internal intercostals. In fact, these muscles are commonly strengthened with spinal cord patients to assist with their breathing

QUESTION 103

Strengthening which of the following muscles will help increase mouth opening for a patient with temporomandibular joint dysfunction?

A. Lateral pterygoid

B. Medial pterygoid

C. Temporalis

D. Masseter

Rationale: A. The lateral pterygoid is one of the main muscles used for mouth opening

QUESTION 104

When working on balance and core exercises with a patient, the quadriceps would _MOST LIKELY_ be recruited with which of the following activities?

A. A large perturbation from a posterior to an anterior direction

B. Medial-lateral weight-shifting

C. Reaching forward outside of the patient's base of support with the feet stationary

D. Catching a weighted ball at the chest thrown from an anterior direction

Rationale: D. A weighted ball thrown at the chest from an anterior direction could cause the knees to buckle if the quadriceps did not contract

QUESTION 105

The ability for a test to correctly identify those with the disease refers to which of the following terms of research?

A. Reliability

B. Validity

C. Sensitivity

D. Specificity

Rationale: C. A high degree of sensitivity helps correctly identify those with the disease

QUESTION 106
Which of the following statements describes the purpose of a control group in a research project?
A. To test the hypothesis
B. To test the experimental criteria
C. To be a group that does not receive the experimental criteria
D. To have more participants in the study

Rationale: C. The control group is the group of subjects who do not receive the experimental intervention and is used for comparison to the experimental group

QUESTION 107
A patient has decreased sensation along the middle finger of the right hand. Which of the following dermatomes is involved?
A. C5
B. C6
C. C7
D. C8

Rationale: C. The C7 dermatome covers this area

QUESTION 108
During respiratory rehabilitation, which of the following motions would you expect to feel as you palpate a patient's anterior rib cage during inhalation?
A. Outflare of the ribs
B. Depression of the ribs
C. Inflare of the ribs
D. Inferior movement of the ribs

Rationale: A. During inspiration, the upper ribs 2 to 7 move ventral/superior. The lower ribs outflare

QUESTION 109
While working in the home setting, the patient exhibits jugular distention and reports a 4-lb weight gain in the last 24 hours. Which of the following diagnoses could you suspect the patient is experiencing?
A. Diabetes mellitus
B. Ascites
C. Varicose veins
D. Right ventricular congestive heart failure

Rationale: D. A patient with chronic congestive heart failure is susceptible to rapid weight gain, particularly when the heart and kidneys become overwhelmed with interstitial peripheral edema. The cause of the weight gain may be due to high potassium or sodium in the blood. The kidneys also may not be able to excrete excessive blood elements effectively. All of these signs relate to chronic ventricular heart failure

QUESTION 110
A patient in cardiac rehab begins to complain of chest pains, shortness of breath, and exhibiting signs of diaphoresis. The patient's blood pressure is 180/150. What is the most concerning about this blood pressure reading?
A. The reading indicates an acute cardiac coronary situation.
B. It is the blood pressure category of hypertensive crisis.
C. The elevated blood pressure is due to exercise intensity.
D. The blood pressure level is of moderate concern.

Rationale: A. If a patient with an acute coronary syndrome and his or her pulse pressure is less than the normal 40 to 60 mm Hg, this may indicate large-vessel arteriosclerosis.

Pulse pressure is sometimes a stronger indicator of cardiovascular events than systolic blood pressure and diastolic blood pressure (Hillegass, 2001) (Bangalore, S. et al. 2009, Oxford Academic, https://academic.oup.com/eurheartj/article/30/11/1395/640726)

QUESTION 111
You are scheduled to administer an intermittent compression pump for a patient currently receiving hospice care secondary to metastatic breast cancer. Which of the following statements would be most concerning relative to this patient and administration of the physical modality?
 A. Ensuring that the patient has adequate kidney function relative to interstitial edema.
 B. Lymphedema is a contraindication to the use of intermittent compression therapy.
 C. Ensuring that the compression will not fracture the fragile bones of the patient.
 D. Ensuring the proper patient education is provided.

Rationale: B. Mechanical or intermittent compression therapy may overwhelm dysfunctional kidneys. The question states the patient has metastatic breast cancer but does not designate the metastasized areas. With proximity to the breasts, cancer most commonly will spread to the bones, lungs, liver, and lymph nodes before affecting the kidneys. Compression garments and compression wraps are accepted modalities for patients with metastatic concerns. An intermittent compression pump is also an acceptable modality if warranted by a patient. Lymphedema is not a contraindication for the use of intermittent compression therapy

QUESTION 112
You are working with a patient with active methicillin-resistant *Staphylococcus aureus* of the sputum. How can you most effectively minimize transmission of the disease?
 A. Practice standard universal precautions
 B. Practice droplet precautions
 C. Practice contact precautions
 D. Practice airborne precautions

Rationale: B. Per the Centers for Disease Control and Prevention (CDC), the viscosity of sputum would correlate to that of practicing droplet precautions

QUESTION 113
Of the following, which laboratory test will help to determine whether a patient has previously had or is having a myocardial infarction?
 A. Cardiac enzymes blood level
 B. Pulse oxygenation level
 C. Cardiac catheterization
 D. ECG imaging study

Rationale: A. Elevation of blood cardiac enzymes is an indication of an acute coronary syndrome or myocardial infarction

QUESTION 114
You are working with a patient who has a 35% valve pumping function of the heart. Which of the following considerations does the noted percentage represent?
 A. Ejection fraction percentage
 B. Preload percentage
 C. Afterload percentage
 D. Stroke volume percentage

Rationale: A. The left ventricular end-diastole pressure (LVEDP) and stroke volume (SV) provide an indication and percentage ratio of the volume of blood ejected by the left ventricle per contraction relative to the volume of blood received by the left ventricle during diastole (O'Sullivan et al., 2019)

QUESTION 115

You are about to enter the room to provide therapy services to a patient with restrictive lung disease who is currently hospitalized and scheduled for a lung transplant. What type of room would you expect to be entering?

A. A room with positive air pressure

B. A room with negative air pressure

C. A room requiring the use of personal protective equipment (PPE) for contact precautions

D. A room with no special considerations

Rationale: A. A hospital room with positive air pressure will help avoid transmission of pathogens into a hospital room upon opening the door to the room

QUESTION 116

A patient suffers from gastroesophageal reflux disease (GERD) and lower lobe anterior basal segment pneumonia. Which of the following treatment interventions would be contraindicated?

A. Initiating a progressive ambulation program on a treadmill

B. Assessing tactile fremitus as a result of percussion

C. Administration of percussion with chest therapy

D. Diaphragmatic breathing in a semi-Fowler position

Rationale: C. The administration of percussion with chest therapy would be contraindicated for this patient type

QUESTION 117

A patient in cardiac rehab begins to complain of chest pains, shortness of breath, and exhibiting signs of diaphoresis. Which of the following medications is used for the symptoms the patient is exhibiting?

A. Thrombolytic agent

B. Vasodilator

C. Angiotensin receptor blocker

D. Nitrates

Rationale: D. It is important to understand pharmacologic management and medications concerning various patient conditions. Nitrates are specific vasodilators that decrease preload and afterload, decreasing myocardial work. Nitrates also dilate coronary arteries during an acute coronary syndrome episode (O'Sullivan et al., 2019)

QUESTION 118

You are working with a patient with chronic pulmonary disease. The patient reports that the medications for their condition sometimes cause tachycardia. Which of the following medications has the potential for this adverse reaction?

A. Mucolytic

B. Bronchodilator

C. Nitrate

D. Anti-inflammatory

Rationale: B. Bronchodilators may cause tachycardia for the pulmonary patient secondary to misuse of an inhaler, distribution of inadequate amounts of the medication. The dilation of the bronchial passageways for the cardiac process is stimulated via the sympathetic nervous system (O'Sullivan et al., 2019)

QUESTION 119

You are working with a home health patient. Lung auscultations reveal high-pitched popping sounds. You would document which of the following information related to the auscultation assessment?

A. Inspiratory wheezing

B. Absent lung sounds

C. Diminished breath sounds
D. Inspiratory crackles

Rationale: D. Crackles are normally heard with inspiration and are a high-pitched popping sound (O'Sullivan et al., 2019)

QUESTION 120

The medical record provides pulmonary testing results for a patient who has been newly diagnosed with restrictive lung disease. Which of the following tests provides a patient's most thorough pulmonary status?

A. Baseline dyspnea testing
B. Perceived rate of exertion testing
C. Exercise tolerance testing
D. Arterial blood gas analysis

Rationale: D. Arterial blood gas analysis will provide the physiologic status of a patient's pulmonary function. The other assessment tests are very important to be administered but involve patient perceptions (O'Sullivan et al., 2019)

QUESTION 121

An inpatient recovering from acute coronary syndrome has recently been cleared to get out of bed and ambulate with assistance. The patient is classified at which level of cardiac rehabilitation?

A. Inpatient rehab, level 1
B. Inpatient rehab, level 2
C. Inpatient rehab, level 3
D. Inpatient rehab, level 4

Rationale: B. According to O'Sullivan, Schmitz, and Fulk, 2019, this patient would be classified at phase 1 inpatient rehab, level 2. The patient is hemodynamically stable and may now get out of bed and begin performing monitored functional mobility activities and beginning gait activity

QUESTION 122

You are scheduled to work with a patient who is hospitalized after having a coronary artery bypass graft. The treatment intervention will involve functional mobility and gait training along with vital sign monitoring. This patient should maintain which of the following heart rate percentages throughout the treatment interventions?

A. 50% to 70% maximum heart rate
B. 55% to 75% maximum heart rate
C. 65% to 80% maximum heart rate
D. 75% to 90% maximum heart rate

Rationale: C. According to O'Sullivan, Schmitz, and Fulk, 2019, the patient participating in cardiac rehabilitation requires continued monitoring of vital signs; with a preferred heart rate of 65% to 80% maximum heart rate

QUESTION 123

You are directed to assess the gait pattern tolerance for an outpatient cardiac patient. You would most likely utilize which of the following assessment tests?

A. Dynamic Gait Index
B. Four Square Step Test
C. Chair stand test
D. Performance-Orientated Mobility Assessment

Rationale: A. Although the Tinetti Performance Orientated Mobility Assessment test provides information about a patient's gait tolerance, the Dynamic Gait Index test provides information specific to gait pattern, gait tolerance, and further gait activity requiring dynamic balance

QUESTION 124

A patient who underwent a coronary artery bypass graft (CABG) also has an incision site on the lower extremity where venous tissue was harvested. Which of the following areas relative to a CABG should be monitored by the clinician during a physical therapy treatment session?
A. The proximal humeral region
B. The lateral cervical region
C. The medial wrist region
D. The medial regions of the lower extremity

Rationale: D. Although grafting does occur from the radial and mammary arteries, it also occurs from the saphenous vein in the lower extremity. All of these areas are utilized; however, the best answer possible would involve the medial region of the lower extremity, which involves the saphenous vein regions (O'Sullivan et al., 2019)

QUESTION 125

A patient is encouraged to perform shoulder active range of motion (AROM) in a pain-free range while avoiding flexion greater than 90 degrees. Which of the following surgeries associates most with this prescribed exercise regimen?
A. Coronary artery bypass graft
B. Angiogram
C. Thoracotomy
D. J-tube insertion

Rationale: A. The patient who undergoes a coronary artery bypass graft (CABG) normally has lifting restrictions and range of motion restrictions. The range of motion restrictions encourage limiting shoulder flexion to no higher than 90 degrees relative to pain levels (O'Sullivan et al., 2019)

QUESTION 126

A patient who has chronic bradycardia and a pulse rate that fails to rise with exercise is a potential candidate for which of the following?
A. Pacemaker implantation
B. Heart transplant
C. A prescription for digitalis
D. Cardiac defibrillator implantation

Rationale: A. The signs and symptoms noted indicate pacemaker implantation (O'Sullivan et al., 2019)

QUESTION 127

You are working with a patient who is performing ambulation and balance activities. The patient complains of chronic leg cramps and fatigue with activities. Which of the following medications is the patient most likely taking?
A. Antifibrogenic medication
B. Gastroesophageal reflux disease (GERD) medication
C. Anticoagulant medication
D. Antihyperlipidemic medication

Rationale: D. The signs and symptoms noted are consistent with intermittent claudication of the lower extremities relatable to atherosclerosis

QUESTION 128

The partial thromboplastin time (PTT) laboratory value was assessed for a patient who is considered an increased fall risk. This patient is most likely taking which of the following medications?
A. Anticoagulant medication
B. Antihyperlipidemic medication

C. Nitrate medication
D. Beta-blocker medication

Rationale: A. The PTT laboratory value determines the value of a patient's blood clotting process. A patient who has coagulation concerns will be at risk for falling

QUESTION 129

A patient who presents with an increased anterior-posterior diameter of the chest with decreased expansion capabilities is most likely to have which of the following conditions?
A. Rotoscoliosis
B. Coronary artery bypass grafting
C. Laminectomy secondary to disk herniation
D. Chronic pulmonary dysfunction

Rationale: D. A barrel chest formation is consistent with an anterior-posterior diameter of the chest. A barrel chest formation is commonly seen in patients with chronic pulmonary dysfunction

QUESTION 130

Decreased recruitment of muscle contraction with great toe extension represents dysfunction in which of the following myotome?
A. L3
B. L4
C. L5
D. S1

Rationale: C. Great toe extension is the L5 myotome

QUESTION 131

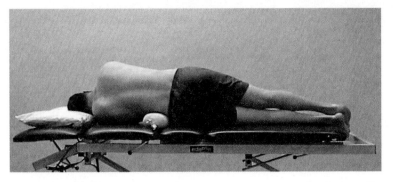

The image above would be the *MOST* appropriate to treat which of the following musculoskeletal conditions?
A. Bilateral hip flexor tightness
B. Left L4-L5 nerve root entrapment
C. Posterior disk herniation
D. Right L4-L5 nerve root entrapment

Rationale: D. Positional distraction of the lumbar spine involves using a small towel roll or pillow on the opposite side of nerve compression to arthrokinematically gap the spine on the affected side. Rotation toward the involved side can further open the foramen

QUESTION 132

When employing the ankle strategy to improve balance, which of the following activities would *BEST* utilize this motor strategy for balance?

A. Large perturbation from a posterior to an anterior direction
B. Medial-lateral weight shifting
C. Reaching forward outside the patient's base of support with feet stationary
D. Catching a weighted ball at the chest from the anterior direction

Rationale: B. Motor strategies include an ankle, hip, and stepping strategy. The ankle strategy involves shifting the center of mass in small increments to control sway and small disturbances. The hip strategy involves the recruitment of hip movement to maintain balance. Stepping strategy is utilized with a large disturbance that requires stepping to avoid falling

QUESTION 133

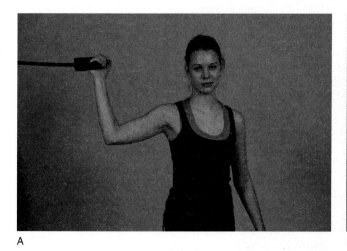
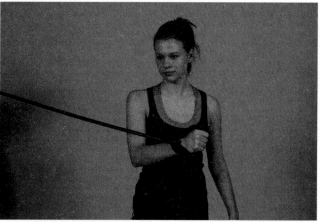

In the image above, which of the following muscle is most specifically being strengthened from image A to image B?

A. Subscapularis
B. Supraspinatus
C. Infraspinatus
D. Biceps

Rationale: A. The motion from Image A to Image B is internal rotation and adduction of the shoulder, which utilizes the subscapularis, teres major, latissimus dorsi, pec major muscles

QUESTION 134

Which of the following characteristics can lead to a circumduction compensation in gait for a person using a transfemoral prosthesis?

A. Weakness in the anterior tibialis.
B. Prosthesis is too loose.

C. Prosthesis is too short.
D. Extension aid is loose.

Rationale: B. A loose prosthesis would cause it to fall out of the socket during the swing
   phase making the leg functionally longer. Circumducting the hip swings the prosthesis
   out to the side to clear it from the ground

QUESTION 135

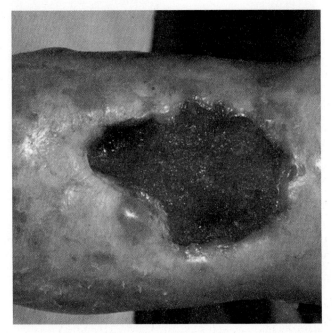

**Which of the following descriptions would be the *MOST* accurate to identify the type of
wound tissue in the image shown above?**
A. Nonviable granulation tissue
B. Viable tissue
C. Viable slough tissue
D. Nonviable eschar tissue

Rationale: B. Granulation tissue is often bright or "beefy" red due to rich vascularization. It
   is viable tissue. Slough is nonviable yellowish tissue, and eschar is nonviable hard, black
   tissue

QUESTION 136

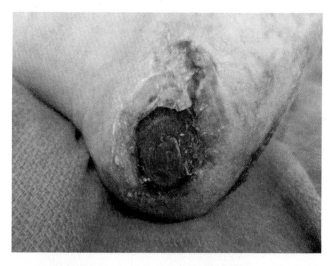

The wound in the image above would be most appropriately classified as which of the following wound stages?
  A. 2
  B. 3
  C. 4
  D. Unstageable

Rationale: Wounds obscured by slough or eschar are unstageable as the extent of tissue damage cannot be visualized or confirmed

QUESTION 137
After observing pistoning of 1/2 in in a patient with a transfemoral prosthesis, which of the following steps would be the most appropriate for you to take?
  A. Refer the patient back to a prosthetist for refitting.
  B. Perform non–weight-bearing exercises for 30 minutes, then recheck if pistoning is still present.
  C. Add a sock layer to the prosthesis.
  D. Continue treatment with only weight-bearing exercises.

Rationale: C. A socket should slip vertically no more than 1/4 in. Sock layers can be added for slippage up to 1/2 in but more than 1/2 in pistoning should be referred back to a prosthetist for refitting

QUESTION 138
You put fingertip pressure into a lower extremity with pitting edema, then document the finding as a 3+ on the pitting edema scale. Which of the following descriptions is consistent with this classification?
  A. A deep indentation that returns to normal within 30 seconds
  B. A slight indentation that returns to normal after 30 seconds
  C. A deep indentation that remains for more than 30 seconds
  D. A slight indentation that returns to normal after 15 seconds

Rationale: A. A 3+ on the pitting edema scale is described as a deeper indentation that returns to normal within 30 seconds. A 1+ is a barely detectable indentation. A 2+ is a slight indentation that returns to normal in 15 seconds. A 4+ is a deep indentation that lasts more than 30 seconds

QUESTION 139
A heel that is too firm can lead to which of the following gait deviations from initial contact to midstance in a patient with a transtibial prosthesis?
A. Circumduction
B. Vaulting
C. Excessive knee flexion
D. Inadequate knee flexion

Rationale: C. A stiff heel cushion can lead to early and excessive knee flexion in the early stance phase of gait

QUESTION 140
A patient who demonstrates knee buckling during the early stance phase of gait would *MOST* benefit from which of the following devices?
A. An ankle-foot orthosis
B. A hip-knee-ankle-foot orthosis
C. A knee-ankle-foot orthosis
D. A posterior leaf spring orthosis

Rationale: C. A knee-ankle-foot orthosis gives stability to the knee in extension during the early stance phase of gait

QUESTION 141
A patient with a transfemoral prosthesis demonstrates abnormal hip abduction during the stance phase of gait on the prosthetic side. Which of the following factors on the prosthetic side could contribute to this compensation?
A. Tight adductor magnus muscle
B. Weak gluteus medius
C. High lateral prosthetic wall
D. High medial prosthetic wall

Rationale: D. Abduction on the prosthetic side in the stance phase can be due to a prosthesis that is too long, the hip joint is abducted, the lateral wall is inadequately adducted, or the medial wall is too sharp or too high

QUESTION 142
Which of the following factors may contribute to excessive knee flexion in the stance phase of gait in a patient with a transtibial prosthesis?
A. The heel cushion is too soft.
B. The socket is too far posterior.
C. The socket is too far anterior.
D. The keel is too long.

Rationale: C. Excessive knee flexion in the stance phase can be due to the shoe heel too high, the heel cushion is too stiff, the socket is excessively flexed, or too far anterior, there is insufficient plantarflexion

QUESTION 143
A patient with a transtibial prosthesis complains of sharp pain in the patellar tendon region during weight-bearing exercises. Which of the following actions would be the *MOST* appropriate for you to take?
A. Cease treatment and contact the supervising physical therapist for a reevaluation.
B. Continue exercises as this response is typical at the patellar tendon.
C. Perform non–weight-bearing exercises for the day and refer to a prosthetist for refitting.
D. Remove the prosthesis to check for irritants, then resume exercise and monitor for continued pain.

Rationale: D. The patellar tendon is a build-up area with a transtibial prosthesis that is pressure-tolerant. Although some redness and mild pressure discomfort in this region may be typical, a sharp pain is not. The PTA can check for an irritant, such as creased socks or liner, then resume exercises and monitor for continued pain. This would be the first step. Referral to the primary physical therapist for reevaluation or the prosthetist is not indicated immediately

QUESTION 144

In a quadrilateral transfemoral prosthesis, a posteromedial concave relief decreases pressure on which of the following sensitive tissues?
A. Obturator nerve
B. Sciatic nerve
C. Rectus femoris muscle
D. Adductor longus tendon

Rationale: B. The adductor longus tendon and obturator nerve have pressure relief from an anteromedial concave relief. The rectus femoris muscle is an anterolateral relief. The sciatic nerve and hamstrings tendon have a posteromedial concave relief

QUESTION 145

Which of the following statements best describes a stage 3 pressure ulcer?
A. Full-thickness loss of skin with visible adipose tissue, undermining and tunneling
B. Partial-thickness loss of skin with exposed dermis
C. Nonblanchable erythema of intact skin with sensation change and discoloration
D. Full-thickness tissue loss with exposure of fascia, muscle, tendon, and bone

Rationale: A. Stage 3 pressure ulcer as defined by the National Pressure Ulcer Advisory Panel is a full-thickness loss of skin where adipose tissue is visible, undermining and tunneling may be present, but fascia, muscle, tendon, ligament, bone are not visible

QUESTION 146

During a treatment session, a clinical instructor measures the same goniometric value for active shoulder flexion as a physical therapist assistant student. Which of the following types of reliability is demonstrated in this example?
A. Test-retest
B. Intrarater
C. Interrater
D. Intraclass correlation

Rationale: C. Interrater reliability establishes whether multiple raters can consistently conduct a test and record results

QUESTION 147

Which of the following statement describes a systematic review of a topic in the research literature?
A. An exhaustive review of multiple databases, references sources, and conferences
B. A literature review of peer-reviewed articles from a set database
C. Summarizing literature from a set number of years to establish a current database of information
D. A review of multiple textbooks compiling information from a variety of authors

Rationale: A. A systematic review should consist of exhaustive reviews of multiple databases, conference proceedings, review of references of studies identified, communication with multiple authors

QUESTION 148

During a supine to sit transfer, a patient becomes light-headed, pale, and diaphoretic. Which of the following actions should the PTA take *NEXT*?
A. Check the patient's oxygen saturation.
B. Educate the patient in pursed-lip breathing while sitting at the edge of the bed
C. Place the patient back in supine with head slightly higher than feet.
D. Contact the nurse for a medical emergency

Rationale: C. These are symptoms of orthostatic hypotension and can occur in patients who have been immobilized or in a recumbent position for extended periods. Orthostatic hypotension can be the result of decreased venous return from the lower extremities. Placing the patient supine with their feet elevated can help with venous return

QUESTION 149
A patient begins to complain of dizziness and has increased postural sway after transitioning from sit to stand. Which of the following conditions should the PTA be concerned about?
A. Benign paroxysmal positional vertigo
B. Orthostatic hypertension
C. Meniere disease
D. Orthostatic hypotension

Rationale: D. Symptoms of orthostatic hypotension include dizziness, light-headedness, nausea, paleness, diaphoresis

QUESTION 150
Which of the following statements should be documented in the Assessment section of a SOAP note?
A. Patient complains of 5/10 pain in the shoulder with the home exercise program.
B. Soft tissue mobilization performed at the piriformis muscle for 5 minutes.
C. Patient became fatigued after two sets of step-up exercises.
D. Add an additional set of push-ups at the next visit.

Rationale: C. Assessment data consist of information about the patient's progress, treatment effectiveness, completion of goals set by the PT in the initial evaluation, changes recommended in the plan of care (POC), and goals completed for the individual treatment sessions

QUESTION 151
Which section of a SOAP note is the *MOST* appropriate to document the statement "The patient stated he lifted a 10-lb bag of flour overhead without pain"?
A. Subjective
B. Objective
C. Assessment
D. Plan

Rationale: A. Subjective data include the patient's feedback on information relevant to the diagnosis. Common verbs are "states, reports, indicates" when used to describe patient's feedback on relevant data such as pain, the progress of activity level, and any response after the last treatment session

QUESTION 152
You take a goniometric measurement of knee flexion before and after treatment. Which section of a SOAP note should this information be documented?
A. Subjective
B. Objective
C. Assessment
D. Plan

Rationale: B. Objective data include any information that can be reproduced or observed by someone else with the same training. Information also includes measurements and tests and objective observations from treatment, such as improvement from pre- to posttreatment

QUESTION 153
Which of the following descriptions is consistent with a macerated wound?
A. Red, warm, and swollen
B. Ecchymosis, shiny, and edematous
C. Wrinkled, pale, and soft
D. Yellow, uneven, and firm

Rationale: C. Macerated skin is boggy, white or pale, soft and wrinkled due to overexposure to moisture

QUESTION 154
Which of the following dressings would be the most appropriate for a wound with heavy, foul-smelling, greenish exudate?
A. Transparent film
B. Hydrocolloid
C. Foam
D. Calcium alginate

Rationale: D. Calcium alginates absorb heavy drainage and can be used with infected wounds. The foul-smelling, greenish color of this wound suggests infection.

QUESTION 155
When performing a home safety assessment, which of the following modifications would be the most important for the PTA to address with a fall-risk patient who uses a front-wheeled walker for mobility?
A. Install a raised commode chair
B. Remove throw rugs
C. Provide chairs with armrests
D. Rearrange furniture

Rationale: B. While each modification would be helpful for a person who is a fall risk, removing dangerous throw rugs that can get caught in a front-wheeled walker would be the most important for this scenario. Furniture would need to be rearranged if they create obstacles

QUESTION 156
During treatment, a patient has a sudden onset of headache, labored breathing, and becomes flushed with skin warm to the touch. Pulse is strong but rapid, and no diaphoresis is present. Which of the following actions should the PTA take *NEXT*?
A. Lay the patient supine with feet elevated.
B. Place a cold compress on the patient's head.
C. Seek immediate emergency medical attention.
D. Provide the patient with a sugary snack.

Rationale: C. This scenario describes heatstroke, an emergency medical condition, and emergency care should be sought as quickly as possible and is, therefore, the *FIRST* step in patient care

QUESTION 157
During treatment, a diabetic patient has a sudden onset of profuse sweating, shakiness, shallow breathing, and double vision. Which of the following actions is the *MOST* appropriate if the patient is conscious?
A. Provide the patient with a sugary snack.
B. Call for immediate medical assistance.
C. Lay the patient in a Trendelenburg position.
D. Allow the patient to rest and return to treatment when symptoms subside

Rationale: A. In a diabetic patient, signs of hypoglycemia include sudden onset of pale, moist skin, shakiness, sweating, tingling sensation in the mouth, and double vision. Although not a medical emergency, the patient should be quickly given some form of sugar, and all exercise and treatment should stop for the day.

QUESTION 158
Which of the following minimum measurement (in inches) is appropriate for door width in a skilled nursing facility?
A. 32
B. 38
C. 44
D. 50

Rationale: B. Minimum door width should be 32 in, but 36-in width is preferable

QUESTION 159
A contractor constructing a wheelchair-accessible ramp in a skilled nursing facility should utilize which of these measurements?
A. 4 in high, 4 ft long
B. 5 in high, 6 ft long
C. 3 in high, 2 ft long
D. 6 in high, 12 ft long

Rationale: A. Wheelchair-accessible ramps should be no more than 1-in rise to 1 ft of vertical rise (length)

QUESTION 160
You are about to perform a sensory examination on a patient recovering from an upper extremity burn. Which of the following would be the best predictor of altered sensation?
A. The extent of any hypertrophic scarring
B. The presence of a skin graft
C. The depth of the burn injury
D. The percentage of the body surface affected

Rationale: C. The depth of the burn appears to be the best predictor

QUESTION 161
You are about to perform a series of manual muscle tests for a patient's trapezius muscle. In which of the following positions should the patient be in to test the left lower trapezius muscle?
A. Right sidelying
B. Left sidelying
C. Prone
D. Supine

Rationale: C. According to Kendall, to test the lower trapezius, the patient should be positioned in prone with the shoulder abducted greater than 120 degrees, and pressure should be applied against the forearm in a direction toward the floor

QUESTION 162
You are working to improve functional tasks with a patient who has right hemiplegia. You ask the patient to brush his teeth but notice that the patient puts the toothpaste directly in his hair instead of the toothbrush. How would you document this finding?
A. Constructional apraxia
B. Ideational apraxia
C. Conceptual apraxia
D. Ideomotor apraxia

Rationale: B. A patient with ideational apraxia finds it difficult to follow a sequence of movements, such as getting dressed, brushing teeth, or bathing

QUESTION 163
You are about to instruct a patient with a transfemoral amputation in residual limb wrapping. Which of the following bandages would be the most appropriate?
A. Two-inch
B. Four-inch
C. Six-inch
D. Eight-inch

Rationale: C. The 6-in wrap would be the most appropriate as it adequately covers the larger surface area of the residual limb in a patient with a transfemoral amputation

QUESTION 164

Your student is performing a quantitative gait analysis. If the student measures the number of steps taken by the patient in a 30-second period, which of the following is the student measuring?

A. Velocity
B. Cadence
C. Acceleration
D. Distance

Rationale: B. Cadence is defined as the number of steps taken by a person per unit of time

QUESTION 165

You have been asked to develop an osteoporosis screening tool for a retirement community. Which of the following would be the most cost-effective and reliable to incorporate?

A. Central DXA
B. Urinalysis screening
C. Measuring height
D. Dietary analysis

Rationale: C. Of the choices listed, measuring a person's height would be the most cost-effective and reliable method to screen for osteoporosis

QUESTION 166

You are supervising an exercise program for a cardiac patient during an activity that uses an energy expenditure of approximately 4 METs. Which of the following activities would best describe this MET level?

A. Walking on a level surface at 1 mi/h
B. Walking on a level surface at 2 mi/h
C. Walking on a level surface at 3 mi/h
D. Walking on a level surface at 4 mi/h

Rationale: C. A 4 MET activity would be walking on a level surface at 3 mph. Other appropriate activities would be bicycling at 6 mi/h or playing golf while pulling a walking cart

QUESTION 167

You are reviewing the various intravenous (IV) lines and monitors encountered in a hospital setting. What is the primary purpose of an arterial line?

A. To measure pulmonary artery pressure
B. To measure right arterial pressure
C. To measure blood pressure
D. To measure heart rate and oxygen saturation

Rationale: C. An arterial line (also referred to as an art-line or a-line) is a thin catheter inserted into an artery to monitor blood pressure directly and obtain samples for arterial blood gas analysis

QUESTION 168

You decide to use proprioceptive neuromuscular facilitation (PNF) techniques to improve a patient's bed mobility skills. What would be your initial command if you use rhythmic initiation (RI) to assist the patient in learning to roll from supine to prone?

A. "Help me roll you over."
B. "Stop me from rolling you over."
C. "Slowly rollover by yourself?"
D. "Relax, and let me move you."

Rationale: D. RI begins with the clinician passively moving the patient, which is usually followed by active-assisted movement, active movement, and finally, resisted movement

QUESTION 169
You use the proprioceptive neuromuscular facilitation (PNF) technique of hold-relax (H-R) to increase a patient's shoulder range of motion. Which type of contraction is used at the endpoint of the patient's available range of motion?
A. Eccentric
B. Isometric
C. Concentric
D. Isokinetic

Rationale: B. The H-R technique uses an isometric contraction at the end of the patient's available range of motion. The patient is then instructed to relax as the clinician moves the extremity into the newly gained range

QUESTION 170
You are providing gait training to a patient with hemiplegia. The patient has been ambulating with an ankle-foot orthosis (AFO), but today you notice that the patient's involved foot frequently catches the ground during the initial swing phase of gait. Which muscle should be the focus of a lower extremity strengthening program to treat this problem effectively?
A. Hamstrings
B. Iliopsoas/rectus femoris
C. Gluteus maximus
D. Gluteus medius

Rationale: B. The muscles involved with foot clearance during the initial swing phase are the dorsiflexors and the hip flexors. In the absence of the dorsiflexors, the hip flexors must be strengthened to allow for foot clearance.

QUESTION 171
You decide to use the D1 extension proprioceptive neuromuscular facilitation (PNF) technique to improve a patient's wrist extension. If you resist the patient's elbow extension to help improve the ability of the patient to extend the wrist, which of the following is this an example of?
A. Quick stretch
B. Reciprocal inhibition
C. Irradiation
D. A and B

Rationale: C. The principle behind irradiation occurs when the strong component of a pattern results in irradiation, or overflow, of impulses from the stronger muscle group to the weaker muscle group

QUESTION 172
You are treating a patient who has suffered a cardiovascular accident (CVA) 3 weeks ago using the Brunnstrom method. According to Brunnstrom, if the patient is beginning to show the ability to produce movement patterns outside of limb synergies, in which stage of recovery is the patient?
A. Stage 2
B. Stage 3
C. Stage 4
D. Stage 5

Rationale: C. According to Brunnstrom stages of recovery, individuals showing the ability to produce movement patterns outside of limb synergies fall into stage 4.

QUESTION 173
You are working with the patient to improve their bed mobility. Which of the following exercises would be the most beneficial for increasing hip stability?
 A. Trunk rotations in the hooklying position
 B. Straight-leg raises
 C. Bridging
 D. None of the above

Rationale: C. Bridging exercises increase the strength of the low back muscles and the hip extensors

QUESTION 174
You are documenting short-term goals for a patient who sustained a traumatic brain injury 4 weeks ago. A goal of being able to transfer from tall kneeling to half-kneeling with supervision is an example of which of the following?
 A. Controlled stability
 B. Mobility
 C. Stability
 D. Controlled mobility

Rationale: D. Controlled mobility is the motor control stage when a patient can demonstrate mobility while simultaneously maintaining postural stability

QUESTION 175
You discuss obtaining subjective information from a patient with your student and emphasize the need to avoid leading questions with a patient. Which of the following questions would not be considered to be leading?
 A. Is your pain worse in the morning?
 B. Does your pain decrease with rest?
 C. Does walking alter your pain in any way?
 D. Does the pain get worse when you bend your elbow?

Rationale: C. This type of question avoids putting words in a patient's mouth

QUESTION 176
You treat a patient who recently underwent a total knee replacement and has difficulty achieving the last 10 degrees of knee extension. You want to use a joint mobilization technique. Which of the following mobilization techniques could be used to help achieve the last 10 degrees of extension?
 A. A posterior glide of the tibia on the femur
 B. An inferior glide of the patella
 C. An anterior glide of the tibia on the femur
 D. A medial glide of the patella

Rationale: C. Based on the shape of the articulating surfaces, an anterior glide of the concave tibial plateau on the convex femur could be used to help achieve the last 10 degrees of knee extension

QUESTION 177
You are reviewing a patient's chart, and you note that the patient is taking a drug via enteral administration. Which of the following is an example of enteral administration?
 A. Injection
 B. Oral
 C. Inhalation
 D. Topical

Rationale: B. Enteral administration involves the esophagus, stomach, and small and large intestines (ie, the gastrointestinal [GI] tract). Other examples of enteral administration include sublingual (dissolving the drug under the tongue) and rectal

QUESTION 178

You are assessing the strength of a patient with a C6 spinal cord injury using manual muscle testing. Which of the following muscles would not be innervated based on the patient's level of injury?

A. Subclavius
B. Brachialis
C. Triceps
D. Teres minor

Rationale: C. The triceps muscle is innervated by the radial nerve (C7-C8)

QUESTION 179

You review a patient's chart admitted to the hospital with a cerebrovascular accident (CVA) and Broca aphasia. Compromise to which of the following arteries is involved with Broca aphasia?

A. Basilar artery
B. Posterior cerebral artery
C. Anterior cerebral artery
D. Middle cerebral artery

Rationale: D. Broca area, located in the left hemisphere, receives its blood supply from the middle cerebral artery

QUESTION 180

Which of the following positions would be best to lengthen the biceps muscle fully?

A. Shoulder flexion, elbow flexion, supination
B. Shoulder extension, elbow extension, pronation
C. Shoulder flexion, elbow extension, supination
D. Shoulder extension, elbow flexion, pronation

Rationale: B. The biceps brachii muscle flexes the elbow and shoulder and supinates the forearm; therefore, the opposite motions would fully lengthen the muscle: elbow and shoulder extension with forearm supination

QUESTION 181

A PTA treating a patient taking nitroglycerin should be aware of a temporary decrease in which of the following measurements?

A. Heart rate
B. Respiratory rate
C. Blood pressure
D. Oxygen saturation

Rationale: C. Nitrates will increase heart rate but decrease blood pressure with exercise. There is no direct abnormal effect on oxygen saturation or respiratory rate

QUESTION 182

A patient demonstrates 3-/5 strength with hip flexion during data collection. Which of the following characteristics of gait would likely result from this finding?

A. Increased stride length
B. Decreased step length
C. Increased cadence
D. Decreased step width

Rationale: B. Hip flexion strength is needed to advance the limb forward during terminal stance to initial contact. A lack of hip flexion due to weakness will result in a decreased step length

QUESTION 183

A patient with a positive Thomas test would likely demonstrate the *MOST* difficulty during which of the following phases of gait on the ipsilateral side?

A. Initial contact

B. Midstance

C. Loading response

D. Terminal stance

Rationale: D. A positive Thomas test indicates decreased hip flexor length (Dutton, p. 597), which will manifest at terminal stance when the hip must attain hyperextension

QUESTION 184

A patient with unilateral quadriceps weakness and fair balance would most benefit from which of the following assistive devices?

A. Straight cane

B. Hemi-walker

C. Front-wheeled walker

D. Quad cane

Rationale: C. The straight cane, quad cane, and hemi-walker only provide unilateral stability, and this patient has fair balance, which would require greater stability provided by the front-wheeled walker

QUESTION 185

A patient in a wheelchair is most susceptible to pressure ulcers developing in which of the following regions?

A. Sacrum

B. Greater tuberosity

C. Elbows

D. Malleoli

Rationale: A. When sitting in a wheelchair, the ischial tuberosities, sacrum, coccyx, scapula, posterior knee, plantar surface of feet are areas of increased pressure and vulnerable to skin breakdown

QUESTION 186

Which of the following abnormal wheelchair fit can increase vulnerability for pressure ulcers at the ischial tuberosities?

A. A seat that is too high

B. A seat that is too low

C. A seat that is too narrow

D. A seat depth that is too short

Rationale: B. A low seat height will cause the knees to elevate and thighs to rise off the seat surface, which increases the load on the buttocks and ischial tuberosity

QUESTION 187

Which of the following materials is the most appropriate for a patient who desires a wheelchair seat cushion that is lightweight, moldable to fit a custom seat, and allows a variety of stiffnesses?

A. Foam

B. Air

C. Viscous fluid

D. Elastomer

Rationale: A. Foam cushions are lightweight, inexpensive, come in many stiffnesses, and can be carved, molded, and cut to fit

QUESTION 188
Your goal is to improve a patient's ability to use the lift pressure relief strategy to unweight the buttocks while using a wheelchair. Which of the following muscles would be the most important to strengthen?
A. Deltoids
B. Biceps
C. Triceps
D. Extensor carpi radialis longus

Rationale: C. The lift pressure relief involves unweighting the buttocks by pushing on the armrests of the wheelchair and lifting the buttocks off the seat. This motion includes elbow extension utilizing the triceps

QUESTION 189
A stage IV pressure injury would be described by which of the following statements?
A. Full-thickness loss of skin with adipose tissue visible. Fascia, tendon, and muscle are not exposed
B. Intact skin with localized nonblanchable erythema
C. Partial-thickness skin loss with exposed dermis. Adipose, fascia, tendon, and muscle are not visible
D. Full-thickness loss of skin with fascia, tendon, muscle exposed

Rationale: D. A Stage IV pressure injury is described as full-thickness skin and tissue loss with exposed or directly palpable fascia, muscle, tendon, ligament

QUESTION 190
Which percentage of total body surface area is affected if a patient has suffered burns to the anterior portions of bilateral lower extremities?
A. 9%
B. 18%
C. 36%
D. 40%

Rationale: B. The anterior and posterior lower extremity together is 18% of the total body surface area. Anterior-only portions of both lower extremities would be 9% and 9% = 18%

QUESTION 191
Which of the following dressings would be appropriate for an arterial insufficiency with minimum exudate and no infection but needs a moist environment?
A. Calcium alginate
B. Foam
C. Gauze
D. Hydrocolloid

Rationale: D. Hydrocolloids maintain a moist environment, keep bacteria out and moisture in, absorb minimal-to-moderate exudate

QUESTION 192
A PTA works with a patient for 30 minutes, including 10 minutes of manual therapy and 20 minutes of therapeutic exercise. The PTA documents 45 minutes of treatment. This error in the documentation would be defined by which of the following terms?
A. Fraud
B. Malpractice
C. Overuse
D. Misdemeanor

Rationale: A. Fraud includes billing for services not provided, overcharging, the substitution of lesser qualified providers, forgery, and the provision of unnecessary services

QUESTION 193

Which of the following special tests would help reinforce the findings of a positive Lachman test?
A. McMurray
B. Apley
C. Thomas
D. Pivot shift

Rationale: D. The Lachman, anterior drawer, and pivot shift special tests are all indicators of anterior cruciate ligament (ACL) deficiency if the test is positive (Dutton, p. 641)

QUESTION 194

With a patient following total hip arthroplasty using a posterolateral approach, which of the following activities should be avoided?
A. Weight shifting side to side in standing
B. Leaning forward to don shoes in sitting
C. Ambulating on stairs
D. Walking down a ramp

Rationale: B. Total hip arthroplasty precautions with a posterolateral approach avoid hip flexion over 90 degrees, hip adduction across the midline, and hip internal rotation. Leaning forward in sitting would place the hip beyond 90 degrees of flexion

QUESTION 195

Following a total knee arthroplasty, a patient complains of pain with ankle dorsiflexion and has warmth and swelling in the region of the posterior lower leg. What should be the PTA's next step in treatment?
A. Continue treatment as this is a normal response following surgery.
B. Gently progress stretching of the gastrocnemius to restore range of motion and decrease pain.
C. Cease exercise and utilize cryotherapy in the posterior lower leg.
D. Cease exercise and contact the supervising physical therapist and/or physician.

Rationale: D. Pain and tenderness in the posterior lower leg with warmth, swelling, and limited ankle dorsiflexion are signs of a deep vein thrombosis, which is a medical emergency

QUESTION 196

You are discussing with your student the function of the various naturally occurring chemicals in the body. Which of the following chemicals is stimulated to act as a vasoconstrictor by a decrease in arterial pressure?
A. Angiotensin
B. Epinephrine
C. Norepinephrine
D. Histamine

Rationale: A. Angiotensin is a protein hormone that causes blood vessels to constrict to maintain blood pressure and fluid balance

QUESTION 197

You are reviewing the chart of a patient who is on a waiting list for a heart transplant. The patient recently received a right ventricular assistive device (RVAD) due to persistent ventricular failure. In which two structures would the tubes for this device be located?
A. Right atrium and pulmonary artery
B. Left atrium and pulmonary artery
C. Right atrium and aorta
D. Left atrium and aorta

Rationale: A. An RVAD functions to pump blood from the right atrium (or right ventricle), where one of the tubes is located, into the pulmonary artery, where the other two was located

QUESTION 198
You are examining a 3-month-old infant when the infant suddenly becomes unresponsive. Which of the following is the most appropriate location to check the infant's pulse?
A. Brachial artery
B. Popliteal artery
C. Radial artery
D. Carotid artery

Rationale: A. The most reliable location to palpate an infant's pulse is the brachial artery

QUESTION 199
You are reviewing the brachial plexus with your student. Which of the following muscles would not be involved with an injury to the posterior cord of the brachial plexus?
A. Infraspinatus
B. Latissimus dorsi
C. Teres major
D. Subscapularis

Rationale: A. The infraspinatus muscle is innervated by the suprascapular nerve (C4-C6) that extends from the superior trunk of the brachial plexus

QUESTION 200
You are reviewing the various support structures of the knee joint complex and their respective functions with your student. Which of the following does not serve as a secondary restraint to the posterior cruciate ligament (PCL)?
A. Medial collateral ligament (MCL)
B. Popliteus tendon
C. Lateral collateral ligament (LCL)
D. Iliotibial band (ITB)

Rationale: D. The iliotibial band serves as a secondary restraint to the anterior cruciate ligament (ACL), not the PCL.

Exam References and Resources

Biel A. *Trail Guide to the Body*. Boulder, CO; Books of Discovery; 2014.

Bircher W. *Documentation for Physical Therapist Assistants*. Philadelphia, Pennsylvania; F.A. Davis Company; 2018.

Dutton M. *Orthopaedics for the Physical Therapist Assistant*. Burlington, Massachusetts; Jones & Bartlett Learning; 2019.

Gresham B. *Concepts of Evidence-Based Practice for the Physical Therapist Assistant*. Philadelphia, Pennsylvania; F.A. Davis Company; 2016.

Hamm R. *Text and Atlas of Wound Diagnosis and Treatment*. New York, NY; McGraw-Hill Education; 2019.

Magee D, Manske R. *Orthopedic Physical Assessment*. New York, NY; Elsevier; 2018.

Martin ST, Kessler M. *Neurologic Interventions for Physical Therapy*. Philadelphia, Pennsylvania; Saunders; 2015.

O'Sullivan S. *Physical Rehabilitation*. Philadelphia, Pennsylvania; F.A. Davis Company; 2019.

Page C. *Management in Physical Therapy Practices*. 2nd ed. Philadelphia, Pennsylvania; F.A. Davis Company; 2015.

Pierson S, O'Shea R, Washington R. *Pierson and Fairchild's Principles & Techniques of Patient Care*. 6th ed. New York, NY; Elsevier; 2018.

Raffensperger M. *Orthopedic Interventions for the Physical Therapist Assistant*. Philadelphia, Pennsylvania; F.A. Davis Company; 2020.

Samuels V. *Foundation in Kinesiology and Biomechanics*. Philadelphia, Pennsylvania; F.A. Davis Company; 2018.

Saunders HD. Lumbar traction. *J Orthop Sports Phys Ther*. 1979;1(1):36-45.

Index

Note: Page numbers followed by *b* indicate boxed material; those followed by *f* indicate figures; those followed by *t* indicate tables.